FIFTH EDITION

Glass's
Office
Gynecology

FIFTH EDITION

Glass's Office Gynecology

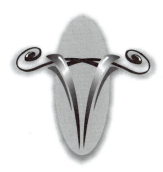

MICHÈLE G. CURTIS, M.D.

Assistant Professor
Department of Obstetrics, Gynecology, and Reproductive Sciences
University of Texas–Houston
Lyndon B. Johnson General Hospital
Houston, Texas

MICHAEL P. HOPKINS, M.D.

Chairman, Department of Obstetrics & Gynecology
Akron General Medical Center
Professor, Department of Obstetrics & Gynecology
Northeastern Ohio Universities College of Medicine
Akron, Ohio

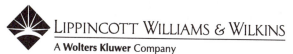

LIPPINCOTT WILLIAMS & WILKINS
A **Wolters Kluwer** Company
Philadelphia · Baltimore · New York · London
Buenos Aires · Hong Kong · Sydney · Tokyo

Editor: Charles W. Mitchell
Managing Editor: Grace E. Miller
Marketing Manager: Peter Darcy
Production Editor: Bill Cady
Design Coordinator: Mario Fernandez

Printed in the United States of America

First Edition 1976   Third Edition 1988   Fifth Edition 1998
Second Edition 1981   Fourth Edition 1993

Library of Congress Cataloging-in-Publication Data

Glass's office gynecology / [edited by] Michèle G. Curtis, Michael P. Hopkins — 5th ed.
    p.   cm.
    Rev. ed. of : Office gynecology / edited by Robert H. Glass. 4th ed. c1993.
    Includes bibliographical references and index.
    ISBN 0-683-30201-9
    1. Gynecology.   I. Glass, Robert H., 1932– .   II. Curtis, Michèle G.   III. Hopkins, Michael P.
    [DNLM: 1. Genital Diseases, Female.   2. Ambulatory Care.   WP 140 G549 1999]
RG103.034   1999
618.1—dc21
DNLM/DLC
for Library of Congress   98-3829
                                                           CIP

99 00 01 02
2 3 4 5 6 7 8 9 10

To Curt, Jessica, and Rachael
Michèle G. Curtis

To my wife, Mary Kay
Michael P. Hopkins

The 20 years that have elapsed since the first edition of this book was published have been marked by a progressive trend away from hospital-based gynecology and toward ambulatory care. Even in vitro fertilization and, to a limited extent, laparoscopy can now be accomplished in an office. Moreover, the greatest part of gynecologic practice has always been office based. My goal in editing the first four editions of *Office Gynecology* was to present up-to-date, concise, and practical information for all those interested in the delivery of health care in an outpatient setting. With this fifth edition, Drs. Curtis and Hopkins have taken on the responsibilities of editorship and have ably followed the same goal. At the same time they have reenergized the book by enlisting new authors for all but one chapter and by adding new subjects that enlarge the focus of the book. I am delighted that *Office Gynecology* is in their capable hands and that it will continue to be a valuable guide not only for gynecologists but also for family practitioners, internists, house officers, medical students, nurses, nurse practitioners, and nurse midwives.

Robert H. Glass, M.D.
Mill Valley, California

Women's health care is an all-encompassing discipline that crosses many fields of medicine. Virtually every physician is somehow involved regardless of their practice specialty. Gynecologic care not only is one important aspect in the overall health care of women but often serves as the catalyst for a physician office visit. Thus not only the gynecologist but also the pediatrician, family medicine physician, and internist routinely serve the health care needs of women.

Despite this broad office practice, the exposure to gynecologic care in medical schools and residency is almost exclusively surgical in nature and oriented to the inpatient setting. When training is completed, many physicians must reorient their practice patterns to the office setting. This text is designed to help address that problem with each chapter providing valuable information specific to office practice. Each chapter has been authored by clinicians knowledgeable in their field with a clinical and practical focus. A review of the literature is provided along with integrated concepts for cross-reference. The text presents a comprehensive coverage of problems across the spectrum.

The fifth edition is a comprehensive update of Dr. Glass's previous edition. All the chapters have been extensively revised, with new chapters added based on the changing demands of the modern gynecologic office practice. New chapters provide up-to-date information on the following: office diagnosis and management of HIV; the diagnosis and management of hereditary cancer; and psychopharmacology for the office. The newly released Centers for Disease Control and Prevention (CDC) recommendations for pelvic inflammatory disease are also included. Measurement instruments are included for office evaluation of anxiety, depression, and premenstrual syndrome. A new chapter covers the scourge of domestic violence in detail, along with a body map for the office recording of data. Clinical notes at the end of each chapter highlight important points for quick office reference.

We are excited and pleased to bring forward the fifth edition of *Glass's Office Gynecology*. We hope you find it comprehensive, easy to read, and a quick reference source in the office.

ACKNOWLEDGMENTS

This book is a result of hard labor, support, and encouragement from several key people we would like to thank wholeheartedly. We are most appreciative of the support and encouragement given by Dr. Glass for this comprehensive revision and update of his classic text. Our thanks to Charley Mitchell, senior editor at Williams & Wilkins, who had enough faith in us to ask us to do this project. We would like to express our gratitude to Grace Miller, managing editor at Williams & Wilkins, who was there to coax, cajole, and keep things on track. The talent of Shelly Overholt, senior medical student at the University of Texas–Houston is greatly appreciated. She worked diligently and tirelessly with us and, through her efforts, made a substantial contribution for which we are most thankful. Finally, our sincerest thanks to our families for their love, support, and understanding at all times.

Tracey A. Banks, M.D.
Attending
Department of Obstetrics and Gynecology
St. Francis Hospital
Blue Island, Illinois

Andrew Berchuck, M.D.
Professor
Division of Gynecologic Oncology
Department of Obstetrics and Gynecology
Duke University Medical Center
Durham, North Carolina

Abbey B. Berenson, M.D.
Associate Professor
Pediatric and Adolescent Gynecology
Department of Obstetrics and Gynecology
University of Texas Medical Branch at Galveston
Galveston, Texas

Molly A. Brewer, D.V.M., M.D.
Assistant Professor
Department of Gynecology
University of Texas Health Science Center, Houston
MD Anderson Cancer Center
Houston, Texas

John R. Brumsted, M.D.
Professor of Obstetrics and Gynecology
University of Vermont
Burlington, Vermont

Michael Carney, M.D.
Associate Physician, Division of Gynecologic Oncology
Department of Obstetrics and Gynecology
Duke University Medical Center
Durham, North Carolina

Francisco J. Garcini, M.D., Ph.D.
Instructor
Department of Obstetrics, Gynecology, and Reproductive Sciences
The University of Texas—Houston
Lyndon B. Johnson General Hospital
Houston, Texas

William K. Graves, M.D.
Clinical Professor
Department of Obstetrics, Gynecology & Reproductive Services
University of Texas Medical School at Houston
Houston, Texas

Gretchen Gross, L.I.C.S.W., A.C.S.W., N.C.A.C.
Licensed Clinical Social Worker
Division of Reproductive Endocrinology and Infertility
University of Vermont
The Vermont Center for Reproductive Medicine
Fletcher Allen Health Care
Burlington, Vermont

Daniel P. Guyton, M.D.
Professor and Chair, Department of Surgery
Northeastern Ohio Universities College of Medicine
Rootstown, Ohio
Chairman, Department of Surgery
Akron General Medical Center
Akron, Ohio

Hunter Hammill, M.D.
Associate Professor
Department of Pediatrics
Department of Family & Community Medicine
Baylor College of Medicine
Houston, Texas

Kathleen F. Harney, M.D.
Assistant Professor of Obstetrics, Gynecology, and Pediatric/
    Adolescent Gynecology
Tufts University School of Medicine
New England Medical Center
Boston, Massachusetts

Andrew W. Helfgott, M.D.
Associate Professor
Department of Obstetrics and Gynecology
University of Florida College of Medicine
Sacred Heart Hospital
Pensacola, Florida

Michael P. Hopkins, M.D.
Chairman, Department of Obstetrics & Gynecology
Akron General Medical Center
Professor, Department of Obstetrics & Gynecology
Northeastern Ohio Universities College of Medicine
Akron, Ohio

Nicolette S. Horbach, M.D.
Associate Clinical Professor of Obstetrics and Gynecology
George Washington University Medical Center
Innova Fairfax Hospital
Washington, D.C.

Justin P. Lavin, Jr., M.D., F.A.C.O.G.
Chief, Department of Maternal Fetal Medicine
Akron General Medical Center
Akron, Ohio
Professor of Obstetrics and Gynecology
Northeastern Ohio University College of Medicine
Rootstown, Ohio

John C. Petrozza, M.D.
Assistant Professor
Division of Reproductive Endocrinology
Tufts University School of Medicine
New England Medical Center
Boston, Massachusetts

Karen Poley, M.D.
Clinical Instructor
Department of Obstetrics and Gynecology
Tufts University School of Medicine
New England Medical Center
Boston, Massachusetts

Judy Sandella, R.N.C., N.P., M.S.
University of Texas Health Science Center, Houston
MD Anderson Cancer Center
Houston, Texas

Alma Sbach, M.S.N., C.S., F.N.P.
University of Texas Health Science Center, Houston
MD Anderson Cancer Center
Houston, Texas

Melanie K. Snyder, M.D.
Instructor
Akron General Medical Center
Northeastern Ohio Universities College of Medicine
Department of Obstetrics and Gynecology
Rootstown, Ohio

John F. Steege, M.D., F.A.C.O.G.
Chief, Division of Gynecology
Department of Obstetrics and Gynecology
The University of North Carolina at Chapel Hill
Chapel Hill, North Carolina

Meir Steiner, M.D., Ph.D., F.R.C.P.C.
Professor of Psychiatry & Biomedical Sciences
McMaster University
Director, Women's Health Concerns Clinic
St. Joseph's Hospital
Hamilton, Ontario
Canada

John W. Stewart, Jr., M.D.
Assistant Professor
Department of Obstetrics and Gynecology
Northeastern Ohio University College of Medicine
Rootstown, Ohio
Director of Fetal Evaluation
Department of Obstetrics and Gynecology
Akron General Medical Center
Akron, Ohio

John M. Storment, M.D.
Clinical Instructor
Division of Reproductive Endocrinology and Infertility
University of Vermont School of Medicine
The Vermont Center for Reproductive Medicine
Burlington, Vermont

Steven Strong, M.D.
Obstetrician/Gynecologist
Physician's Group of the Woodlands
Woodlands, Texas
Clinical Assistant Professor
Department of Family Medicine
University of Texas Medical Branch at Galveston
Galveston, Texas

Moshe S. Torem, M.D., F.A.P.A.
Chairman, Department of Psychiatry & Behavioral Sciences
Akron General Medical Center
Akron, Ohio
Professor and Chair, Department of Psychiatry
Northeastern Ohio Universities College of Medicine
Rootstown, Ohio

William F. Ziegler, D.O.
Clinical Instructor
Department of Obstetrics and Gynecology
University of Vermont
The Vermont Center for Reproductive Medicine
Burlington, Vermont

Andrea L. Zuckerman, M.D.
Assistant Professor of Obstetrics, Gynecology, and Pediatric/Adolescent Gynecology
Tufts University School of Medicine
New England Medical Center
Boston, Massachusetts

CONTENTS

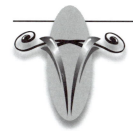

CHAPTER 1

Pediatric and Adolescent Gynecology

ANDREA L. ZUCKERMAN
KATHLEEN F. HARNEY

Both pediatric and adolescent patients often have gynecologic problems. Often pediatricians are not comfortable with gynecologic disorders and gynecologists are not comfortable with pediatric and adolescent patients. Therefore, these patients do not always receive the care and attention they need. Pediatric gynecologic examinations differ from adult exams in that they require more patience and different instruments. Adolescent exams can be performed similarly to adult exams, but careful preparation of the adolescent must be done before starting the exam and different problems must be considered in this population.

EXAMINATION OF PEDIATRIC AND ADOLESCENT PATIENTS

All newborns should undergo a genital examination to determine whether they have normal external genitalia and a vagina present. Patients do present at 18 years of age with vaginal agenesis, never having had an examination of their genitalia previously. If examination of the child's genitalia is performed during routine pediatric appointments, she is less likely to suffer embarrassment during her exams in her adolescent years and congenital anomalies will be diagnosed before puberty.

When examining a young child, it is important to put the child at ease, and often it is helpful to distract the child during the exam. Allow the child to touch and look at all instruments that will be used. The exam should be discussed with the child and her parent or guardian before beginning. It is helpful to look in her ears and listen to her heart, just as you would for a nongynecologic exam. This is part of the exam she is comfortable with and it may put her at ease. Palpation of the breasts with Tanner staging (Fig. 1.1) *and* an abdominal exam should be performed. A child should never be forced into a gynecologic exam; postponing this part of the exam until a return visit may allow the girl to develop a relationship with a new practitioner, ultimately making the examination easier to perform. If an examination needs to be performed immediately, it may be done under anesthesia to minimize traumatization. It is important to inform the parents that an examination will not change the child's hymen unless a vaginoscope or speculum is used. If either instrument is used, the hymenal configuration may change, but this has no implications for her future health or sexuality.

A parent or guardian is usually in the room at the child's head during a gynecologic exam to ease anxiety. The exam should include visualization of the external genitalia and vagina and, in some cases, a rectoabdominal exam. Different positions are used to help visualize the pediatric vagina, such as the frog-leg position or knee-to-chest position. Older children can often be placed in the lithotomy position using stirrups or by straddling the caretaker's legs. A speculum is not used in the pediatric patient unless the child is very cooperative and can tolerate the exam. If it is

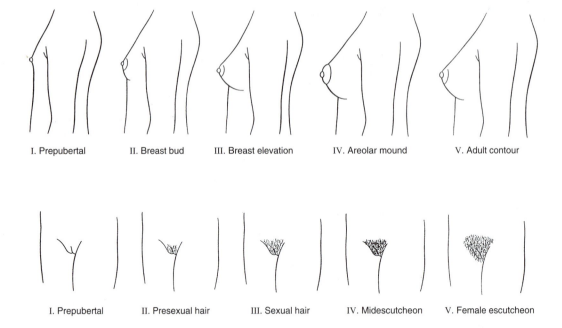

I. Prepubertal   II. Breast bud   III. Breast elevation   IV. Areolar mound   V. Adult contour

I. Prepubertal   II. Presexual hair   III. Sexual hair   IV. Midescutcheon   V. Female escutcheon

FIGURE 1.1. Tanner staging of thelarche and pubarche is helpful for diagnosing premature or delayed aspects of puberty. (Reprinted with permission from Speroff L, Glass RH, Kase NG. Clinical Gynecologic Endocrinology and Infertility. 5th ed. Baltimore: Williams & Wilkins, 1994:378–379.)

necessary to thoroughly examine the vagina, as in the case of undiagnosed vaginal bleeding in a young child, an exam under anesthesia should be performed with the use of a vaginoscope.

When examining the hymen and vagina in a supine position, it is helpful to pull anteriorly and laterally on the labia majora of the child; in knee-to-chest position, pull laterally and posteriorly on the labia majora. These maneuvers open the hymen and allow better visualization. The knee-to-chest position is best for providing visualization of the cervix but requires greater cooperation from the child. For those children whose hymen is redundant, making it difficult to see inside the vagina, Valsalva maneuvers are frequently helpful in opening the hymen. Use of a colposcope is helpful for magnification of the vulva and vagina if one is available; if not, an otoscope or ophthalmoscope can be a useful light source for the vaginal exam.

If a vaginal infection needs to be ruled out, a culture using a moistened Calgi swab (a very small cotton swab, like those used in obtaining urethral cultures in men) should be placed in the vagina after discussion with the patient. Children respond best if they are shown the Calgi swab before the exam begins. The normal-sized cotton swab used in adult women is too large and abrasive, especially when placed in a dry vagina, and is more likely to lead to hymenal changes such as clefts, strictures, or evidence of trauma.

Normal findings in the prepubertal child differ from the adolescent. The labia minora are underdeveloped until the production of estrogen, and the clitoris is small. The newborn is under the influence of maternal hormones, and the effects usually resolve within the first 6 to 8 weeks of life. The most common findings seen in the newborn female are vulvar edema, vaginal discharge and/or bleeding, and breast enlargement. About 10% of newborns will have some withdrawal bleeding.

Approximately two thirds will have a breast discharge similar to colostrum in the neonatal period. These findings are much less pronounced in the premature infant, although their clitoris is relatively large. This is not a cause for concern.

The hymen of newborn infants is usually protruding at the introitus as a result of thickening and enlargement. It may stay thick and enlarged for up to 2 years after birth. The main three normal variants of hymen configuration are annular (circumferential), crescentic, and fimbriated (folded) (Fig. 1.2*A*) (1). Congenital anomalies of the hymen (Fig. 1.2*B*) include imperforate (lacking fenestration), microperforate (with only a small opening into the vagina), cribriform (with multiple small openings), and septate (with a soft-tissue divider forming two openings). In a study by Berenson et al. (1), all newborns who were examined had some hymenal tissue present, and most had annular hymens. Of note, clefts, which are splits in the rim of the hymen, are normally in the anterior hymenal ring. However, those found in the posterior position indicate the occurrence of trauma. This is an important finding for the evaluation of possible sexual abuse (1).

Congenital hymenal anomalies are managed surgically, wherein a needle-tipped cautery is used to resect the extra hymenal tissue. The procedures are quick and easily performed with mask anesthesia, but some parents prefer to wait until the child is older. Patients respond better to the surgery if performed before pubertal development.

Neonates may present with a hymenal polyp or "tag." This is secondary to the high levels of maternal estrogen and will resolve spontaneously. If they persist or the child's parents are overly concerned, resection can be performed in the operating room, but this should be combined with vaginoscopy to rule out a vaginal mass.

Examination of the adolescent should not be rushed. A careful history with special attention to sexual activity and any gynecologic problems should be addressed.

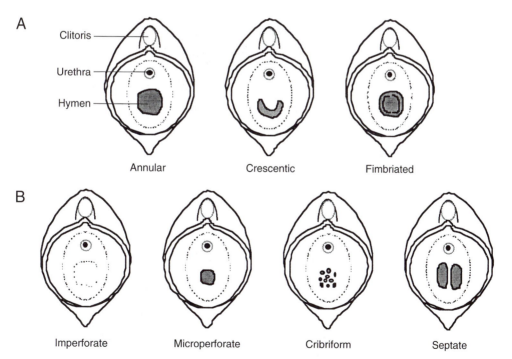

FIGURE 1.2. **A.** Normal variants of hymen configuration are annular (circumferential), crescentic, and fimbriated (folded). **B.** Congenital anomalies of the hymen include imperforate, microperforate, cribriform, and septate.

Adolescence is a time of transition that is very difficult for many patients, and they will frequently have specific concerns regarding development, sexual intercourse, and sexuality. Teens require a health care provider who will spend time with them and answer questions without the patient feeling rushed or criticized.

The examination of the adolescent should include a breast exam and Tanner staging. The pelvic exam should be discussed with the patient (with a demonstration of the speculum) before beginning. It is helpful during the pelvic exam to ask permission for each step of the exam, giving the adolescent a sense of control. A Huffman-Graves speculum is designed to allow easy inspection of the cervix in adolescents. It is as narrow as a Pedersen speculum but as long as a Graves speculum; hence, it is the speculum that most patients tolerate best during their first pelvic exam (Fig. 1.3). In a prepubertal child, the size ratio of the uterine corpus compared with the cervix is 1:3, in the pubertal child it is 1:1, and in the adult woman it is 3:1. Patients who have never been sexually active and who have a tight hymenal ring should undergo a one-finger (rather than two-finger) bimanual exam. Occasionally, it will not be possible to do a bimanual exam, and a rectal examination may have to be done instead.

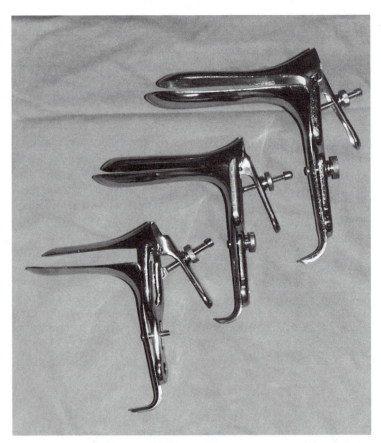

FIGURE 1.3. Speculums for use in the pediatric and adolescent populations are shorter and narrower. The *speculum* on the *bottom* is a Pedersen speculum, which is narrow and short. The *middle speculum* is a Huffman speculum, specially designed to fit the adolescent vagina. The *speculum* on *top* is a Graves speculum, which will cause great discomfort in the adolescent and may even be uncomfortable for the nulliparous, but nonvirginal, woman.

VULVOVAGINITIS

Vulvovaginitis, defined as an inflammatory process involving the vagina and vulva, accounts for approximately 70% of prepubertal gynecologic complaints. The process itself may begin in either the vagina or vulva and spread to the other site. Prepubertal girls are particularly susceptible to vulvovaginal problems for a number of reasons. Poor hygiene and lack of estrogenization of the vaginal epithelium are probably the two most important factors contributing to an increased susceptibility to inflammation and infection. In addition, the prepubertal labia do not cover the entire vestibule and there is a short distance from the anus to the vagina, predisposing young girls to vulvovaginitis (2).

The characteristic symptoms of vulvovaginitis include vulvar pruritus, pain, burning, vaginal discharge (mucopurulent or purulent), and dysuria. Vaginal bleeding may also be a presenting symptom, although other causes such as trauma and a foreign object need to be considered. Typical findings on physical exam may include erythema, excoriations, discharge, blood, cracks or fissures, or even lichenification if the irritation has been chronic. A rash may be present secondary to an infection (e.g., *Staphylococcus*) or a dermatitis (e.g., poison ivy). The differential diagnosis of prepubertal vulvovaginitis includes infectious and noninfectious etiologies, but most commonly no specific cause can be found (Table 1.1). Cultures should be per-

TABLE 1.1. **Differential Diagnosis of Prepubertal Vulvovaginitis**

INFECTIOUS CAUSES
Respiratory pathogens
Group A β-hemolytic streptococcus
S. pneumoniae
N. meningitides
S. aureus
H. influenzae

Enteric pathogen
Shigella

Sexually transmitted (some may be acquired perinatally)
Gardnerella vaginalis
Neisseira gonorrhoeae
Chlamydia trachomatis
Herpes simplex
Human papilloma virus
Trichomonas vaginalis

Others
Candida
Enterobiasis vermicularis (pinworm)

NONINFECTIOUS CAUSES
Foreign body
Poor hygiene
Lichen sclerosus
Psoriasis
Seborrhea
Contact dermatitis
Persistent exposure to urine

formed to rule out infectious agents. This may be done using a saline-moistened Calgi swab inserted gently through the hymenal opening. A wet prep should be done as well, looking for mycotic organisms, *Trichomonas,* parasitic ova, and red and white blood cells. If bleeding is present, attempts should be made to visualize the vagina and cervix to rule out a foreign body.

Infectious Causes

Infectious vulvovaginitis in the prepubertal female may be due to nonsexually transmitted or sexually-transmitted organisms. Respiratory organisms are often involved, and a history of recent respiratory or ear infections should be sought. Pathogens may include group A β-hemolytic streptococci, *Streptococcus pneumoniae, Neisseria meningitidis, Staphylococcus aureus,* or *Haemophilus influenzae.* Group A β-hemolytic streptococcal infection usually presents 7 to 10 days after an upper respiratory infection and may cause vaginal bleeding or a blood-tinged discharge with pronounced irritation of the vulva and perianal area. Treatment is with penicillin (Pen-Vee K, Veetids) 25 to 50 mg/kg per day divided two to four times a day (up to 125 to 250 mg four times a day) for 10 days. *Haemophilus* vaginitis may result in a greenish vaginal discharge and can be treated with amoxicillin (Amoxil, Polymox) 20 to 40 mg/kg per day divided three times a day (up to 250 to 500 mg three times a day) for 7 days. Of the enteric organisms causing vulvovaginitis, *Shigella* is the most common and may in fact cause a bloody vaginal discharge. Diarrhea is absent in most patients. The recommended treatment is trimethoprim/sulfamethoxazole (Bactrim, Septra) 40/200 per 5 mL liquid dosed at 5 mL/10 kg per dose twice a day (up to 10 mL twice a day) for 7 days. Candidal vulvovaginitis is rare in prepubertal girls, and its presence should make one suspicious for diabetes or immunosuppression. Recent antibiotic use may also elicit candidal infection. Initial treatment is with an antifungal cream. Human papilloma virus (HPV) can be a cause and may be transmitted either neonatally or via sexual abuse (3). Pinworm (*Enterobiasis vermicularis*) may also cause vulvovaginitis; physical exam in this case may reveal anal excoriations, and symptoms include vulvar and anal pruritus. The perianal pruritus is typically worse at night. Pinworm is a common entity among children in day care and school. Treatment is oral mebendazole (Vermox) 100 mg in a single dose to everyone in the household over 2 years old. This drug has not been extensively studied in children under 2 years old, so the risks and benefits must be weighed. It is a category C drug for pregnancy.

In any prepubertal female with vulvovaginal symptoms, care must be taken to rule out sexually transmitted organisms as a causal factor (including *Neisseria gonorrhoeae, Chlamydia trachomatis,* herpes simplex virus, HPV, and *Trichomonas vaginalis*) and to rule out sexual abuse, especially in children under the age of consent. The relationship between *Gardnerella vaginalis* (bacterial vaginosis) and sexual abuse in the pediatric patient is not clear. In the prepubertal female, the primary site of a sexually transmitted disease is the vagina, not the cervix, so a vaginal culture should be performed.

Chlamydia may be perinatally acquired and may persist in the vagina for up to a year before being cleared by the immune system. The diagnosis of *Chlamydia* should always be made by cell culture technique because the ELISA test for chlamydia is often falsely positive in the prepubertal child. The findings of either *N. gonorrhea* or *C. trachomatis* should prompt evaluation for sexual abuse, and the patient should be treated to cover both organisms. For the child weighing less than 45 kg, the recommended treatment for *N. gonorrhea* is a single dose of ceftriaxone (Rocephin) intramuscularly using 125 mg if the child weighs less than 45 kg and using 250 mg for those weighing 45 kg or more. If the child is 8 years or older, she should also receive oral doxycycline (Vibramycin, Doryx) 100 mg twice a day for 7 days to cover for *Chlamydia*. The recommended treatment for *C. trachomatis* in the child younger than 8 years is erythromycin ethyl succinate 50 mg/kg per day divided two or four times a day (up to 400 mg four times a day) for 10 days.

Herpes simplex virus (both type I and II), HPV, and *Trichomonas* are usually sexually transmitted when seen in prepubertal girls. It is possible that the child with oral herpes infection (type I or II) may spread it to her genitalia with her hands. The possibility of abuse must, however, be explored. Genital warts can be transmitted by perinatal exposure, close physical contact, or sexual abuse. The amount of time after birth that a perinatally acquired infection may present is not known. Genital warts that appear in the first or second year of life are generally thought to represent perinatal infection. As the age of the child at diagnosis of HPV infection increases, the suspicion of abuse should also rise. Over 50% of children with anal or genital warts have a history of sexual abuse (4, 5). *Trichomonas* is uncommon in prepubertal girls outside the newborn period because the organism prefers an estrogenic environment. The diagnosis is often made on a wet prep, but cultures are more sensitive. Fomites for *Trichomonas,* such as wet towels, have been demonstrated, but if the organism is found in a child, sexual abuse is extremely likely. Treatment for *Trichomonas* in the child is oral metronidazole (Flagyl) 15 mg/kg per day three times a day (up to 250 to 750 mg three times a day) for 7 to 10 days.

Cases of suspected sexual abuse should be handled by a health care team familiar with the evaluation of the prepubertal child. A careful exam, including the use of a colposcope, should be performed (Table 1.2).

Other systemic illnesses and infections may also affect the vulva, including measles, chicken pox, Kawasaki's disease, scarlet fever, and Crohn's disease, and should be considered in the differential diagnosis for vulvovaginal complaints.

Noninfectious Causes

In noninfectious cases, a vaginal culture usually reveals normal vaginal flora, including lactobacilli, diphtheroids, *Staphylococcus epidermidis*, α streptococci, and

TABLE 1.2. Documentation of Physical Findings when Sexual Abuse Is Suspected in a Child

PERINEUM/LABIA

Document the location of lacerations, abrasions, erythema, and bruising and note any discharge.

In the vestibule, look for erythema and note any lesions around the urethra.

In the posterior fourchette, look for labial adhesions, neovascularization, and friability.

HYMEN

Note the configuration (see Fig. 1.2) and the appearance of the edges (thin and sharp, thickened, rolled, projections or notches, vascularity).

Measure the horizontal and vertical diameters, noting which position the child was in at that time.

VAGINA

If visualized, comment on ridges, rugae, and discharge.

If not visualized, note why.

Gram-negative enteric organisms such as *Escherichia coli* (6). Nonspecific vulvo-vaginitis is most likely secondary to irritants. Poor hygiene may contribute to the etiology, and stool or toilet paper may be offending agents. The vulva can also become inflamed in response to chemical irritants such as strong soaps, perfumed or dyed toilet paper, detergents, or bubble baths. Vulvitis may be worse in obese girls or in those with urinary incontinence.

Primary vulvar diseases such as lichen sclerosus, seborrhea, psoriasis, and contact dermatitis may also cause symptoms. Rarely, congenital anomalies, such as an ectopic ureter, in which the ureter drains into the vagina, may be the underlying abnormality leading to recurrent vulvovaginitis secondary to persistent exposure to urine.

Once infectious causes have been ruled out, primary treatment of noninfectious vulvovaginitis includes removing any irritants. Improved hygiene is very important, including demonstration of proper wiping technique (from front to back only). Avoidance of soaps, perfumes, and strong detergent in addition to wearing cotton underwear, avoiding tight jeans or leotards, and changing from wet bathing suits or leotards are all important behavioral practices to recommend. Sitz baths of warm water or warm water with baking soda, colloidal oatmeal, or cornstarch are usually curative and soothing. Wet compresses with Burrow's solution may be helpful in cases of "weepy" vulvar lesions. Antibiotics such as amoxicillin (Amoxil, Polymox) or a cephalosporin may be used in complicated or recurrent cases for 10 days (2). For persistent cases, low-dose antibiotics may need to be used for up to 2 months. Hydrocortisone cream 0.5 to 1.0% may be used on the vulva to decrease inflammation.

Vulvovaginal complaints in adolescents follow along the lines of those seen in adults (see Chapter 6), with a few special considerations. Physiologic leukorrhea, which typically begins 6 months before menarche, may irritate the vulva. Yeast, bacterial vaginosis, and retained tampons are other common causes of vulvovaginitis in the adolescent. Any evaluation of an adolescent should include a history to screen for risk factors for sexually transmitted disease and a pelvic exam. Counseling on the prevention of infections should be part of every visit with adolescents.

LICHEN SCLEROSUS

Lichen sclerosus is a dystrophic lesion of the vulva of unknown etiology. A classic presentation in the prepubertal female would be complaints of vulvar pruritus, irritation and dysuria, and occasional frank bleeding from persistent rubbing. Typically, the vulva would appear white and atrophic. Lichen sclerosus has been described as having a "parchment paper" appearance. At times, the area may show an increase in erythema and vascular markings, although repetitive exams show hypopigmentation in an hourglass shape involving the labial, clitoral, and perianal regions. Those lesions with pronounced vascular markings may bruise easily and produce bloody blisters that are prone to secondary infection(s). The diagnosis in the prepubertal child is usually made clinically and rarely requires a biopsy.

Treatment is initially supportive, with the removal of all irritants and the use of a protective emollient (such as A&D ointment). A sedating antihistamine given at night may help to alleviate scratching. Avoidance of straddle sports (e.g., bicycle riding) is also beneficial. The next step is short-term use of a topical steroid (e.g., hydrocortisone 1.0 to 2.0%). Testosterone cream (useful in postmenopausal patients) is not recommended in children because of the possibility of virilization. Laser therapy has been attempted and has shown some promise (7). Lichen sclerosus resolves spontaneously or improves during puberty in more than 50% of these patients.

LABIAL ADHESIONS

Labial adhesions, complete or partial fusion of the lower labia minora, are a fairly common complaint in the prepubertal girl. The patients typically present between 6 months and 6 years of age, with most cases occurring before the age of 2 years. The etiology of labial adhesions is not known, but it is presumed that the low estrogen state is a contributing factor. In fact, labial adhesions are not seen in the neonate, probably because the maternal estrogens are still high in the newborn circulation. Inflammation of the vulvar tissue from local irritation, trauma, and infection is probably a contributing factor to labial adhesions as well.

Clinically, the vagina may appear "absent" with a thin smooth membrane covering the vaginal opening. Most patients will be asymptomatic, the problem having been discovered by a parent. Some girls have poor drainage of vaginal secretions and interference with urination, sequestration of urine, or, in rare cases, acute urinary retention that requires immediate attention. Others present with recurrent urinary tract infections. Patients may complain of dysuria or recurrent vulvar or vaginal infections.

Mild asymptomatic cases may simply be followed, as they will resolve at puberty with the increase in systemic estrogen. If more severe or if the parent is anxious for treatment, topical estrogen cream applied directly over the central raphe of the adhesions twice daily for 2 to 3 weeks will separate most adhesions (8). After separation, daily use of an emollient (e.g., Desitin or A&D ointment) will keep the labia separated. Good perineal hygiene is important in these patients. In cases where medical treatment fails or acute urinary retention exists, surgical separation of adhesions is necessary. Although the adhesions separate easily, it should never be done in the office without anesthesia (viscous lidocaine [Xylocaine 2%]) because it is extremely painful for the child.

PREPUBERTAL VAGINAL BLEEDING

Vaginal bleeding in childhood is a relatively rare and, for parents, alarming condition that requires immediate attention to rule out significant pathology. It may be secondary to a number of processes, including exogenous hormones, inflammation or infection, trauma, foreign body, genital tract neoplasm, or urologic pathology (Table 1.3) (9). Another possible etiology, precocious puberty, is discussed in the next section.

TABLE 1.3. Causes of Prepubertal Vaginal Bleeding

Exogenous hormones
Inflammation or infection
Trauma
Foreign body
Urologic pathology
Genital tract neoplasm

Exogenous Hormones

Genital bleeding in the prepubertal female may represent bleeding from the endometrium. Such bleeding may be seen in the first few weeks of life as the result of estrogen withdrawal as the maternal hormones are cleared from the newborn's circulation. No treatment is necessary and the condition is self-limiting. Iatrogenic causes, such as the use of estrogen cream for the treatment of labial adhesions, may also lead to prepubertal bleeding (10). A careful history should be taken to exclude ingestion of prescription hormone pills.

Isolated precocious menarche without any other signs of pubertal development is rare but has been reported. Isolated episodes of vaginal bleeding are suspected to be due to elevations in plasma estradiol as a result of transient ovarian activity and possibly to an increased sensitivity of the endometrium to estrogens (11). In these cases, one sees normal pubertal development at the appropriate age with subsequent normal fertility and attainment of expected height (12). These patients should, of course, be followed closely for any signs of true precocious puberty.

Inflammation and Infection

Some studies suggest that as many as 45% of cases of prepubertal vaginal bleeding may be attributable to infection or inflammation (13). Of the specific infectious etiologies, *Shigella* has been associated with a bloody vaginal discharge and bloody diarrhea. Vaginitis caused by group A β-hemolytic *Streptococcus* often results in vaginal bleeding. Condylomata acuminata (venereal warts) are seen in the pediatric population, most often associated with sexual abuse. These exophytic lesions, which may be vaginal or vulvar in location, may be extremely friable and present with vaginal bleeding. Lichen sclerosus and vulvovaginitis, discussed earlier in this chapter, may also have vaginal bleeding as a presenting symptom.

Trauma

Trauma may result in a vulvar hematoma and/or laceration with subsequent vaginal bleeding. Such injuries are fairly common with bike riding and other activities, especially in the summer months. Important in the evaluation of trauma is exclusion of the possibility of sexual abuse; the physician should evaluate the injury for compatibility with the story. Of equal importance is determination of the extent of the injury and whether it requires an examination under anesthesia or surgical repair. In the case of an injury that is penetrating or if hymenal injury cannot be excluded, care must be taken to ensure that the peritoneal cavity was not penetrated. This may require examination under anesthesia. Catheterization and rectal exam must be done to evaluate the integrity of the bladder and bowel. Many vulvar hematomas may be managed nonsurgically with the use of ice, observation, and serial hemoglobin measurements to ensure that the hematoma is stable. Placement of a Foley catheter is often necessary in these cases because significant swelling may occur and obstruct the urethral outflow (14).

Foreign Bodies

Foreign bodies placed in the vagina by a small child are a common cause for childhood vaginal bleeding. They usually result in a foul-smelling, bloody vaginal discharge. The presentation may look suspicious for sexual abuse if changes are seen in the posterior aspect of the hymen. Usually, the child will not acknowledge or recall placing a foreign body in her vagina. The most common foreign body reported by most series is toilet paper; other common objects are pen caps, safety pins, coins, and hair pins. Most foreign bodies are not radiopaque, so x-ray studies are often not helpful.

Management in the office using a local anesthetic and nasal speculum may be possible in some patients; however, a child should never be forced to undergo an exam, and complete visualization of the cervix and vagina is preferable. Visualization via vaginoscopy may reveal a foreign body or simply a reactive area of the vaginal mucosa, since frequently the foreign body will have been spontaneously expelled or removed by the child. In most cases of prepubertal vaginal bleeding, examination under anesthesia with vaginoscopy should be performed to visualize the entire vaginal canal. Irrigation may be helpful in flushing out small foreign bodies, especially those in the lower third of the vagina. Larger objects may require use of forceps. The presence of vaginal excrescences may help to differentiate vaginal bleeding due to a foreign body versus sexual abuse (15). Recurrences of vaginal foreign bodies are common, so the parent(s) and child should be counseled regarding proper perineal hygiene.

Urologic Pathology

Disorders of the urinary tract may initially present as "vaginal bleeding." Patients with urinary tract infections and gross hematuria may present to the pediatric gynecologist with complaints of vaginal bleeding. Urethral prolapse, a complete circular eversion of the urethral mucosa, presents as a painless bleeding annular lesion above the vaginal entrance. Urethral prolapse may be seen secondary to trauma or medical conditions that lead to an increase in intraabdominal pressure (e.g., constipation leading to straining). The average age of children with urethral prolapse is 5 years old. Therapy consists of frequent sitz baths, estrogen cream, and, in the presence of infection, topical or oral antibiotics. With these measures, urethral prolapse will usually resolve in 4 to 6 weeks. Where possible, the underlying cause should be treated. Urethral prolapse requires surgical intervention if medical therapy fails, if the prolapsed tissue becomes necrotic, or if there is acute urinary retention. An indwelling catheter should be used for 24 hours postoperatively. Rarer urologic abnormalities such as urethral neoplasms may also present as vaginal bleeding.

Genital Tract Neoplasms

Genital tract tumors often present with vaginal bleeding and should be completely excluded in any case of prepubertal vaginal bleeding. Benign vaginal polyps should be removed and examined pathologically to exclude malignancy (16). Other benign tumors of the vulva and vagina that may occur in children and adolescents include hemangiomas, simple hymenal cysts, paraurethral duct cysts, teratomas, or even benign granulomas. Hemangiomas of the capillaries usually resolve with puberty and require no intervention. Cavernous hemangiomas may bleed extensively if injured, so surgical intervention is warranted. A paraurethral duct cyst may distort the urethra, and surgical treatment is recommended. Teratomas present as midline, cystic perineal masses. They are usually benign, but because recurrence is likely, a large margin of healthy tissue is excised at the time of surgery.

Cancer of the genital tract is rare in prepubertal girls; unfortunately, these tumors often carry a poor prognosis. They are more common in girls less than 4 years old. The most common malignant tumors of the prepubertal vagina include the embryonal rhabdomyosarcoma (more commonly known as sarcoma botryoides) and adenocarcinoma of the vagina; both may present with vaginal bleeding. Sarcoma botryoides is the most common malignancy of the lower genital tract in girls and appears as a friable polypoid tumor originating from the anterior vagina. The tumor arises in the submucosal tissues and spreads beneath the vaginal epithelium. This causes the vaginal mucosa to bulge into a series of polypoid growths. Definitive diagnosis requires a biopsy of the lesion. A combination of surgery, chemotherapy, and radiotherapy offers the best treatment success to these patients. Clear-cell adenocarcinoma of the vagina, a rare malignancy, is associated with in utero exposure to diethylstilbestrol. Endodermal sinus tumor of the vagina is a rare germ cell tumor with a poor outcome. Granulosa theca cell tumors of the ovary are the most common tumor, producing signs of precocious puberty. These may present as an abdominal mass (and abdominal pain) because the ovaries are at the pelvic brim in the prepubertal patient. Surgery consisting of a unilateral salpingo-oophorectomy is usually curative (17).

PUBERTAL ABNORMALITIES

Puberty is the development of secondary sexual characteristics and the attainment of reproductive capabilities (18). The changes seen during puberty are secondary to increased secretion of adrenal androgens followed by increased secretion of ovarian steroids (19). The regulation of these hormones is controlled by gonadotropin-releasing hormone (GnRH) secretion from the hypothalamus. GnRH is secreted in a pulsatile fashion and this stimulates pulsatile release of luteinizing hormone (LH) and follicle-stimulating hormone (FSH) from the anterior pituitary gland (20).

Puberty begins with thelarche (breast development) in 85% of girls. The remainder of patients experience pubarche (pubic and axillary hair development) first (18). Breast development begins with a gradual increase in unopposed estrogen (20). Initially, estrogen levels are low, but they rise with pubertal development. At times, breast development is unilateral, although it ultimately progresses to bilateral development (21). Pubarche usually follow thelarche by about 6 months (22). An acceleration in the rate of growth ("growth spurt") accompanies, or precedes, the development of secondary sex characteristics. Often, an early hallmark of onset of accelerated growth is a sudden increase in shoe size. In early puberty, girls grow 4 to 5 cm (1.5 to 2 inches) per year. This skeletal growth is initiated by very low levels of estrogen. During the growth spurt, maximal growth velocity is approximately 9 cm (3.5 inches) per year and occurs in girls around age 12 years (22). By the time maximal growth velocity is reached, about 90% of final adult height has been achieved. Most girls reach maximal growth velocity 2 years after thelarche and approximately 1 year before menarche. Menarche (onset of menstruation) follows the peak of the growth spurt and occurs at a mean age of 12.8 years (23). After menarche, growth slows and usually no more than 6 cm (2.5 inches) is further achieved. Puberty is complete once positive feedback of estrogen on the pituitary and hypothalamus has occurred, inducing ovulation.

The entire normal pubertal process usually occurs over 18 months to 6 years (23). The timing of puberty appears to be largely genetic, although factors such as geographic location, health, nutrition, and psychological factors play a role (23). Pubertal abnormalities include many types of both precocious and delayed puberty, delayed being the more common (22).

Premature Thelarche

Normal thelarche occurs between 8 and 13 years with a mean age of 9.5 years (22) and represents the first sign of increased ovarian estradiol production (24). Premature thelarche is defined as breast development before 8 years old and must be differentiated from precocious puberty (25). It may be unilateral or bilateral. Approximately 10% of patients with premature thelarche will progress to precocious puberty, whereas the remainder regress and undergo puberty at a normal time (25, 26). Premature thelarche before 2 years old is more common than in later childhood years, and most of these cases will regress completely and without any long-term sequelae (27, 28); bone age in these patients is equal to chronologic age, and vaginal smears fail to show any estrogen effect. Surgical biopsy is not warranted. However, when premature thelarche occurs after 2 years old, it more frequently persists and often is a sign of early and precocious puberty. Patients who experience persistent premature thelarche frequently have accelerated bone age (28). All patients with premature thelarche show an elevation in their FSH and LH levels (28).

The pathophysiology of premature thelarche is still unclear. It is believed to result from a transient increase in estrogen secretion (such as from a follicular cyst), increased sensitivity of the breast to estrogen, ingestion of estrogen via food contamination, or from activation of the hypothalamic-pituitary-ovarian axis, causing increased secretion of FSH (25). Premature thelarche usually lasts 6 months to 6 years, although it may persist. It is bilateral in about half of reported cases (27). One study on premature babies with very-low birth weight showed an 8.7% increased risk of premature thelarche compared with a normal population (29). This was thought to be caused by damage to the hypothalamic-pituitary-ovarian axis.

Because most precocious thelarche cases are self-limiting, treatment is not recommended (30). Patients should be followed carefully every 6 months until resolution, because progression to full precocious puberty may occur.

Precocious Adrenarche and Pubarche

Adrenarche begins with the maturation of the zona reticularis of the adrenal glands, leading to an increase in adrenal gland secretion of dehydroepiandrosterone (DHEA), dehydroepiandrosterone sulfate (DHEA-S), and androstenedione (18, 31). This in turn stimulates pubic and axillary hair development (pubarche) and acne (18). Adrenarche occurs independently of gonadarche (maturation of the gonads and secretion of sex steroids), but they are temporally related in most cases (18, 32). Gonadarche typically occurs 2 years after adrenarche.

Premature adrenarche is the secretion of adrenal androgens before age 8, and most cases occur after age 6 (31, 33, 34). It may be due to an adrenal enzyme deficiency or a tumor (e.g., Sertoli-Leydig cell tumor). Measurement of 17-hydroxyprogesterone is usually adequate to exclude an adrenal enzyme deficit, specifically 21-hydroxylase deficiency. In patients with advanced bone age or circulating androgens consistent with late puberty or adulthood, an adrenocorticotropic hormone stimulation test should be performed. Precocious adrenarche does not progress into precocious puberty (18, 34). Gonadotropin levels are at prepubertal levels, whereas adrenal androgen levels are at pubertal levels. Premature adrenarche may accelerate bone maturation or growth but does not lead to short adult stature (14). Typically, premature adrenarche patients reach pubic Tanner stages II and III without any breast development (31).

Premature adrenarche and pubarche are seen more commonly in certain ethnic backgrounds such as blacks and Hispanics. Causes include precocious puberty, enzyme deficiencies such as congenital adrenal hyperplasia, heightened sensitivity to adrenal androgens, or androgen-secreting ovarian tumors (33–35).

DHEA-S, produced entirely from adrenal DHEA, is a useful marker of adrenarche (32). Congenital adrenal hyperplasia is screened with the dexamethasone suppression test and an 8 AM 17-hydroxyprogesterone level (33). These tests must be done in the morning because of diurnal variation.

It is recommended to follow patients every 6 to 12 months from the onset of precocious pubarche and/or adrenarche until late adolescence or early adulthood because these patients are at increased risk for menstrual irregularity, hirsutism, acne, and polycystic ovarian disorder (26). No other long-term sequelae appear to result from premature pubarche and adrenarche.

Precocious Menarche

Premature menarche is the development of cyclic vaginal bleeding without other signs of secondary sex characteristic development (36). Once other causes of prepubertal vaginal bleeding (discussed earlier in chapter) have been excluded, this diagnosis can be made. This condition is thought to be secondary to transient estrogen production from premature follicular development or it may result from heightened endometrial sensitivity to low estrogen levels. Estradiol levels are prepubertal, and vaginal smears fail to show estrogen effect. Adult height is not compromised in these patients, and their eventual menstrual patterns and fertility are not adversely affected.

Precocious Puberty

Precocious puberty is defined as pubertal development in girls before the age of 8, which is 2.5 standard deviations (SDs) below the mean age of pubertal onset (22). It usually progresses from premature thelarche to menarche (as in normal puberty), since the breasts respond faster to estrogen than the endometrium. The incidence of precocious puberty is 1 in 5,000 to 1 in 10,000 (18) and is more common in girls than boys at a ratio of 23:1 (22, 30, 35). The etiology, however, is discovered more frequently in boys than in girls. In girls older than 4 years, a specific etiology for true precocious puberty is usually not found, whereas in younger girls, a central nervous system (CNS) lesion is often present.

There are two main categories of precocious puberty: central (which is GnRH dependent) and peripheral (which is GnRH independent) (Table 1.4). In either case, ovulation occurs and so can pregnancy (36).

TABLE 1.4. Precocious Puberty Types and Causes

CENTRAL (GnRH DEPENDENT)
Idiopathic
CNS tumors
Hydrocephaly
CNS injury secondary to trauma or infection
CNS irradiation
Neurofibromatosis
PERIPHERAL (GnRH INDEPENDENT)
Hormone-excreting tumor of adrenal glands or ovaries
Gonadotropin-producing tumors
Congenital adrenal hyperplasia
McCune-Albright syndrome
Severe hypothyroidism
Exogenous estrogens
Follicular cysts of the ovary

Central Precocious Puberty

Central, or true, precocious puberty is caused by activation of the hypothalamic-pituitary-ovarian axis, leading to secretion of gonadotropins and ovarian sex steroids (37). Idiopathic activation of this axis is the most common cause of central precocious puberty in girls, comprising about 80% of cases (18, 30). Central precocious puberty can also be caused by tumors of the CNS (most commonly congenital hamartomas of GnRH neurons [35]), hydrocephaly, CNS injury from trauma or infections, CNS irradiation, and neurofibromatosis. CNS lesions cause about 15% of central precocious puberty cases (36). When the diagnosis of true precocious puberty is made, radiographic imaging of the CNS with either computed tomography (CT) or magnetic resonance imaging (MRI) is done. Patients with known CNS lesions or a history of CNS irradiation and true precocious puberty should have growth hormone levels drawn in their evaluation.

Patients with central precocious puberty have a disinhibited GnRH pulse generator, leading to LH and FSH levels in the pubertal range and ratio. The LH and FSH levels may fluctuate, so multiple samples (e.g., every 30 minutes for several hours) may be necessary. A GnRH stimulation test in girls with central precocious puberty shows a pubertal response, with LH levels rising three times above baseline and elevating greater than FSH levels (38). The pattern of pubertal development and its chronologic progression are normal, albeit at an abnormally early age.

Peripheral Precocious Puberty

Peripheral, or pseudoprecocious, puberty is the result of secretion of sex steroids by peripheral sources such as a hormone-secreting tumor of the adrenal gland or ovaries, gonadotropin-producing tumors, congenital adrenal hyperplasia, McCune-Albright syndrome (polyostotic fibrous dysplasia of the long bones, cafe au lait spots, and peripheral precocious puberty), and severe hypothyroidism (18, 22, 35, 37). Exogenous estrogen in the form of medications, skin creams, or ingestion of estrogen-treated animal meat (particularly poultry) must be excluded. Peripheral precocious puberty can be either isosexual (same-sex development) or heterosexual (masculinizing development).

Hypothyroidism may cause peripheral precocious puberty. With severe hypothyroidism, elevated FSH levels (36) and delayed bone growth are usually seen. The elevated FSH induces the formation of ovarian cysts and estrogen production. The occurrence of primary hypothyroidism and precocious puberty has been associated with galactorrhea and pituitary enlargement as well. This premature puberty is reversible with thyroid hormone replacement (39).

McCune-Albright syndrome causes peripheral precocity via autonomously functioning cysts of the ovary. Diagnosis is based on the skin pigmentation changes and demonstration of bone lesions or pathologic fractures. However, in this condition, the order and progression of pubertal development does not necessarily follow the normal path (22). Vaginal bleeding is the first sign of puberty in most patients. Testolactone (Teslac), an androgenic agent, appears to be effective treatment (36). Prognosis for girls with McCune-Albright is not good. Most achieve reduced adult heights secondary to premature epiphyseal closure and pathologic fractures. Most suffer menstrual irregularities and are infertile.

Follicular cysts are the most common gonadal cause of peripheral precocious puberty (22). These follicular cysts may occur spontaneously or result from benign ovarian tumors, inducing the surrounding tissue to produce estrogen. Ovarian cysts tend to be recurrent, so surgical excision is not usually helpful. Treatment with medroxyprogesterone acetate (Provera, Cycrin) may inhibit estrogen production

TABLE 1.5. Workup of Precocious Puberty

History and physical, including pelvic/rectoabdominal examination if possible
Vaginal maturation index
Lab tests: estradiol, thyroid function tests, testosterone, progesterone, β-hCG,
   adrenal androgen levels
Ultrasound of abdomen/pelvis or MRI
Bone age assessment

and FSH release, ultimately causing the cyst(s) to regress. Testolactone (Teslac), which inhibits aromatase and hence peripheral production of estrogen, may also be useful. Juvenile granulosa cell tumors are another gonadal cause; these are almost always unilateral and usually present at an early stage (22). With peripheral precocious puberty, the prolonged or repeated exposure of the CNS to estrogen may culminate in superimposed central precocious puberty as well. In these cases, treatment of the peripheral cause may not be sufficient to arrest pubertal development and addition of a GnRH agonist may be required.

The evaluation of patients suspected to have precocious puberty, central or peripheral, includes a complete history with close attention to any past or current medical problems, medications ingested, family history of precocious puberty, and ethnic background. Careful questioning on the type of development, timing of development, and rapidity of progression are helpful. A complete physical examination should focus on height and weight (plotted on a growth curve), vital signs, neurologic evaluation including vision, examination of the skin (focusing on pigmentation and signs of virilization such as acne and hirsutism), thyroid, abdomen, and Tanner staging of the breasts and pubic hair (21). Some patients will allow a pelvic examination or a rectoabdominal examination. A vaginal smear for maturation index can be obtained and is helpful in quantifying the amount of estrogen present. Patients with peripheral precocious puberty do not have elevated LH and FSH levels (unless the cause is hypothyroidism). They will show a prepubertal response to a GnRH stimulation test with FSH levels remaining higher than LH levels (18). Laboratory tests should include estradiol, thyroid function tests, testosterone, progesterone, human chorionic gonadotropin (hCG), and adrenal androgen levels. An ultrasound of the abdomen and pelvis is performed to better assess the adrenals and ovaries and to rule out a tumor or cyst(s). Imaging studies, MRI being the most sensitive (37), should be done in all patients under 6 years old and should be considered for patients 6 to 8 years old (Table 1.5).

In addition to its role in bone mineral density, estrogen is important for the maturation and growth of bones during puberty. The diagnostic evaluation of precocious puberty includes a bone age to look for accelerated growth: a radiograph of the nondominant hand is compared with appropriate tables of normal bone (such as those in Greulich and Pyle) to determine chronologic ages (18). A bone age of 11 years usually corresponds with breast development, whereas a bone age of 13 years corresponds with menarche (23). Any bone age greater than 2 SDs above the mean indicates accelerated bone maturation (18). Patients with precocious puberty begin their growth spurt at a shorter height than normal and also undergo premature closure of the epiphyseal plates. Thus, the end height that these patients attain is less than if they began their growth spurt at a normal age and height (30, 35, 39). One quarter to one third of girls with untreated precocious puberty will attain adult heights less than 150 cm (5 feet) (40).

Patients with precocious puberty should undergo treatment to ensure attainment of normal adult height and to return to prepubertal status to prevent the psychological and social issues incurred with puberty. Patients with untreated precocious puberty are physiologically capable of becoming pregnant (36). Treatment of peripheral precocious puberty is aimed at treating the underlying cause, as is also true when a cause of central precocious puberty can be found.

Treatment of central precocious puberty with a long-acting GnRH agonist results in arrest of pubertal development and return of estradiol levels to prepubertal levels (22, 41). Pediatric patients tolerate the GnRH agonist therapy very well. Predicted adult height can be increased by 5 to 10 cm (2 to 4 inches) by treatment with a slow-release GnRH agonist in a dose of 0.3 mg/kg every 4 weeks (22). A decrease in bone mass has been noted with this treatment (40–42), but preliminary studies show children undergoing treatment with a GnRH agonist still exhibit an increase in bone mineral density and growth consistent with rates normal for their chronologic age (42). Correct dosing of the GnRH agonist can be ascertained by an abbreviated GnRH stimulation test, which should show suppressed LH and FSH levels (38). Treatment should be stopped when patients reach an appropriate age for puberty, good height prognosis is attained, or if the family desires treatment stopped. In older girls with precocious puberty, the degree of bone age advancement and rapidity of progression of the pubertal process are key issues in determining initiation, continuation, and cessation of therapy. If therapy is not initiated, or stopped, the amount of compromise in final adult height (based on calculated decreases in predicted adult height) must be fully addressed with the patient and her family. Once treatment is stopped, pubertal development occurs more quickly than in normal children. Menarche typically occurs just over a year after treatment is stopped (42). Women with a history of precocious puberty do not have an increased risk for or incidence of premature menopause.

Delayed Puberty

Delayed puberty is defined as the absence of any secondary sexual characteristics by age 13, which is 2.5 SDs from the mean, or no menarche by age 15; it occurs in about 3% of children (19, 22, 35, 43, 44). It can be classified by the status of the secondary sexual characteristics. The etiology of pubertal delay may be constitutional, anatomic, or secondary to hypergonadotropic or hypogonadotropic hypogonadism (Table 1.6) (19). Patients with delayed puberty of any cause will have low estrogen levels, and bone age may be delayed to ages 11 or 12 years. If the bone age is more severely delayed, hypothyroidism and growth hormone deficiency should also be considered (22).

Eugonadism

Patients categorized with eugonadism have normal gonadotropin levels but nevertheless present with pubertal delay or amenorrhea. On physical examination, patients may be found to have an anatomic cause of amenorrhea; müllerian anomalies are addressed in "Congenital Anomalies," below. If a normal vagina is found, the patient should be assessed for estrogen production to rule out chronic anovulation or polycystic ovarian syndrome. Assessment of estrogen levels can be accomplished in two ways. A vaginal smear may be performed by gently rolling a cotton swab on the lateral vaginal walls and then rolling the cotton swab onto a slide without overlapping the rows. Once the slide dries, it should be stained with, for example, urine sedistain for 1 minute before examination under a microscope. If greater than 30% of the cells seen are superficial cells, the patient has adequate estrogen production. However, if parabasal and intermediate cells predominate, the patient is hypoestro-

TABLE 1.6. Delayed Puberty: Types and Causes

CONSTITUTIONAL

ANATOMIC
Imperforate hymen
Transverse vaginal septum
Vaginal agenesis (most common anatomic defect)
Uterine didelphys with longitudinal vaginal septum

EUGONADISM
Chronic anovulation
Polycystic ovarian disease

HYPERGONADOTROPIC HYPOGONADISM
Chromosomally competent
Gonadal agenesis
Testicular feminization (androgen insensitivity)
Swyer's syndrome
Premature ovarian failure secondary to autoimmune disease, chemotherapy,
  irradiation
Resistant ovary syndrome

Chromosomally incompetent
Turner's syndrome (most common in this category)

HYPOGONADOTROPIC HYPOGONADISM
Constitutional
CNS tumors (craniopharyngiomas, pituitary adenomas)
Illicit drug use, esp. marijuana
Eating disorders
Excessive exercise
Stress
Chronic illness, including endocrinopathies
Kallmann's syndrome
Isolated gonadotropin deficiency
Pituitary destruction

DELAYED PUBERTY WITH VIRILIZATION
Enzyme deficiency (e.g., 21-hydroxylase deficiency)
Neoplasm
Male pseudohermaphroditism

genic. The second test for estrogen levels is the progestin challenge test. Patients are given medroxyprogesterone acetate (Provera), 10 mg/day for 12 days, and should have a normal withdrawal bleed within 1 week after stopping the progestin if they have adequate estrogen production (22).

Another cause of eugonadism with primary amenorrhea is androgen insensitivity (also called testicular feminization). In this case, patients have a 46,XY karyotype but are phenotypically female due to an androgen receptor defect. The gonads are normal testicles, usually intraabdominal. Testosterone levels are elevated to the normal male range, patients attain tall stature, and breast development occurs because of aromatization of androgens to estrogens and a small amount of estrogen production by the testes. The breasts are abnormal because there is little actual glandular tissue, the nipples are small, and the areolae are pale in color. Patients' quantity of pubic hair ranges from normal to none, depending on whether the androgen receptor defect is complete or partial. An inguinal hernia is present in over 50% of these patients. The labia minora are usually poorly developed, and the vagina is a short, blind pouch. A vaginal smear in these patients may be normal, but they do not have a uterus or cervix. Because there is no dysgenesis, the gonads should be retained until after puberty to allow growth and breast development but then should be removed because they can undergo malignant transformation (22). After removal of the gonads, patients should be placed on estrogen therapy to maintain the secondary sex characteristics (22).

Patients with incomplete androgen insensitivity will exhibit signs of virilization, and removal of the gonads is done once the diagnosis is made to prevent malignant transformation. Fortunately, this variant is rare.

Congenital Anomalies

The uterus and upper two thirds of the vagina originate from the müllerian or paramesonephric ducts (45), and congenital anomalies are found in this system in 2 to 3% of women (46). The müllerian system is closely related to the urinary system embryologically; thus, anomalies found in one system obligate a close evaluation of the other system. Both the metanephric duct, which is the embryologic origin of the ureters, kidneys, and bladder, and the paramesonephric duct originate from the mesonephric or wolffian duct (47). The müllerian ducts fuse to form the uterus and upper vagina. They also fuse with the urogenital sinus to form the vaginal plate. Initially, the vaginal plate is solid but canalization occurs to result in a normal vagina (47).

Patients with an imperforate hymen may present as a neonate, prepubertal child, or during puberty. Bulging may be seen in the area of the hymen from a collection of mucus (a mucocolpos) in the prepubertal child or of blood (hematocolpos) in the pubertal child. Patients with hematocolpos may complain of cyclic crampy pain, and physical exam reveals normal secondary sexual characteristics. Correction is made surgically.

Hematocolpos, hematometra, and even hematoperitoneum can also result from a transverse vaginal septum, although this is much more rare than an imperforate hymen. On exam, a transverse vaginal septum will usually not bulge with Valsalva maneuvers, although an imperforate hymen will. An ultrasound examination will show a normal uterus and cervix, although they may be dilated with the accumulation of menstrual blood. Repair of this defect is also surgical but is much more complicated than that of the imperforate hymen. Care must be taken not to cause stenosis of the vagina. Postoperatively, patients often need to use vaginal dilators to prevent stricture of the vagina (45).

An adolescent with an anatomic defect may also present with complaints of cyclic crampy pain, often with progressively worsening dysmenorrhea, but with all the milestones of puberty met (48). These patients must be evaluated for a duplication of the müllerian system in which the müllerian bulbs fail to fuse. Patients may have a uterine didelphys with a longitudinal vaginal septum and a hemiobstructed vagina; these patients may complain of urinary retention and have a unilateral vaginal mass on examination. Ultrasound reveals a pelvic mass secondary to a hematocolpos. This has at times been mistaken for a germ cell tumor. Because this anomaly is almost always associated with renal agenesis on the side of the hemiobstruction, a renal ultrasound should be performed when this diagnosis is considered. There is an increased incidence of endometriosis secondary to the obstruction that usually regresses after surgical relief of the obstruction (48). MRI may be the most useful radiographic study to illustrate the exact nature of the anatomic defect(s) and help in the planning of surgical repair(s).

The two-part surgical repair of this condition first involves drainage of the hematocolpos by making an incision into the vaginal septum over the obstruction. This incision should be large enough to remain open until the second surgery is performed. The second surgery is resection of the longitudinal vaginal septum with care being given to avoid the bladder and rectum. An intraoperative hysterosalpingogram should be performed to rule out any connection between the two uterine cavities. A laparoscopy may be performed to evaluate for endometriosis (46), but in most cases, any endometriosis present resolves after adequate drainage of the hemiobstruction (49). A unicornuate uterus with a noncommunicating but functional horn may present similarly, and these patients also usually have renal agenesis (46).

The most common anatomic anomaly causing primary amenorrhea is that of vaginal agenesis or Mayer-Rokitansky-Kuster-Hauser syndrome. The incidence is approximately 1 in 5000 (50). It is second only to gonadal dysgenesis as a cause for primary amenorrhea. Often, the diagnosis is missed until the late teenage years when patients present with primary amenorrhea. Demonstration of a normal female karyotype is important to rule out some types of male pseudohermaphroditism. As discussed in the section above, androgen insensitivity presents similarly and should be ruled out. MRI is a very useful radiologic study to aid in the diagnosis of vaginal agenesis.

Most patients with vaginal agenesis have no functioning endometrial tissue within the uterine bulbs or remnants, although a few patients will have some (47). It is rare to see a normal uterus, but there have been a few reported cases of pregnancy after a connecting surgical procedure has been performed. Vaginal agenesis patients have a normal 46,XX karyotype and exhibit normal development of secondary sex characteristics and ovarian function. Urinary and renal anomalies such as pelvic kidney and renal agenesis are common, occurring in approximately 40% of patients. Skeletal anomalies such as scoliosis and wedge vertebrae are also common and occur in about 12% of patients (45, 47). Growth and development overall are normal.

Treatment of vaginal agenesis consists of the creation of a neovagina. This can be accomplished through the use of molds (Frank dilators) or through surgery. Patients are fitted with a dilator and shown where to place it. They then wear spandex underwear and sit on a bicycle seat, preferably a racing bike seat, to hold pressure on the mold. Patients must be cautioned to position the mold carefully so accidental dilation of the urethra does not occur. Patients should be encouraged to use the molds from 20 minutes up to 2 hours a day (to the point of modest discomfort) and to return to the office for frequent examinations and refitting of the molds. An adequate vagina can be attained in a few months time. Plastic syringe covers can be used in lieu of the commercially available dilators. A more in-depth description of the use of dilators can be found in the 1971 article by Wabrek et al. (51).

Some patients, however, prefer to undergo surgical creation of a neovagina. The most common surgical procedure is called a McIndoe (45). This procedure uses a split-thickness skin graft over a mold. A space is surgically created between the urethra and rectum, with care not to enter either. The mold is sewn in place and removed after 1 week, using cautery to remove any granulation tissue seen. Postoperatively, patients must use a mold to prevent scarring and stenosis of their neovagina. Operative treatment is usually reserved for patients in whom dilator usage is unacceptable or has failed or if a well-formed uterus is present and surgery will preserve fertility.

Hypergonadotropic Hypogonadism

In evaluating patients with delayed puberty and hypogonadism, it is important to check gonadotropin levels. FSH and LH levels are secreted in a pulsatile fashion, and thus levels may vary (22), but if they are found to be elevated on several occasions, the patient has hypergonadotropic hypogonadism. Hypergonadotropic hypogonadism may be divided into chromosomally competent and chromosomally incompetent categories. Patients, therefore, must have a karyotype checked (22, 44).

Chromosomally Competent. Patients with hypergonadal hypogonadism can have a karyotype of either 46,XY or 46,XX. Patients with 46,XY genotype but female phenotype have either Swyer's syndrome or testicular feminization (androgen insensitivity). Of the two, androgen insensitivity is more common. It is discussed in more detail earlier in the chapter (see Eugonadism). With Swyer's syndrome, gonadal dysgenesis is present. Patients have streak gonads with a Y cell line and thus are at risk of developing gonadal malignancies (incidence more than 25%); the gonads should be removed once the patient is diagnosed. These patients have a vagina and uterus because they cannot produce müllerian-inhibiting substance, but they experience pubertal delay and need treatment with estrogen to undergo female secondary sexual characteristic development (22).

Elevated FSH and LH levels are markers for ovarian failure, whether it be prematurely or menopausally. Karyotype 46,XX patients with premature ovarian failure may present with pubertal delay or primary or secondary amenorrhea. They have normal internal and external female genitalia and may attain normal height if pubertal delay does not occur. Autoimmune types of thyroid disease or Addison's disease may produce concomitant premature ovarian failure, most likely because of an autoimmune response to the ovaries themselves. Other causative agents include chemotherapy, irradiation, and resistant ovary syndrome or Savage syndrome (despite high levels of gonadotropins, the ovary does not respond secondary to a receptor or postreceptor defect). Evaluation includes an autoimmune workup with thyroid function tests, an 8 AM cortisol level, calcium, phosphorous, and antinuclear antibody assay (22); an adrenocorticotropic hormone stimulation test may be needed to rule out Addison's disease.

Patients with autoimmune or idiopathic premature ovarian failure may attain reproductive capabilities. There are reported cases of pregnancies in patients, so appropriate precautions should be undertaken when pregnancy is not desired, although patients should be told that the likelihood of a spontaneous pregnancy is low. These patients are candidates for donor oocyte assisted reproduction.

Hypergonadotropic hypogonadism may be caused by previous treatment for childhood cancers. Both radiation therapy and chemotherapy may lead to premature ovarian failure. Radiation therapy will affect patients differently depending on their age at treatment, the dose of treatment, the location of treatment, and whether they had a prophylactic oophoropexy. The younger the patient at the time of radiation, the less likely she is to suffer premature ovarian failure. This may be secondary to ovarian resistance because the ovary in a prepubertal child has less stimulation of follicles than a postpubertal patient (20). Those patients receiving 2000 to 3000 rads of abdominal or spinal radiation are less likely to have normal ovarian function after treatment. Oophoropexy is a procedure in which the ovaries are surgically tacked behind the uterus to shelter them from radiation (20). Radiation to the head can also lead to premature ovarian failure by affecting pituitary and hypothalamic function (20).

Chemotherapy may lead to premature ovarian failure via ovarian fibrosis and follicle destruction (52). Once again, the age at exposure influences the ovary's likelihood of functioning, with the prepubertal ovary showing the most resistance to chemotherapy (20, 35, 52, 53). The amount of chemotherapy also affects future gonadal function (53). Some patients may have normal gonadal function initially but develop premature ovarian failure at a later date. Postpubertal patients who receive chemotherapy and later develop amenorrhea have not been shown to regain ovarian function (53).

Patients with a history of childhood cancer and treatment should be evaluated for delayed puberty if no development has occurred by age 13, or sooner if concerns about premature ovarian failure exist. Evaluation of height, weight, and development are crucial to the evaluation. Measurement of FSH determines whether the patient has ovarian failure (FSH level more than 40 mIU/mL) or if she is hypogonadal with a low FSH. Some patients may regain ovarian function up to 5 years after chemotherapy, but it is extremely rare for this to occur beyond 5 years (20).

Chromosomally Incompetent.   Of patients with hypergonadal hypogonadism, one half will have Turner's syndrome (22). Although this is one of the more common chromosomal abnormalities among live births, most fetuses with Turner's syndrome are aborted spontaneously (54). Turner's syndrome is the most frequent cause of premature ovarian failure. The absence of an X chromosome causes premature atresia of ovarian follicles and skeletal malformations. Most of these girls have ovarian failure at birth secondary to follicular atresia that occurred in utero.

The stigmata of Turner's syndrome include short stature, webbed neck, high arched palate, low posterior hairline, and lymphedema (22). They are at risk for renal and cardiac malformations. Approximately 40 to 50% of patients have a cardiac anomaly such as coarctation of the aorta, bicuspid aortic valve, pulmonic valve anomalies, and/or a dilated aorta. Hypertension is common in these patients, as is diabetes mellitus, obesity, and thyroid disease (22, 54). Patients should be screened regularly for diabetes, thyroid disease, hypertension, and lipid abnormalities and given periodic echocardiograms.

Turner's syndrome patients may have a single X cell line (45,XO) or may be mosaic (e.g., 45,XO/46,XX). Patients who have undergone some pubertal development are mosaic for a 46,XX cell line, whereas patients who do not undergo any pubertal development may or may not be mosaic. There are reported pregnancies in cases of mosaic Turner's syndrome. Some patients have cell lines with Y material present and hence have gonadal dysgenesis. These patients are at risk of developing virilization at puberty and gonadal tumors such as gonadoblastoma or dysgerminoma (22, 54). If the gonads are left in place, approximately 15% of these patients develop a malignancy. Thus, it is recommended to remove the gonads upon finding a Y cell line. Upon requesting a karyotype in patients with Turner's syndrome, one must request that at least 40 cells are examined to rule out the presence of a Y cell line.

Once a patient is diagnosed with Turner's syndrome, treatment of the pubertal delay should be undertaken. If a child is diagnosed at an early age, treatment with growth hormone can be initiated. Some studies show attainment of greater adult height when patients are treated with both recombinant growth hormone and oxandrolone (Oxandrin), an anabolic steroid (22). Untreated adults with Turner's syndrome attain a mean height of 143 cm (57 inches) (54). Often, pubic hair will develop spontaneously (35). Treatment with low-dose estrogen allows breast development to occur. Patients are begun at a dose of conjugated estrogen (Premarin) 0.3 mg/day or estradiol (Estrace) 0.5 mg/day for approximately 6 months to a year to stimulate skeletal growth without inducing premature epiphyseal closure. The dose is then increased to 0.625 to 1.25 mg/day of Premarin or 1 to 2 mg/day of Estrace until adequate breast development occurs. Progestin therapy is then initiated for 12 to 14 days of the month to provide endometrial protection. Once through puberty, patients can be placed on a combination oral contraceptive pill for hormone replacement (22).

Hypogonadal Hypogonadism

Hypogonadal hypogonadism (pubertal delay with normal or low levels of FSH and LH) accounts for 31% of patients with pubertal delay (44). These patients do not need karyotyping unless they have an associated congenital anomaly such as Prader Willi syndrome (mental retardation associated with loss of a region of paternal chromosome 15) (22). Constitutional delay because of hypothalamic or pituitary causes is the most frequent cause of pubertal delay in these patients (22, 35, 43). Congenital lesions or acquired lesions such as infection, trauma, or tumors may cause hypogonadal hypogonadism (19, 43).

These patients have a delayed onset of growth spurt and delayed secondary sexual characteristic development. This may be caused by a delay in the reactivation of the GnRH pulse generator (22). Puberty is usually initiated in these patients by the time their bone age reaches 12, although they are chronologically older than 12. If the patient and her parents desire, treatment can be initiated with low-dose estrogen. Once initiated, puberty will usually progress even with discontinuation of the estrogen (22).

Patients with breast development but no menarche by age 15 must be evaluated to rule out eugonadism as discussed above (22). Patients without any breast development by age 13 are hypoestrogenic; however, they may have low, normal, or elevated gonadotropins (22).

The most common types of tumors responsible for hypogonadal hypogonadism include craniopharyngiomas and pituitary adenomas. Craniopharyngiomas are tumors arising from remnants of Rathke's pouch; the capsule or tumor proper may be calcified (22, 24, 35). They interfere with the portal blood flow between the hypothalamus and pituitary gland. They usually become symptomatic (with signs and symptoms of increased intracranial pressure like headache, nausea, vomiting, and visual abnormalities) between the ages of 6 and 14 years (24) and are diagnosed by head imaging studies such as CT or MRI (44). Patients often demonstrate delayed bone age, and diabetes insipidus may be present. Treatment includes surgery and radiation therapy (22, 24). Some patients may present with delayed puberty as a result of the surgical resection of a cranial tumor (24).

Pituitary adenomas should be suspected when prolactin levels are elevated. These patients may present with pubertal delay or primary amenorrhea, and galactorrhea is commonly, although not always, present (35, 55). If the prolactin level exceeds 100 ng/mL, imaging of the sella turcica is indicated. Head imaging studies reveal whether the adenoma is a macroadenoma (greater than 1 cm diameter) or a microadenoma (less than 1 cm diameter). If a macroadenoma is present, surgical excision with postoperative irradiation may be necessary. If a microadenoma is present but the patient is asymptomatic, no treatment is indicated and follow-up imaging in 1 to 2 years recommended. Treatment of symptomatic patients with microadenomas remains medical with bromocriptine (Parlodel). Primary hypothyroidism may also, rarely, cause hypogonadal hypogonadism. These patients often do very well in school, have short stature, and retain their deciduous teeth (24).

Complete pituitary testing should be undertaken to rule out a pituitary etiology in hypogonadal hypogonadism. This includes measurement of thyroid-stimulating hormone, prolactin, LH, FSH, and 8 AM cortisol and growth hormone levels (44). Because growth hormone levels are affected by sleep, exercise, and various foods, the laboratory should be consulted before drawing this sample. Stimulation tests are necessary to completely evaluate pituitary gland function, including a GnRH stimulation test wherein GnRH is given intravenously and LH and FSH levels are measured. If no rise is found in theses levels, a deficiency in LH and FSH may exist. Another stimulation test involves administering thyrotropin-releasing hormone and measuring thyroid-stimulating hormone and prolactin levels. An insulin tolerance test assesses the hypothalamic-pituitary-adrenal axis by inducing hypoglycemia, which should lead to secretion of growth hormone, adrenocorticotropic hormone, and prolactin (22).

Other causes of hypothalamic hypogonadism may be either reversible or permanent (22). Reversible causes include marijuana use, eating disorders, stress, and exercise. Anorexia nervosa must be considered in adolescent girls with pubertal delay or pubertal arrest (22, 43, 44). In severe cases of anorexia nervosa, permanent hypogonadism can be seen. Intensive exercise, such as that seen in ballet dancers and Olympic gymnasts, can also lead to pubertal delay (43, 44). Chronic illnesses, including chronic renal failure, severe asthma, malnutrition, gastrointestinal malabsorption, and thalassemia major, can all lead to pubertal delay (24, 43).

If all pituitary levels are normal upon measurement but the patient has pubertal delay, she is diagnosed with idiopathic hypogonadal hypogonadism or isolated GnRH deficiency (22, 44). This diagnosis is often difficult to differentiate from constitutional delay of puberty. A GnRH stimulation test may be helpful in identifying the location of the deficit. If a patient has a pubertal response (LH levels rising three times above baseline and rising higher than FSH levels), the patient has a deficiency in GnRH. However, if the patient has a prepubertal response (FSH levels remain higher than LH), the patient may have pituitary deficiency. Not all patients with idiopathic hypogonadal hypogonadism, however, respond in a prepubertal fashion to a GnRH stimulation test (44).

A rare cause of hypogonadotropic hypogonadism is Kallmann's syndrome. This is an isolated deficiency of GnRH associated with intracranial anomalies and anosmia and is more common in boys than girls (22, 44). Almost all patients with Kallmann's syndrome have a normal karyotype (44). Estrogen replacement therapy may be used in the initiation and sustenance of secondary sex characteristics. If pregnancy is desired, the patient will require the administration of gonadotropins or pulsatile GnRH for ovulation induction.

The treatment of patients with hypogonadal hypogonadism should focus on treating the underlying etiology whenever possible. Patients with idiopathic hypogonadal hypogonadism should be treated with GnRH given in a pulsatile fashion either subcutaneously or intravenously to initiate puberty (44). All patients with hypogonadal hypogonadism may be treated with low-dose estrogen therapy to initiate skeletal growth and breast development. Patients should initially be given unopposed estrogen in low doses to prevent premature epiphyseal closure, increasing the dose after 6 to 9 months and continuing until breast development reaches adequate size. A progestin may then be added (44).

OVARIAN MASSES

Benign

Most ovarian cysts found in adolescents are benign. Functional ovarian cysts are found in 20 to 50% of cases (56), and most are simple follicular cysts. Corpus luteum and theca lutein cysts may be complex cysts seen on ultrasound but are also benign. Theca lutein cysts are the least common and are usually bilateral. Corpus luteum cysts have normal endocrine function and may persist in progesterone secretion. These cysts usually spontaneously resolve in 1 to 2 months. Cysts that persist beyond this time often require surgical intervention.

Ovarian cysts in adolescents can be followed and managed conservatively. However, once a cyst reaches 10 cm, the risk of torsion markedly increases and surgery is recommended. Patients with acute abdominal pain and an ovarian cyst need to be evaluated for cyst rupture or ovarian torsion. If torsion occurs, quick progression to surgery is important to preserve ovarian tissue. Rupture of a corpus luteum cyst may result in hemoperitoneum and may require surgical intervention to control the bleeding.

Malignant

Children and adolescents are at risk for developing gynecologic malignancies. The most common of these are the germ cell tumors, although the most common germ cell tumor is the benign, mature cystic teratoma. Germ cell tumors are classified by cell types and comprise approximately 2% of ovarian tumors, although they account for 60% of ovarian tumors in the pediatric and adolescent age groups. Characteristically, these tumors grow rapidly. Patients present early with an enlarging abdominal girth, abdominal pain, and torsion. Adolescents may be found to have an adnexal mass, but in children the ovaries are intraabdominal in location so they present with an abdominal mass. Frequently, these tumors bleed into themselves and cause patients to present with an acute abdomen. Specific tumor markers are often elevated, including α-fetoprotein, β-hCG, and lactate dehydrogenase. These tumors are aggressive but respond well to chemotherapy. Survival has markedly improved with further refinement of chemotherapy regimens (57).

There are three common types of germ cell tumors: dysgerminomas, immature teratomas, and endodermal sinus tumors. Dysgerminomas are most common in women under the age of 30 years, and in 10 to 15% of cases are bilateral (58). Dysgerminomas rarely have elevated tumor markers. Careful examination of the pathology must be undertaken to rule out a mixed germ cell tumor. Dysgerminomas are the only radiosensitive tumor, although systemic chemotherapy is now regarded as the treatment of choice, with the obvious advantage being potential preservation of fertility.

Immature teratomas resemble the mature teratoma or dermoid. However, there are immature elements, usually composed of neural tissue, within the tumor. They are most common in 10 to 20 year olds. Usually, immature teratomas are unilateral, although frequently the opposite ovary contains a mature teratoma. Postoperative chemotherapy is recommended for all patients except those with stage 1a, grade 1 disease.

Endodermal sinus tumors, or yolk sac tumors, are the third most frequent malignant germ cell of the ovary and often enlarge rapidly. Usually, patients present with a short history of an enlarging abdominal mass and pain (59). The tumor growth rate of endodermal sinus tumor is probably the fastest of any human malignancy; thus, endodermal sinus tumors represent a surgical and therapeutic emergency. The median age for presentation is 18 years. Frequently, patients have an elevated α-fetoprotein level. All patients with endodermal sinus tumors receive either adjuvant or therapeutic chemotherapy.

Rarer forms of germ cell tumors include embryonal carcinoma, choriocarcinoma, and polyembryoma. Embryonal carcinoma often occurs in the pediatric population with the median age at presentation being 14 years. Frequently, patients demonstrate isosexual (characteristic of the same sex) precocious puberty. Serum hCG and α-fetoprotein levels are often elevated. Choriocarcinoma can be difficult to differentiate from pregnancy-induced choriocarcinoma. Although as a pure germ cell tumor it is extremely rare, it frequently is part of a mixed germ cell tumor. Serum hCG levels are elevated in these patients. Polyembryoma is a very rare germ cell tumor and is almost exclusively part of a mixed germ cell tumor. Prognosis of the mixed germ cell tumors depends on the germ cell tumor type that has the worst prognosis. All specimens should be carefully examined by an expert in gynecologic pathology to rule out a mixed germ cell tumor (57).

Treatment of germ cell tumors should be conservative surgery (58). Even if the tumor involves both ovaries, fertility is possible with donor oocytes. Adequate staging should be performed. Postoperative chemotherapy is required in most cases except very well-differentiated stage 1 tumors.

ACUTE PELVIC PAIN

The differential diagnosis of acute abdominal pain in the adolescent is similar to that for adult women. It includes ovarian cysts with rupture and torsion, pelvic inflammatory disease (PID), ectopic pregnancies, and nongynecologic causes such as appendicitis.

Pelvic Inflammatory Disease

PID is an infectious process that involves the upper genital tract: the uterus, fallopian tubes, and ovaries. Teenagers account for 16 to 20% of the 1 million plus cases of PID each year in the United States. Although the overall incidence of PID seems to be stabilizing, it continues to increase in adolescents (60). Adolescents are at a threefold greater risk for developing PID than women aged 25 to 29, in part because of risk-taking behavior (61–64). Risk factors include multiple sexual partners and failure to use barrier methods of contraception; it is most commonly acquired through sexual transmission.

Long-term sequelae can and do occur in this population and include tubal scarring, leading to an approximately 10% higher rate of infertility and a 6- to 10-fold increase in ectopic pregnancies (61, 65). The risk of infertility increases at all ages for increasing severity of the disease and with increasing numbers of episodes. A leading cause of maternal mortality in the United States is ectopic pregnancy, and adolescents aged 15 to 19 have the highest mortality in this group. Nongonococcal infection seems to predispose patients more to ectopic pregnancy. Thus, adolescents should be treated with antibiotics even if the diagnosis of PID is unclear.

The U.S. Centers for Disease Control and Prevention has issued guidelines for the diagnosis and treatment of PID (Tables 1.7 and 1.8) (62). Diagnosis is by physical examination and laboratory findings. Patients usually experience abdominal and pelvic pain, vaginal discharge, and fever. On examination, the lower abdomen may be tender with the presence of adnexal tenderness on pelvic exam. Abnormal cervical secretions are present. Laboratory findings include elevated white blood cell count and sedimentation rate and positive cultures for sexually transmitted diseases such as chlamydia and gonorrhea. Frequently, however, the cultures are negative. Laparoscopy is considered the gold standard for diagnosing PID because direct cultures can be obtained and the fallopian tubes can be visualized. Endometrial biopsy has been used to support a clinical diagnosis of PID. The finding of plasma cell endometritis has a sensitivity of 89% and a specificity of 67%, compared with laparo-

TABLE 1.7. Diagnostic Criteria for PID

ALL THREE OF THESE REQUIRED FOR DIAGNOSIS
Lower abdominal tenderness
Adnexal tenderness
Cervical motion tenderness

ONE OR MORE OF THESE INCREASES THE SPECIFICITY OF THE DIAGNOSIS
Fever (oral temperature > 38.3°C [>101.8°F])
Abnormal cervical or vaginal discharge
Elevated erythrocyte sedimentation rate
Elevated C-reactive protein level
Infection with *Neisseria gonorrhoeae* or *Chlamydia trachomatis*

ONE OR MORE OF THESE MAY BE USED TO MAKE A PRESUMPTIVE DIAGNOSIS OF PID
Histopathologic evidence of endometritis on endometrial biopsy
Tubo-ovarian complex, thickened tubes with/without free pelvic fluid on sonography or other imaging tests
Laparoscopic abnormalities consistent with PID

Reprinted from MMWR Morb Mortal Wkly Rep 1998;47(RR-1):80.

TABLE 1.8. Inpatient[a] Treatment of PID

REGIMEN A[b]
Cefoxitin (Mefoxin) 2 g IV q 6 hr *or* cefotetan (Cefotan) 2 g IV q 12 hr
plus
Doxycycline (Vibramycin) 100 mg IV or PO q 12 hr

REGIMEN B[b]
Clindamycin (Cleocin) 900 mg IV q 8 hr
plus
Gentamicin (Garamycin) 2 mg/kg IV or IM loading dose followed by 1.5 mg/kg IV q 8 hr

Reprinted from MMWR Morb Mortal Wkly Rep 1998;47:82–83.
[a]Although PID may be treated on an outpatient basis, the Centers for Disease Control and Prevention recommend hospitalization for adolescents because compliance with outpatient therapy is unpredictable in this population.
[b]These regimens are to be used until at least 48 hours after the patient demonstrates substantial clinical improvement. They may then be changed to doxycycline (Vibramycin) 100 mg PO BID for a total of 14 days of treatment. IF tubo-ovarian abscess is present, many health care providers use clindamycin (Cleocin) 900 mg TID for continued therapy instead of doxycycline.

scopically detected salpingitis (66). Ultrasound cannot confirm or exclude simple PID but is helpful in diagnosing tubo-ovarian abscesses.

PID is treated with antibiotics, either as an inpatient or outpatient. Compliance is often an issue in adolescents, and thus young patients with suspected PID should be hospitalized for antibiotic treatment. Other reasons patients should be admitted include uncertain diagnosis, suspected tubo-ovarian abscess, and unreliability (62). Adolescents have a higher incidence of developing tubo-ovarian abscesses than their adult counterparts; one study documented a 20% incidence of tubo-ovarian abscesses in adolescent girls with PID (67). Antibiotic therapy should be for 10 to 14 days in patients with tubo-ovarian abscesses. If improvement in symptoms and findings does not occur, surgical or CT-guided drainage can be performed.

CLINICAL NOTES

Examination of Pediatric and Adolescent Patients

- Communication, techniques, positioning, and instruments are different for the child's exam compared with an adult.
- Look for congenital anomalies and deformities and signs of abuse.
- The exam may have to be done under sedation or anesthesia.
- The adolescent exam is similar to the adult exam but involves more patient education regarding development, sexuality, and sexually transmitted diseases.

Vulvovaginitis

- Can present with vulvar pruritus, pain, burning, vaginal discharge, dysuria, and vaginal bleeding.
- Infectious causes include respiratory organisms, enteric organisms, sexually transmitted organisms, yeast, viruses, and nematodes.
- Noninfectious causes are usually related to poor hygiene or chemical irritants

Lichen Sclerosus

- A dystrophic vulvar lesion of unknown etiology.
- Can present with vulvar pruritus, irritation, dysuria, and bleeding.
- Diagnosis is clinical and treatment is conservative.

Labial Adhesions

- No treatment is required; if symptomatic, topical estrogen cream usually resolves it.

Prepubertal Vaginal Bleeding

- Differential diagnosis includes exogenous hormones, inflammation and infection, trauma, foreign bodies, urologic pathology, and genital tract neoplasms.

Pubertal Abnormalities

- Premature thelarche (breast development)—usually self-limiting.
- Precocious adrenarche (elevated adrenal gland secretions) and pubarche (pubic and axillary hair development)—follow every 6 to 12 months because of increased risk of menstrual irregularity, hirsutism, acne, and polycystic ovarian syndrome.
- Precocious menarche—cyclic vaginal bleeding without ovulation due to transient estrogen production.
- Precocious puberty (pubertal development before 8 years old).
  — Central: usually idiopathic in girls but can be caused by CNS tumor, hydrocephaly, CNS trauma, and neurofibromatosis; treat underlying cause; treat idiopathic with GnRH agonist.
  — Peripheral: causes include hormone-secreting tumor of adrenals or ovaries, congenital adrenal hyperplasia, McCune-Albright syndrome, and severe hypothyroidism; treat underlying cause.
  — Workup: history, physical including pelvic, laboratory tests (LH, FSH, GnRH stimulation test, estradiol, thyroid-stimulating hormone), ultrasound, MRI (definitely if less than 6 years old; consider if 6 to 8 years old), bone age studies.
- Delayed puberty.
  — Absence of secondary sex characteristics by age 13 or absence of menarche by age 15.
  — Categories include eugonadism, congenital anomalies, hypergonadotropic hypogonadism (both chromosomally competent and incompetent), and hypogonadotropic hypogonadism.

Ovarian Masses

- Benign masses are usually cysts or benign germ cell tumors. Treat conservatively unless more than 10 cm (increased risk of torsion) or persistence more than 2 months.
- Malignant masses are usually germ cell tumors (usually dysgerminomas, immature teratomas, or endodermal sinus tumors). Treatment is surgical, usually with adjuvant chemotherapy.

Acute Pelvic Pain

- PID is more common in adolescents than adults and is more likely to be complicated by a tubo-ovarian abscess. Teens with PID are at greater risk for infertility and ectopic pregnancy than adults with PID. Always treat the adolescent with antibiotics, even if diagnosis cannot be confirmed.

References

1. Berenson A, Heger A, Andrews S. Appearance of the hymen in newborns. Pediatrics 1991;87:458–465.
2. Ryan K, Berkowitz R, Barbieri R. Pediatric and adolescent gynecology. In: Ryan KJ, ed. Kistner's Gynecology. 6th ed. St. Louis: Mosby, 1995:571–632.
3. Bradshaw K, Hairston L, Kass-Wolff J. Pediatric and adolescent gynecology. In: Cunningham FG, MacDonald PC, Gant NF, et al., eds. Williams Obstetrics. 20th ed. Stamford, CT: Appleton & Lange, 1997:1–14.
4. American Academy of Dermatology Task Force on Pediatric Dermatology. Genital warts and sexual abuse in children. J Am Acad Dermatol 1984;11:529–530.
5. Shelton TB, Jerkins GR, Noe HN. Condylomata acuminata in the pediatric patient. J Urol 1986;135:548–549.
6. Winter J, Good A, Simmons P. Vulvovaginitis in children. Part 1. Postgrad Obstet Gynecol 1994;14:1–7.
7. Davis AJ, Goldstein DP. Treatment of pediatric lichen sclerosus with the CO_2 laser. Adolesc Pediatr Gynecol 1989;2:103–105.
8. Aribarg A. Topical oestrogen therapy for labial adhesions in children. Br J Obstet Gynaecol 1975;82:424–425.
9. Sanfilippo J, Wakim N. Bleeding and vulvovaginitis in the pediatric age group. Clin Obstet Gynecol 1987;30:653–661.
10. Hill NC, Oppenheimer LW, Morton KE. The aetiology of vaginal bleeding in children. A twenty year review. Br J Obstet Gynaecol 1989;96:467–470.
11. Blanco-Garcia M, Evain-Brion D, Roger M, et al. Isolated menses in prepubertal girls. Pediatrics 1985;76:43–47.
12. Murram D, Dewhurst J, Grant DB. Premature menarche: a follow-up study. Arch Dis Child 1983;58:142–156.
13. Imai A, Horibe S, Tamaya T. Genital bleeding in premenarcheal children. Int J Gynaecol Obstet 1995;49:41–45.
14. Pediatric gynecologic disorders. ACOG Tech Bull 1995;201:1–6.
15. Pokorny S. Long-term intravaginal presence of foreign bodies in children. J Reprod Med 1994;39:931–935.
16. Farghaly S. Gynecologic cancer in the young female: clinical presentation and management. Adolesc Pediatr Gynecol 1992;5:163–170.
17. Breen J, Bonamo J, Maxson W. Genital tract tumors in children. Symposium on Pediatric and Adolescent Gynecology. Pediatr Clin North Am 1986;28:355–366.
18. Merke DP, Cutler GB. Evaluation and management of precocious puberty. Arch Dis Child 1996;75:269–271.
19. Malasanoa TH. Sexual development of the fetus and pubertal child. Clin Obstet Gynecol 1997;40:153–167.
20. Jones KP. Gynecologic issues in pediatric oncology. Clin Obstet Gynecol 1997;40:200–209.

21. Simmons PS. Diagnostic considerations in breast disorders of children and adolescents. Pediatr Adolesc Gynecol 1992;19:91–102.

22. Layman LC, Reindollar RH. Diagnosis and treatment of pubertal disorders. Adolesc Med 1994;5:37–55.

23. Speroff L, Glass RH, Kase NG. Abnormal puberty and growth problems. In: Clinical Gynecologic Endocrinology and Infertility. 5th ed. Baltimore: Williams & Wilkins, 1994.

24. Reindollar RH, McDonough PG. Etiology and evaluation of delayed sexual development. Pediatr Clin North Am 1981;28:267–286.

25. Pasquino AM, Pucarelli I, Passeri F, et al. Progression of premature thelarche to central precocious puberty. J Pediatr 1995;126:11–14.

26. Rosenfield RL. Invited commentary: Are adrenal and ovarian function normal in true precocious puberty? Eur J Endocrinol 1995;133:399–400.

27. Winter JT, Noller KL, Zimmerman D, et al. Natural history of premature thelarche in Olmsted County, Minnesota, 1940 to 1984. J Pediatr 1990;116:278–280.

28. Pasquino AM, Tebaldi L, Cioschi L, et al. Premature thelarche—a follow up study of 40 girls: natural history and endocrine findings. Arch Dis Child 1985;60:1180–1192.

29. Nelson KG. Premature thelarche in children born prematurely. J Pediatr 1983;5: 756–758.

30. Brook CGD. Precocious puberty. Clin Endocrinol 1995;42:647–650.

31. Morris AH, Reiter EO, Geffner ME, et al. Absence of nonclassical congenital adrenal hyperplasia in patients with precocious adrenarche. J Clin Endocrinol Metab 1989;69: 709–715.

32. Sklar CA, Kaplan SL, Grumbach MM. Evidence for dissociation between adrenarche and gonadarche: studies in patients with idiopathic precocious puberty, gonadal dysgenesis, isolated gonadotropin deficiency, and constitutionally delayed growth and adolescence. J Clin Endocrinol Metab 1980;51:548–556.

33. Siegel SF, Finegold DN, Urban MD, et al. Premature pubarche: etiological heterogeneity. J Clin Endocrinol Metab 1992;74:239–247.

34. Miller D, Emans SJ, Kohane I. Follow-up study of adolescent girls with a history of premature pubarche. J Adolesc Health 1996;18:301–305.

35. Ghali K, Rosenfield RL. Disorders of pubertal development: too early, too much, too late, or too little. Adolesc Med 1994;5:19–35.

36. Styne DM, Grumbach MM. Disorders of puberty in the male and female. In: Yen S, Jaffe R, eds. Reproductive Endocrinology. 3rd ed. Philadelphia: WB Saunders, 1991:511–554.

37. Kornreich L, Horev G, Daneman D, et al. Central precocious puberty: evaluation by neuroimaging. Pediatr Radiol 1995;25:7–11.

38. Loughlin JS. GnRH analog treatment of precocious puberty. Semin Reprod Endocrinol 1993;11:143–153.

39. Anasti JN, Flack MR, Froehlich J, et al. A potential novel mechanism for precocious puberty in juvenile hypothyroidism. J Clin Endocrinol Metab 1995;80:276–279.

40. Murram D, Dewhurst J, Grant DB. Precocious puberty: a follow-up study. Arch Dis Child 1984;59:77–78.

41. Antoniazzi F, Bertoldo F, Zamboni G, et al. Bone mineral metabolism in girls with precocious puberty during gonadotropin-releasing hormone agonist treatment. Eur J Endocrinol 1995;133:421–417.

42. Oostdijk W, Rikken B, Schreuder S, et al. Final height in central precocious puberty after long-term treatment with a slow release GnRH agonist. Arch Dis Child 1996;75: 292–297.

43. Albanese A, Stanhope R. Investigation of delayed puberty. Clin Endocrinol. 1995;43: 105–110.

44. Layman LC. Idiopathic hypogonadotropic hypogonadism: diagnosis, pathogenesis, genetics, and treatment. Adolesc Pediatr Gynecol 1991;4:111–118.

45. Meyers RL. Congenital anomalies of the vagina and their reconstruction. Clin Obstet Gynecol 1997;40:168–180.

46. Tridenti G, Bruni V, Ghiardini G, et al. Double uterus with a blind hemi-vagina and ip-

silateral renal agenesis: clinical variants in three adolescent women: case reports and literature review. Adolesc Pediatr Gynecol 1995;8:201–207.

47. Griffin JE, Edwards C, Madden JD, et al. Congenital absence of the vagina. The Mayer-Rokitansky-Kuster-Hauser syndrome. Ann Intern Med 1976;85:224–236.

48. Maneschi M, Maneschi F, Incandela S. The double uterus associated with an obstructed hemivagina: clinical management. Adolesc Pediatr Gynecol 1991;4:206–210.

49. Sanfilippo JS, Wakim NG, Schikler KN, et al. Endometriosis in association with uterine anomaly. Am J Obstet Gynecol 1986;154:39–43.

50. Altchek A. Pediatric and adolescent gynecology. Comp Ther 1995;21:235–241.

51. Wabrek AJ, Millard PR, Wilson WB Jr, et al. Creation of a neovagina by the Frank nonoperative method. Obstet Gynecol 1971;37:408.

52. Gershenson DM. Menstrual and reproductive function after treatment with combination chemotherapy for malignant ovarian germ cell tumors. J Clin Oncol 1988;6:270–275.

53. Rivkees SA, Crawford JD. The relationship of gonadal activity and chemotherapy-induced gonadal damage. JAMA 1988;259:2123–2125.

54. Saenger P. Clinical review 48: The current status of diagnosis and therapeutic intervention in Turner's syndrome. J Clin Endocrinol Metab 1993;77:297–301.

55. Badawy SZ, Marshall L, Refaie A. Primary amenorrhea-oligomenorrhea due to prolactinomas in adolescent and adult girls. Adolesc Pediatr Gynecol 1991;4:27–31.

56. Emans SJ, Goldstein DP. Ovarian masses. In: Emans SJ, ed. Pediatric and Adolescent Gynecology. 3rd ed. Boston: Little, Brown and Company, 1990.

57. Germa JR, Perira JM, Barnadas A, et al. Sequential combination chemotherapy for malignant germ cell tumors of the ovary. Cancer 1988;61:913–918.

58. Gordon A, Lipton D, Woodruff JD. Dysgerminoma: a review of 158 cases from the Emil Novak Ovarian Tumor Registry. Obstet Gynecol 1981;58:497–504.

59. Athanikar N, Saika TK, Ramkrishan G, et al. Aggressive chemotherapy in endodermal sinus tumor. J Surg Oncol 1989;40:17–20.

60. Shafer MA, Sweet RL. Pelvic inflammatory disease in adolescent females. Pediatr Clin North Am 1989;36:513.

61. Westrom L. Incidence, prevalence, and trends of acute pelvic inflammatory disease and its consequences in industrialized countries. Am J Obstet Gynecol 1980;138:880.

62. Handsfield HH, Holmes KK, Berg AO, et al. The Centers for Disease Control and Prevention: sexually transmitted diseases treatment guidelines. MMWR Morb Mortal Wkly Rep 1993;42:75–80.

63. McCormack WM. Pelvic inflammatory disease. N Engl J Med 1994;330:115–118.

64. Sweet RL. Pelvic inflammatory disease: prevention and treatment. Mod Med 1987;55:64–70.

65. Hillis S, Black C, Newhall J, et al. New opportunities for Chlamydia prevention: applications of science to public health practice. Sex Transm Dis 1995;22:197–202.

66. Paavonen J, Aine T, Teisala K, et al. Comparison of endometrial biopsy and peritoneal fluid cytologic testing with laparoscopy in the diagnosis of acute pelvic inflammatory disease. Am J Obstet Gynecol 1985;151:645–650.

67. Cromer BA, Brandstetter LA, Fischer RA, et al. Tuboovarian abscess in adolescents. Adolesc Pediatr Gynecol 1990;3:21–24.

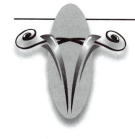

C H A P T E R   2

Care of the Perimenopausal and Postmenopausal Woman

FRANCISCO J. GARCINI
STEVEN STRONG

The cessation of menstruation because of the retirement of ovarian function defines menopause. It is a retrospective diagnosis and is based on the absence of menses for 12 months or greater. The median age of menopause in the United States is 51 years, occurring between the ages of 47 and 55 years in greater than 90% of women and before 40 years in only 1% (1, 2). The perimenopause, or climacteric, encompasses the transition from the reproductive stage of life to the postmenopausal state. The median age for the onset of the perimenopause is 47 years and lasts an average of 4 years. This period of waxing and waning ovarian function is often characterized by menstrual irregularity, hot flushes, emotional lability, and vaginal atrophy. The age at which a woman experiences menopause is influenced by genetic factors, with mothers and daughters tending to experience menopause at the same age, and cigarette smoking, which lowers the age of menopause by 1 to 2 years. Living at high altitudes and undernourishment also predispose a woman toward an earlier menopause. There is no correlation between the age of onset of menarche and the age of onset of menopause.

The impact of menopause on society has increased substantially as a result of our aging population. By the year 2000, 33% of American women will be menopausal. The largest growing segment of the U.S. population is women over the age of 75 (3). With this significant increase in life expectancy, there is an increasing number of women that will live well past menopause. In fact, based on a life expectancy of 85 years, women will spend an estimated 33% of their lives in the menopausal state. It is imperative that health care providers understand the changing health care risks of the menopausal woman to maximize the health and productivity of their patients.

PHYSIOLOGY OF MENOPAUSE

A woman's supply of ovarian follicles, 300,000 at puberty, is steadily depleted during her reproductive years through ovulation and attrition. In the perimenopause, as fewer and fewer follicles grow during each cycle, there is a decrease in the amount of inhibin produced. Decreased inhibin leads to an elevation in follicle-stimulating hormone (FSH), which gradually rises to greater than 10 times normal by 1 to 3 years after menopause. Inhibin production is not affected by exogenous estrogen so that administration of estrogen replacement cannot suppress the increase in FSH. Therefore, FSH levels cannot be used to titrate hormone replacement therapy (HRT) doses.

Estradiol levels may remain in the normal range until follicular development ceases, although the concentrations of estrogen and progesterone in these cycles is less than that found in cycles of younger women (4–6). It is not uncommon for women to complain of hot flushes while still exhibiting normal levels of FSH and continued, albeit often irregular, menstruation. However, a woman's symptoms often serve as her own best bioassay. It is important to understand that FSH levels fluctuate greatly during the perimenopausal period and that blood tests reflect the hormonal state at the moment in time they are drawn. The symptoms of hot flushes, when not due to other physiologic clauses, result from ebbs in estrogen levels, thus leading to vasomotor instability.

With the cessation of menses, FSH levels plateau within the first year. Although some women have an increase in luteinizing hormone (LH) before menopause, for most women, the LH levels remain normal before menopause but increase and plateau during the first year of the climacteric (4–6).

Menopause is associated with a decrease in ovarian secretion of testosterone and androstenedione. For most postmenopausal women, testosterone levels are much less than the mean levels found in younger women. The adrenal glands serve as a source of the androgen precursors dehydroepiandrostenedione and dehydroepiandrostenedione sulfate. Although these levels decrease with age, this is independent of menopause (7, 8).

For about 90% of postmenopausal women, most circulating estradiol is from the peripheral aromatization of androgens (9, 10). Estrone, which is peripherally converted from androstenedione, accounts for most circulating estrogen after menopause. Although estradiol production ceases almost entirely in the postmenopausal ovary, approximately 10 to 20 pg/mL of estradiol is present as a result of conversion from estrone.

SEQUELAE OF MENOPAUSE

In the early stages of menopause women may complain of hot flushes, night sweats, insomnia, emotional lability, and/or short-term memory loss. They may also complain of vaginal atrophy and dyspareunia. Later, these women may experience urge and/or stress incontinence and notice some thinning of the skin. Late in menopause they may manifest osteoporosis, coronary heart disease, or even Alzheimer's disease.

Menstrual Irregularity

In the 2 years immediately preceding the onset of menopause, over 90% of women report abnormalities in their menstrual cycles. Menstrual cycles in the perimenopausal woman may initially be ovulatory, but with time, anovulation becomes more frequent. As the number of recruited follicles decreases, the production of inhibin also decreases. This leads to an increase in FSH levels, inducing a rapid maturation of remaining follicles and ultimately resulting in a shortened follicular phase. This excess in FSH stimulation may produce sufficient estrogen to cause an LH surge and normal luteal phase. As the follicles are depleted, however, the amount of estrogen produced is insufficient to induce an LH surge, and anovulation results. In some women, this anovulation results in amenorrhea, menorrhagia, and/or metrorrhagia. Although fertility is declining during the perimenopausal time period, pregnancy is still possible. For women over the age of 35 who are in good health or have well-controlled medical problems and do not smoke, oral contraceptives may provide an ideal method to regulate menstrual cycles while providing contraception.

Hot Flushes

Although the exact pathophysiologic process of hot flushes is unknown, their occurrence is related to the drop of estrogen levels. Hot flushes are most prevalent in the first 2 years after menopause and lessen over time for most women (11). It would seem that for most women, hot flushes begin before menopause. The frequency, duration, and intensity of hot flushes vary from woman to woman.

Approximately 10 to 15% of women have very frequent and severe hot flushes (12). Hot flushes last an average of 3 to 6 minutes, although they may be of shorter or much longer duration. Although the frequency of hot flushes decreases over time for most women, some women continue to experience them for decades after menopause (13) (Table 2.1). For some women, specific trigger events are associated with the occurrence of hot flushes, including stress, heat, alcohol, caffeine, or spicy foods (12, 14). There is no association between hot flushes and socioeconomic factors (14). There is some evidence that heavier women suffer fewer hot flushes than thinner women (15). For many women, there is a prodromal feeling of anxiety, tingling, or pressure in the head just before a hot flush (12). Studies have shown that preceding the hot flush, there is an increase in core temperature from 0.5 to 2°F. The trigger for this increase in core basal body temperature is not currently known. The increase in body temperature and subsequent hot flush are associated with an LH surge. This LH surge, however, is not the precipitating cause of the hot flush but a concurrent event, since hypophysectomized women also experience hot flushes.

Hot flushes occur more frequently at night and may prevent a woman from spending adequate time in rapid eye movement sleep. In addition to this, sleep efficiency is lower. As a result, the patient may wake up feeling tired. This is thought to contribute to many of the psychological complaints reported in the immediate menopausal time period. It is noteworthy that although 75% of North American women suffer from hot flushes, this phenomenon is seen in only 25% of Japanese women (16). This may be related to the increased amount of soy (a rich source of plant phytoestrogens) in the Japanese diet. Although conclusive evidence is still pending, initiatives are currently underway investigating soy as a potential estrogen supplement.

Hot flushes can be physically draining and have significant negative effects on the woman's work, family, and social relationships. The available therapies do not relieve all hot flushes for all women, although they do decrease the frequency, intensity, and/or duration for most. Estrogen, oral or transdermal, is the most effective treatment for hot flushes, and its effect is usually immediate. For women who

TABLE 2.1. Clinical Picture in a Hot Flush

Symptom	Description
Core temperature	Decreases (0.1–0.9°C) minutes after hot flush starts
Sensation	Sudden feeling of heat and sometimes anxiety
Heart rate	Increases (5–35 bpm) may be felt as palpitations
Finger skin temperature	Rises rapidly (1–7°C) and slowly declines after hot flush ends
Cutaneous blood flow	Increase; observed as flushing
Sweating	Often profuse, rapid onset
Sleeping problems	Increase in nighttime awakenings associated with hot flushes (night sweats)

are unable or choose not to take estrogen or for women in whom estrogen does not ameliorate their hot flushes even at high doses, other modes of therapy are available.

Medroxyprogesterone acetate (MPA; Provera), 150 mg intramuscularly, has been shown to decrease the number of hot flushes, and its major side effect is abnormal bleeding (17). The oral form (20 to 80 mg/day) is associated with fewer side effects (18). Megestrol acetate (Megace), 20 to 80 mg/day orally, is also effective in treating hot flushes.

Clonidine (Catapres), an α-adrenergic agonist, has been used to treat hot flushes. One study demonstrated a dose-response relationship between clonidine (0.1, 0.2, and 0.4 mg/day orally) and a decrease in hot flushes (19). Side effects such as dry mouth, nausea, and dizziness increased with increase in dose.

Nonpharmacologic approaches may be considered in the treatment of hot flushes, although definitive data proving efficacy are lacking for most. These would include maintenance of a cool ambient temperature, use of vitamin E, acupuncture, exercise, and dietary elimination of suspected triggers of hot flushes.

Complaints of hot flushes in the presence of normal cyclic menses reflect episodes of either insufficient or sudden drops in estrogen level during the transition from the reproductive years to the menopausal state. The use of supplemental estrogen is useful in these instances. Unopposed physiologic doses of estrogen may be given while monthly withdrawal bleeding occurs with the addition of a cycled progestin when menstruation ceases. Alternatively, a low-dose combined oral contraceptive pill may be used.

Genitourinary Symptoms

Vaginal Atrophy and Dyspareunia

Estrogen deprivation after menopause or castration results in atrophy of the vaginal mucosa. Without estrogen, the vaginal walls shorten and narrow, and the urethral meatus "moves" closer to the introitus, rendering the urethra more susceptible to trauma and/or infection. With the loss of estrogen, the vaginal pH increases, and this results in a decrease in lactobacilli concentration. This loss of lactobacilli allows increased proliferation of organisms in endocervical glands, the vagina, and the perineum. This may manifest as a chronic vaginal discharge and pruritus. Shrinkage in the thickness of the vaginal walls and loss of vaginal lubrication may precipitate complaints of vaginal irritation and dyspareunia. This dyspareunia may ultimately interfere with the woman's normal sexual function and ability to maintain an intimate relationship. Because many elderly women are hesitant to discuss sexual issues, this complaint may not be volunteered by the patient but should be solicited by the health care provider (20). Although oral and parenteral estrogen replacement is effective in alleviating vaginal atrophy, there are two alternatives for women who cannot or will not take systemic estrogen: topical estrogen or an estrogen-containing pessary. Estrogen vaginal cream (1 to 2 g) is applied nightly for 1 to 2 weeks and 0.5 to 1 g is applied three nights a week thereafter. With this method, a local estrogenic effect is achieved by topical absorption but systemic absorption is minimal.

An alternative method involves the use of Estring, a vaginal pessary that is imbued with estrogen. The pessary is placed into the vagina. The estrogen is released slowly, thus resulting in a localized estrogen effect on the vaginal walls and genitourinary tissues.

If a hyperplastic dystrophy is diagnosed, corticosteroids (0.25% fluocinolone acetonide [Synalar]) are used until the pruritus resolves. The patient is then changed to a hydrocortisone-based steroid because long-term use of fluorinated steroids may cause atrophy of the treated tissues.

Urinary Incontinence

Urinary incontinence is a common problem in postmenopausal women and may be due to genuine stress incontinence, urge incontinence, or a mixed incontinence. Tissues of the lower urinary tract, intimately associated with the genital tract during embryologic development, are also under the direct influence of estrogen. Atrophy of the bladder mucosa predisposes toward irritability of the detrusor muscle, both by direct action of urine on afferent nerve endings and by increasing the incidence of recurrent cystitis. Urge incontinence is usually described as a sudden overwhelming need to urinate, allowing only a few moments or minutes before spontaneous voiding occurs. It is the most common type of incontinence in elderly women and the most common problem associated with hypoestrogenic atrophy of the genitourinary tract. For these women, replacement of estrogen results in thickening of the bladder mucosa and may result in improvement, if not complete resolution, of these symptoms.

Instability of the detrusor results in uncontrollable bladder emptying and may follow from central nervous system conditions such as stroke, Parkinson's disease, Alzheimer's disease, or tumors. Hypoestrogenic atrophy, bladder infection, fecal impaction, diabetic neuropathy, and spinal cord lesions may also cause detrusor instability.

Pelvic relaxation and resultant urethrovesical prolapse bring about genuine stress urinary incontinence. An increase in intra-abdominal pressure with cough or Valsalva is applied to the bladder dome and exceeds the pressure in the displaced urethrovesical junction. This creates a pressure gradient and results in the spontaneous loss of small amounts of urine, often without any urge to void. The most common cause is pelvic floor relaxation, although it may result from abdominal tumors or chronic pulmonary disease (i.e., chronic cough). Although estrogen deprivation does not cause pelvic relaxation, estrogen appears to improve symptoms of genuine stress urinary incontinence, likely by action on the urethral mucosa.

Overflow incontinence occurs with obstruction or impaired sensation. The bladder is hypotonic and distended. It may occur secondary to neurogenic injury or use of anticholinergic or antidepressant medications. (For more information on the evaluation and treatment of incontinence, see Chapter 16.)

Cardiovascular Disease

Heart disease is the leading killer of postmenopausal women, causing 500,000 deaths annually in the United States (Fig. 2.1). Among American women, 46% of all deaths are due to cardiovascular disease, and 50% of these are due to coronary artery disease (CAD). Other than hypertension, the most common cardiovascular diseases are CAD, congestive heart failure, and chronic atrial fibrillation. In the United States, a woman has a 23% lifetime risk of dying from ischemic heart disease (21). Although studies indicate that most American women perceive breast cancer as the most significant health threat facing them, more women die from cardiovascular disease each year than from all cancers combined (22, 23).

Before menopause, women enjoy relative protection from heart disease with mortality rates that are threefold lower than those for men. Although both sexes have an increase in the incidence of cardiovascular disease with increasing age, this increase is more pronounced in women after menopause such that the female to male ratio becomes 2:1 at age 50 and 1:1 beyond age 65 (24). This is thought to result in large part from the loss of estrogen.

Traditionally, most studies addressing heart disease included large cohorts of

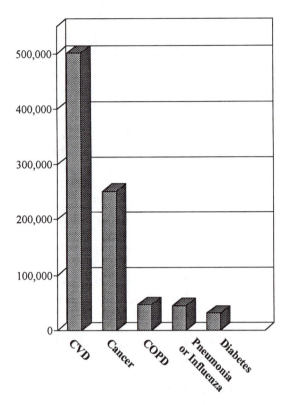

FIGURE 2.1. Leading causes of death for women in 1993. *CVD,* cardiovascular disease; *COPD,* chronic obstructive pulmonary disease. (Reprinted with permission from the American Heart Association. 1997 Heart and Stroke Facts: Statistical Update. Dallas, TX: American Heart Association, 1996.)

men and only small numbers of women. Unfortunately, the results of these studies were extrapolated from men to women, and it has only been within the past 5 to 7 years that an appreciation of gender differences regarding cardiovascular disease has developed. Distinct differences exist between men and women in the manifestation of cardiovascular disease, response to the therapy, and prognosis. In patients with CAD, 65% of women present initially with angina compared with only 35% of men (25). Mortality within 1 year after a myocardial infarction is 39% in women compared with 31% in men (26). Chest pain is more difficult to interpret in women. In women with typical angina, CAD is present in only 35 to 65%, and in those with atypical chest pain, CAD is present in less than 20% (27). Women tend to have milder symptomatology despite the more severe disease, are less likely to be referred until their disease is more advanced, and are less likely to have advanced procedures performed (28–30). Even when surgically treated, differences still remain. Women with severe angina who undergo coronary artery bypass surgery experience less pain relief and have a higher rate of subsequent myocardial infarction.

Risk Factors for Cardiovascular Disease in Women
The risk factors for cardiovascular disease in women are similar to those found in men—family history, hypertension, lipid disorders, smoking, obesity, and diabetes—although differences in these risk factors are found. Women have a greater prevalence for obesity than men. Levels of low-density lipoprotein (LDL) increase abruptly

in women after ages 50 to 55, whereas the decrease in high-density lipoprotein (HDL) occurs more steadily (31). It is known that a 1% increase in total cholesterol increases the risk of CAD by 2%, and a 1% decrease in HDL cholesterol increases CAD risk by 2 to 4.7% (32). Hypertension is a major risk factor for CAD, although its impact is stronger in women than in men. For women, both increased diastolic and systolic levels in blood pressure are independent risk factors (33). Among all risk factors, cigarette smoking is the most preventable risk for cardiovascular disease and CAD in women (34). Currently, about 30% of American women smoke, and it is estimated that in the next decade, the number of women smokers will surpass the number of male smokers (35). Smoking is more than additive to diabetes, hypertension, and dyslipidemias in the impact on cardiovascular disease and CAD. Cessation of smoking can cause an estimated 50 to 70% decrease in the risk of CAD. Diabetes mellitus accelerates the process of atherosclerosis and increases the risk of coronary ischemia, especially in women (36). Diabetes can be considered a more aggressive cardiovascular disease factor in women than in men because diabetic women have a fourfold increase in the incidence of cardiovascular disease than diabetic men. The two strongest independent risk factors for cardiovascular disease for women are age and HDL level.

Estrogen Effects on Cardiovascular Disease

Estrogen replacement therapy (ERT)/HRT has been shown through clinical, observational, and autopsy studies to have a definitive benefit in lowering the relative risk for cardiovascular disease in women. Some studies demonstrated a 50% reduction in the risk of CAD for women who use HRT or ERT (37–43). In addition, it has been shown to lower the risk of death and future cardiovascular events in women with established CAD. Mechanisms for this protective effect are being elucidated and include alterations in lipids and lipoproteins, inhibition of formation and progression of atherosclerosis, possible stabilization and/or regression of plaque formation, and direct endothelial and vascular smooth muscle effects.

Estrogen increases the level of HDL and lowers the levels of LDL. These beneficial alterations, which are associated with a decreased risk of CAD, are blunted by the addition of a progestational agent. The Postmenopausal Estrogen/Progestin Interventions trial was a randomized, placebo-controlled, double-blind study with an intention-to-treat analysis designed to study the overall lipid impact for women on estrogen and progestin compared with those on estrogen only or placebo (44). There were several subgroups of hormone regimens in the study, with one arm receiving estrogen only. Other arms of the study received estrogen and progestational agents in various regimens, or placebo. This study demonstrated that in all groups of women (both those on estrogen alone and those on estrogen with progesterone), there was a statistically significant increase in HDL levels and a statistically significant decrease in LDL levels. This was not the case with the placebo group. This study put to rest the questions regarding the net balance effect for women taking estrogen and progestational agents. Although estrogen has a positive impact on the lipid profile, this accounts for only 25 to 50% of estrogen's beneficial effect on the cardiovascular system (39). Given that most estrogen benefits come from other pathways and the new pharmacologic agents known as selective estrogen receptor modulators (SERMs), it is imperative that clinicians understand the pathophysiology of atherosclerosis and the other mechanisms of estrogen on the cardiovascular system (Table 2.2).

Uptake of LDL from the bloodstream into the vessel wall initiates the formation of an atherosclerotic plaque. For LDL to be taken up by endothelial cells, it first must

TABLE 2.2. Factors Affecting Plaque Growth[a]

LIPIDS
↑ LDL oxidation
↑ LDL uptake

ENDOTHELIAL FUNCTION
↓ Nitric oxide
↑ Endothelin
↓ PGI_2
↑ Thromboxane
↑ Adhesion molecule
↑ Cytokines

OTHER
↑ Insulin

[a]An ↑ in any of these factors promotes/increases the formation of plaque(s).

be oxidized. Estrogen exerts some of its positive cardiovascular benefit by acting as an antioxidant, thereby inhibiting plaque formation. Estrogen may also modify the effects of specific cytokines and hence prevent further sequestration of macrophages into atherosclerotic lesions, leading to an arrest of the progression of (the) fatty streaks. Estrogen is also known to decrease smooth muscle hyperplasia, endothelial hyperplasia, and collagen and elastin deposition (45, 46).

Estrogen is known to increase the production of vasodilators (nitric oxide and prostacyclin [PGI_2]) while decreasing levels of vasoconstrictors such as thromboxane. A decrease in fibrinogen and plasminogen activator inhibitor-1 levels, factors associated with arterial clotting, have been demonstrated with estrogen use (47). Estrogen exerts an inotropic effect on the heart muscle, leading to an increase in stroke volume and end diastolic pressure (48, 49). Estrogen has also been shown to decrease insulin and mean glucose levels and to improve insulin resistance (50).

Clinically, the presence of estrogen may allow diseased vessels to function similarly to normal vessels. In one study, men and women with angiographically proven CAD received an infusion of acetylcholine with a resultant vasoconstriction. Both these groups then received an intravenous infusion of 17β-estradiol followed by a second acetylcholine infusion 20 minutes later. The men continued to show a constrictive response, whereas the women demonstrated a dilatory response similar to that observed in normal vessels (51).

Further evidence for estrogen cardiac benefit can be seen in a study by Rosano et al. (52) where 11 postmenopausal women with CAD, not on estrogen, were examined. The women performed a treadmill exercise test 40 minutes after receiving either sublingual estradiol or placebo. They were then crossed over on a later day. All women experienced chest pain on exertion after receiving placebo, whereas only 6 of 11 women reported chest pain on exertion after receiving 17β-estradiol sublingually. In all 11 women, a 1-mm depression in the ST segment was seen with exertion after placebo. With estradiol, 7 of 11 women demonstrated a 1-mm ST segment of depression with the exertion, but the time to 1-mm ST segment depression and the total exercise time was increased in all patients in this group.

A beneficial effect of ERT for women already suffering from heart disease has been established (53, 54). Sullivan et al. (55) looked at the effect of estrogen therapy on 10-year survival of three cohorts of women: no or minimal CAD, moderate CAD, and severe CAD (defined as left main coronary artery stenosis, greater than or equal to 50%, or other major coronary artery stenosis greater than or equal to 70%). Women with severe CAD had the greatest benefit in terms of 10-year survival compared with the other cohorts.

Another cardiovascular condition that may be influenced by the presence of estrogen is syndrome X, as described by Kemp. The overwhelming number of patients with syndrome X are women. These patients have intermittent pain on exertion but normal coronary arteries on angiography. Although their cardiac prognosis is good, the disease often places significant limitations on daily activities. An additional feature of this syndrome is an abnormal hyperemic response (i.e., occlusion and subsequent release of a vessel does not manifest a normal sequence of rapid vasodilation and increase in oxygen consumption in the immediate reperfusion time period). This abnormal hyperemic response has been inferred by some to signify that it is specifically the microvasculature that is diseased in these patients, hence accounting for the normal angiography. In a study by Sarrel et al. (56), women with syndrome X who were placed on estrogen showed a statistically significant improvement in their symptoms and a hyperemic response that more closely resembled that of normal control subjects. This is of great interest because this has been a difficult and somewhat recalcitrant disease to treat.

Stroke

Although several studies show that ERT/HRT lowers the risk of stroke in postmenopausal women, only one showed an increased risk (37, 57–59). Most studies demonstrate no increase in the risk of stroke with the use of ERT/HRT. Although there is some evidence that women may benefit from the daily use of aspirin, this benefit may be offset by an increased risk for hemorrhagic stroke (60).

Osteoporosis

Osteoporosis is a significant health problem in the United States, affecting more than 25 million women. There are over 1.3 million fractures per year due to osteoporosis, and the annual health care costs due to osteoporosis are estimated to be $12 to 13 billion. Health care costs in the United States associated with osteoporosis lag only behind the costs associated with congestive heart failure, the leading expense in annual health care costs (61). Osteoporosis is defined as a systemic skeletal disease leading to a loss in the quantity of bone and not a deficiency or metabolic problem with the quality of the bone. This loss in bone mass increases the risk of fractures secondary to increased bone fragility. There are two basic types of bone: trabecular and cortical. Trabecular bone is found in appendicular structures and the axial spine. Although it constitutes only 20% of the skeletal mass, it accounts for 80% of the bone turnover and is eight times more metabolically active than cortical bone. Cortical bone, found in the shafts of long bones and pelvis, accounts for 80% of the skeletal mass but only 20% of bone turnover.

To understand osteoporosis, one needs to understand the natural history of bone mass in women. Peak bone density is reached at approximately 30 to 35 years of age. Subsequent to that there is a loss of about 0.5 to 1% of bone mass per year. During the perimenopausal time period, however, this loss increases to 1 to 2% per year. At the time of menopause, with the cessation of estrogen production, this rate increases to 2 to 3% per year, with accelerated bone loss continuing over the next 5 to 10 years. This accelerated phase is resistant to calcium supplementation in the absence of estrogen.

Bone is constantly being remodeled at the sight of microscopic fractures. Bone resorption is mediated by specialized cells, osteoclasts. This process takes approximately 5 to 7 days. With the formation of a microarchitectural pit in the bone, another cell type, the osteoblast, moves in and lays down the matrix to form new bone. This process takes approximately 1 to 3 months. If insufficiently filled, the net result is that of bone loss, with the activity of the osteoclast and resultant absorption faster than the rate of formation. With a decrease in estrogen, there is an increase in the number of remodeling sites. This leads to a decrease in skeletal mass, and it is thought that with the loss of estrogen, the amount of bone resorbed exceeds that of bone formed and replaced (62). In menopausal women, this becomes manifest as a loss of connectivity among the trabeculae of bone and a resultant increase in bone fragility.

There are multiple risk factors for osteoporosis. The most commonly cited are small body size, fair skin, Asian or Caucasian race, and a family history of osteoporosis. Women who have history of excess thyroid medications, glucocorticoid steroid use, anticonvulsants, heparin, and other medications are also at increased risk for osteoporosis (Table 2.3). Postmenopausal women not on estrogen and women who have undergone surgical menopause are also at increased risk. Patients who are physically inactive, current or past cigarette smokers, or women with diets low in dairy products or sources of calcium are also at increased risk. It is estimated that the average North American woman's diet incorporates only 500 to 900 mg of calcium per day (far below the recommended daily allowance).

When evaluating a woman for osteoporosis, alternate disease states that may lead to a decreased bone loss must be ruled out by history, physical examination, and appropriate laboratory tests. These diseases may include multiple myeloma, hyperthyroidism, or hypoparathyroidism (for a complete listing, see Table 2.4). Laboratory tests in the workup for osteoporosis should include a complete blood count, calcium, phosphorus, and alkaline phosphatase (for other laboratory tests, see Table 2.5).

Various methods of bone mass measurement are available. These include quantitative computed tomography (CT), single x-ray absorptiometry, radiographic absorptiometry, and dual x-ray absorptiometry. Ultrasound has recently been approved as a screening tool for determining bone mineral density. Dual x-ray absorptiometry, however, is currently the gold standard for the measurement of bone mineral density and bone mass measurement. It is a rapid test that has good accuracy and precision. It requires no specific oral or intravenous contrast agent and can be done in an office setting. Results of a dual x-ray absorptiometry include a T

TABLE 2.3. Medications That May Contribute to Secondary Osteoporosis

Glucocorticoids
Anticonvulsants
Gonadotropin-releasing hormone agents
Thyroid hormone
Methotrexate
Cyclosporine
Heparin
Aluminum antacids
Isoniazid
Lithium

TABLE 2.4. Causes of Secondary Osteoporosis

ENDROCRINE
Hypogonadism
   Premenopausal hypogonadism
Hypercortisolism
Hyperthyroidism
Hyperparathyrodism
Diabetes mellitus (type I)

MARROW DISORDERS
Lymphoma
Multiple myeloma
Disseminated carcinoma
Chronic alcoholism

GASTROINTESTINAL
Gastrectomy
Malabsorption
Primary biliary cirrhosis
Anorexia nervosa
Severe malnutrition

CONNECTIVE TISSUE DISEASE
Marfan's syndrome
Ehlers-Danlos syndrome

MISCELLANEOUS
Immobilization
Chronic obstructive pulmonary disease
Radiation treatment
Rheumatoid arthritis
Osteogenesis imperfecta

TABLE 2.5. Laboratory Tests in the Workup of Osteoporosis[a]

Complete blood count (CBC)
Erythrocyte sedimentation rate (ESR)
Serum calcium, phosphorus, alkaline phosphatase, proteins, and creatine levels
Liver function tests
Thyroid function tests
Urine calcium and creatinine
Glucose and protein content of urine

[a]For patients with uncomplicated osteoporosis, these tests should be normal. Abnormalities suggest the presence of a secondary disease process.

score and a Z score. The T score is the standard deviation above or below the peak bone mass of young adult women of the same ethnicity as the patient. The Z score is the standard deviation above or below the bone mass of same aged women of same ethnicity. The T score is used for the diagnosis of osteoporosis. The World Health Organization defines osteoporosis as a T score greater than or equal to 2.5 standard deviations below the mean. Severe osteoporosis is defined as greater than 2.5 standard deviations below the mean. Indications for obtaining a bone mineral density measurement include estrogen deficiency (not on HRT/ERT), metabolic abnormalities, x-ray-diagnosed osteopenia, long-term glucocorticoid therapy, or mild asymptomatic primary hyperparathyroidism. Another indication for testing is when a woman will base her decision to use estrogen or not on the test results.

Estrogen has long been recognized as both a preventive and treatment modality for osteoporosis. Its mechanisms of action are not entirely clear, although specific receptors for estrogen have been identified in the osteoblast cell line (63, 64). Estrogen may also exert its bone-protective effect through a reduction in cytokines such as interleukin-1 and interleukin-6, known stimulators of bone resorption (65). Use of estrogen in postmenopausal women is associated with rapid normalization of bone resorption and formation (66).

The rate of bone loss is accelerated in the immediate period (first 5 to 7 years) after menopause. After this period, the loss continues but at a slower rate. The earlier therapy is started, the more bone mass and structure are preserved. Estrogen has been shown to decrease the risk of hip fracture by up to 50% and of vertebral fractures by up to 75% (67, 68). The minimum bone-protective dose of estrogen for most women is 0.625 mg of conjugated estrogen (Premarin) or its equivalent (69–71). Transcutaneous delivery of estrogen has also been demonstrated to be effective in preventing bone loss (72). The clinical question of whether it is ever too late to start estrogen therapy for osteoporosis is often raised. A recent Rancho Bernardo study demonstrated that estrogen therapy initiated after the age of 65 increases bone mineral density in a statistically significant manner (73). Hence, it is never too late to start estrogen therapy for the treatment of osteoporosis.

There are two U.S. Food and Drug Administration (FDA)-approved agents for the prevention of osteoporosis: estrogen and alendronate (Fosamax). Both agents are inhibitors of bone absorption and show a statistically significant decrease in the incidence of osteoporosis for women using one for preventive therapy. The bone formed in patients taking alendronate has been shown to be biochemically and histologically normal. In the randomized, double-blind, placebo-controlled early postmenopausal intervention cohort study, alendronate was compared with estrogen/progestin therapy and placebo regarding efficacy in preventing bone loss. There was no significant difference between estrogen/progestin and alendronate (Fosamax), 5 mg/day orally, in preventing bone loss (74). It is a useful drug in preventing osteoporosis in women unable or unwilling to take ERT. Studies have shown an additive effect in the increase of bone mineral density for patients receiving either estrogen or alendronate and use of supplemental calcium.

Fosamax must be taken with a full glass of water on an empty stomach upon arising in the morning. It is imperative that the patient remain upright for 30 minutes after ingestion of the drug. This practice prevents side effects like esophageal irritation. There have been recent reports of esophageal ulceration in a small number of patients. The patient should refrain from eating or drinking anything in the 30 minutes after ingestion because any food or drink will inhibit the absorption of the active ingredients of the Fosamax and hence preclude any beneficial effect. Contraindications to alendronate include abnormalities of the esophagus, the inability to stand or sit upright for at least 30 minutes, or any hypersensitivity to the drug.

In the treatment of osteoporosis there are several recognized and improved agents, including estrogens, calcitonin, and bisphosphonates. All have been shown to have a statistically significant impact on reducing the incidence of vertebral fractures. Estrogen and alendronate (Fosamax) have also demonstrated a statistically significant reduction in female neck fractures (75). The treatment dose of alendronate for osteoporosis is 10 mg/day.

Calcitonin in the injectable form has been used for years in the treatment of osteoporosis and is known to increase bone mineral density. It has been shown to decrease the incidence of fracture in the hip, vertebrae, and forearm (76). It is purported to have an analgesic effect and relieve the pain associated with new or chronic fractions from osteoporosis (77). Injectable calcitonin's primary associated side effect is flushing. Because the parenteral form is not practical for long-term use, a newer delivery modality (nasal spray, Miacalcin) has been introduced and approved for the treatment of postmenopausal osteoporosis. This is given as 200 IU (two puffs/day) in one nostril, alternating nostrils daily. There is evidence that it increases bone mineral density in the vertebral spine and decreases the incidence of vertebral fractures (78). Studies are forthcoming regarding its effect on hip fractures. Miacalcin is for use in women who are 5 years or more past the onset of menopause. This agent has not been proven to be efficacious in women before that time. The most common side effect is rhinitis.

In the years immediately after menopause and the loss of estrogen, calcium has little effect on bone (79). Calcium is known to be beneficial for patients with osteoporosis past the first 5 to 7 years of menopause. Various forms of calcium supplementation are available. The carbonate forms must be taken with foods, although the citrate forms do not. The recommended dosage is 1000 mg/day for women on estrogen replacement and 1500 mg/day for women not on estrogen (80, 81).

Vitamin D is also recommended for patients with osteoporosis and for the prevention of osteoporosis. It is particularly recommended for the elderly, who may spend very little time outside, hence limiting their sun exposure (82–84). The recommended dosage for patients over age 65 is 600 IU/day. Dosages should not exceed 1000 IU/day.

An often overlooked modality for the treatment of osteoporosis is weightbearing exercise. Of concern is a potential increase in the fracture rate with exercise in patients already suffering from osteoporosis. One study demonstrated in a group of elderly patients that with the appropriate exercise regimen, this is not a major concern (85). It should be noted that exercise increases muscle mass and strength and balance, thus decreasing the propensity to fall.

Cognitive Function

Estrogen has been shown to have an impact on central nervous system function in many animal studies. Its impact on the human central nervous system is only now beginning to be researched and understood. Psychiatric disorders increase in prevalence with each decade of life (86). The incidence of depression in older women is approximately 10% (87). Depression in the elderly more frequently presents as somatic and vegetative symptoms and may be incorrectly attributed to "senility." Underlying medical disorders such as anemia, vitamin D deficiency, and hypothyroidism may present as depression. In addition, medications (e.g., propanolol or methyldopa, sedatives or hypnotics) may produce depression. Patients may be depressed to an extent that causes interference with memory and cognitive function. This must be distinguished from true dementias. Vascular dementia accounts for about 20 to 25% of dementia cases in the elderly (88). Diagnosis is often made by history and confirmed on CT. Focal neurologic signs are usually present.

Of recent interest is the effect of estrogen on the prevention and/or treatment of Alzheimer's's disease. Alzheimer's's disease is a degenerative process of the brain causing a slow progressive loss of mental function. It is a major public health problem. Currently there are 4 million people afflicted with Alzheimer's disease in the United States. Forty percent of patients over the age of 80 are affected (89). It is the leading cause of loss of independence and institutionalization of the elderly. The prevalence of Alzheimer's disease is greatest in those patients over the age of 85, and this is currently the fastest growing segment of the population in America (89–91). The prevalence of Alzheimer's disease is greater in women than in men of the same age, and the prevalence doubles every 4.5 years after the age of 60. This is a consistent finding regardless of ethnicity or culture. It is usually sporadic, although it may be transmitted as an autosomal dominant trait (88). Several studies demonstrated a 50 to 60% reduction in the risk of Alzheimer's disease in women who have taken ERT/HRT (92–95). Although small in numbers, another study demonstrated that estrogen had a significant improvement in memory in women with Alzheimer's when compared with those women with Alzheimer's disease who did not receive estrogen. Although this improvement in memory was somewhat modest, the overall effect of receiving estrogen was to delay the progression of Alzheimer's disease by approximately 2 years (96).

Kantor et al.'s study (97) found that women with Alzheimer's disease who received conjugated estrogen (Premarin) had an improvement in their communica-

TABLE 2.6. Mechanisms of Estrogen's Action on Brain Function

Stimulates the expression of neurotrophic factors
Protects neurons from β-amyloid toxicity (in vitro)
Stimulates axonal regeneration and synaptogenesis (in vivo)
Maintains viability of neurons in culture
Increases regional cerebral blood flow
Stimulates production of neurotransmitters acetylcholine and serotonin

tions and self-care abilities over the first year of therapy, with some decline in these skills later on. However, the estrogen therapy did allow a maintenance of independence for an additional 2 years compared with patients receiving placebo.

Further evidence that estrogen maybe helpful in the treatment in Alzheimer's disease is seen in a study where women with Alzheimer's disease were treated with conjugated estrogen (Premarin) and compared with placebo. Women receiving estrogen had improvement in the Hasegawa dementia scale and Mini-Mental State Examination scores over a period of 5 months compare with women with Alzheimer's disease who received placebo (98).

A recent double-blind placebo-controlled trial was conducted in which patients diagnosed with Alzheimer's disease received conjugated estrogen (Premarin) and progesterone every 3 months or placebo (99). The outcome measure of this study was the clinician interview-based impression scale. The patient and the caregiver were interviewed by a clinician who was blinded to treatment and to any objective measures of cognitive function. Of those women receiving conjugated estrogen (Premarin), 80% showed improvement. The placebo group showed no improvement.

The mechanisms of estrogen's action on brain function at the molecular level are only now beginning to be understood (Table 2.6). It is known that estrogen stimulates the expression of neurotrophic factors within the central nervous system (100). Estrogen has also been demonstrated to stimulate neuronal regeneration and synaptogenesis and to maintain viability of neurons in culture (101). Physiologically, it has been demonstrated to increase regional cerebral blood flow (102).

DIAGNOSING MENOPAUSE

In trying to determine when a woman has completed the transition between perimenopause and menopause, an FSH level is drawn. For women on oral contraceptives, it is recommended that the FSH level be drawn on days 5 to 7 of the pill-free week. If the FSH level is elevated and consistent with menopausal levels, contraception is no longer necessary. Oral contraceptives may be discontinued and the patient switched to a menopausal hormonal regimen. For women not on oral contraceptives (and with no contraindications), initiation of HRT is indicated. The evaluation for the initiation of HRT should include a history and physical examination, including pelvic and breast examination.

HORMONE REPLACEMENT THERAPY

Estrogen

Conjugated equine estrogen (Premarin) is the gold standard by which other estrogenic agents are compared. It has been in use for over 50 years and has been used in most scientific studies. Continued research demonstrated that some of the estrogenic components found in Premarin may be quite site specific in their impact. A typical estrogen regimen consists of 0.625 mg/day of conjugated equine estrogens.

Transdermal estrogen has been shown to be beneficial for women. Its primary indication is in those women who prefer to take this mode of ERT. Transdermally administered 17β-estradiol is available in 4- and 8-mg dose patches delivering 50 and 100 µg/day, respectively. These patches are changed every 3 days (Estraderm). Recently, a transdermal delivery system requiring only weekly changes was developed (Climara). Recommended areas of application of the patch are the lower abdomen or the buttocks. Delivery of the estrogen via the transdermal route has certain theoretic advantages (103). By bypassing gastrointestinal tract absorption and hepatic portal circulation (first-pass effect), lower doses of the hormone are required. In addition, by avoiding first-pass effect, changes in lipoprotein metabolism, bile composition, and induction and alteration of liver and coagulation protein can be avoided (104). Thus, this mode of delivery can be potentially beneficial to women who smoke cigarettes or have migraine headaches, hypertriglyceridemia, hepatobiliary disorders, or history of thromboembolism (105).

Selective Estrogen Receptor Modulator

With increasing knowledge of the interaction between estrogen, estrogen receptors, adaptor proteins, and the nucleus, there have been intensive efforts to create the "perfect estrogen." Increasing evidence supports the idea that estrogen has specific sites of action and that these actions are determined by the chemical structure of the estrogen, the adaptor proteins that are present, and the receptor to which it binds. Intense efforts are currently underway to develop estrogens that would selectively interact or modulate specific receptors at specific sites.

Tamoxifen was initially hailed as an estrogen with all the benefits and none of the risks of estrogen. However, although initially thought to have no stimulatory affect on the endometrium, this has been shown to be wrong.

The newest SERM is raloxifene (Evista), and although there is evidence that it increases bone mineral density above that of placebo, its effects are modest at best compared with conjugated estrogen (Premarin). Newer SERMs are under investigation and research. These would also include the phytoestrogens (naturally occurring estrogens that are found in plants, particularly soy). A benefit of the current development investigation of SERMs is the explosion of knowledge that has occurred in the basic science arena and is extending into the clinical arena regarding the effects and the potential uses of estrogen and estrogenic agents.

Progestins

The use of unopposed estrogen increases the risk of endometrial cancer in postmenopausal women. Multiple studies showed that the use of progestin in combination with estrogen can protect against endometrial cancer (106). This protective effect is postulated to be mediated by progestins by reducing the number of estradiol receptors in the endometrium and by stimulating the activity of endometrial estradiol 17β-dehydrogenase (converting estradiol to estrone).

Many types of progestins can be used for combination hormone therapy. Most women taking combination therapy in the United States are on a regimen that uses oral MPA. Usual dosages include 10 mg MPA/day for the first 14 days of the month (for sequential dosing) or 2.5 mg/day (for continuous dosing).

Alternatively, 200 mg micronized progesterone per day for the first 14 days (sequential) or 200 mg daily (continuous) may be used in lieu of MPA. This preparation is becoming increasingly available in pharmacies in the United States. A third choice for continuous therapy could be norethindrone acetate, 0.35 mg daily.

Regimens

Unopposed Estrogen

Women without a uterus may receive estrogen alone. There does not appear to be any physiologic benefit to adding a progestational agent for these women. It should be remembered that women that do have a uterus and receive unopposed estrogen have an increase in their risk of endometrial hyperplasia and endometrial carcinoma. As previously discussed, this increase in risk is canceled by the addition of a progestational agent. It does not, however, abrogate entirely the risk of endometrial carcinoma. It is important to remember that endometrial carcinoma does occur in women who have not received unopposed estrogen.

For women who refuse progestational agents, there is the option of unopposed estrogen use with yearly endometrial biopsy sampling. Extensive counseling about the risk incurred by unopposed estrogen on the endometrium should be given to the patient and informed consent obtained for this particular regimen.

Sequential HRT

Previous regimens of sequential HRT prescribed estrogen for days 1 through 25 of each month and a progestational agent for days 16 through 25. This created a 5- to 6-day hiatus at the end of the month where no hormonal agents were ingested. This was a regimen derived on theoretic grounds and not based on strict scientific evidence. This regimen is rather cumbersome to explain and difficult for patients to remember (there is nothing momentous on the 16th of each month that normally occurs in women's lives). Therefore, a more convenient regimen is the use of estrogen on a daily continuous basis. The progestational agent is taken on days 1 to 12 of each month. The original regimen of progestational use called for 10 mg of Provera or its equivalent for 10 days. Recent studies demonstrated, however, that the dose necessary to protect the endometrium is 70 mg/month. The current regimen that most practitioners now use is that of a progestational agent at 5 mg/day for either 12 to 14 days each month. The sequential regimen is recommended for women in the first 2 to 3 years of menopause to minimize any breakthrough bleeding (Table 2.7).

TABLE 2.7. Sequential Program for Postmenopausal Hormone Therapy[a]

> **DAILY ESTROGEN**
> 0.625 mg conjugated estrogens, or
> 0.625 mg estrone sulfate, or
> 1.0 mg micronized estradiol
>
> **MONTHLY PROGESTIN**
> 5 mg medroxyprogesterone acetate, or
> 0.7 mg norethindrone, or
> 200 mg micronized progesterone given daily for 2 weeks every month
>
> ---
> [a]Combined with calcium supplementation (500 mg with a meal) and vitamin D (400 IU in winter months and 600 IU for women over age 70).

TABLE 2.8. Continous Combination Program for Postmenopausal Hormone Therapy[a]

DAILY ESTROGEN
0.625 mg conjugated estrogens, or
0.625 mg estrone sulfate, or
1.0 mg micronized estradiol

DAILY PROGESTIN
2.5 mg medroxyprogesterone acetate, or
0.35 mg norethindrone, or 100–200 mg micronized progesterone

[a]Combined with calcium supplementation (500 mg with a meal) and vitamin D (400 IU in winter months and 600 for women over age 70).

Continuous Combined HRT

Continuous combined HRT (Table 2.8) was developed in an attempt to avoid a withdrawal bleed each month. This is particularly attractive for the older menopausal patient. In this regimen, estrogen is administered on a daily basis in conjunction with a daily dosage of 2.5 to 5 mg of Provera or its equivalent. With this regimen, the overall effect is to convert the endometrium to an atrophic state and eliminate any withdrawal bleeding.

By the end of the first year, most women become amenorrheic on this regimen, with a higher percentage becoming amenorrheic in the second subsequent year. Breakthrough bleeding during the first 6 months of this regimen is quite common. Bleeding arising after the sixth month may require further investigation with either endometrial biopsy and/or transvaginal ultrasound, with or without hysterosonography. The continuous combined regimen is not recommended for those patients within 2 years of the onset of menopause because there seems to be a higher incident of breakthrough bleeding.

CONTRAINDICATIONS FOR ESTROGEN THERAPY

Contraindications for HRT include undiagnosed abnormal uterine bleeding, active disease involving estrogen-sensitive tumors, and metabolic disorders such as acute vascular thrombosis or acute liver disease.

Metabolic Disorders

It should be recalled that oral contraceptives contain a pharmacologic level of estrogen, whereas hormone replacement regimens contain a physiologic level of estrogen. As a result of this, the contraindications for ERT are not the same as for oral contraceptive use. There is no contraindication to the use of ERT for women with hypertension or diabetes. Given the cardioprotective effect of estrogen, there may be an actual indication for estrogenic use in these patients.

Although oral contraceptive agents have been shown to increase thromboembolic potential in women, this has not been proven to be the case with ERT. There are several recent studies that suggested an increase in thromboembolic disease and/or pulmonary embolism in women on ERT, but there are several flaws with these studies. If ERT does increase thromboembolic risk, the clinical significance of this increase in risk is questionable.

As previously discussed, transdermal estrogen delivery may be the mode of choice for postmenopausal women with special medical conditions. The patient should be counseled carefully with special attention to weighing risks versus benefits.

Breast Cancer

Although breast cancer is an emotionally charged issue and is perceived by a large number of women to be the number one health risk in the menopausal state, it accounts for 3% of deaths in women. It is erroneously perceived as the leading cancer killer among women. Lung cancer is the number one cause of cancer deaths among women 45 to 80 years of age; after age 80, it is exceeded by colon cancer deaths.

Although there has been an increase in the incidence of breast cancer since 1983, this reflects an increase in the diagnosis of carcinoma in situ; of significance is that the mortality rate has remained stable (107, 108). The media and the medical community have clouded the issue of breast cancer with the ongoing debate regarding the role of estrogen and initiation of breast cancer. Clinical studies showed no definitive link between the use of HRT and the onset of breast cancer. Of interest is the finding that the 5-year survival rate for women with a history of ERT and a diagnosis of breast cancer is greater than the 5-year survival rate of women with a diagnosis of breast cancer and no previous use of estrogen replacement (109, 110).

The risk of developing breast cancer increases with a woman's age (Table 2.9) and is significantly related to her decade in life (111). The media commonly quotes that women have a lifetime risk of developing breast cancer of one in eight (23). This must be seen, however, from the prospective of the decade that the woman occupies. For example, a woman aged 40 has a 1.6% risk of developing breast cancer over the next 10 years. The same woman at age 40 has a 10.3% risk of developing breast cancer by the age of 80.

TABLE 2.9. Risk of Breast Cancer by Age[a]

Age (yr)	Odds
25	1 in 19,608
30	1 in 2525
35	1 in 622
40	1 in 217
45	1 in 93
50	1 in 50
55	1 in 33
60	1 in 24
65	1 in 17
70	1 in 14
75	1 in 11
80	1 in 10
85	1 in 9
Lifetime/85+	1 in 8

[a]Data are from the National Cancer Institute.

Several epidemiologic analyses of ERT and the relative risk of breast cancer have been done. Overall, there does not appear to be a significant increase in the risk of breast cancer in women taking ERT (112). Additionally, it must be realized that if in fact there is a risk, the risk is made tolerable by the numerous benefits regarding osteoporosis and heart disease.

Estrogen replacement after breast cancer treatment is controversial. There are currently some small prospective studies being done on the use of ERT after diagnosis of breast cancer. Preliminary results are encouraging, with no increase in the incidence of recurrence. Patients with a history of breast cancer who are inquiring about ERT should seek consultation from their gynecologist and oncologist and should be counseled in great detail. Ultimately, however, the decision is up to the individual patient.

Endometrial Cancer

Patients with history of stage I low-grade adenocarcinoma of the endometrium can be placed on an estrogen replacement regimen without fear of recurrence of disease (113–118). There is some controversy as to how long one should wait before starting these patients on HRT, with some authors favoring immediate treatment. Because most recurrences occur within the first 2 years, it would be reasonable to offer HRT to patients with a 2-year disease-free interval. Insufficient information is available to make recommendations for patients with history of high-grade tumors or advanced disease.

GENERAL CARE OF THE MENOPAUSAL WOMAN

Preventive Medicine

Regularly scheduled disease prevention and screening should become part of the routine care of the patient. In addition to their annual pelvic examinations and Papanicolaou (Pap) smears, women ages 40 to 65 should have a mammography every 1 to 2 years after age 40 and yearly after age 50 (women at increased risk for breast cancer should begin yearly screening at age 40). Cholesterol screening should be performed every 5 years, fecal occult blood screening should be done annually, and sigmoidoscopy should be done every 3 to 4 years after age 50. Women in the perimenopause or who are menopausal (not on HRT) and with increased risk factors for osteoporosis should be offered a screening test for bone density if the results of the test have clinical relevance to the patient's treatment or prevention of osteoporosis.

For women 65 and older, Pap smears should be performed every 2 years and if three negative consecutive tests are obtained, they can then be performed at the discretion of the patient and the physician. These women should continue to receive annual breast and pelvic examinations, however. Mammograms and screening for fecal occult blood should be offered on a yearly basis. Thyroid (thyroid-stimulating hormone) and cholesterol screening should be offered every 5 years, and sigmoidoscopy every 4 years. Height and weight measurements, urinalysis, and hemoglobin levels should be surveyed on an annual basis in this age group. Annual vision test and screening for glaucoma (tonometry) should be offered as well. The pneumococcus vaccine (Pneumovax) should be offered to all patients over the age of 65 (Table 2.10).

TABLE 2.10. Preventive Screening for Well Women

	Age (yr)		
	40–49	50–59	60–69
COMPLETE HISTORY AND PHYSICAL EXAMINATION	q 5 yr	q 5 yr	q 2 yr
Smoking, alcohol, drug use, weight, height, blood pressure	q visit	q visit	q visit
Breast, pelvic, rectal/occult blood examination	q 1 yr	q 1 yr	q 1 yr
Pap smear	q 1 yr	q 1 yr	q 1 yr
Hearing assessment	q 10 yr	q 10 yr	q 1 yr
Visual assessment	q 10 yr	q 10 yr	q 1 yr
IMMUNIZATIONS			
Tetanus-diptheria booster	q 10 yr	q 10 yr	q 10 yr
Influenza immunization			after 65, q yr
Pneumovax			1 at 65 yr
LABORATORY WORK			
Lipid profile	q 5 yr	q 5 yr	q 5 yr
Sexually transmitted disease	High risk only		
Tuberculosis screen	High risk only		
Hematocrit or hemoglobin	q 10 yr	q 10 yr	q 10 yr
Thyroid assessment (TSH)	1 at 45 yr		q yr
SPECIAL ITEMS			
Proctosigmoidoscopy		q 3 yr	q 3 yr
Mammography baseline at 35	q 2 yr	q yr	after 65q 2 yr
REGULAR COUNSELING	Nutrition, smoking, exercise, breast and skin self-examinations, sexual practices, dental health, injury prevention		

TSH; thyroid-stimulating hormone.

SPECIAL GYNECOLOGIC ISSUES FOR THE POSTMENOPAUSAL WOMAN

Pelvic Mass

Adnexal masses in the postmenopausal woman should be highly suspect for malignancy until proven otherwise (particularly complex masses greater than 5 cm). The workup should include a thorough rectovaginal examination, pelvic ultrasound, CA-125 level, and a CT if clinically indicated.

Abnormal Uterine Bleeding

All postmenopausal women with abnormal bleeding must be evaluated carefully to rule out organic disease. Evaluation should include a careful history and physical (which includes a pelvic examination and thorough examination of the vulva, vagina, and cervix). A Pap smear should be performed as well.

Pathologic findings in a Pap smear should be followed appropriately. Abnormal pathology or obvious lesions may require a colposcopic examination with or without cervical biopsies. An endocervical curettage should be performed if indicated.

The absence of findings in the above tests should prompt the physician to investigate intrauterine sources for the bleeding. This evaluation should include an endometrial biopsy. If bleeding persists, a repeat endometrial biopsy should be performed. Inability to perform an endometrial biopsy secondary to cervical os stenosis is a indication for a diagnostic fractional dilatation and curettage. Alternatively, the stenosis can be relieved with the use of the loop electrosurgical excision procedure, provided that the stenosis is limited to the external cervical os (119). Hysterosonography or hysteroscopy can be done as part of the workup of persistent bleeding to rule out the presence of endometrial polyps.

Transvaginal ultrasonography can be used as an alternative to an endometrial biopsy in the initial workup of abnormal bleeding in a postmenopausal woman receiving continuous combined estrogen-progestin replacement therapy (Fig. 2.2). Finding of an endometrium greater than 4 mm would warrant further investigation by endometrial biopsy, whereas an endometrium less than 4 mm can be followed with annual sonograms (120, 121).

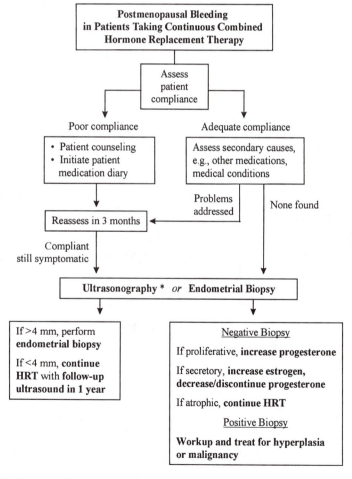

FIGURE 2.2. Workup of postmenopausal bleeding in patients taking continuous combined HRT. *Asterisk* indicates ultrasonography, if available, with or without hysterosonography. Some physicians prefer to proceed directly to endometrial biopsy.

CLINICAL NOTES

Perimenopause

- Menopause is a retrospective diagnosis and is based on the absence of menses for 6 to 12 months.
- The age at menopause is influenced by genetic factors, cigarette smoking, living at high altitudes, and undernourishment. It is not related to the age at menarche.

Sequelae of Menopause

Hot Flushes

- Administration of estrogen replacement will not suppress the increased FSH of menopause. FSH levels cannot be used to titrate ERT/HRT doses.
- It is not uncommon for women to complain of hot flushes while still menstruating and exhibiting normal levels of FSH.
- Menstrual cycles in the perimenopausal women may initially be ovulatory, but with time, anovulation becomes more frequent. Pregnancy is still possible in the perimenopausal state.
- The frequency of hot flushes decreases over time for most women, but some women continue to experience them (many) years after the menopause.
- Estrogen is the most effective treatment for hot flushes.
- Alternative therapies for hot flushes include progestational agents (Provera, 150 mg intramuscularly every month or 20 to 80 mg orally every day) or Clonidine (0.1 to 1.5 mg/day).

Genitourinary Symptoms

- Estrogen deprivation results in vaginal atrophy. This may manifest as vaginal irritation and/or dyspareunia.
- Treatment of vaginal atrophy is systemic, with oral or parenteral estrogen, or topical, with a cream or estrogen-containing pessary.
- Urge incontinence is the most common problem associated with hypoestrogenic atrophy of the genitourinary tract. Replacement of estrogen results in thickening of the bladder mucosa and may result in improvement, if not complete resolution, of symptoms.

Cardiovascular Disease

- Heart disease is the number one killer of postmenopausal women in the United States. American women have a 23% lifetime risk of dying from ischemic heart disease.
- A 1% increase in total cholesterol increases the risk of CAD by 2%; a 1% decrease in HDL increases the risk of CAD by 2 to 4.7%.
- In women, increased diastolic and/or systolic blood pressures are independent risk factors for CAD.
- The use of ERT/HRT reduces the risk of CAD in postmenopausal women by approximately 50%.

Osteoporosis

- Peak bone mass is achieved at age 35 or so. In the perimenopausal period, bone is lost at 0.5 to 1% per year. At the time of menopause, the rate increases to 2 to 3% per year for 5 to 7 years thereafter. It then slows, but continues.
- Risk factors for osteoporosis include small body size, fair skin, family history, use of certain medications, physical inactivity, past or current smokers, diets low in calcium, and certain medical diseases.
- Dual x-ray absorptiometry is the gold standard for diagnosing osteoporosis. The T score is used for the diagnosis. A T score greater than or equal to a 2.5 standard deviations below the mean constitutes osteoporosis.

- FDA-approved agents for the medical prevention of osteoporosis can be achieved with the use of estrogen, alendronate (Fosamax, 5 mg/day), or raloxifene (Evista, 60 mg/day).
- FDA-approved agents for the treatment of osteoporosis include estrogen, alendronate (Fosamax, 10 mg/day), and nasal calcitonin (Miacalcin, 200 IU/day).
- Vitamin D (600 IU/day) is recommended for patients over 65 with and without osteoporosis.

Cognitive Function

- The incidence of depression in older women is about 10%. Depression in the elderly more frequently presents as somatic vegetative symptoms and may be incorrectly attributed to senility.
- Underlying medical disorders any present as depression in the elderly.
- Vascular dementia accounts for about 20 to 25% of dementia cases in the elderly.
- Alzheimer's disease is twice as common in women over age 70 than in men. Several studies demonstrated a 50 to 60% reduction in the risk of Alzheimer's disease in women who have taken ERT/HRT.

Diagnosing Menopause

- To determine if an amenorrheic woman is menopausal, an FSH level is drawn. For perimenopausal women on oral contraceptives, the FSH level is drawn on days 5 to 7 of the pill-free week.

Hormone Replacement Therapy

Regimens

- Unopposed estrogen may be used in women without a uterus. In women with a uterus, use of unopposed estrogen increases their risk of endometrial hyperplasia and uterine cancer.
- Sequential HRT is given as a daily estrogen and progesterone on days 1 to 12 each month. Withdrawal bleeding is expected to occur with this regimen.
- Continuous combined estrogen is given as a daily estrogen and daily progesterone (2.5 or 5 mg of Provera).

Contraindications for Estrogen Therapy

- Contraindications for estrogen include undiagnosed abnormal uterine bleeding, current breast cancer or uterine cancer, acute vascular thrombosis, or acute liver disease.
- There is no contraindication to the use of estrogen in postmenopausal women with hypertension, diabetes, or heart disease.
- The role of estrogen as a risk factor for the development of breast cancer is controversial, although there are studies indicating an improvement in 5-year survival rates among breast cancer patients with a history of previous estrogen use.
- Patients with a history of stage I low-grade adenocarcinoma may be placed on estrogen replacement without increasing their risk of recurrent disease.

General Care of the Menopausal Woman

- Regularly scheduled disease prevention and screening should be determined by the patient's history and significant health risks for her age group.

Special Gynecologic Issues for the Postmenopausal Woman

- Adnexal masses in the postmenopausal woman should be suspected for malignancy until proven otherwise.
- Abnormal bleeding in the postmenopausal woman *must* be evaluated. This may initially be done with endometrial biopsy, transvaginal ultrasound (with or without hysterosonography), or both.

References

1. Krailo MD, Pike MC. Estimation of the distribution of age at natural menopause from prevalence data. Am J Epidemiol 1983;117:356.
2. Coulam CB, Adamson SC, Annegers JF. Incidence of premature ovarian failure. Obstet Gynecol 19086;67:604.
3. National Center for Health Statistics. Advisory report of final mortality statistics. 1991, Monthly Vital Statistic Report, 42 (2). Hyattsville, MD: Public Health Service, 1993.
4. Sherman BM, West JH, Korenman SG. The menopausal transition: analysis of LH, FSH, estradiol, and progesterone concentrations during menstrual cycles of older women. J Clin Endocrinol Metab 1976;42:629–636.
5. Metcalf MG, Donald RA, Livesey JH. Pituitary-ovarian function in normal women during the menopausal transition. Clin Endocrinol 1981;14:245–255.
6. Metcalf MG. The approach of menopause: a New Zealand study. N Z Med J 1988;101:103–106.
7. Zumoff B, Rosenfeld RS, Strain GW, et al. Sex differences in the twenty-four-hour mean plasma concentrations of dehydroisoandrosterone (DHA) and dehydroisoandrosterone sulfate (DHAS) and the DHA to DHAS ratio in normal adults. J Clin Endocrinol Metab 1980;51:330–333.
8. Carlstrom K, Brody S, Lunell NO, et al. Dehydroepiandrosterone sulphate and dehydroepiandrosterone in serum: differences related to age and sex. Maturitas 1988;10:297–306.
9. Longcope C, Hunter R, Franz C. Steroid secretion by the postmenopausal ovary. Am J Obstet Gynecol 1980;138:564–568.
10. Judd HL, Judd GE, Lucas WE, et al. Endocrine function of the postmenopausal ovary: concentration of androgens and estrogens in ovarian and peripheral blood. J Clin Endocrinol Metab 1974;39:1020–1024.
11. Voda AM. Climacteric hot flash. Maturitas 1981;3:73–90.
12. Kronenberg F. Hot flashes: epidemiology and physiology. Ann N Y Acad Sci 1990;592:52–86.
13. Feldman BM, Voda AM, Gronseth E. The prevalence of hot flash and associated variables among perimenopausal women. Res Nurs Health 1985;8:261–268.
14. Gannon L, Hansel S, Goldwin J. Correlates of menopausal hot flashes. J Behav Med 1987;10:277–285.
15. Erlik Y, Meldrum DR, Judd HL. Estrogen levels in postmenopausal women with hot flashes. Obstet Gynecol 1982;59:403–407.
16. Lock M. Ambiguities of aging: Japanese experience and perceptions of menopause. Cult Med Psychiatry 1986;10:23–46.
17. Bullock JL, Massey FM, Gambrell RD Jr. Use of medroxyprogesterone acetate to prevent menopausal symptoms. Obstet Gynecol 1975;46:165–168.
18. Albrecht BH, Schiff I, Tulchinsky D, et al. Objective evidence that placebo and oral medroxyprogesterone acetate therapy diminish menopausal vasomotor flushes. Am J Obstet Gynecol 1981;139:631–635.
19. Laufer LR, Erlik Y, Meldrum DR, et al. Effect of clonidine on hot flashes in postmenopausal women. Obstet Gynecol 1982;6055:583–586.
20. Thompson B, Hart SA, Durno D. Menopausal age and symptomatology in a general practice. J Biosoc Sci 1973;5:71–72.
21. Advance report of final mortality statistics, 1989. Monthly Vital Stat Rep 1992;40(suppl 2):1–47.
22. National Center for Health Statistics. Vital Statistics of the United States. Publication no. 96–1101. Washington, DC: Public Health Service, 1992:2A.
23. Miller et al., eds. SEER Cancer Statistics Review 1973–1993. National Cancer Institute, 1997.
24. Manson JE, Tosteson H, Ridker PM, et al. The primary prevention of myocardial infarction. N Engl J Med 1992;326:1406–1416.

25. Kannel WB, Feinleib M. Natural history of angina pectoris in the Framingham study. Prognosis and survival. Am J Cardiol 1972;29:154–163.
26. American Heart Association. Heart and Stroke Facts. Dallas: American Heart Association National Center, 1993.
27. Detry JR, Kapita BM, Cosyns J, et al. Diagnostic value of history and maximal exercise electrocardiography in men and women suspected of coronary heart disease. Circulation 1977;56:756.
28. Ayanian JZ, Epstein AM. Differences in the use of procedures between women and men hospitalized for coronary heart disease. N Engl J Med 1991;325:221–224.
29. Maynard C, Litwin PE, Marin JS, et al. Gender differences in the treatment and outcome of acute myocardial infarction. Arch Intern Med 1992;152:972–976.
30. Kahn SS, Nessim S, Gray KR, et al. Increased mortality of women in coronary artery bypass surgery: evidence for referral bias. Ann Intern Med 1990;112:561–567.
31. Jensen J, Nilas L, Christiansen C. Influence of menopause on serum lipids and lipoproteins. Maturitas 1990;12:321–331.
32. Chen Z, Peto R, Collins R, et al. Serum cholesterol concentration and coronary heart disease in a population with low cholesterol concentration. Br Med J 1991;303:276–282.
33. Van der Giezen AM, van Kessel JGS-G, Schouten EG, et al. Systolic blood pressure and cardiovascular mortality among 13,740 Dutch women. Prev Med 1990;19:456–465.
34. Bush TL, Comstock CW. Smoking and cardiovascular mortality in women. Am J Epidemiol 1983;118:480–488.
35. LaCroiz AZ, Lang J, Scherr P, et al. Smoking and mortality among older men and women in three communities. N Engl J Med 1991;324:1619–1625.
36. Kannel WB, Wilson PW, Zhang TJ. The epidemiology of impaired glucose tolerance and hypertension. Am Heart J 1991;121:1268–1273.
37. Boysen G, Nyboe J, Appleyard M, et al. Stroke incidence and risk factors for stroke in Copenhagen, Denmark. Stroke 1988;19:1345–1353.
38. Criqui MH, Suwarez L, Barrett-Connor E, et al. Postmenopausal estrogen use and mortality. Am J Epidemiol 1988;128:606–614.
39. Bush TL, Barrett-Connor E, Cowan LD, et al. Cardiovascular mortality and noncontraceptive use of estrogen in women: results from the Lipid Research Clinics Program Follow-up Study. Circulation 1987;75:1102–1109.
40. Falkeborn M, Persson I, Adami HO, et al. The risk of acute myocardial infarction after oestrogen and oestrogen-progestogen replacement. Br J Obstet Gynecol 1992;99:821–828.
41. Psaty BM, Heckbert SR, Atkins D, et al. The risk of myocardial infarction associated with the progestins in postmenopausal women. Arch Intern Med 1994;154:1333–1339.
42. Stampfer MJ, Willett WC, Colditz GA, et al. A prospective study of postmenopausal estrogen therapy and coronary heart disease. N Engl J Med 1985;313:1044–1049.
43. Wolf PH, Madans JH, Finucane FF, et al. Reduction of cardiovascular disease-related mortality among postmenopausal women who use hormones: evidence from a national cohort. Am J Obstet Gynecol 1991;164:489–494.
44. PEPI Trial Writing Group. Effects of estrogen or estrogen/progestin regimens on heart disease risk factors in postmenopausal women: the Postmenopausal Estrogen/Progestin Interventions (PEPI) Trial. JAMA 1995;273:199–208.
45. Gerhard M, Ganz P. How do we explain the clinical benefits of estrogen? From bed side to bench. Circulation 1995;92:5–8.
46. Sullivan JM. Hormone replacement therapy in cardiovascular disease: the human model. Br J Obstet Gynaecol 1996;103(suppl 13):50–67.
47. Scarabin PY, Kopp CV, Bara L, et al. Factor VII activation and menopausal status. Thrombosis Res 1990;57:227–234.
48. Schaible TF, Malhotra A, Ciambrone G, et al. The effects of gonadectomy on left ventricular function and cardiac contractile proteins in male and female rats. Circ Res 1984;54:38–49.
49. Ganger KF, Vyas S, Whitehead M, et al. Pulsatility index in internal carotid artery in relation to transdermal oestradiol and time since menopause. Lancet 1991;338:839–842.

50. Barrett-Connor E, Laasko M. Ischemic heart disease risk in postmenopausal women: effects of estrogen use on glucose and insulin levels. Arteriosclerosis 1990;10:531–53.

51. Reis SE, Gloth ST, Blumenthal RS, et al. Ethinyl estradiol acutely attenuates abnormal coronary vasomotor responses to acetylcholine in postmenopausal women. Circulation 1994;89:52–60.

52. Rosano GM, Rosano C, Sarrel PM, et al. Beneficial effect of oestrogen on exercise-induced myocardial ischaemia in women with coronary artery disease. Lancet 1993;342: 133–136.

53. Henderson BE, Paganini-Hill A, Ross RK. Decreased mortality in users of estrogen replacement therapy. Arch Intern Med 1991;151:75–78.

54. Newton KM, LaCroix AZ, McKnight B, et al. Estrogen replacement therapy and prognosis after first myocardial infarction. Am J Epidemiol 1997;145:269–277.

55. Sullivan JM, Vander Zwaag R, Hughes JP, et al. Estrogen replacement and coronary artery disease. Effect on survival in postmenopausal women. Arch Intern Med 1990;150: 2557–2562.

56. Sarrel PM, Lindsay D, Rosano CM. Angina and normal coronary artery in women: gynecological findings. Am J Obstet Gynecol 1992;167:467–421.

57. Finucane FF, Madams JH, Bush TL, et al. Decreased risk of stroke among postmenopausal hormone users. Results from a National cohort. Arch Intern Med1993;153: 73–79.

58. Grodstein F, Stampfer MJ, Manson JE, et al. Postmenopausal estrogen and progestin use and the risk of cardiovascular disease. N Engl J Med.1996;335:453–461.

59. Wilson PW, Garrison RJ, Castelli WP. Postmenopausal estrogen use, cigarette smoking, and cardiovascular morbidity in women over 50: The Framingham Study. N Engl J Med 1985;313:1038–1043.

60. Hennekens CH. Aspirin in the treatment and prevention of cardiovascular disease. Annu Rev Public Health 1997;18:37–49.

61. Ray NF, Chan JK, Thamer M, et al. Medical expenditures for the treatment of osteoporotic fractures in the United States in 1995: report from the National Osteoporosis Foundation. J Bone Miner Res 1997;12:24–35.

62. Parfitt AM. Bone remodeling: relationship to the amount and structure of bone, and the pathogenesis and prevention of fractures. In: Riggs BL, Melton LJ, eds. Osteoporosis: Etiology, Diagnosis, and Management. New York: Raven Press, 1988:45–93.

63. Komm BS, Terpening CM, Benz DJ. Estrogen binding, receptor mRNA, and biologic response in osteoblast-like osteosarcoma cells. Science 1988;241:81–84.

64. Eriksen EF, Colvard DS, Berg NJ, et al. Evidence of estrogen receptors in normal human osteoblast-like cells. Science 1988;241:84–86.

65. Jilka RL, Hangoc G, Girasole G, et al. Increased osteoclast development after estrogen loss-mediation by interleukin-6. Science 1992;257:88.

66. Christiansen C, Christensen MS, McNair P, et al. Prevention of early postmenopausal bone loss. Controlled 2 year study in 315 normal females. Eur J Clin Invest 1980;10:273–279.

67. Riis BJ, Thomsen K, Strom V, et al. The effect of percutaneous estradiol and natural progesterone on post menopausal bone loss. Am J Obstet Gynecol 1987;156:61–65.

68. Consensus Development Conference. Prophylaxis and treatment of osteoporosis. Am J Med 1991;90:107–110.

69. Horsman A, Jones M, Francis R, et al. The effect of estrogen dose on postmenopausal bone loss. N Engl J Med 1983;309:1405–1407.

70. Christensen MS, Hagen C, Christiansen C, et al. Dose-response evaluation of cyclic estrogen/gestagen in postmenopausal women: placebo controlled trial of its gynecologic and metabolic actions. Am J Obstet Gynecol 1982;144:873–879.

71. Lindsay R, Hart CM, Clark DM. The minimum effective dose of estrogen for prevention of postmenopausal bone loss. Obstet Gynecol 1983;63:759–763.

72. Ribot C, Tremollieres F, Pouilles J. Cyclic Estraderm TTS 50 plus oral progestogen in the prevention of postmenopausal bone loss over 24 months. In: Christiansen C, Overgaard K, eds. Osteoporosis 1990. Vol. 2. Copenhagen: Osteopress ApS, 1990:1995–1998.

73. Schneider D, Barrett-Connor EL, et al. Timing of postmenopausal estrogen for optimal bone mineral density, the Rancho Bernardo study. JAMA 1997;277:543–547.

74. McClung M, Clemmesen B, Daifotis A, et al. Alendronate prevents postmenopausal bone loss in women without osteoporosis. A double-blind, randomized, controlled trial. Alendronate Osteoporosis Prevention Study Group. Ann Intern Med 1998;128:253–261.

75. Black DM, Cummings SR, Karpf DB, et al. Randomized trial of effect of alendronate on risk of fracture in women with existing vertebral fractures. Fracture Intervention Trial Research Group. Lancet 1996;348:1535–1541.

76. Overgaard K, Riis BJ, Christiansen C, et al. Nasal calcitonin for treatment of established osteoporosis. Clin Endocrinol 1989;30:435–442.

77. MacIntyre I, Stevenson JC, Whitehead MI, et al. Calcitonin for prevention of post-menopausal bone loss. Lancet1988;1:900.

78. Fioretti P, Gambacciani M, Taponeco F, et al. Effects of continuous and cyclic nasal calcitonin administration in ovariectomized women. Maturitas 1992;15:225.

79. Heaney RP, Recker RR, Saville PD. Menopausal changes in calcium balance performance. J Lab Clin Med 1978;92:953–963.

80. Hasling C, Charles P, Jensen FT, et al. Calcium metabolism in postmenopausal osteoporosis: the influence of dietary calcium and net absorbed calcium. J Bone Miner Res 1990;5:939.

81. NIH Consensus Development Panel on Optimum Calcium Intake. Optimal calcium intake. JAMA 1994;272:1942.

82. Tilyard MW, Spears GFS, Thomson J, et al. Treatment of postmenopausal osteoporosis with calcitriol or calcium. N Engl J Med. 1992;326:357.

83. Ooms ME, Roos JC, Bezemer PD, et al. Prevention of bone loss by vitamin D supplementation in elderly women: a randomized double-blind trial. J Clin Endocrinol Metab 1995;80:1052.

84. Chapuy MC, Arlot ME, Duboeuf F, et al. Vitamin D3 and calcium to prevent hip fractures in elderly women. N Engl J Med 1992;327:1637.

85. Chow RK, Harrison JE, Brown CF, et al. Physical fitness effect on bone mass in post-menopausal women. Arch Phys Med Rehabil 1986;67:231.

86. Butler RN. The geriatric patient. In: Usdin G, Lewis JM, eds. Psychiatry in General Medical Practice. New York: McGraw Hill, 1979.

87. Blazer D. Depression in the elderly. N Engl J Med 1989;320:164.

88. Schneck SA. Aging of the nervous system and dementia. In: Schrier RW, ed. Clinical Internal Medicine in the Aged. Philadelphia: WB Saunders, 1982:29–40.

89. Evans DA, Scherr PA, Cook NR. Estimated prevalence of Alzheimer's disease in the United States. Milbank Mem Fund Q 1990;68:267–268.

90. Brumback RA, Leech RW. Alzheimer's disease: pathophysiology and the hope of therapy. J Okla State Med Assoc 1994;83:103–111.

91. Jorm AF, Korten AE, Henderson, AS. The prevalence of dementia: a quantitative integration of the literature. Acta Psychiatr Scand 1987;76:465–479.

92. Brenner DE, Kukull WA, Stergachis A, et al. Postmenopausal estrogen replacement therapy on the risk of Alzheimer's disease: a population-based case-control study. Am J Epidemiol 1994;140:262–267.

93. Morrison A, Resnick S, Corrada M. A prospective study of estrogen replacement therapy and the risk of developing Alzheimer's disease in the Baltimore longitudinal study of aging. Neurology 1996;469(suppl 2):a435–a436.

94. Paganini-Hill A, Henderson VW. Estrogen deficiency and risk of Alzheimer's disease in women. Am J Epidemiol 1994:140:256–261.

95. Paganini-Hill A, Henderson VW. Estrogen replacement therapy and risk of Alzheimer's disease. Arch Intern Med 1996;156:2213–2217.

96. Caldwell BM. An evaluation of psychological effects of sex hormone administration in aged women. J Gerontol 1954;9:168–174.

97. Kantor HI, Michael CM, Shore H. Estrogen for older women. Am J Obstet Gynecol 1973;116:15.

98. Ohkura T, Isse K, Akazawa K, et al. Low-dose estrogen replacement therapy for Alzheimer disease in women. J North Am Menop Soc 1994;1:125–130.

99. Birge SJ. The role of estrogen in the treatment of Alzheimer's disease. Neurology 1997; 48(suppl 7):S36–S41.

100. Singh M, Meyer EM, Simpkins JW. The effect of ovariectomy and estradiol replacement on brain-derived neurotrophic factor messenger ribonucleic acid expression in cortical and hippocampal brain regions of female Sprague-Dawley rats. Endocrinology 1996;136:2320–2324.

101. Brinton RD, Tran J, Profitt P, et al. 17β-Estradiol increases the growth and survival of cultured cortical neurons. Neurochem Res 1997;22:1339–1351.

102. Ohkura T, Teshima Y, Isse K, et al. Estrogen increases cerebral and cerebellar blood flows in postmenopausal women. Menopause 1995;2:13–18.

103. Chetkowski RH, Meldrum DR, Steingold KA, et al. Biologic effects of transdermal estradiol. N Engl J Med 1986;314:1615.

104. Nachtigall LE. Emerging delivery systems for estrogen replacement: aspects of transdermal and oral delivery. Am J Obstet Gynecol 1995;173:993–997.

105. Lufkin EG, Ory SJ. Relative value of transdermal and oral estrogen therapy in various clinical situations. Mayo Clin Proc 1994;69:131–135.

106. Grady D, Gebretsadik T, Kerlikowske K, et al. Hormone replacement therapy and endometrial cancer risk: a metanalysis. Obstet Gynecol 1995;85:304–313.

107. Miller BA, Feuer EJ, Hakney BF. Letter. N Engl J Med 1992;327:1756–1757.

108. Harris JR, Lippman ME, Veronesi U, et al. Breast cancer. N Engl J Med 1992;327:319–328.

109. Bergkvist L, Adami H, Persson I, et al. Prognosis after breast cancer diagnosis in women exposed to estrogen and estrogen-progestin replacement therapy. Am J Epidemiol 1989; 130:221–228.

110. Willis DB, Calle EE, Miracle-Mahill HL, et al. Estrogen replacement therapy and risk of fatal breast cancer in a prospective cohort of postmenopausal women in the United States. Cancer Causes Control 1996;7:449–557.

111. Feuer EJ, Wun LM, Boring CC, et al. The lifetime risk of developing breast cancer. J Natl Cancer Inst 1993;85:892–897.

112. Dupont WD, Page DL. Menopausal estrogen replacement therapy and breast cancer. Arch Intern Med 1991;151:67–72.

113. Creasman WT. Estrogen replacement therapy: is previously treated cancer a contraindication? Obstet Gynecol 1991;77:308.

114. Creasman WT. Recommendations regarding estrogen replacement therapy after treatment of endometrial cancer. Oncology 1992;6:23–26.

115. Creasman WT, Henderson D, Hinshaw W, et al. Estrogen replacement therapy in the patients treated for endometrial cancer. Obstet Gynecol 1996;67:326–330.

116. Lee RB, Burke TW, Park RC. Estrogen replacement therapy following treatment for stage I endometrial carcinoma. Gynecol Oncol 1990;36:189.

117. Baker DP. Estrogen replacement therapy in patients with previous endometrial carcinoma. Comp Ther 1990;16:28.

118. Collins J, Donner A, Allen LH, et al. Oestrogen use and survival in endometrial cancer. Lancet 1980;2:961–964.

119. Curtis M. The use of the loop electrosurgical excision procedure (LEEP) in relieving stenosis of the external cervical os. J Gynecol Surg 1996;12:201–203.

120. Bakos O, Smith P, Heimer G. Transvaginal ultrasonography for identifying endometrial pathology in postmenopausal women. Maturitas 1995;20:181–189.

121. Karlsson B, Granberg S, Wikland M, et al. Transvaginal ultrasonography of the endometrium in women with postmenopausal bleeding: a Nordic multicenter study. Am J Obstet Gynecol 1995;172:1488–1494.

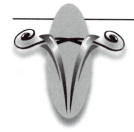

C H A P T E R 3

Contraception

WILLIAM K. GRAVES

HISTORY

In the first third of the century, most American physicians and medical societies were either indifferent or in vigorous opposition to family planning. In 1916, Margaret Sanger opened the first U.S. birth control clinic in Brooklyn. This was in violation of laws passed through Congress and various state legislatures that forbade the distribution of contraceptive information and/or devices. The New York City Vice Squad closed Sanger's clinic and jailed her. Sanger persisted and continued to win additional public support for her organization, which later became Planned Parenthood (1). In 1937, Dr. Robert Dickinson succeeded in persuading the American Medical Association to pass a resolution acknowledging the importance of contraception and calling for its teaching in medical schools (2).

After World War II, most physicians caring for women, who were not bound by moral constraint, were offering contraceptive counseling and fitting diaphragms. But it was not until the 1950s and 1960s that physicians progressively became involved in family planning efforts. General physician participation increased sharply after introduction of the oral contraceptive (OC) pill for prescription in 1960.

Until the early 1960s, it continued to be unlawful to prescribe or discuss contraceptive information with women in the states of Connecticut and Massachusetts. In 1962, C. Lee Buxton, the Chairman of Obstetrics and Gynecology at Yale University Medical School, publicly fitted a woman with a diaphragm in the New Haven Planned Parenthood Clinic. He was arrested, and this led to litigation (*Griswold v Connecticut*) that eventually resulted in the overthrow of the restrictive law by the Supreme Court in 1965 (3).

Although there are no perfect contraceptive methods, there are several types available: behavioral, mechanical, and hormonal. It is up to the patient to decide which method is best for her, barring any contraindication to her choice.

NATURAL FAMILY PLANNING

Natural family planning, also known as the rhythm method or periodic abstinence, encompasses four techniques: the calendar rhythm method, basal body temperature method, cervical mucus method, and symptothermal method. All are based on the fact that pregnancy is possible for only about 7 days of the menstrual cycle (4). The calendar technique requires the woman to record the length of her menstrual cycle for several months. She then subtracts 19 days from her shortest cycle and 9 days from her longest cycle to determine her fertile period. She then abstains from intercourse during that time. For example, if a woman's cycle averages 27 to 31 days, her fertile period would start on day 8 (27 − 19 = 8) and end on day 22 (31 − 9 = 22). This method is not recommended for women whose cycle is less than or equal to 25 days or if it varies by more than 8 days between cycles.

The determination of temperature is a way of estimating the day of ovulation in each cycle. A special thermometer is available that determines if there is a rise in basal body temperature. With the rise in progesterone that follows ovulation, there is an increase in the basal body temperature of 0.5 to 1°F. The woman must check the temperature upon awakening, but *before* arising, and records the reading on a graph. Abstinence from intercourse starts on the first day of menses and continues until there is at least a 3-day duration, consecutively, of elevated basal body temperature. This technique requires a fairly long period of abstinence. It is worth remembering that weekends, which often involve later hours and arising later, will tend to cause an elevation of the basal temperature, which may approach 0.4 or 0.5°F, so that only persistence of the elevation in following days is a certain determinant that ovulation has occurred. It is also useful to remember that the progesterone-induced temperature elevation begins only *after* ovulation, which is why its usefulness is mainly retrospective.

In addition to the basal body temperature, the time of ovulation can be identified by the amount and consistency of cervical mucus, and in this case imminent ovulation can be anticipated before it occurs. Endogenous levels of estrogen and progesterone directly influence the quantity and quality of cervical mucus. Women are taught to recognize these changes. Abstinence is used during the menses and then may be used every other day until the first appearance of a larger amount of very thin, slippery mucus. After that, abstinence resumes until 4 days after the last day the almost liquid-like discharge was present. Ovulation can also be determined in advance by urinary measurements of luteinizing hormone and estradiol, but this often requires the expense of three to four determinations per cycle.

The symptothermal method relies on both calendar calculations and cervical mucus changes to approximate when the fertile period begins and, with the use of the basal body temperature and changes in the cervical mucus, to determine when it ends.

The failure rate of natural family planning is usually estimated as 20 to 30% per year, and a principal reason for this is that sperm, after ejaculation, may have a longevity up to 6 to 8 days in the fallopian tube or in the fluid in the pelvic peritoneal cavity (5). In addition, strict compliance with abstinence may be unreliable, and misinterpretations of cervical mucus changes may occur. One study showed no increase in the spontaneous abortion rate associated with natural family planning (6).

LACTATIONAL AMENORRHEA METHOD

The contraceptive effect of lactation has been recognized for a long time, but specific knowledge concerning the degree and duration of this effect is lacking. A quoted consensus statement from 1988 emphasized that women are protected against another pregnancy during the first 6 months postpartum, provided they are not using significant supplement (7). Lactational amenorrhea method pregnancy rates were 2.9 and 5.9 per hundred women at 6 and 12 months in women supplementing with formula, but when no supplement was used, the pregnancy rate was 0.7 at 6 months (8). A study in Pakistan of 391 women who were breast feeding and were amenorrheic until 6 months postpartum had a pregnancy rate of 0.6%; the pregnancy rate was 1.1% at 1 year (9). It is obvious that if menstrual periods resume, the risk of conception is increased, but lactation still appears to provide some additional protection against pregnancy, perhaps by imperfect ovulation or endometrial response.

ORAL CONTRACEPTIVES

Many observers regard the development and availability of the OC pill as a medical milestone of this century, second in importance only to the development and use of antibiotics. Although 80% of reproductive-aged women report past or current pill usage, only about 20% of women of reproductive age currently use an OC (10). Part of this figure may be secondary to the increased popularity of sterilization of one of the partners, recent increased popularity of the intrauterine device (IUD) as a contraceptive, and/or lack of current contraceptive need.

In selecting patients for whom combined OCs are appropriate, a careful history and physical examination are done to ensure the woman has no contraindications to OC use. Absolute contraindications include, but are not limited to, history of thromboembolic disorders or deep vein thrombophlebitis, undiagnosed vaginal bleeding, known or suspected pregnancy, and markedly impaired liver function. For a complete list of absolute contraindications, see Table 3.1. Other disorders that are relative contraindications to the use of OCs are listed in Table 3.2.

In choosing an OC, the optimal formulation comprises the lowest effective dose with the lowest potency and least incidence of side effects. OCs alter protein, lipid, and carbohydrate metabolism. All combination OCs with less than 50 µg estrogen use ethinyl estradiol as the estrogenic component. It is unusual to start a woman on an OC with more than 30 to 35 µg of ethinyl estradiol. Among the progestins, there are those related to norethindrone or levonorgestrel. With the exception of the new progestins

TABLE 3.1. Absolute Contraindications to Oral Contraceptive Use

Thrombophlebitis/thromboembolic disorders
History of deep vein thrombophlebitis or thromboembolic disorders
Cerebral vascular or coronary artery disease
Known or suspected breast cancer
Known or suspected endometrial cancer or estrogen-dependent neoplasm
Abnormal uterine bleeding of unknown etiology
Cholestatic jaundice of pregnancy or jaundice with prior oral contraceptive use
Hepatic adenomas, carcinomas, or benign liver tumors
Known or suspected pregnancy
Markedly impaired liver function
Benign or malignant liver tumor that developed during previous use of oral
   contraceptives or other estrogen-containing products

TABLE 3.2. Relative Contraindications to Oral Contraceptive Use

Migraine or vascular headache
Cardiac or renal dysfunction
Blood pressure ≥ 90 mm Hg diastolic or ≥ 160 mm Hg systolic
Major depressive disorder
Varicose veins
Smoker ≥ 30 years old
Sickle cell disease or sickle cell–hemoglobin C disease
History of cholestatic jaundice during pregnancy
Hepatitis or mononucleosis during past year
Breast feeding
Asthma
First-degree family history of nonrheumatic cardiovascular disease (fatal or nonfatal)
   or diabetes at <50 years old
Use of drugs known to interact with oral contraceptives
Ulcerative colitis

(desogestrel, gestodene, and norgestimate), the levonorgestrel progesterones are more potent on an equal weight basis than those related to norethindrone. The three newer progestins referred to are related chemically to levonorgestrel but have greater progestational activity and are less androgenic than levonorgestrel. For a more in-depth comparison of the various OCs, refer to Table 3.3.

OCs are usually started on either the first day of menses or the Sunday thereafter. If started after the fifth day of menstruation, however, OCs may not inhibit ovulation. The benefit of starting the pill on a Sunday is that for most women, their subsequent periods occur early to mid week and are usually completed by the weekend. For information regarding missed pills, see Table 3.4.

If starting OCs after a pregnancy, the time necessary to wait to start the pill depends on the gestational age achieved. For pregnancies extending beyond the 28th week, a 2- to 3-week delay between delivery and OC initiation is advised to decrease the risk of postpartum thrombophlebitis. For pregnancies ending between 13 and 28 weeks gestation, a delay of 1 week is recommended. For pregnancies ending before the 13th week of gestation, OCs may be started immediately. For women who are nursing, the combination OC is not recommended because it decreases the quantity of milk. Progestin-only minipills are preferred for lactating women seeking oral hormonal contraception.

Systemic Effects

Cerebrovascular

Cerebrovascular events (i.e., stroke, cerebral thrombosis or hemorrhage, or subarachnoid hemorrhage) may be increased in OC users. Most cerebrovascular accidents suffered by OC users are arterial ischemic attacks rather than venous thrombosis or cerebral hemorrhage. A recent study found that the odds ratio for ischemic stroke among *current* low-dose users of OCs was 1.18 after adjusting for additional risk factors for stroke. The adjusted odds ratio for hemorrhagic stroke was 1.14. For hemorrhagic stroke, there is a positive relationship between current OCs and smoking, with these odds ratios being placed at 3.64 (11). In other control studies, the odds ratios for hemorrhagic stroke among current OC users compared with former users and never users was also very low (1.1, 1.5, and 0.89, respectively) (11–13). A more recent study among 1.1 million reproductive-aged women who were current users of OCs did not have a significantly increased risk of either ischemic or hemorrhagic stroke. These studies indicate the estrogen formulation of current low-dose OCs, less than 50 µg, is associated with a small and barely discernible, if any, risk of stroke in the woman who does not smoke. Women who develop persistent headaches and/or transient hemiparesis while using OCs should discontinue them immediately. Women who suffer a stroke while using OCs should undergo a thorough evaluation for other possible causes, including antiphospholipid syndrome or defects in coagulation.

Migraine and Headache

It is estimated that 20 to 30% of reproductive-aged women have migraines. Simplistically, migraines may be divided into two groups: classic or common. Estimates put the incidence of classic migraine in women of reproductive age at 5%. There are two case-control studies that show women with classic migraines have an increased risk for stroke (14, 15). Patients with classic migraine headaches associated with neurologic symptoms that precede or accompany the headache (scotomata, transient hemianopsia, or paresthesias) should not use OCs. If the woman's migraines suggest or are known to have concurrent transient ischemia attacks associated with them, combination OCs should not be used. A progestin-only method is probably the better choice.

TABLE 3.3. Composition and Activities of Oral Contraceptives

	Progestin and Dose (mg)	Estrogen and Dose (μg)	Activity		
			Endometrial	Progestational	Androgenic
MONOPHASIC					
Brevicon	Norethindrone 0.05	EE 35	I	L	L
Demulen	Ethinyl diacetate 1.0	EE 50	L	H	L
Demulen 1/35	Ethinyl diacetate 1.0	EE 35	L	H	L
Desogen	Desogestrel 0.15	EE 30	I	H	L
Genora 1/35	Norethindrone 1.0	EE 35	I	I	I
Genora 1/50	Norethindrone 1.0	M 50	I	I	I
Levlen	Levonorgestrel 0.15	EE 30	I	I	I
Loestrin 1.5/30	Norethindrone 1.5	EE 30	L	I	I/H
Loestrin 1/20	Norethindrone 1.0	EE 20	L	I	I/H
Lo/Ovral	Norgestrel 0.3	EE 30	I	I	I
Modicon	Norethindrone 0.5	EE 35	I	L	L
Nelova 1/35E	Norethindrone 1.0	EE 35	I	I	I
Nelova 0.5/35E	Norethindrone 0.5	EE 35	I	L	L
Nordette	Levonorgestrel 0.15	EE 30	I	I	I
Norethin 1/35E	Norethindrone 1.0	EE 35	I	I	I
Norethin 1/50M	Norethindrone 1.0	M 50	I	I	I
Norinyl 1/35	Norethindrone 1.0	EE 35	I	I	I
Norinyl 1/50	Norethindrone 1.0	M 50	I	I	I
Norlestrin 1/50	Norethindrone 1.0	EE 50	I	I	I
Norlestrin 2.5	Norethindrone 2.5	EE 50	H	H	H
Ortho-Cept	Desogestrel 0.15	EE 30	I	H	L
Ortho-Cyclen	Norethindrone 0.25	EE 35	L	L	L
Ortho-Novum 1/35	Norethindrone 1.0	EE 35	I	I	I
Ortho-Novum 1/50	Norethindrone 1.0	M 50	I	I	I
Ovcon 35	Norethindrone 0.4	EE 35	I	L	L
Ovcon 50	Norethindrone 1.0	EE 50	H	H	H
Ovral	Norgestrel 0.5	EE 50	H	H	H
MULTIPHASIC					
Jenest 7/14 days	Norethindrone 0.5/1.0	EE 35/35	I	I	I
Ortho-Novum 7/7/7 7/7/7 days	Norethindrone 0.5/0.75/1.0	EE 35/35/35	I	I	I
Ortho-Novum 10/11 10/11 days	Norethindrone 0.5/1.0	EE 35/35	L	L	L
Tri-Cyclen 7/7/7 days	Norgestimate 0.18/0.215/0.25	EE 35/35/35	L	L	L
Tri-Levlen 6/5/10 days	Levonorgestrel 0.05/0.075/0.125	EE 30/40/30	I	L	I
Tri-Norinyl 7/9/5 days	Norethindrone 0.5/1.0/0.5	EE 35/35/35	I	I	I
Triphasil 6/5/10 days	Levonorgestrel 0.05/0.075/0.125	EE 30/40/30	I	L	I
PROGESTIN ONLY					
Micronor	Norethindorne 0.35	None	L	L	L
Nor-QD	Norethindrone 0.35	None	L	L	L
Ovrette	Norgestrel 0.075	None	L	L	L

EE, ethinyl estradiol; H, high; I, intermediate; L, low; M, mestranol.

TABLE 3.4. Instructions for Patients Who Missed an Oral Contraceptive Pill

Consecutive Pills Omitted	Time in Cycle	Instructions to Patient[a]
1	Any time	Take missed pill immediately and next one at regular time.
2	First 2 weeks	Take 2 pill QD for next 2 days, then resume taking pills on regular schedule.
2	Third week	Take 1 pill QD until last day of third week. Dispose of placebos and begin new pack next day.
≥3	Any time	Take 1 pill QD until last day of that week. Dispose of placebos and begin new pack next day.

[a]Additional contraceptive measures should be used as soon as the omission of oral contraceptive pills is discovered. These additional measures should be used for at least 7 days.

For women with common migraine, there is no evidence of any serious adverse effects induced by OCs. The Walnut Creek study was unable to demonstrate a higher frequency of migraine headache in pill users compared with nonusers (16). However, Ryan (17) reported different results with two groups of 20 migraineurs taking 50 μg ethinyl estradiol and 500 mg norgestrel in alternate 2-month periods for 4 months total. He reported that 12 of 40 improved, whereas 28 in 40 worsened while on medication. The study was not blinded, and the steroid doses were inappropriate by today's standards. Because of the limited and conflicting literature with as many as one third of migraineurs noting improvement with OC use, pill trial and individualization would seem appropriate. Women who note improvement in their migraine frequency and/or intensity while on OCs may further benefit with elimination of the pill-free interval.

Headache is a subjective complaint and is common even among patients not taking OCs. If a patient using an OC with a progestin of high or medium androgenic activity complains of headaches during the cycle when biologically active pills are taken, a change to a progestin-containing pill with lower androgenic activity may be helpful. If this does not help, or if the headaches worsen, an alternate form of contraception may be needed. If headaches occur predominately in the pill-free time period, it is most likely due to the withdrawal of estrogen. In this instance, daily use of a monophasic OC may be helpful. The multiphasic OCs may cause breakthrough bleeding if use continuously.

Seizure Disorder
The incidence of epilepsy in the general population is approximately 1%. There are several considerations for the epileptic patient desiring oral contraception: the effect on epilepsy of OCs, the tendency of most antiepileptic drugs to decrease steroid concentrations in most women, and the concerns about unintended pregnancy in a population where good contraceptive control is particularly important (18). The induction of hepatic microsomal enzymes by most antiepileptic drugs may accelerate the metabolism of OCs. Breakthrough bleeding may be the earliest sign of this process. The effectiveness of OCs therefore is lessened, and a higher hormonal dose for adequate contraception may be needed. Additionally, OCs induce hepatic enzymes and may result in lower concentrations of antiepileptic drugs. Theoretically, an increase in seizure frequency may result. To date, there has been no demonstrated exacerbation of epileptic seizures by OCs (19, 20). Epilepsy in pregnancy is

associated with increased teratogenic risk and maternal and fetal injury secondary to seizures. Benzodiazepines and valproic acid do not reduce steroid levels; the remainder of antiepileptic drugs, including phenytoin, do so (21).

Cardiovascular

Almost all excess mortality in OC users is due to cardiovascular disease, most from myocardial infarction. The morbidity and mortality of cardiovascular diseases in OC users is related to the estrogen content and progestin dose and activity of the pill. The cardiovascular disease risk with OC use is most prevalent in women over 35 years of age who smoke and who have used OCs for long periods of time.

Deep Vein Thrombosis

For most women, use of a low-dose OC does not result in a hypercoagulable state. A cohort study of 200,000 women enrolled in the Michigan Medicaid population demonstrated no increased risk in venous thrombosis in women taking less than 50-μg estrogen preparations (22). Others demonstrated, however, even with OCs containing less than 50 μg of estrogen, a fourfold increased relative risk in venous thromboembolic disease in OC users compared with nonusers (23, 24). In these studies and others, the possibility was raised that the newer progestational agents, desogestrel and gestodene, may exacerbate the risk of venous thromboembolic disease. However, the evidence does not currently support changing a woman's OCs with the newer progestins nor ceasing to prescribe them. Personal history of deep vein thrombosis (DVT) is a contraindication for all estrogen-containing OCs, although studies suggest that this risk decreases with decreasing estrogen dose. Alternative contraceptive methods for these women should be used. Women with a family history of thromboembolic disease should undergo evaluation for antithrombin III deficiency, protein C or S deficiency, or activated protein C resistance. These are rare but can be familial secondary to a mutation in the factor V Leiden gene. A woman who develops a DVT while on OCs should be evaluated for these deficiencies. There are currently no studies to show that the 20-μg estrogen dose OCs are associated with a lower risk of venous thromboembolic disease than the 30- to 35-μg dose pills.

Hypertension

Two issues arise when considering oral contraception in hypertensive patients: the extra load that would be imposed on the system by a pregnancy and the risk of adverse circulatory effects caused by the pill. Patients with mild hypertension, defined as 140 to 159 over 90 to 99, which is controlled by hygienic measures such as smoking cessation, weight loss, exercise, and restriction of salt and alcohol, are suitable candidates for low-dose OCs. This is also true when "moderate" pharmacologic measures such as diuretics or β-blockers are required. Only low-dose OCs, less than 50 μg, should be used. Prudence would suggest following these women every 3 months (25). If hypertension is uncontrolled, OCs should not be used because they may worsen it.

A history of pregnancy-induced hypertension or preeclampsia does not increase a woman's risk of hypertension on OCs. Occasionally, OCs may cause an idiosyncratic increase in blood pressure. This may occur in up to 8% of patients with either borderline or established hypertension (26). When this occurs, it is usually mild to moderate, with a 10 to 20 mm Hg increase in diastolic pressure and a 20 to 40 mm Hg increase in systolic blood pressure. This may occur at any time. Surveillance of blood pressure in women on OCs is advised.

Lipids

Estrogens are known to increase high-density-lipoprotein (HDL) levels and decrease low-density-lipoprotein (LDL) levels. Oral estrogens are also known to increase triglyceride levels. Androgens and androgenic progestins depress HDL levels and increase LDL levels, changes associated with increased risk of atherosclerosis. Although data are incomplete, there is no evidence of increased risk of cardiovascular disease with OC use in moderately hypercholesterolemic women. Women under 35, in the absence of uncontrolled hypertension, diabetes, or other OC contraindications, may consider OC use, even with LDL cholesterol levels as high as 160 mg/dL (27). There may be additional benefits from the newer lower gonane progestins. Therefore, women with hypercholesterolemia should be given OCs with progestins of low androgenicity. If a woman's triglycerides are above 350 mg/dL or in patients with familial hypertriglyceridemia, OCs should be avoided because they may precipitate pancreatitis and/or adversely affect the patient's risk for cardiovascular disease.

Angina and Coronary Atherosclerosis

OCs do not stimulate the atherosclerotic process and may actually inhibit plaque formation. One study of women less than 50 years of age who had experienced myocardial infarction found that the incidence of angiographically confirmed coronary atherosclerosis in non-OC users was almost twice that of OC users (79 versus 36%, respectively) (28). In addition, there is no increase in the incidence of cardiovascular disease secondary to atherosclerosis in past users of OCs. However, smoking, when combined with OC use, markedly increases the risk of atherogenesis (29). Women with known angina and suspected atherosclerosis but with no history of prior myocardial infarction or additional risk factors may safely use low-dose OCs (30).

Mitral Valve Prolapse

In general, OCs can be safely used by women with mitral valve prolapse who are symptom free. OC use should be limited to mitral valve prolapse patients with an echocardiographic-confirmed diagnosis but without mitral regurgitation. A history of thrombotic complications requires another contraceptive method. Long-acting progestins such as injection or implants are safe to use and may provide increased fibrinolytic activity.

Diabetes

Young diabetic women who are free of retinopathy, nephropathy, hypertension, or other complicating vascular disease(s) are appropriate candidates for low-dose contraceptives. It is the progestin component of OCs that is antagonistic to insulin. A formulation with the lowest androgenic potential such as gonane progestins should be selected to avoid an increase in insulin resistance. Women with a history of gestational diabetes during their last pregnancy can safely take low-dose OCs. The incidence of frank diabetes developing within 3 years of pregnancy is no higher in women taking these low doses than in those using nonhormonal contraceptive methods (31).

Lupus

Because the estrogen components of OCs may increase their flare-ups, combination OCs are contraindicated (32). It is possible that OCs containing 20 to 25 μg ethinyl estradiol might alter this dictum, but does anyone want to conduct the trial?

Interactions with Other Drugs

Antimicrobial agents can interact with the pharmacokinetics and efficacy of sex steroid hormones present in OCs (33, 34). Rifampicin (Rifampin) has been shown to decrease circulating levels of ethinyl estradiol, resulting in OC failures (35). Certain antibiotics, particularly penicillins and their derivatives and tetracyclines, may diminish the effectiveness of OCs. It is suggested that additional contraceptive measures are used while using these drugs. Other drugs have been implicated in diminishing the efficacy of OCs, but these data are anecdotal. A current drug history should be taken when prescribing OCs, and new medications should be reported by the user. For a brief list of various drugs and their interactions with OCs, refer to Table 3.5.

Perimenopausal Women and Oral Contraceptives

The transition period of changing hormone patterns, or perimenopausal state, begins about 5 to 10 years before the actual menopause. According to the census bureau of 1990, from 1975 to 1990, the number of women in the age range of 35 to 44 increased about 60%. Characteristics of the perimenopause are irregular cycles, changes in both the volume and the duration of bleeding, and, for approximately half the women, the onset of variable vasomotor symptoms. The perimenopausal period is characterized by an increased incidence of anovulatory cycles, resulting in an unopposed estrogen state. This predisposes to dysfunctional uterine bleeding, possible endometrial hyperplasia, and a poorly documented, but frequently observed, accelerated growth of uterine myomata. Although the fertility of women has markedly diminished by age 45, pregnancy is still possible. This is reflected in the fact that the pregnancy termination rate in women 40 to 50 years of age is exceeded only by those women under 15 years of age. There continues to be a need for con-

TABLE 3.5. Interactions of Drugs and Oral Contraceptives

Drug	Mechanism of Action	Management Options
Hydantoins Barbiturates Primidone (Mysoline) Carbamazepine (Tegretol)	Liver enzyme induction	Alternate drug or use a pill regimen with 50 μg estrogen
Rifampin (Rimactane)	Liver enzyme induction	Use additional contraceptive measures or use a pill regimen with 50 μg estrogen
Certain antibiotics Penicillins and derivatives Tetracyclines Sulfonamides Metronidazole (Flagyl) Nitrofurantoin (Macrodantin)	Possibly diminished enterohepatic circulation of ethinyl estradiol	Use additional contraceptive measures
Griseofulvin (Fulvicin, Grifulvin)	Liver enzyme induction	Use additional contraceptive measures

traception for sexually active women over age 40 or 45. Aside from permanent sterilization, OCs should be the method of choice for women who do not smoke cigarettes to regulate menstrual periods and to provide contraception. These women often do well on the lowest estrogen dose of 20 μg. To determine if the patient has become truly menopausal and can be changed from OCs to hormone replacement therapy (HRT), the follicle-stimulating hormone level should be checked on the sixth or seventh day of the pill-free week. If it is more than 25 mIU/mL, the OCs may be discontinued and HRT may begin. If menses resumes without OCs, the patient can decide to use OCs again. If breakthrough bleeding occurs on HRT, consideration can be given to using OCs again for an additional 6 months to 1 year in lieu of HRT. This is, of course, in the absence of any other causes of abnormal bleeding.

Oral Contraceptives and Cancer

Breast Cancer

There has been no greater deterrent to the more widespread and appropriate use of OCs than concern about the possibility of increasing the risk of cancer in women. Perhaps the greatest concern growing out of the epidemiologic studies of breast cancer has been the possible effects of OC administration (36). Although some have found a small increase in the risk of breast cancer among current users of OCs (relative risk = 1.3), once OCs are discontinued, this risk declines over 10 years until the risk becomes identical to never users (37). The overwhelming majority of studies do not find an association between OC use and increased relative risk of breast cancer. Overall, the risk of breast cancer in women who take OCs up to the age of 55 years appears to be no different from that of nonusers (38). The largest controlled study on the relationship of OCs in breast cancer was conducted by the Centers for Disease Control and Prevention. The results showed no added risk linked to OC use at a younger age, before a first pregnancy, or in women with benign breast disease or a family of history of breast cancer. In other words, the addition of OCs to these increased risk groups did not increase the incidence (39). OC users who develop breast cancer have lower stage tumors and a lower incidence of positive lymph nodes than control subjects. Their tumors also tend to be more localized (40). OC use by women with a family history of breast cancer in a first-degree relative does not increase her risk of breast cancer (41).

It appears that OCs may actually protect against benign breast disease, although most of these data are derived from higher dose OCs (42, 43). In one case-control study of low-dose OCs, the use of a low-dose OC before the first term pregnancy decreased the risk of benign nonproliferative disease but did not significantly affect the risk of proliferative disease. Because OCs produce effects mimicking pregnancy, it has been suggested that the risk of developing breast cancer may be similar to pregnancy. It is known that pregnancy imparts a degree of lifetime protection against breast cancer, but it is also true that pregnancy actually increases the short-term risk of breast cancer in women under 45 years of age. The protective effects do not become apparent until years later. This may be the same pattern we are starting to see with OC use (44).

Cervical Cancer

Based on its risk factors (the number of sexual partners and age of first coitus, exposure to certain types of human papilloma virus), cervical cancer is considered by many to be a sexually transmitted disease. Although earlier studies suggested that OCs increased the risk of preinvasive and invasive cervical disease, three large, well-controlled, newer studies are more reassuring (45–47).

Adenocarcinoma of the cervix seems to be a different story. A case-control study in Los Angeles suggested a pill-associated increased risk for this neoplasm (48). Another study was comprised of larger numbers of women with adenocarcinoma and with hospital-based case control subjects from 10 hospitals in 12 countries. The control subjects were matched for sexual behavior factors. This study showed a statistically increased relative risk of 1.6 (confidence interval, 1.2 to 2.1) in ever users, and this increased in long-term users (49). Although adenocarcinoma represents only 10% of invasive cervical cancer cases, clinicians need to be aware of this possible association. Although some clinicians advocate Papanicolaou (Pap) smears every 6 months in women at high risk for squamous cell carcinoma of the cervix or women with a history of long-term OC use, there is currently no evidence that this is beneficial.

Endometrial Cancer

Because of their progestin content, OCs have a clear protective effect against endometrial cancer. In a World Health Organization study, a review of data from 130 cases and 835 matched control subjects showed a nearly 50% reduction in the risk of endometrial cancer in women who had ever used OCs (50). This protective effect has been shown to persist for up to 20 years after discontinuation of OCs (51). The relative risk of endometrial cancer declines with increasing duration of OC use up through 10 years of use. There does not appear to be any loss of protection with use of low-dose OCs versus high-dose OCs (52). Other studies showed a similar protective effect but not necessarily for short-term use (under 2 years). Young women with irregular menses suggestive of anovulatory cycles and women with polycystic ovarian syndrome are predisposed to developing endometrial cancer. The use of OCs in these patients can protect the endometrium and help to regulate their cycles.

Ovarian Cancer

As with endometrial cancer, protection from ovarian cancer may persist for up to 20 years after discontinuation of OCs (53). In addition, the degree of protection is directly related to the duration of OC use. For women who use OCs for 10 years or more, there is an 80% reduction in their risk for ovarian cancer. There does not appear to be any diminution in protection with the use of low-dose versus high-dose OCs (54).

Side Effects of Oral Contraceptives

Side effects of OCs are a major source of patient noncompliance and discontinuation. Breast tenderness and nausea, which are estrogen related, are markedly reduced with pills containing less than 50 µg estrogen in current use. When they do occur, they will usually decline after the first 3 months of OCs. Patients who persist with nausea may try taking the OC immediately after a meal rather than at night on an empty stomach. Additionally, changing to a 20-µg pill may help.

Menstrual changes occurring with OC use produce patient anxiety and are a common reason for discontinuation. Breakthrough bleeding or spotting occurs in approximately 25% of users during the first 3 months of OC use. Counseling patients regarding this possibility at the time of initial prescription will alleviate anxiety and should diminish the discontinuation rate. Most breakthrough bleeding resolves after the third month of use. If it continues, the clinician should inquire about the pattern of use. With low-dose OCs, it is important that they be taken at about the same time every day. Consideration should also be given to the presence of a pelvic infection. One study reported an increased prevalence in chlamydial infections among OC users with breakthrough bleeding (55). If the patient is taking the OC correctly and there is no infection, changing to a different progestin-category OC may help. If this is unsuccessful, it may be necessary to switch to a 50-µg OC after ensuring there is not a nonhormonal problem (e.g., an endometrial polyp or submucous fibroid). Failure of withdrawal bleeding may be managed similarly if this causes concern—after pregnancy has been excluded, of course.

The perception of weight gain is a common reason patients, especially adolescents, discontinue OCs. In several studies of OCs using either norgestimate or desogestrel, the maximum mean weight gain after 1 year of use was one half of a pound (56–58). There are few studies comparing lower androgenic progestins with OCs containing high or medium androgenic progestins. One study did fail to find a statistically significant difference in the discontinuation of OCs secondary to perceived weight gain in women using a norgestimate preparation and women using a norgestrel-containing OC (57).

Patients may voice concerns about the potential to induce or aggravate existing acne with OC use. Recent studies showed significant improvement in acne and/or hirsutism in women using OCs with a low androgenic progestin (58, 59).

Benefits of Oral Contraception

Protection against menstrual dysfunction, which is more common in adolescents and women over 40, is provided by the low-dose OC (60). In the adolescent, androgen-related disorders such as acne, hirsutism, and weight gain are benefited by the low-estrogen pill with a gonane progestin. In older women who are nonsmokers, this pill likely improves menstrual dysfunction without cardiovascular, diabetogenic, or other significant metabolic effects. Decreased growth rate of uterine fibroids is also probable with the low-estrogen pill, although precise evidence is lacking. Women using combination OCs benefit from more regular, less painful, and scantier menstrual periods and a decreased risk of ovarian and endometrial cancer (61). The risk of ectopic pregnancy and functional ovarian cysts is also decreased (62). Spread of pelvic inflammatory disease to the fallopian tubes is inhibited, as judged by laparoscopic findings, and other confirmatory studies suggest a reduced risk of upper tract spread from lower tract infection in OC users (63, 64).

Discontinuation of the Pill

After discontinuing OCs, there may be a delay of a few months in the return of ovulatory cycles. If the amenorrhea lasts more than 6 months, evaluation for prolactin-producing tumor or other causes is in order. The combination OC should be stopped 2 weeks before elective major surgery. This is not necessary for minor or outpatient surgery. Although patients are often told to wait until after the first normal menstrual cycle to attempt pregnancy, the only reason for this is to improve dating of the pregnancy. There is no increase in spontaneous abortions or birth defects (chromosomal or nonchromosomal) in patients who conceive while on OCs.

PROGESTIN-ONLY MINIPILL

Three brands are currently available in the United States, two containing 0.35 mg of norethindrone (Micronor, Nor-QD) and one containing 0.075 mg of norgestrel (Ovrette). This level of progestin is not sufficient to suppress gonadotropins, and approximately 40% of patients ovulate. Although the exact mechanism(s) of action are unknown, it is known that the cervical mucus becomes thick and impermeable. In addition, the endometrium is out of phase, inhibiting nidation. The effect on tubal physiology is speculative. The minipill is taken every day, with no pill-free interval.

When initially prescribing the minipill, the patient must be carefully counseled about the importance of taking the pill at the same time of day. Timing should be based on the fact that the change in the cervical mucus requires 2 to 4 hours to take effect and, most importantly, permeability of the cervical mucus increases by 22 hours after the last pill; by 24 hours, sperm penetration is essentially unimpaired. If pregnancy occurs, the clinician must be aware that it is more likely to be an ectopic, although the incidence is still below the incidence of ectopic pregnancy without any contraception. The history of a previous ectopic pregnancy is not a contraindication to the minipill. There are no significant metabolic effects on coagulation factors, carbohydrate metabolism, or lipid levels. There is an immediate return to the woman's baseline level of fertility for her age and circumstances after discontinuation of the pill. Failure rates range from 1.1 to 9.6 per 100 women in the first year of use (65). The failure rate is higher in younger women than in women over 40 and generally varies up to 6% per year of use. This is an excellent method of contraception for women over 40 where the reduced fertility rate adds to the minipill's efficacy.

The minipill should be started on the first day of menses and a backup contraceptive method must be used for the first 7 days because of the possibility of early ovulation. Again, the importance of taking the pill at the same time each day must be emphasized. If a pill is forgotten, a backup method should be used immediately and continued until the pills have been resumed for at least 2 days. If the pill is more than 3 hours late, a backup method should be used for 48 hours (66).

The major side effect of the pill is irregular menstrual bleeding, and this is the major reason why women discontinue the minipill (67). There is a greater tendency toward the development of functional ovarian cysts, and if this is a recurring problem, consideration should be given to a combined OC or Depo-Provera. There is also an increased incidence of acne with a levonorgestrel minipill.

The minipill is particularly useful in lactating women who feel the need for additional contraception. There is no diminution in the quality and/or quantity of the milk produced and the minipill may be started immediately after delivery.

The minipill is obviously a good choice in situations where estrogens are contraindicated, such as lupus erythematosus, diabetes with vascular disease, and some severe varieties of cardiovascular disease. The minipill is a good option for the woman who complains of decreased libido on OCs or who refuses combination OCs secondary to side effects they deem unacceptable, such as breast tenderness, headaches, and nausea. Because of the low dose of progestin, patients should avoid medications that increase liver metabolism, including rifampin and most antiepileptic agents, as discussed previously. There is no measurable impact of the minipill on the coagulation system (68). It can probably be safely used in women with a history of thrombosis, although the package insert carries the same precautions and warnings that apply to combined OCs. Definitive evidence that addresses this issue is still forthcoming.

EMERGENCY CONTRACEPTION

Emergency contraception, also known as postcoital contraception or the "morning-after" pill, has been available for more than 30 years. However, most women are still unaware of this method to prevent unplanned pregnancy, particularly after rape, barrier method failure, or contraceptive omission. Since its availability, various individual steroids, either alone or in combination, were evaluated and shown to be effective in preventing pregnancy after a single unprotected coital act. No drug has received specific marketing approval in the United States for this purpose, but in

Western Europe, the combination of ethinyl estradiol and norgestrel has been marketed specifically for use as a postcoital contraceptive agent. Several treatment regimens are effective and are listed in Table 3.6. Nausea may occur in up to 30 to 50% of patients but is usually not severe, and the prophylactic use of an over-the-counter antinausea preparation such as Dramamine or Benadryl 1 hour before the first dose may be appropriate in women thought to be susceptible. Vomiting may be seen in 15 to 20% of patients. Before the use of emergency contraception, an already existing pregnancy must be ruled out.

Because of infrequent, but demonstrated, prolonged sperm survival of up to 6 or 8 days in the female reproductive tract, any coital episode occurring in the first part of the cycle, the follicular phase, should receive the regimen. The necessity for treatment in a coital episode occurring in the luteal phase in a woman with regular cycles would seem questionable, but decisions concerning patient reliability and degree of concern can be decided individually. As long as the first two pills are taken within 72 hours of unprotected intercourse, the effectiveness is high (0.6% failure rate in 1300 cases with no ectopic pregnancies) (69). Menses should begin within 21 days. If it does not, the patient should seek medical attention for pregnancy testing and evaluation. These regimens are not teratogenic.

A survey of 450 undergraduate and graduate students at a major university showed that awareness and approval of the emergency contraceptive pill were widespread, but the lack of detailed knowledge and uncertainty about health and ethical implications probably contributed to misgivings about the regimen. Students who possessed accurate information, especially those who knew that the therapy is a large dose of regular OCs and that side effects were generally minor, were significantly more likely than others to report favorable attitudes. A few students confused the pills with the abortifacient RU-486 (70). Not only is continuing the dissemination of information among college students desirable, but more widespread publicity involving the general female population should be, and is being, undertaken.

For patients unable to take combination OCs, levonorgestrel alone is an alternative. The patient takes two pills, each 0.75 mg, as soon as possible, but it must be within 48 hours of intercourse. An additional two pills (0.75 mg each) are taken 12 hours later. The failure rate of this method was about 40% in on study (71). Another method of emergency contraception is insertion of a copper IUD (ParaGard T-380A) within 5 to 7 days after exposure. The failure rate associated with this method is less than 1% and provides long-term contraception (72). This method should not be used in cases of rape or possible sexually transmitted disease infection. For further information on emergency contraception, see Table 3.6.

TABLE 3.6. Emergency Contraceptive Regimens

Conjugated estrogens (Premarin) 30 mg BID × 5 days *or* 10 mg QD × 5 days *or* 25 mg IV immediately and again 24 hr later

Ethinyl estradiol (Estinyl) 2.5 mg BID × 5 days *or* 5 mg QD × 5 days

Oral contraceptive regimens[a]

  Ovral 2 tablets immediately and again 12 hr later

  Levlen, Levora, Lo/Ovral, Nordette, Tri-Levlen, or Triphasil 4 tablets immediately and again 12 hr later

[a]In the event of vomiting, the dose must be repeated.

INJECTABLE DEPO-MEDROXYPROGESTERONE ACETATE

Depo-medroxyprogesterone acetate suspension (Depo-Provera; DMPA) is the only injectable contraceptive available in the United States. One hundred fifty milligrams of DMPA is injected every 3 months, and the contraceptive efficacy is very high. Clinical trials reported failure rates ranging from 0 to 0.7 per 100 woman years, with 0.3 per 100 women year being the most accepted incidence. The ideal time to initiate DMPA is within 5 days of the onset of menses or immediately postpartum. If the first injection is given more than 5 days after menses, the patient must use a backup method of contraception for the first 2 weeks. This has been shown to inhibit ovulation for at least 14 weeks so that an injection every 3 months provides a grace period. The efficacy of DMPA is not diminished by other drugs and is not dependent on the patient's weight.

The principle concern is occasional delayed return of fertility after discontinuation. This is not related to the duration of use. After discontinuing DMPA to become pregnant, 50% of women conceive promptly (73). In a small proportion of women, fertility is not reestablished for as long as 18 months after the last injection. Thus, counseling is required before initiation of this method, which is obviously not ideally suited for simple spacing of pregnancy.

The typical side effects concern menstrual changes, particularly with episodes of unpredictable irregular bleeding during the first months of use. With increasing duration of use, these episodes decrease and amenorrhea becomes common. If breakthrough bleeding persists, the next dose of DMPA can be given early or conjugated estrogens (1.25 mg) may be given daily for 10 to 21 days for several cycles. Approximately 50% of women who use DMPA for 1 year report amenorrhea, and this is an advantage for women troubled with increased or irregular periods. By 3 years, approximately 80% of users are amenorrheic. Women may also complain of breast tenderness, weight gain, and/or depression.

Women with sickle cell anemia, congenital heart disease, or those over 35 who smoke are excellent candidates for DMPA. There is no link with cervical cancer, no increase in breast cancer risk, and a decrease in the incidence of anemia. There does not appear to be any relationship between the use of DMPA and the risk of ovarian cancer. One small study suggested a decreased risk of pelvic inflammation disease (74). Depo-Provera is an excellent choice for epileptics because the high progestin levels raise the seizure threshold (75).

Women with a history of long-term use of DMPA have lower bone mineral densities than nonusers, although this has not yet been associated with an increase in fracture rate (76). The effect on lipids has been inconsistent, but the use of DMPA has not been associated with increased risk for myocardial infarction. DMPA has not been found to increase a woman's risk of thrombotic episodes. Women using DMPA may experience a 2- to 3-pound weight gain over several years. It is not teratogenic and is safe for use in lactating women. It may be given immediately postpartum even in women who are breast feeding.

NORPLANT

Levonorgestrel implants (Norplant) consists of six soft plastic implants, 34 × 2 × 2.4 mm each, filled with 36 mg of levonorgestrel. The original overall daily rate of release is 85 μg, which gradually declines to approximately 30 μg by the fifth year of use (77). Insertion and removal of the implants is usually a minor office procedure performed under local anesthesia. The implants should be inserted within 5 to 7 days after the onset of the menstrual period and immediately inhibit ovulation. Circulating progestin levels are sufficient to prevent ovulation in most women using implants. However, there is a degree of luteal activity manifested by low progesterone levels. In addition to impaired oocyte maturation, progestin-induced hostile cervical mucus is sufficient to prevent conception even when ovulation occurs (78, 79). Annual pregnancy rates among implant users average 0.8 per 100 during the entire 5 years of use. There are no weight restrictions for Norplant users, although pregnancy rates for heavier women using Norplant may be higher in years 4 and 5 of use compared with lighter women. The overall pregnancy rate is still less than that of OCs. After removal of the implants, serum progestin levels fall to undetectable amounts within 1 week (80). Because Norplant does not interfere with lactation, it can be inserted immediately postpartum.

Menstrual changes are the most common side effect of implants, and many women will experience an irregular bleeding pattern during the first year after insertion; however, this declines to about one third by the fifth year. During the entire 5 years, 5 to 10% of women experience amenorrhea. Headache is the nonmenstrual side effect that most frequently leads to removal. About 20% of women who discontinue use do so because of headache complaints. Functional ovarian cysts can occur in some women using implants, some as large as 10 cm in diameter. These resolve spontaneously and should be managed expectantly (81).

Acne is the most common skin complaint. Use of topical antibiotics (1% clindamycin solution or gel or topical erythromycin) may help. Norplant has no major impact on the lipid profile, carbohydrate metabolism, coagulation factors, or liver function. Women using medications that induce microsomal liver enzymes (phenytoin, phenobarbital, rifampin, and carbamazepine) have an increased risk of pregnancy secondary to lower blood levels of norgestrel. The most promising future of implant contraception may lie with gonane progestins, which are less androgenic and use a single capsule (82).

INTRAUTERINE CONTRACEPTION

Millions of users worldwide suggest that a properly selected parous patient who has an IUD inserted by an appropriately experienced practitioner constitutes the closest thing to an ideal contraceptive that is currently available. Yet use of the IUD in the United States has declined from 2.2 million in 1981 to 0.7 million in 1988. During the same time period, use of the IUD has increased approximately 28% in the rest of the world (83). The first truly modern IUD was developed in 1962 by Jack Lippes of Buffalo. This was a polyethylene device with a single filament thread as a tail. This quickly became the most widely used IUD by the late 1960s. Also in the late 1960s, several reports appeared of increased coronary artery disease and myocardial infarction in women taking the high-dose OC pill of the time. This received extensive media attention and investigation by a well-publicized U.S. Senate committee on the safety of oral contraception for American women. This probably contributed to the introduction of the Dalkon Shield without adequate clinical trials. Within 3 years of its introduction in 1970, a high incidence of pelvic infection was recognized. This was due to the inappropriate selection of patients and a multifilament tail that provided a pathway for bacteria to ascend from the vagina into the uterus through the normal barrier of cervical mucus. Sales of the device were discontinued in 1975, but a call for removal of devices in place was not issued until the early 1980s. This experience adversely affected the attitude of consumers and health care providers. Lawsuits were extended to the copper devices, most of them successfully defended, but the cost of defense exceeded profit from the sale of the devices. Copper IUDs were withdrawn from the market in 1986. The availability of the progesterone-containing IUD (Progestasert) continued. In 1988, a new copper-containing IUD, with an increased amount of copper added to the arms of the device, began to be marketed as ParaGard (Fig. 3.1).

The "T"-shaped Progestasert releases 65 μg of progesterone per day for more than 1 year. Although the manufacturer recommends replacement in 1 year, significant empirical experience shows that its effectiveness is probably closer to 18 months. The mechanism of action is not an abortifacient for either this or the copper device, which is a common misperception. A sterile inflammatory response to the foreign body in the uterus produces tissue injury of a minor degree but sufficient enough to be spermicidal. In a recent study, interleukin and tumor necrosis factor cytokines in the endometrial cavity were obtained at curettage or at hysterectomy.

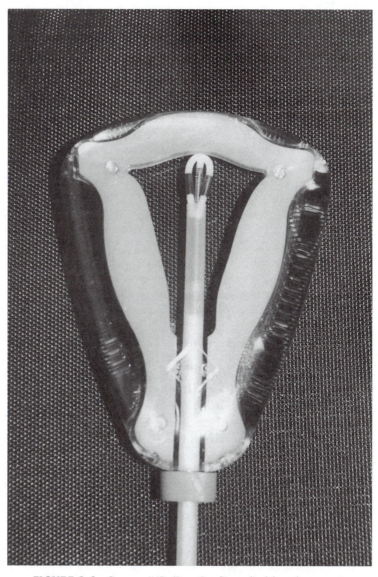

FIGURE 3.1. Copper IUD (ParaGard) readied for placement.

These cytokines were found to be increased in all IUD users. The copper IUD in particular was associated with an increased concentration of endometrial cytokines, and this may well be its significant mechanism of action (84). These changes are thought to be primarily spermicidal in nature, although the inflammatory response also prevents implantation. In addition to increasing local cytokines, the progestin IUD thickens the cervical mucus, creating a barrier to sperm penetration through the cervix. Its proposed major mechanism of action is inhibition of implantation and inhibition of sperm capacitation and survival. Removal of the IUD, particularly when done premenstrually to allow "cleansing" of the endometrium, is followed by normal conception rates for the next cycle and thereafter.

A 1987 review of a first-year trial of experience in parous women showed that in the first year of use, the copper T (Cu T-380A) experienced an expulsion rate of 5% and a removal rate, usually for pain or bleeding, of 14%, whereas the progesterone IUD (ParaGard) experienced an expulsion rate of 2.7% and a removal rate of 9.3% (85). The progesterone IUD may decrease blood flow by 40 to 50% and improve dysmenorrhea so that its use may be preferable in women experiencing heavy or painful periods. The copper IUD is associated with some increase in blood loss and dysmenorrhea. However, the progesterone IUD produces an ectopic pregnancy rate of 6.8 per 1000 women-years, compared with 0.2 for the copper-containing IUD. This is all in contrast with the ectopic pregnancy rate of 3 to 4.5 per 1000 women-years for noncontraceptive users (86, 87). The Progestasert IUD has an annual pregnancy failure rate of 2% for total pregnancies compared with 0.8% for the ParaGard (86). The copper IUD is effective for 10 years, and expulsion rates decrease to 0.4 to 3.7% per year by the 10th year, and the cumulative net pregnancy rate after 7 years of use is 1.5 per 100 women-years (88). The copper T is a more effective and semipermanent device; the progesterone T is better tolerated in the first year of use and is perhaps more suitable for child spacing.

The IUD is recommended for the parous woman in a mutually monogamous relationship with no history of pelvic inflammatory disease and desirous of long-term contraception. IUDs may be used safely in a nulliparous and/or nulligravida woman if both she and her partner are monogamous. The incidence of pain, bleeding, and/or syncope may be higher at the time of insertion in nulliparous women. For a list of contraindications to placement and use of the IUD, refer to Table 3.7. The patient should be cautioned at the time of insertion that if there is a change in that relationship, strong consideration should be given to IUD removal and use of another contraceptive method. If pregnancy occurs with an IUD in place, the device should be removed as soon as possible, whether or not termination or pregnancy continuation is planned. The sooner this is accomplished, the greater the chance that the threads will still be accessible in the enlarging uterus. If there is no evidence of infection and the strings are easily seen, this can be done in the office or clinic setting. Women who become pregnant with an IUD in place have an increased rate of spontaneous abortion (approximately 50%). After removal of the IUD, the spontaneous abortion rate is about 30%. If the IUD cannot be easily removed, a therapeutic abortion should be offered to the patient. The risk of life-threatening septic abortion in the second trimester is increased 20-fold if the IUD is left in utero. If removal of the IUD is being done in an infected pregnant uterus, removal should be accomplished only after intravenous antibiotic blood levels have been achieved. It should be done in area where emergency measures are available, in case septic shock ensues. Studies have not shown any increase in congenital anomalies associated with the IUD in place during pregnancy.

The IUD can be inserted safely at any time after delivery, abortion, or during menses. There is a higher rate of expulsion immediately postpartum, although this

TABLE 3.7. Contraindications to Use of Copper T-380A or Progesterone-Releasing IUD

CONTRAINDICATIONS TO USE OF BOTH
Known or suspected pregnancy
Abnormalities of uterus that distort uterine cavity, including uterus with cavity
  < 6 cm or > 10 cm on sounding
Presence or history of pelvic inflammatory disease or sexually transmitted diseases
Patient or partner has multiple sexual partners
Known or suspected uterus or cervical malignancy, including unresolved abnormal
  Pap smear
Conditions or treatments that increase susceptibility to infection
Genital bleeding of unknown etiology
Genital actinomycoses
Untreated acute cervicitis or vaginitis, including bacterial vaginosis
Postpartum endometritis or septic abortion in past 3 months
Valvular heart disease (may use in mitral valve prolapse, but if mitral regurgitation is
  present, give prophylactic antibiotics at time of insertion)
Anticoagulant therapy
Severe anemia
Severe dysmenorrhea and/or menstruation (more significant contraindication for
  copper IUD than for progesterone IUD)

CONTRAINDICATIONS SPECIFIC TO COPPER T-380A IUD
Wilson's disease
Known allergy to copper

can be decreased with high fundal placement. Insertion of the IUD during the period of lactational amenorrhea has the advantage of not being associated with a spotting problem often encountered during the first cycle after insertion. The usually atrophic endometrium tolerates the IUD very well. While menstruating, the ideal time for insertion is at the end of a menstrual period or within 2 to 3 days thereafter. For women at low risk of occult sexually transmitted diseases, there is probably no benefit of prophylactic antibiotics before insertion of the IUD. Most believe that administration of doxycycline (Doryx, Vibramycin, 200 mg) 1 hour before insertion may give some protection against insertion associated pelvic infection. Directions for placement of the copper and progesterone IUDs are found in Appendices 3.1 and 3.2.

The patient is to check for the IUD string monthly, and the practitioner checks for it at the time of gynecologic examination. If it is not present, an ultrasound should be done to confirm intrauterine location. If the ultrasound does not show it, a flat-plate abdominal radiograph is done. If the IUD is intraabdominal/extrauterine, it must be physically retrieved. An intraabdominal IUD can cause serious problems, including bowel obstruction or perforation. Removal should be done as soon as possible after the diagnosis is made. Copper IUDs in particular elicit a strong inflammatory response that may make laparoscopic removal quite difficult. Perforations of the uterus usually occur at the time of insertion, so it is important to identify the strings a few weeks afterward.

To remove an IUD, the strings are grasped with either a ring forceps or uterine dressing forceps and firm traction is exerted. If the string(s) cannot be seen, a cytobrush in the endocervical canal may help in extracting them. If further maneuvers are necessary, a paracervical block should be given. Visualization of the IUD with sonography or hysteroscopy may be necessary to facilitate removal.

DIAPHRAGM

The diaphragm can be an effective method of contraception. Diaphragm failure rates for the first year are estimated at 13 to 23% (89). When used faithfully, the failure rate is probably closer to 6%. The diaphragm is fitted by the practitioner in the office, preferably using actual diaphragms rather than rings. There are three types of diaphragms: the flat metal spring, all-flex arcing type, or hinged arcing type. Sizes range from 50 to 105 mm in diameter with most women using a size between 65 and 80 mm. To fit the diaphragm, place the middle finger against the vaginal wall and posterior cul de sac. Lift the hand anteriorly until the index finger is against the back of the symphysis pubis. Mark this point with the thumb to approximate the necessary diameter of the diaphragm. Insert the corresponding ring or diaphragm. Both the practitioner and patient are to assess the fit. If it is too tight, a smaller size is chosen. If it is expelled with increased intraabdominal pressure, a larger size is needed. The practitioner should instruct and observe the patient in the insertion process and check for proper placement.

Although recommended for use with a spermicidal agent, there have been no adequate studies to determine if the efficacy is different with or without these agents (90). Spermicides may increase the risk of *Escherichia coli* bacteriuria by changing the natural vaginal flora (91). The diaphragm should be placed no more than 6 hours before intercourse. It should be left in the vagina for about 6 hours afterward but no more than 24 hours after coitus. Additional spermicide should be placed intravaginally without removing the diaphragm for each additional episode of intercourse. After it is removed, it should be washed with soap and water, rinsed, and dried. Powders should never be used on the diaphragm. Periodic checks for leaks should be done. The diaphragm should not be exposed to light or extreme temperatures during storage.

The incidence of urinary tract infections among diaphragm users is about twice that of women using OCs. This may be due to pressure on the urethra with the diaphragm in place (92). Voiding after intercourse is helpful in avoiding urinary tract infection. A single postcoital dose of prophylactic antibiotics may also be used. There are some parous women with relaxation of the anterior vaginal wall in whom proper fitting is difficult, although the flat-spring diaphragm may be tried in such instances. Well-motivated, properly fitted, and instructed women find the diaphragm a very acceptable method of contraception. The diaphragm reduces the incidence of sexually transmitted diseases and cervical neoplasia, presumably by reducing acquisition of HPV and other pathogens (93). With a change in weight greater than 10 pounds, the woman may need to be refitted with a diaphragm of another size.

CERVICAL CAP

The Femcaps, a silicone rubber cap shaped like a sailor's hat, was introduced in 1990 and seems superior to the cavity rim cervical cap, Prentif, which comes in four sizes: 22, 25, 28, and 31 mm. This represents the internal diameter of the rim. The dome covers the cervix and the rim fits snugly into the vaginal fornices. The brim adheres and conforms to the vaginal walls. Approximately 50% of women can be properly fitted. Women with a long cervix, short cervix, or one that is too anterior may not be suitable candidates for the cap. Spermicidal cream or a jelly is applied to the inside and then it is positioned over the cervix by hand or with a special applicator. The cap should be inserted no less than 20 minutes and no more than 4 hours before intercourse. The device is removed up to 48 hours after insertion but no sooner than

6 hours after intercourse. After insertion and after each act of coitus, the cervix should be checked to ensure it is covered. Pressure is exerted on the rim to break the seal and remove it. The advantage of the cap is that is supplies a barrier method similar to the diaphragm but is suitable in women who have anterior vaginal wall relaxation. It is about as effective as the diaphragm but is harder to fit and properly insert. Squatting seems to be the best position for both insertion and removal. In a study of 121 women, 5 became pregnant. Of these, two reported dislodgement of the cap during intercourse and the other three did not use the device on several occasions (94). Another multicenter study found a first-year pregnancy rate of 11.3 per 100 women, although women with near perfect use in the first year had a pregnancy rate of only 6.1 per 100 women (95). The device has several advantages over currently available barrier contraceptive devices. The silicone rubber material is nonallergenic, durable, and easy to clean. The Femcaps design fits the cervical anatomy better and accommodates physiologic or arousal changes, making it superior to the cavity rim device.

The cap must be fitted to the size of the cervix by the practitioner. Most nulliparous women use a size 22 and parous women usually require a size 25. The cervix size should be estimated by both inspection and palpation before fitting. The cap is compressed between the thumb and forefinger and placed through the introitus with the dome facing outward. It is pushed over the cervix and the dome indented to create suction. The dome should stay compressed for a few seconds and should not be easily dislodged with lateral pressure on the rim. Before use, the cap should be filled one third with spermicidal jelly or cream. The use of the cervical cap is not associated with an increased incidence of cystitis.

CONDOMS

Condoms are the third most popular contraceptive method used by married couples in the United States, after sterilization and OCs. First-year failure rates with condom use are reported to be 8 to 15% (88). Contraceptive failure rates are lower in women over the age of 30 years, those who seek to prevent pregnancy rather than delay it, and women of higher socioeconomic status and level of education. Use of the condom by highly motivated couples has a failure rate of 2 to 4% (96). The use of a spermicide decreases the failure rate in event of breakage. If it does break, leak, or spill, spermicidal agent should be quickly placed into the vagina. The risk of breakage is about 3%, although water-based lubricants may reduce this risk. Petroleum-based lubricants markedly decrease the strength of condoms, even with only brief exposure times. There are two types of condoms: latex and "natural skin," made of lamb's intestine. Allergic reactions to latex or chemicals in the latex can occur, either immediately or as delayed reactions. It is important to place the condom before any genital contact occurs. Uncircumcised men must pull the foreskin back before placement. Before unrolling and applying the condom, air should be squeezed out of the reservoir and the tip of the condom should extend beyond the end of the penis. The condom must be withdrawn before loss of the erection. The principle disadvantage to the use of the condom relates to an interruption of sexual foreplay, which can be minimized by incorporating its application during foreplay. Some men are unable to maintain an erection with the use of the condom and this makes it unsatisfactory.

For women with multiple sexual partners, use of condoms either as a single method of contraception or in combination with other methods should be encouraged to reduce the risk of sexually transmitted diseases. In addition to the decreased transmission of *Neisseria gonorrhoeae* and *Chlamydia trachomatis*, transmission of the herpes virus, the human immunodeficiency virus (HIV), and the human papilloma virus are also strikingly decreased when condoms are used.

FEMALE CONDOM

The female condom was approved by the U.S. Food and Drug Administration in 1994 (Fig. 3.2). There are several studies that evaluated its use and effectiveness. One study included female employees of two hospitals in Cape Town, South Africa. Twenty-three of 52 participants used all 10 of the devices issued to them, 21 stated that they or their partner(s) did not enjoy using the method, and an additional 9 had other problems with it. Sexual responsiveness, however, was the same or better

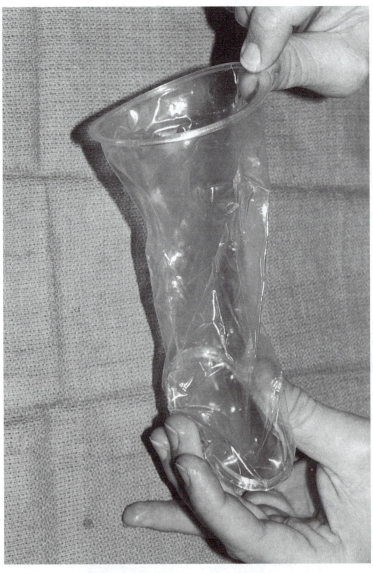

FIGURE 3.2. Female condom.

in 52% and overall acceptability was 52%. Compared with the male condom, 50% of the women and 44% of their partners considered the device as good or better than the male condom (97).

Another study from Kenya used a questionnaire comparing the acceptability of the female condom and the latex male condom in a sample of low-risk women receiving care from private obstetrician/gynecologists in Nairobi. Eighty-five percent of all subjects who completed the questionnaires reported they liked using the female condom, and more than two thirds of all of the women liked the female condom as much or better than the male condom. Fifty-five percent of the women would use the device in the future if it was available. The least-liked features were that it was too large for easy insertion, messy to handle, and reduced sensation. Use tended to become more acceptable as experience was gained (98). In the initial U.S. trial, there was a pregnancy rate of 15% in 6 months, although, with perfect use, the pregnancy rate is probably 3% (99). Another reported problem is that the device is noisy.

This limited experience provides preliminary data indicating that the female condom is a fairly acceptable method for some couples but suggests further research into safety, cost effectiveness, and hindrances to acceptability. A clear advantage is that it is a female-controlled contraceptive and provides protection against sexually transmitted diseases, including HIV. Sufficient numbers have not been obtained to accurately reflect its contraceptive effectiveness. Directions regarding placement of the female condom can be found in Appendix 3.3.

SPERMICIDES

Spermicides are supplied as jellies, creams, foams, melting suppositories, foaming tablets, and soluble films. These are chemical agents that inactivate sperm in the vagina before entrance into the cervix. Aerosol foams offer the best protection because the jellies and melting suppositories provide poor intravaginal distribution (100). The spermicide must be applied 10 to 30 minutes before intercourse. The jelly, cream, and foam preparations last up to 80 minutes. The tablets and suppositories are good for 1 hour or less. Most use nonoxynol-9 in concentrations ranging from 2.7 to 12.5%. Nonoxynol-9 is not absorbed from the vagina. Other agents include Octoxynol-9 and Menfegol. Most preparations contain 60 to 100 mg of these agents per vaginal application. The use of spermicides does not increase the risk for spontaneous abortion, birth defects, or low birth weight (101). Failure rates vary widely from less than 1% to nearly 33% in the first year of use. Failure rates of approximately 20% per year are most typical (88). The regular use of spermicide may increase vaginal colonization with *E. coli*. This may increase the risk of *E. coli* bacteriuria after intercourse (102). If this occurs, voiding immediately after intercourse and/or use of a prophylactic single dose of antibiotics may prove helpful. The most common minor side effect is allergy, occurring in 1 to 5% of users. The solution here is to change products. It should be noted parenthetically that vaginal douches are ineffective contraceptives, even those containing spermicidal agents. Postcoital douching is too late to prevent the ingress of sperm into the cervix.

FEMALE STERILIZATION

Sterilization is one of the most common methods of contraception in the United States. Most procedures are done in an outpatient surgical setting, although some are done in private offices. The mortality rate for sterilization is 1.5 per 100,000 procedures. This is lower than the mortality associated with childbirth (10 per 100,000)

(103). The average failure rate is one to four per 1000 procedures, with the actual rate being operator, patient, and technique dependent. Patients under 35 have a higher failure rate, as do women who are not lactating at the time of the procedure. Techniques that rely on more equipment have a higher failure rate secondary to technical problems (104, 105).

With sterilization currently being readily available, careful consideration and counseling is in order. This is particularly true of women under 30, and the procedure should generally be limited to the patient who is presumably in a long-term relationship. These criteria are obviously not the case when a disease is present that could be worsened by the complication of subsequent pregnancy. The median age at sterilization is 30, and there is a higher incidence of regret in women sterilized before age 30 and among those who divorce and remarry. In certain ethnic cultures, a woman incapable of bearing children may be considered "damaged" to some degree. The question needs to be asked: "What if something happened to your husband or your relationship, or to one of your children, would this change your mind?" The decision should be regarded as irrevocable, and unseemly optimism for the possibility of uncomplicated reversal should be faced with facts of insurance payments, the increase in risk of ectopic pregnancy, and the greatly diminished chance of success in the event of any type of cauterization procedure. An informed consent should state the risk of failure and the increased rate of ectopic pregnancy in that event.

At the present time, nearly all tubal sterilization procedures in this country are with the Pomeroy method in conjunction with cesarean section, immediate postpartum partial salpingectomy, or via laparoscopy. An interval minilaparotomy approach would certainly be appropriate if the patient's history or pelvic findings suggested the possibility of significant pelvic adhesions and perhaps distortion of anatomy.

Failures of sterilization are associated with a higher rate of ectopic pregnancies, with the incidence dependent on the surgical procedure originally performed. Bipolar cauterization has a higher incidence of ectopic pregnancy associated with failures than mechanical occlusion (106). The overall risk for ectopic pregnancy in sterilized women, however, is still lower than if they were not sterilized. A recently published multicentered, prospective, cohort study involving 10,685 women was reported from the U.S. Collaborative Review of Sterilization (CREST) in the literature. The CREST data show that failures continue beyond the first year; by 5 years, more than 1% of women had a sterilization failure, and by 10 years, 1.8% failed (107). It is well known that the risk of ectopic pregnancy after tubal sterilization is greatly increased. Another study found 7.3 tubal pregnancies per 1000 procedures and found that bipolar tubal coagulation before the age of 30 had a probability of ectopic pregnancy 27 times greater than women of similar age who underwent postpartum partial salpingectomy. This also showed that a history of tubal sterilization does not rule out the possibility of ectopic pregnancy, even 10 years after the procedure (108).

The first suggestion of a "posttubal syndrome" was in 1951 (109). The CREST multicenter prospective study on this subject showed that of patients interviewed immediately before and again after sterilization for up to 5 years, 35% report higher levels of menstrual pain, 49% reported very heavy increase in menstrual flow, and 10% reported increased spotting between periods. This was at the fifth year; the first year showed a lesser degree of pain and hypermenorrhea (110). It is obvious that aging of the cohort may be a factor, as well as the fact that it takes such changes a significant time to develop. In similar paired studies of poststerilization on women conducted several years apart, Rulen et al. (111, 112) and De Stephanou et al. (113, 114) showed an increased prevalence of pain in the latter studies. These reports do not make patient counseling about the long-term menstrual effects of tubal sterilization an easy task.

There have been anecdotal reports about the prevalence of hysterectomy after sterilization. Hillis et al. (115) reported that the cumulative probability of undergoing hysterectomy by 14 years after sterilization was 17%. The highest likelihood occurred among women who reported a history of endometriosis or noted prolonged bleeding before sterilization. Not surprisingly, women with gynecologic disorders were at greater risk of hysterectomy than women without these disorders. Women may be reassured that there is no detrimental effect on sexual response associated with tubal sterilization (116).

CLINICAL NOTES

- To use the calendar technique of natural family planning, subtract 19 days from the shortest cycle length and 9 days from the longest cycle length. The woman then abstains from intercourse during those days of her cycle.
- Using basal body temperature allows women to determine that ovulation has occurred; it is a retrospective form of natural family planning that allows prospective estimates on when ovulation is most likely to occur.
- The symptothermal method of natural family planning combines the use of basal body temperature changes with cervical mucus changes to determine the period of fertility.
- Lactation provides some, but not complete, protection from ovulation and subsequent pregnancy.
- Delay the start of OCs for 2 to 3 weeks after pregnancies of more than 28 weeks gestation. Delay the start of OCs for 1 week for pregnancies lasting more than 13 weeks but less than 28 weeks. There is no need to delay the start of OCs for pregnancies that lasted less than 13 weeks.
- The risk of stroke in a nonsmoking woman under 35 years of age using OCs is minimal.
- OCs should not be used in women with a history of classic migraines or migraines associated with transient ischemic attacks.
- OCs may be used in women with common migraines. Some women will notice improvement, some worsening, and some no change in frequency and/or intensity of attacks.
- In epileptics who desire OCs, the 50-μg dose may be necessary to provide adequate contraception.
- Women with known antithrombin III deficiency, protein C or S deficiency, or activated protein C resistance should not be placed on OCs. A woman who develops a deep vein thrombosis while on OCs should be evaluated for these disorders as a reflection of factor V Leiden mutation.
- Patients with controlled hypertension are eligible for the use of OCs. A history of pregnancy-induced hypertension or preeclampsia does not preclude the use of OCs.
- OCs should be avoided in women with triglycerides higher than 350 mg/dL or a familial hypertriglyceridemia.
- Diabetic women free of complicating vascular diseases and with good glucose control are candidates for OC use.
- OCs are useful agents for the control of irregular bleeding commonly seen in the perimenopausal time period and to provide contraception, barring any contraindications.
- OCs are known to decrease ovarian and uterine cancer. There is no long-term increase in breast cancer. The effect on adenocarcinoma of the cervix is still being elucidated.
- The progestin-only minipill is ideal for contraception in lactating women and for women who have contraindications to the combination contraceptives.
- With use for 1 year, 50% of women receiving DMPA report amenorrhea.
- The most common clinical complaints associated with Norplant are irregular bleeding, headaches, depression, bloating, and acne.
- The copper IUD is effective for 10 years. It may cause increased menstrual loss and dysmenorrhea.

- The progesterone IUD is effective for 1 year. It may cause irregular bleeding.
- The diaphragm must be placed no more than 6 hours before intercourse and should be removed no sooner than 6 hours afterward. It may cause increased frequency of urinary tract infections in some women.
- The cervical cap is not associated with an increased incidence of cystitis but may be more difficult for some patients to adequately place.
- Women who are sterilized before age 30 or who divorce and remarry have the highest incidence of regret about the procedure.
- Failure of sterilization is associated with a higher rate of ectopic pregnancies.

Placement of the Copper IUD

1. Can be inserted whenever pregnancy has been reliably excluded, including immediately postpartum or after abortion.
2. Confirm uterine size and position on examination.
3. Clean cervix and upper vagina with antiseptic.
4. Apply topical anesthesia or paracervical block to cervix; place tenaculum on anterior lip of cervix for traction (if uterus is extremely retroverted, placing tenaculum on posterior lip of cervix may be more helpful).
5. Sound the uterus; do not place IUD if uterus sounds to less than 6 cm or greater than 9 cm.
6. Document IUD lot number in chart and open IUD package, keeping contents sterile.
7. Wear sterile gloves; load the IUD into the insertion tube with the arms of the "T" folded *downward* into tube; do not leave the IUD in the insertion tube with the arms folded for more than 5 minutes.
8. Insert solid tube into bottom of insertion tube until it touches the bottom of the IUD.
9. Adjust the flange of the insertion tube to depth of uterus and to the plane in which the arms will open. Make sure the horizontal arms and long axis of the flange lie in the same horizontal plane.
10. Place insertion tube into cervix/uterus until it touches fundus of uterus. The flange should be at the cervix. Hold solid rod stationary and retract the insertion tube no greater than 0.5 inch to release the arms.
11. Hold insertion tube still and remove solid rod only. After the solid rod is out, remove the insertion tube. Cut threads 2.5 to 4 cm beyond os. Measure and record the length of the strings.

Placement of Progesterone IUD

1. Able to insert in latter part of menstrual period or for 1 to 2 days after menses has finished. If being used postpartum, uterine involution must be complete. It is not to be placed immediately postabortion or postpartum.
2. Confirm uterine size and position on examination.
3. Clean cervix and upper vagina with antiseptic.
4. Apply topical anesthesia or paracervical block to cervix; place tenaculum on anterior lip of cervix for traction (if uterus is extremely retroverted, placing tenaculum on posterior lip of cervix may be more helpful).
5. Sound the uterus; do not place IUD if uterus sounds to less than 6 cm or greater than 9 cm.
6. Document IUD lot number in chart and open IUD package, keeping contents sterile.
7. Use the cocking device to fold the arms against the stem by pressing insert straight down on a solid surface. Do not leave cocked for more than 5 minutes.
8. Adjust the inserting tube for the curvature of the uterus; if anteverted, the numbers face up, if retroverted, the numbers face down.
9. Check that the thread-retaining plug at the end of the tube is secure.
10. Wear sterile gloves; place into cervix/uterus until it reaches fundus. The number at the cervix on the inserter should equal the depth noted on the sounding of the uterus.
11. Hold the arm of the inserter still and squeeze the wings of the thread-retaining plug to remove it.
12. Withdraw inserter. Measure shorter of the two threads. The IUD is at the fundus if the length of the shorter thread is equal to the difference between 9 cm and the uterine depth in centimeters noted on sounding. Cut other thread usual length and record.

Placement of the Female Condom

1. After removing condom from package, check to make sure the lubrication is spread evenly inside the pouch from the bottom to the top. If more lubricant is necessary, add two drops from the additional lubricant that is supplied. (Some women may need more than two drops.)
2. Check that the inner ring is at the bottom closed end of the pouch.
3. Hold the condom with the open end hanging down toward the ground. Squeeze the inner ring with your thumb and middle finger. It should look like a long, narrow "O."
4. With the other hand, separate the labia so the vagina is accessible. The hand holding the condom pushes the inner ring and pouch up into the vagina until the entire inner ring is just behind the pubic bone. (This is the same placement one uses for a diaphragm.) The condom should be inserted straight into the vagina; in other words, it should not be twisted. There should be about 1 inch of the open end outside the vagina.
5. During sex, the outer ring may move from side to side, which is normal. If it begins to slide or slip, more lubricant should be added. If it seems noisy during sex, add more lubricant.
6. If the outer ring begins to be pushed into the vagina, a new condom should be placed with extra lubricant around the opening of the pouch or on the penis.
7. To remove the condom, squeeze and twist the outer ring, keeping the sperm and semen inside the pouch. The condom is not designed to be flushed down a toilet and must be placed in the trash. It should *not* be reused.
8. A new condom must be used with every act of sex.
9. The female condom should not be used at the same time as a male condom. If used simultaneously, both products will not stay in place.

References

1. Wardell D. Margaret Sanger: birth control's successful revolutionary. Am J Public Health 1980;70:191.
2. Gordon L. Woman's Body, Woman's Right: A Social History of Birth Control in America. New York: Grosman, 1976:262.
3. Speert H. Obstetrics and Gynecology in America: A History. Baltimore: Waverly Press, 1980:162.
4. Brown JB, Blackwell LF, Billings JJ, et al. Natural family planning. Am J Obstet Gynecol 1987;157:1082.
5. Brown JB, Holmes J, Barker G. Use of the home ovarian monitor in pregnancy avoidance. Am J Obstet Gynecol 1991;165:2008.
6. Roetzer J. Natural family planning and pregnancy outcome. Int J Fertil 1988;33 (suppl):40.
7. Bohler E. Breast feeding as family planning in a global perspective. Tidsskr Nor Laegeforen 1997;117:701.
8. Kennedy KI, Visness CM. Contraceptive efficacy of lactational amenorrhea. Lancet 1992;330:227.
9. Kazi A, Kennedy KI, Visness CM, et al. Effectiveness of the lactational amenorrhea method in Pakistan. Fertil Steril 1995;64:717.
10. Abma JC, Chandra A, Masher WD, et al. Fertility, family planning, and women's health: new data from the 1995 National Survey of Family Growth. Vital Health Stat 23 1997; 19:1–114.
11. Longstreth WT, Nelson LM, Koepsell TD, et al. Subarachnoid hemorrhage and hormonal factor in women: a population-based case-control study. Ann Intern Med 1994; 121:168.
12. Thorogood M, Mann J, Murphy M, et al. Fatal stroke and use of oral contraceptives: findings from a case-control study. Am J Epidemiol 1992;136:35.
13. Hannaford PC, Croft PR, Kay CR. Oral contraception and stroke. Evidence from the Royal College of General Practitioners' Oral Contraception Study. Stroke 1994;25:935.
14. Tzourio C, Tehindrazanarivelo A, Iglesias S, et al. Case-control study of migraine and risk of ischaemic stroke in young women. BMJ 1995;310:830.
15. Carolei A, Marini C, De Matteis G, et al. History of migraine and risk of cerebral ischaemia in young adults. Lancet 1996;347:1503.
16. Ramcharan S, Pellegrin FA, Ray FM, et al. The Walnut Creek Contraceptive Drug Study. A prospective study of the side effect of oral contraceptives. III. An interim report: a comparison of disease occurrence leading to hospitalization or death in users and nonusers of oral contraceptives. J Reprod Med 1980;25:345.
17. Ryan RE. A controlled study of the effect of oral contraceptives on migraine. Headache 1978;17:250.
18. Crawford P, Chadwick DJ, Martin C, et al. The interaction of phenytoin and carbamazepine with combined oral contraceptive steroids. Br J Clin Pharm 1990;30:892.
19. Mattson RH, Rebar RW. Contraceptive methods for women with neurologic disorders. Am J Obstet Gynecol 1993;168:2027.
20. Mattson RH, Cramer JA, Darney PD, et al. Use of oral contraceptives by women with epilepsy. JAMA 1986;256:238.
21. Back DJ, Orme ML. Pharmacokinetic drug interactions with oral contraceptives. Clin Pharmacokinet 1991;18:472.
22. Gerstman BB, Piper JM, Tomita DK, et al. Oral contraceptive estrogen dose and the risk of deep venous thromboembolic disease. Am J Epidemiol 1991;133:32.
23. Spitzer WO, Lewis MA, Heinemann LA, et al. Third generation oral contraceptives and risk of venous thromboembolic disorders: an international case-control study. BMJ 1996;312:83.
24. Poulter N, et al. Venous thromboembolic disease and combined oral contraceptives: results of an international multicenter case control-study. Lancet 1995;346:1575.
25. Speroff L, Darney PD. A Clinical Guide for Contraception. 2nd ed. Baltimore: Williams & Wilkins, 1994:56.

26. Tsai CC, Williamson HO, Kirkland BH, et al. Low dose oral contraception and blood pressure in women with a past history of elevated blood pressure. Am J Obstet Gynecol 1985;151:28.

27. Knopp RH, LaRosa JC, Burman RT Jr. Contraception and dyslipidemia. Am J Obstet Gynecol 1993;168:1994.

28. Engel HJ, Engel E, Lichtlen PR. Coronary atherosclerosis and myocardial infarction in young women—role of oral contraceptives. Eur Heart J 1983;4:1.

29. Mileikowsky GN, Nadler JL, Huey F, et al. Evidence that smoking alters prostacyclin formation and platelet aggregation in women who use oral contraceptives. Am J Obstet Gynecol 1988;159:1547.

30. Sullivan JM, Lobo RA. Considerations for contraception in women with cardiovascular disorders. Am J Obstet Gynecol 1993;168:2006.

31. Kjos SL, Shoupe D, Douyan S, et al. Effect of low-dose oral contraceptives on carbohydrate and lipid metabolism in women with recent gestational diabetes: results of a controlled, randomized, prospective study. Am J Obstet Gynecol 1991;163:32.

32. Jungers P, Dougados M, Pelissier C, et al. Influence or oral contraceptive therapy on the activity of systemic lupus erythematosus. Arthritis Rheum 1982;25:618.

33. Shenfield GM, Griffin JM. Clinical pharmacokinetics of contraceptive steroids: an update. Clin Pharmacokinet 1991;20:15.

34. Orme ML. The Third SK&F Prize Lecture, University of London, December 1981. The clinical pharmacology of oral contraceptive steroids. Br J Clin Pharm 1982;14:31.

35. Back DJ, Breckenridge AM, Crawford FE, et al. The effect of rifampicin on the pharmacokinetics of ethinyl-estradiol in women. Contraception 1980;21:135.

36. Kelsey JL, Berkowitz GS. Breast cancer epidemiology. Cancer Res 1988;48:5615.

37. Collaborative Group on Hormonal Factors in Breast Cancer. Breast cancer and hormonal contraceptives: further results. Contraception 1996;54(3 suppl):1.

38. Thomas DB. Oral contraceptives and breast cancer: review of the epidemiologic literature. Contraception 1991;43:596.

39. Cancer and Steroid Hormone Study Group. Oral-contraceptive use and the risk of breast cancer. The Cancer and Steroid Hormone Study of the Centers for Disease Control and the National Institute of Child Health and Human Development. N Engl J Med 1986;315:405.

40. Caygill CP, Hill MJ. Oral contraceptives and breast cancer. Lancet 1989;1:1258.

41. Murray PM, Stadel BV, Schlesselman JJ. Oral contraceptive use in women with a family history of breast cancer. Obstet Gynecol 1989;73:977.

42. Ory H, Cole P, MacMahon B, et al. Oral contraceptives and reduced risk of benign breast disease. N Engl J Med 1976;294:419.

43. Brinton La, Vessey MP, Flavel R, et al. Risk factors for benign breast disease. Am J Epidemiol 1981;113:203.

44. Herbst AL, Berek JS. Impact of contraception on gynecologic cancers. Am J Obstet Gynecol 1993;168:1980.

45. Parazzini F, La Vecchia C, Negri E, et al. Oral contraceptive use and invasive cervical cancer. Int J Epidemiol 1990;19:259.

46. Brinton LA. Oral contraceptives and cervical neoplasia. Contraception 1991;43:581.

47. Kjaer SK, Engholm G, Dahl C, et al. Case-control study of risk factors for cervical squamous-cell neoplasia in Denmark. III. Role of oral contraceptive use. Cancer Causes Control 1993;4:513.

48. Ursin G, Peters RK, Henderson BE, et al. Oral contraceptive use and adenocarcinoma of the cervix. Lancet 1994;344:1390.

49. Thomas DB, Ray RM. Oral contraceptives and invasive adenocarcinomas and adenosquamous carcinomas of the uterine cervix. Am J Epidemiol 1996;44:281.

50. Thomas DB. The WHO Collaborative Study of Neoplasia and Steroid Contraceptives: The influence of combined oral contraceptives on risk of neoplasms in developing and developed countries. Contraception 1991;43:695.

51. Jick SS, Walker AM, Jick H. Oral contraceptives and endometrial cancer. Obstet Gynecol 1993;82:931.

52. CDC/National Institute of Health and Development. Combination oral contraceptive use and the risk of endometrial cancer. JAMA 1987;257:796.

53. Rosenberg L, Palmer JR, Zauber AG, et al. A case-control study of oral contraceptive use and invasive epithelial ovarian cancer. Am J Epidemiol 1994;139:654.

54. CDC/National Institute of Child Health and Development. The Cancer and Steroid Hormone Study: The reduction of ovarian cancer associated with oral contraceptive use. N Engl J Med 1987;316:650.

55. Krettek SE, Arkin SI, Chaisilwattana P, et al. *Chlamydia trachomatis* in patients who used oral contraceptives and had intermenstrual spotting. Obstet Gynecol 1993;81:728.

56. Anderson FD. Selectivity and minimum androgenicity of norgestimate in monophasic and triphasic oral contraceptives. Acta Obstet Gynecol Scand Suppl 1992;156:15–21.

57. Corson SL. Efficacy and clinical profile of a new oral contraceptive containing norgestimate: U.S. clinical trials. Acta Obstet Gynecol Scand Suppl 1990;152:25–31.

58. Bilotta P, Favilli S. Clinical evaluation of a monophasic ethinyl estradiol/desogestrel containing oral contraceptive. Arzneimittelforschung 1988;38:932

59. Palatsi R, Hirvensalo E, Liukko P, et al. Serum total and unbound testosterone and sex hormone binding globulin (SHBG) in women acne patients treated with two different oral contraceptives. Acta Derm Venereol Suppl (Stockh) 1984;64:517.

60. Sulak PJ, Haney AF. Unwanted pregnancies: understanding contraceptive use and benefits in adolescents and older women. Am J Obstet Gynecol 1993;168:2042.

61. Vessey M, Metcalf A, Wells G, et al. Ovarian neoplasms, functional cysts, and oral contraceptives. BMJ 1987;294:1518.

62. Lanes AF, Birmann B, Walter MM, et al. Oral contraceptive type and functional ovarian cysts. Am J Obstet Gynecol 1992;166:956.

63. Wolner-Hanssen P, Svensson L, Mardh PA, et al. Laparoscopic findings and contraceptives use in women with signs and symptoms of acute salpingitis. Obstet Gynecol 1985; 66:233–238.

64. Ryden G, Fahraeus L, Molin L, et al. Do oral contraceptives influence the spread of acute pelvic inflammatory disease in women with gonorrhea? Contraception 1979;20:149.

65. Trussell J, Hatcher RA, Cates W Jr, et al. Contraceptive failures in the United States: an update. Stud Fam Plann 1990;21:51.

66. Speroff L, Darney PD. A Clinical Guide for Contraception. 2nd ed. Baltimore: Williams & Wilkins, 1992:109.

67. Broome M, Fotherby K. Clinical experience with the progestin-only pill. Contraception 1990;42:489.

68. Fotherby K. The progestogen only pill and thrombosis. Br J Fam Plann 1989;15:83.

69. Yuzpe AA, Smith RP, Rademaker AW. A multicenter clinical investigation employing ethinyl estradiol combined with dl-norgestrel as contraceptive agent. Fertil Steril 1982;37:508.

70. Harper CC, Ellertson CE. The emergency contraceptive pill: a survey of knowledge and attitudes among students at Princeton University. Am J Obstet Gynecol 1995;173:1438.

71. Ho PC, Kwan MS. A prospective randomized comparison of levonorgestrel with the Yuzpe regimen in post-coital contraception. Hum Reprod 1993;8:389.

72. Glasier A. Emergency postcoital contraception. N Engl J Med 1997;337:1058.

73. Schwallie PC, Assenze JR. The effect of depo-medroxyprogesterone acetate on pituitary and ovarian function, and the return of fertility following its discontinuation: a review. Contraception 1974;10:181.

74. Gray RH. Reduced risk of pelvic inflammatory disease with injectable contraceptives. Lancet 1985;1:1046.

75. Mattson RH, Cramer JA, Caldwell BV, et al. Treatment of seizures with medroxyprogesterone acetate. Neurology 1984;34:1255.

76. Cundy T, Reid OR, Roberts H. Bone density in women receiving depot medroxyprogesterone for contraception. BMJ 1991;303:13.

77. Robertson DN, Sivin I, Nash HA, et al. Release rates of levonorgestrel from Silastic capsules, homogeneous rods and covered rods in humans. Contraception 1983;27:483.

78. Shoupe D, Horenstein J, Mishell D, et al. Characteristics of ovarian follicular development in Norplant users. Fertil Steril 1991;55:766.
79. Croxatto HB, Diaz S, Salvatierra AM, et al. Treatment with Norplant subdermal implants inhibits sperm penetration through cervical mucus in vitro. Contraception 1987;36:193.
80. Croxatto HB, Diaz S, Pavez M, et al. Clearance of levonorgestrel from the circulation following removal of Norplant subdermal implants. Contraception 1988;38:509.
81. Sivin I, Diaz S, Holma P, et al. A four-year clinical study of Norplant implants. Stud Fam Plann 1983;14:184.
82. Olsson S-E, Odlind V, Johansson E. Clinical results with subcutaneous implants containing 3-keto desogestrel. Contraception 1990;42:1.
83. Population Crisis Committee. Access to birth control: a world assessment. Population Briefing Paper 19, Washington, DC, 1986.
84. Ammala M, Nyman T, Strengell L. Effect of intrauterine contraceptive devices on cytokine messenger ribonucleic acid expression in the human endometrium. Fertil Steril 1995;63:773.
85. Sivin I, Schmidt F. Effectiveness of IUDs: a review. Contraception 1987;36:55.
86. Franks AL, Beral V, Cates W Jr. Contraception and ectopic pregnancy risks. Am J Obstet Gynecol 1990;63:1120.
87. Sivin I. Dose and age-dependent ectopic pregnancy risk with intrauterine contraception. Obstet Gynecol 1991;78:291.
88. WHO Special Programme of Research, Development and Research Training on Human Reproduction: Task Force on the Safety and Efficacy of Fertility Regulating Methods. The TCu380A, TCu220C, Multiload 250, and Nova T IUDs at 3, 5 and 7 years of use—results from three randomized multicenter trials. Contraception 1990;42:151.
89. Grady WR, Haywood MD, Yagi J. Contraceptive failure in the United States. Estimates from the 1982 National Survey of Family Growth. Fam Plann Perspect 1986;18:200.
90. Craig S, Hepburn S. The effectiveness of barrier methods of contraception with and without spermicide. Contraception 1982;26:347.
91. Gooton TM, Hillier S, Johnson C, et al. *Escherichia coli* bacteriuria and contraceptive method. JAMA 1991;265:64.
92. Fuhn SD, Lathan RH, Roberts P, et al. Association between diaphragm use and urinary tract infections. JAMA 1986;254:240.
93. Wright WH, Vessey MP, Kenward B, et al. Neoplasia and dysplasia of the cervix uteri and contraception: a possible protective effect of the diaphragm. Br J Cancer 1978; 38:273.
94. Shihata AA, Trussell J. A new female intervaginal barrier contraceptive device. Preliminary clinical trial. Contraception 1991;44:11.
95. Richwald MA, Greenland S, Gerber MM, et al. Effectiveness of the cavity rim cervical cap: results of a large clinical study. Obstet Gynecol 1989;74:143.
96. Trussell J, Hatcher RA, Kates W Jr, et al. Contraception failure in the United States: an update. Stud Fam Plann 1990;21:51.
97. Sapire KE. The female condom (Femidon)—a study of user acceptability. S Afr Med J 1995;85:1081.
98. Runinjo JK, Steiner M, Joanis C, et al. Preliminary comparison of the polyurethane female condom with the latex male condom in Kenya. East African Med J 1996;73:101.
99. Trussell J, Sturgen K, Strickler J, et al. Comparative contraceptive efficacy of female condom and other barrier methods. Fam Plan Perspect 1994;26:66–72.
100. Johnson V, Masters WH. Intravaginal contraceptive study. Phase II. Physiology. West J Surg Obstet Gynecol 1963;71:144.
101. Linn S, Schoenbaum SC, Monson RR. Lack of association between contraceptive usage and congenital malformation in offspring. Am J Obstet Gynecol 1983;147:923.
102. Gooton TM, Hillier S, Johnson C, et al. *Escherichia coli* bacteriuria and contraceptive method. JAMA 1991;265:64.
103. Escobedo LF, Peterson HB, Grubbs GS, et al. Case fatality rate for sterilization in United States hospitals. Am J Obstet Gynecol 1989;160:147.

104. Mosher WE, Pratt WF. Contraceptive use in the United States, 1973–1988. Advance data from vital and health statistics. No 182. Hyattsville, MD: National Center for Health Statistics, 1990.

105. Cheng M, Wong YM, Rochat R, et al. Sterilization failure in Singapore: an examination of ligation techniques and failure rates. Stud Fam Plann 1977;8:109.

106. McCausland A. High rate of ectopic pregnancy following laparoscopic tubal coagulation failure. Am J Obstet Gynecol 1980;136:977.

107. Peterson HB, Xia Z, Hughes JM, et al. The risk of pregnancy after tubal sterilization: findings from the U.S. Collaborative Review of Sterilization. Am J Obstet Gynecol 1996;174:1161.

108. Peterson HB, Xia Z, Hughes JM, et al. The risk of ectopic pregnancy after tubal sterilization. N Engl J Med 1997;336:762.

109. Williams EL, Jones HE, Merrel RE. The subsequent course of patients sterilized by tubal ligation. Am J Obstet Gynecol 1951;61:423.

110. Wilcox LS, Martinez-Schnell B, Peterson, HB, et al. Menstrual function after tubal sterilization. Am J Epidemiol 1992;135:1368.

111. Rulen MC, Turner JH, Dunworth R, et al. Post-tubal sterilization syndrome—a misnomer. Am J Obstet Gynecol 1985;151:13.

112. Rulen MC, Davidson AR, Philliber SG, et al. Changes in menstrual symptoms among sterilized in comparison women: a prospective study. Obstet Gynecol 1989;74:149.

113. De Stephanou F, Huezo CM, Peterson HB, et al. Menstrual changes after tubal sterilization. Obstet Gynecol 1983;62:673.

114. De Stephanou F, Pearlman JA, Peterson HB, et al. Long-term risk of menstrual disturbances after tubal-sterilization. Obstet Gynecol 1985;152:835.

115. Hillis HD, March-Banks, PA, Taylor GP. Tubal sterilization and long-term risk of hysterectomy findings from the U.S. Collaborative Review of Sterilization. The U.S. Collaborative Review of Sterilization Working Group (CREST). Obstet Gynecol 1997; 89:609.

116. Kjer J. Sexual adjustment to tubal sterilization. Eur J Obstet Gynecol 1990;35:211.

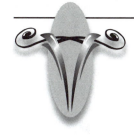

CHAPTER 4

Screening for and Detection of Fetal Disorders During Antepartum Care

JUSTIN P. LAVIN, JR.
JOHN W. STEWART, JR.

In 1914, during an address longer remembered for the quote "Once a cesarean section, always a cesarean section," Edwin Cragin proposed that physicians begin to offer systematic prenatal care (1). His recommendations dealt mainly with the assessment and preservation of maternal health. Fortunately, knowledge and technical expertise have progressed to a point where obstetricians are now also able to assess, and to some degree influence, fetal status. Well-woman or routine gynecologic visits offer an excellent opportunity to begin this process with preconceptual counseling. Otherwise, such care should commence with the initial prenatal visit and continue throughout the antepartum period.

INITIAL GENETIC/TERATOGENIC HISTORY AND COUNSELING

Inquiry and discussions regarding family history, ethnic origin, drug ingestion, and genetic testing often require unusual patience and tact. Some couples regard prior abnormal outcomes with a sense of guilt or failure. Not infrequently, relevant facts have been hidden from others for years. Discussions should be nonjudgmental, and most authorities recommend nondirectional counseling. The patient and her husband should be questioned to determine family history of structural anomaly, metabolic disease, chromosomal abnormality, mental retardation, repetitive abortion, stillbirth, or severe neonatal disease. A family pedigree should be constructed. It is often useful to refresh the patient's memory by specifically mentioning some of the more common disorders outlined in Table 4.1. A number of multifactorial defects should also be included in the family pedigree (Table 4.2).

Ethnic origin should be determined because certain groups are at increased risk for specific problems. For example, individuals of Ashkenazi Jewish, French-Canadian, and/or Cajun descent have a higher risk for Tay-Sachs disease. Persons of Mediterranean, African, Asian, Indian, and/or Pakistani groups are at increased risk for hemoglobin disorders and α- and β-thalassemias.

The age of both parents should be determined. The association between advanced maternal age and increased risk of fetal aneuploidy should be discussed. For women under the age of 30 at the birth of a child, the risk of Down's syndrome is 1 in 1000 to 1700 live births. Women under 30 at the time of childbirth have a risk for all chromosomal anomalies of 1 in 417 to 526 live births (excluding 47,XXX). For women aged 40 at the time of birth, the risk of Down's syndrome is 1 in 105 live births. These women's risk of all chromosomal abnormalities at age 40 is 1 in 65

TABLE 4.1. Conditions Associated with Genetic Risk or Teratogenic Potential to Discuss at Initial Visit

FAMILY HISTORY
Chromosomal disorders
Trisomy 21, 18, 13
Translocations

Metabolic disorders
Cystic fibrosis
Duchenne muscular dystrophy
Tay-Sachs disease
Hemoglobinopathy
Thalassemia

Structural abnormalities
Cardiac malformations
Neural tube defects
Hydrocephalus
Renal or bladder anomalies
Gastroschisis
Omphalocele
Skeletal dysplasias

Miscellaneous
Family history of mental retardation

MATERNAL HISTORY
Age ≥ 35 yr
Diabetes
Congenital adrenal hyperplasia
Phenylketonuria
Repetitive abortion
Medications
Substance abuse

TERATOGEN EXPOSURE
See list of potential and proven human teratogens in Appendix 4.1.

live births (Table 4.3) (2). Paternal age above 40 years has been associated with the occurrence of new autosomal dominant mutations (3).

The occurrence of maternal diseases that may be associated with fetal or newborn malformation or dysfunction such as diabetes, congenital adrenal hyperplasia, or phenylketonuria should be ascertained. Medications should be reviewed so that known or strongly suspected teratogens (see Appendix 4.1) may be substituted with more appropriate agents. Smoking, alcohol, or illegal drug use should be documented.

Women should receive prenatal vitamins containing 0.4 mg of folic acid because this has been associated with a 50% reduction in neural tube defects among the infants of families not at increased risk. Neural tube defects occur when the neural tube fails to close normally during embryogenesis. This may result in anencephaly, spina bifida that includes myelomeningocele or meningocele, and other midline neural defects such as encephalocele. Anencephaly is not compatible with long-term survival, but spina bifida is and may result in hemiparesis, urinary incontinence, and hydrocephalus if untreated. Although it is preferable to begin folic acid preconcep-

TABLE 4.2. Multifactorial Birth Defects[a]

Hydrocephaly, except for Dandy-Walker syndrome and some forms of aqueductal stenosis
Neural tube defects
Cleft lip, with or without cleft palate
Most cardiac defects
Diaphragmatic hernia
Omphalocele
Renal agenesis
Ureteral abnormalities
Posterior urethral valve syndrome
Hypospadias
Müllerian defects
Limb defects, including clubfoot

[a]After one affected child, the recurrence risk is 1–5%. After two affected children, the recurrence risk is higher.

TABLE 4.3. Incidence of Chromosomal Abnormalities in Live Born Infants by Maternal Age[a]

Maternal Age (yr)	Down's Syndrome	All Chromosomal Abnormalities
20	1/1,667	1/526
21	1/1,667	1/526
22	1/1,429	1/500
23	1/1,429	1/500
24	1/1,250	1/476
25	1/1,250	1/476
26	1/1,176	1/476
27	1/1,111	1/455
28	1/1,053	1/435
29	1/1,000	1/417
30	1/952	1/384
31	1/909	1/384
32	1/769	1/322
33	1/625	1/317
34	1/500	1/260
35	1/385	1/204
36	1/294	1/164
37	1/227	1/130
38	1/175	1/103
39	1/137	1/82
40	1/106	1/65
41	1/82	1/51
42	1/64	1/40
43	1/50	1/32
44	1/38	1/25
45	1/30	1/20
46	1/23	1/15
47	1/18	1/12
48	1/14	1/10
49	1/11	1/7

[a]Information regarding 47,XXX for ages 20–32 not available. Adapted from Hook EB. Rates of chromosomal abnormalities at different maternal ages. Obstet Gynecol 1981;58:282–285.

tually, it should at least be given at the first prenatal visit (if this occurs early in the first trimester). Women with a first- or second-degree relative with a neural tube defect, who are diabetic, or who are being treated with valproic acid or carbamazepine are at high risk for having an infant with a neural tube defect. These women should receive a daily dose of 4 mg of folic acid before and during the first trimester. Daily ingestion of this dose has been linked to a reduction in the occurrence of neural tube defects among these high-risk women.

MATERNAL MULTIPLE MARKER SERUM AND OTHER HEMATOLOGIC TESTING

Multiple Marker Testing

Initially, prenatal testing for neural tube defects was confined to families with a prior history of such abnormalities. Amniocentesis was done to measure the level of amniotic α-fetoprotein, a blood component unique to the fetus. This technique diagnoses all cases of fetal neural tube defect except for the 5 to 10% of cases of spina bifida where skin covers the lesion (4). Acetylcholinesterase is concurrently measured to rule out false-positive elevations of fetal α-protein. The baseline risk of a neural tube defect in the United States is one to two per 1000 live births, and in Great Britain it is one to two per 100 live births. With one affected first-degree relative, the risk is elevated 10-fold. However, 90% of neural tube defects occur among individuals with no prior family history (5). Appreciation of these facts led Wald et al. (6) in Great Britain and Milunsky et al. (5) in the United States to propose universal maternal serum α-fetoprotein (MSAFP) screening for neural tube defects.

Although sampling is most accurate when performed between 16 and 18 weeks of gestation, it can be performed between 15 and 22 weeks (5). Most laboratories use a cutoff of 2.5 multiples of the median in singleton pregnancies and 3.5 multiples of the median in twins to define individuals at increased risk for neural tube defects. Approximately 3 to 4% of the population has an elevated value that may or may not be associated with a neural tube defect. There are several reasons why MSAFP may be elevated other than the presence of a neural tube defect: underestimation of gestational age, multiple gestation, threatened abortion, Rh disease, anomalies other than neural tube defects, and fetal demise. If the MSAFP value is elevated but less than 3.0 multiples of the median and the patient is less than 18 weeks, a second sample should be obtained 1 week after the initial screen. Individuals with a second elevated MSAFP value, those with an initial value of at least 3.0 multiples of the median, and/or women who are greater than 18 weeks gestational age at the time of the initial elevated value should undergo a thorough ultrasound examination (5, 6). In most patients, an underlying cause of the elevated MSAFP is identified, but if none is found and if there is inadequate visualization or uncertainty, amniocentesis may be performed for amniotic fluid α-fetoprotein and acetylcholinesterase. In a population of 1000 pregnant women undergoing MSAFP screening, 50 will have a single elevated MSAFP, and of those 50, 1 to 2 will ultimately prove to have a neural tube defect. Women with elevated MSAFP values whose fetuses do not have neural tube defects are still at increased risk for other obstetric complications compared with women with normal MSAFP values. These women have a higher incidence of intrauterine growth retardation, fetal demise, preterm labor, and placental abruption.

In 1984, Merkatz et al. (7) made the fortuitous observation that low MSAFP values were associated with an increased risk of Down's syndrome. This is an important breakthrough because screening for Down's syndrome by amniocentesis is generally offered only to women greater than 35 years of age. Although this group is clearly at increased risk, 80% of Down's syndrome infants are born to women younger than age 35 because of the age distribution of pregnant women (8). There is a wide overlap in the distribution of MSAFP in normal and Down's syndrome pregnancies, although serum values lower than 0.4 multiples of the median significantly increase the risk of Down's syndrome. Rather than using a precise cutoff to separate normal from abnormal, the patient's age-related risk of Down's syndrome is adjusted based on her MSAFP. Amniocentesis is then offered to those women whose individual risk is the same or greater than that of a 35-year-old gravida (i.e., approximately 1 in 270). This approach has resulted in amniocentesis being offered to approximately 5% of pregnant women under age 35 and identifies about 25% of the cases of Down's syndrome occurring in this population (9).

Others reported that elevated maternal serum human chorionic gonadotropin (MShCG) and low maternal serum unconjugated estriol (MSE_3) are also associated with an increased risk of Down's syndrome (10, 11). In 1988, Wald et al. (12) proposed combining MSAFP, MShCG, MSE_3, and maternal age to predict the risk of Down's syndrome. This approach has been referred to as multiple marker or triple screen testing. Approximately 6.0 to 7.2% of pregnant women screened have an abnormal result in all three markers. After correction for gestational age and multiple gestation by ultrasound, 3.2 to 4.1% of women have been offered an amniocentesis, and 57 to 91% of cases of Down's syndrome have been identified (13–15). In some women, all three markers are decreased and have been found to be at increased risk for fetal trisomy 18 (16). Individuals with abnormal multiple marker results subsequently found to have fetuses with normal karyotypes are at increased risk for premature labor and intrauterine growth restriction (17). The use of two markers instead of three or other chemical markers has been reported, but this is not as widely accepted. In addition, further studies are required to evaluate their accuracy and cost efficiency.

Presently, multiple marker testing should be offered to all gravidas under 35 years old on a voluntary basis. The patient should be informed that the testing is for *screening* for an increased risk of a neural tube defect, Down's syndrome, or trisomy 18. It should be made clear that these tests are not diagnostic of these conditions. The possible need for further testing should be introduced and discussed as well. To date, this approach has not been applied to a large number of women greater than age 35. Chromosomal abnormalities are more common in this age group, and a maternal serum screen is less likely to detect chromosomal abnormalities than amniocentesis or chorionic villus sampling. As a result, most authorities do not recommend the triple screen for Down's syndrome screening in women over age 35. It may be offered, however, to those women who are unwilling to accept the risk of an invasive procedure or who wish to have additional information before making a decision regarding amniocentesis or chorionic villus sampling (18).

Screening for Disorders of Hemoglobin Formation

Initial attempts at screening for hemoglobin disorders in the United States were largely confined to the use of solubility tests such as the Sickledex for the detection of hemoglobin S. The ever-widening ethnic diversity of the American population and the resultant presence of other abnormalities of hemoglobin formation have led to the realization that this alone is no longer appropriate (19). Although a complete discussion of hemoglobin disorders is beyond the scope of this chapter, women at risk (as defined in Table 4.4) should be screened with a complete blood count with red blood cell indices. Individuals of Asian or Mediterranean descent who are found to have a hemoglobin level less than 11 g/dL, a mean corpuscular volume less than 80 fl, or a mean

TABLE 4.4. Screening for Disorders of Hemoglobin Formation

GROUPS AT RISK
Couples of African, Asian, or Mediterranean descent

TESTING
All at-risk patients should be screened
If of African descent, perform hemoglobin electrophoresis.
If of Asian or Mediterranean descent, check complete blood count with red blood
    cell indices.
  If microcytic, hypochromic anemia with normal iron stores, perform
    hemoglobin electrophoresis.

Hemoglobin electrophoresis abnormal in mother
Test the father of the fetus with hemoglobin electrophoresis.
  If father's hemoglobin electrophoresis is also abnormal, offer amniocentesis or
    chorionic villus sampling for fetal diagnosis.
  If father's test is normal, no further testing.

Hemoglobin electrophoresis normal in mother
If mother is of African or Mediterranean descent, no further testing.
If mother is of Asian descent, DNA testing of mother for α-globulin abnormalities.
  If mother's DNA test is positive, test DNA of father for a α-globulin abnormalities.
  If father's DNA test is positive, offer amniocentesis or chorionic villus sampling
    for fetal diagnosis.

corpuscular hemoglobin less than 27% with normal iron stores and women of African descent should undergo a hemoglobin electrophoresis. If they are found to have hemoglobin AS, AC, SS, SC, other abnormal hemoglobins, or hemoglobin A_2 more than 3.5%, their partner should be tested to rule out an abnormality of hemoglobin formation. If no hemoglobinopathy is detected and the woman is of Asian descent, DNA testing for α-globin abnormalities should be performed. If the patient is found to have α-thalassemia, her partner should be tested to determine if he is positive for α-thalassemia. If the couple is found to be at risk for α-thalassemia or if a woman is found to be at risk and her partner refuses to be tested, prenatal diagnosis by amniocentesis or chorionic villus sampling for DNA analysis should be offered (19, 20).

Screening for Tay-Sachs Disease

Tay-Sachs disease is an autosomal recessive disorder caused by a deficiency of the hex-A form of the enzyme hexosaminidase. This abnormality leads to a lysosomal storage disorder with the accumulation of GM_2 gangliosides in the central nervous system, resulting in severe neurologic disease and death in early childhood. Individuals of Eastern European Jewish descent (Ashkenazi) have been reported to have a carrier frequency of 1 in 30. The carrier frequency in the non-Jewish population has been found to be 1 in 150 to 300. People of French-Canadian and Cajun descent also have been reported to have elevated carrier frequencies (21, 22).

In the nonpregnant state and in the absence of oral contraceptive use, carrier screening is performed on serum. Serum assays should not be used during pregnancy or while consuming oral contraceptives because they may falsely classify the woman as a carrier (23). Screening must be done on leukocytes. Most laboratories report hex-A levels as a percentage of hexosaminidase activity. The hex-A activity in noncarriers is generally more than 60% and in carriers is usually less than 55% (24).

DNA testing of the α-subunit gene for Tay-Sachs disease is also available but should be reserved for couples who consistently have inconclusive results on serum and leukocyte testing (23).

Recently, the American College of Obstetricians and Gynecologists (ACOG) has recommended serum screening of couples from high-risk groups or with a positive family history. If only one member of the couple is at high risk, he or she should be screened and the partner tested only if the screen is positive. Ambiguous results or positive tests in individuals not at high risk should be confirmed by molecular analysis. If both members of a couple test positive, genetic counseling and prenatal diagnosis should be offered (23).

Screening for Other Metabolic Disorders

During the past decade, the proliferation of molecular biology has made it possible to screen for a myriad of genetic disorders. Usually, either direct DNA analysis or linkage analysis by restriction fragment length is used. At present, such testing is usually offered only to couples with a positive family history of inherited disease, including cystic fibrosis, Duchenne muscular dystrophy, α- and β-thalassemia, most forms of hemophilia, Huntington's chorea, adrenal 21-hydroxylase deficiency, and adult-onset polycystic kidney disease. However, physicians must be cognizant that the same clinical disease may be manifested by individuals with a large number of different mutations. This makes screening technically difficult and less than 100% accurate. Formal genetic counseling should always precede such screening. Obstetricians usually enlist the aid of geneticists or genetic counselors to assist with the care of these families.

INVASIVE PROCEDURES FOR FETAL DIAGNOSIS

Indications for amniocentesis and chorionic villus sampling include advanced maternal or paternal age, parental chromosomal defect, previous child with a chromosomal abnormality, previous stillborn or abortus that did not receive chromosomal analysis, and exposure to radiation or chemotherapy in first or early second trimester (Table 4.5).

Amniocentesis

The clinical use of second-trimester amniocentesis became widespread during the latter 1970s and early 1980s. Several collaborative studies suggested that the period of 15 to 17 weeks after the last menstrual period is the safest gestational age and a 20- to 22-gauge needle is optimal (24–27). The fetal loss rate appears to be approximately 0.5% higher among women who underwent amniocentesis than among control subjects in the American and Canadian trials (25, 26). It was 1.6% higher in

TABLE 4.5. Indications for Prenatal Cytogenetic Studies

Advanced maternal age (≥35 years of age at time of child birth)
Advanced paternal age (≥40 years of age)
Parental translocation, inversion, or aneuploidy
Previous child with a chromosomal abnormality
Previous stillborn or abortus that did not receive chromosomal analysis
Exposure to radiation or chemotherapeutic agents in first and/or early second trimester

a large British-European trial (27). However, it was subsequently recognized that in the latter study, a higher percentage of the procedures were performed because of an elevated MSAFP, which carries an inherently higher risk for pregnancy loss. After correction for this factor, the loss rate in the British-European report was similar to those observed in the other large national studies (25). Approximately 1% of women experience temporary bleeding, leakage of amniotic fluid, or cramping after the procedure. Infection rates are less than 1% (25–27).

Midtrimester amniocentesis is usually performed with real-time ultrasound guidance to allow simultaneous visualization of needle placement and evaluation of the fetus. Some clinicians prefer the "free-hand" technique, whereas others prefer to use a transducer-attached fixed "needle guide." There have not been any large studies to evaluate the benefit of one technique over the other. Most studies are carried out for cytogenetic diagnosis because the mother is greater than 35 years old, there is an increased risk of Down's syndrome on the basis of multiple marker testing, or a structural anomaly has been detected on ultrasound. The diagnostic accuracy of amniocentesis is over 99%, and culture failures are rare (25–27). Results are usually available within 2 weeks. Some laboratories report results more rapidly.

Another common indication for amniocentesis is to determine amniotic fluid α-fetoprotein and acetylcholinesterase levels as part of an evaluation for a neural tube defect. This usually occurs when there is an abnormally elevated MSAFP with no identifiable etiology or when there is an inconclusive ultrasound diagnosis of neural tube defect. This indication has become less frequent as experience with ultrasound increases (28). Because the level of α-fetoprotein is substantially higher in fetal blood, contamination of the specimen with minute amounts of fetal blood may result in spuriously elevated results. This can be avoided by testing the fluid for hemoglobin and acetylcholinesterase. Acetylcholinesterase is present in the amniotic fluid of all pregnancies affected by neural tube defects where no skin covers the defect. If the specimen is positive for hemoglobin, negative for acetylcholinesterase, and there are no clearly abnormal ultrasound findings, it can be assumed to be falsely positive. In the absence of hemoglobin and acetylcholinesterase, other causes of elevated amniotic α-fetoprotein such as abdominal wall defects, dermatologic disorders, or Finnish nephrosis should be considered.

To facilitate earlier prenatal diagnosis, several groups studied the use of early amniocentesis (i.e., at 11 to 14 weeks after the last menstrual period). Pregnancy loss rates ranged from 1.5 to 3.3% (29–34). Given the varying gestational ages at which the procedures have been performed, the lack of control groups, and so on, it is somewhat difficult to place these data in perspective. Some authors expressed the opinion that the procedure is quite safe, others suggested that it is riskier than midtrimester amniocentesis, and still others called for a randomized trial to further evaluate the issue (29–34). The diagnostic accuracy associated with this technique appears to be high, and the false mosaicism that can be seen with chorionic villus sampling is exceptionally rare (35). Some authors expressed the opinion that the procedure is technically more difficult before 12 weeks, but most believe that if a physician has prior experience with midtrimester amniocentesis, it is easier to perform early amniocentesis than chorionic villus sampling. Although there are limitations to the current state of knowledge, early amniocentesis appears to be a reasonable alternative for those women desiring early diagnosis.

Chorionic Villus Sampling

In the latter 1980s, chorionic villus sampling was developed as a technique to facilitate prenatal diagnosis in the late first or early second trimesters (36, 37). Chorionic villi are derived from the same embryonic origin as the fetus and therefore reflect the genetic status of the fetus. They may be sampled by a transcervical, transabdominal, or transvaginal approach, although the latter is rarely used. The transvaginal approach is used for posterior placentas and/or a retroflexed uterus and is done with a spinal needle. In the transcervical approach, the specimen is obtained by placing a catheter through an aseptically prepared cervix and aspirating the villi. The transabdominal approach is similar to amniocentesis, but the needle is directed into the placenta. Transcervical and transabdominal approaches have been reported to be approximately equal in risk (38, 39). Some investigators believe the abdominal approach is technically easier and better accepted by patients because it is less uncomfortable (39). The safety and diagnostic accuracy of transcervical chorionic villus sampling have been evaluated in several individual centers and on a more widespread basis in two large American and Canadian multicenter trials (35, 38, 40).

Cytogenetic diagnosis has been obtained in approximately 98% of women. Approximately 1% of patients require repeat chorionic villus sampling or midtrimester amniocentesis because of unusual mosaicism, culture failure, or contamination (41). Cramping and spotting after the procedure are relatively common, but significant maternal infection or other serious complications have been very rare (35–37). The pregnancy loss rate—including elective terminations because of abnormal results, spontaneous abortions, stillborns, and neonatal deaths—has been reported as 0.6 to 0.8% higher than that found among women undergoing midtrimester amniocentesis, although this is not statistically significant (35, 36).

In the early 1990s, a number of authors reported clusters of infants with limb reductions after chorionic villus sampling (42–44). A workshop sponsored by the National Institute of Child Health and Development and ACOG concluded that there did appear to be an association of oromandibular-limb hypogenesis with chorionic villus sampling. This association was thought to be stronger with procedures performed before 10 weeks gestation, and opinion was divided regarding procedures performed between 10 and 12 weeks gestation (45). Subsequent to this workshop, a large American case-control study showed no overall increased risk of limb reduction, but there was an increased risk of transverse digital deficiency (46). A multinational World Health Organization study involving 138,996 infants born after chorionic villus sampling showed no increase in limb disorders (47). ACOG has concluded that chorionic villus sampling is relatively safe and accurate but has recommended that until further information is available, it should not be performed before 10 weeks gestation and that there may be a risk of transverse digital deficiency on the order of 1 in 3000 (37). Indications for chorionic villus sampling are very similar to those previously discussed for amniocentesis. However, α-fetoprotein levels can not be determined by this method, and because methylation patterns are different in chorionic villi and fetuses, chorionic villus sampling is also not an appropriate modality for the evaluation of fragile X syndrome (48, 49).

Other Invasive Techniques

When an anomaly is detected later in pregnancy, cordocentesis or funipuncture is a rapid technique to obtain fetal blood for karyotype or other testing. In most instances, this technique is used after 20 weeks gestation. Before that gestation, it is technically more difficult to perform because of the small cord size. During cordocentesis, a needle is inserted transabdominally into the umbilical vein. Blood is aspirated and rapidly tested using either the Kleihauer-Betke test or determining the mean corpuscular value to ensure that it is fetal blood. Indications for cordocentesis include the need for a rapid karyotype or DNA analysis, determination of fetal blood type, fetal hemoglobin level, fetal platelet count, and/or for evaluation of infection such as cytomegalovirus or toxoplasmosis. A 98% success rate has been reported when cordocentesis is performed. The risk of fetal loss as a result of the procedure is approximately 0.5 to 1% (50). However, the risk has been found to be substantially higher if the fetus is extremely hydropic or thrombocytopenic (51).

Nicolini et al. (52) suggested an alternative technique of obtaining fetal blood from the hepatic vein. In their report, 91.1% of the fetuses were successfully sampled (unfortunately, the success rate in the control subjects undergoing cordocentesis of the umbilical vein was not described), and procedure-related fetal loss rate was low. Others described the use of cardiocentesis (i.e., insertion of a needle into the fetal heart to sample fetal blood). This procedure appears to carry a fetal loss rate of 5.6 to 6.5%. The authors suggested that it should be offered in highly selected cases when a high probability of fetal hemoglobinopathy exists and when cordocentesis is not technically possible (53). At the present time, experience with the last two techniques is limited to a few centers.

There are a few hereditary fetal skin conditions that require analysis of fetal tissue for diagnosis. Originally, this was accomplished by fetoscopy, but this procedure is associated with a relatively high fetal loss rate. Recently, the use of ultrasound-guided fetal skin sampling was reported (54). The authors reported a high rate of success and no fetal complications in a relatively small sample.

ULTRASOUND

A detailed description of the use of ultrasound to establish prenatal genetic diagnosis far exceeds the limitations of this chapter. The following comments are intended to provide the reader with a brief overview of the general scanning technique and to discuss a few of the more common indications for targeted ultrasound (Table 4.6).

During prenatal ultrasound, attention should be directed not only to growth, but also toward anatomy. The skull should be evaluated to rule out anencephaly, to look for frontal notching (the so-called "lemon sign"), and to determine if an encephalocele (an extrusion of brain tissue through a skull defect) is present (55, 56). Identification of a cystic hygroma, nuchal fold thickening (more than 5 mm), nuchal band, or choroid plexus cyst(s) may be indications of a chromosomal abnormality (56). An attempt should be made to visualize the face to rule out abnormal ocular dimensions or clefts that may suggest more complex congenital or chromosomal anomalies (57). The brain should be evaluated with attention to the width of the lateral, third, and fourth ventricles to rule out ventriculomegaly. This may be associated with infection, a wide variety of congenital syndromes, and/or chromosomal abnormalities. The shape of the cerebellum should be determined. A narrow crescent shape (the so-called "banana sign") may suggest a neural tube defect. The presence of an abnormally wide cisterna magna may suggest a chromosomal problem (56).

The chest and abdominal walls should be visualized to determine if they are intact and to rule out abdominal wall defects such as gastroschisis or omphalocele (58). Many cardiac malformations may be detected by evaluation of the heart, particularly the more severe defects. An attempt should be made to visualize all four cardiac chambers, their relative size and relationship to each other, and the motion of the cardiac valves (59). Evaluation of the aortic root in addition to the four chambers, a so-called five-chamber view, may improve the sensitivity for detecting malformations (60). The cardiac axis should be determined. Left axis deviation of greater than 75° is associated with a high rate of both cardiac and extracardiac anomalies (61). The diaphragm should be visualized to determine if it is intact. Defects or

TABLE 4.6. Common Conditions Amenable to Screening with Ultrasound

NEURAL TUBE DEFECTS
Meningomyelocele
Anencephaly
Encephalocele
Ventriculomegaly
Intracranial hemorrhage
Other structural anomalies

CARDIAC
Structural abnormalities
Arrhythmias
Pericardial effusion

CHEST
Diaphragmatic hernia
Cystic adenomatoid malformation (hamartoma)
Pleural effusion
Pulmonary sequestration

ABDOMINAL WALL DEFECTS
Gastroschisis
Omphalocele

GASTROINTESTINAL
Duodenal atresia
Bowel obstruction
Meconium ileus and peritonitis
Ascites

GENITOURINARY
Vesicoureteral reflux or obstruction
Bladder outlet obstruction
Polycystic kidney disease
Renal agenesis

SKELETAL
Skeletal dysplasias
Hypomineralization disorders
Fractures

abdominal contents in the chest suggest a diaphragmatic hernia (62). The stomach should be visualized to determine that it is on the left side, normal in size, and that there is no "double bubble" sign that may indicate duodenal atresia. Dilated loops of bowel may suggest obstruction. Hyperechoic bowel, which is as acoustically dense as the surrounding bone, may be associated with chromosomal abnormalities or cystic fibrosis (63).

The bladder should be identified. If absent, it may be a sign of renal dysfunction. If abnormally large, it should be observed for emptying to rule out bladder outlet obstruction. The location, size, shape, and acoustic consistency of the kidneys should also be evaluated. Significant dilation of the central renal collecting system suggests vesicoureteral reflux or obstruction. If the dilation is bilateral, the ureters are bilaterally dilated, and this is accompanied by an enlarged, thickened bladder, one should consider the possibility of bladder outlet obstruction (64, 65).

The skeleton should be examined to determine the degree of mineralization, size, and shapes of various bones to rule out skeletal dysplasias and hypomineralization states (66).

If anomalies are suspected, the patient should be referred to a center experienced in the evaluation of fetal anatomic defects for targeted ultrasound examination, also called a level II ultrasound (67). Depending on the specific anomaly identified, patients are often offered amniocentesis or cordocentesis to rule out a chromosomal disorder. Additional testing with DNA analysis or biochemical evaluation may also be done. It is important to recognize that even very experienced ultrasonographers have not been able to recognize all anomalies, and patients should be counseled about this.

The effect of routine ultrasound on the diagnosis of congenital anomalies among a large population of low-risk patients has been evaluated in the Routine Antenatal Diagnostic Imaging with Ultrasound study (68). Among the women randomized to routine ultrasound, 35% of anomalous fetuses were identified versus 11% among the control subjects. There was no significant effect, however, on the rate of therapeutic abortion or survival among infants with potentially treatable anomalies (68). Because of this, the authors concluded that routine ultrasound could not be justified using these grounds. Others questioned this conclusion and continue to advocate routine ultrasound.

One of the most common indications for targeted ultrasound is evaluation of an elevated MSAFP (55). Ultrasonographic examination of the skull has been reported to rule out anencephaly with nearly 100% accuracy when performed using standard sonographic techniques after 14 weeks gestation (69, 70). Nicolaides et al. (56) determined that a very high proportion of fetuses with spina bifida can be identified by cranial abnormalities, including a biparietal diameter that is small for gestational age, ventriculomegaly, presence of a lemon sign, obliteration of the cisterna magna, and/or presence of a banana sign. Careful attention should be directed to the spine on lateral views to determine that it is parallel and on transverse cuts to rule out a protruding sac or splaying of the posterior ossific centers. Negative findings have been reported to reduce the risk of a neural tube defect by at least 95% (56, 67).

When the ultrasound examination is complete, the patient should be counseled regarding the clinical findings, the statistical observations outlined above, and the prognosis for any defects that have been detected. She can then make decisions as to whether or not she wishes to undergo amniocentesis for further evaluation, continue the pregnancy, or consider termination. In the absence of abnormal ultrasound findings, it is wise to counsel the patient about rare dermatologic and renal problems that may not be detected on ultrasound. More importantly, she should be counseled about the increased risk of preterm delivery and intrauterine growth restriction associated with an elevated MSAFP (17).

Women are frequently referred for ultrasound as an adjunct to amniocentesis for advanced maternal age or when multiple marker testing reveals an increased risk of aneuploidy. Several second-trimester ultrasound findings have been reported to improve the detection of fetuses with Down's syndrome, including nuchal thickening, a short femur, a short humerus, pyelectasis, echogenic bowel, choroid plexus cysts, a hypoplastic middle phalanx of the fifth digit, a wide space between the first and second toe, a two-vessel umbilical cord, and shortened long bones in relation to the biparietal diameter (71, 72). Some authors suggested that a normal genetic ultrasound can be used to recalculate the risk for having a fetus with Down's syndrome (73). Although their work is extremely promising, others found a normal scan to be less reassuring (74). Additionally, there has not been a great deal of experience with this technique in the general obstetric community. Currently, ACOG does not advocate ultrasound as a reliable screen for Down's syndrome.

Patients are referred for targeted examination because of suspected renal malformations on the basis of oligohydramnios or a family history of genetically transmitted kidney disease. Examination should be performed as outlined above. Unilateral vesicoureteral reflux or obstruction or bilateral reflux with normal bladder function and amniotic fluid has generally been associated with good outcome, and most authorities recommend conservative observation to term (64). Women whose fetuses are found to have bladder outlet obstruction should be referred to a center with experience in the evaluation of fetal renal function and shunting procedures. Most fetuses with infantile polycystic kidney disease have been recognized by mid-pregnancy because of the development of oligohydramnios. They, and other fetuses with early onset oligohydramnios, have a very poor prognosis because of associated pulmonary hypoplasia (64).

Known or suspected abdominal wall defects may be referred for level II sonography. Patients with omphalocele have relatively high rates of abnormal karyotypes and should be offered amniocentesis or cordocentesis for chromosomal analysis (75). Infants with gastroschisis, however, have low rates of karyotypic abnormalities and, unless other malformations are present, do not require invasive testing. Generally, patients with either of these defects are followed conservatively to term. High rates of preterm labor and birth have been reported with both anomalies. There has been considerable controversy regarding the proper mode of delivery (58). At present, the trend has been toward vaginal delivery.

CLINICAL NOTES

History and Counseling

- A family pedigree should be constructed in the initial genetic/teratogenic historical intake.
- Ethnic origin should be determined because certain groups are at increased risk for specific problems.
- The age of *both* parents is important in assessing for fetal genetic risk(s).
- Maternal diseases should be listed because some (e.g., diabetes, phenylketonuria) may be associated with fetal malformation or dysfunction.

Multiple Marker Testing

- The baseline risk for a neural tube defect in the United States is one to two per 1000 live births. Most (90%) of all neural tube defects occur in families with no previous history. With one affected first-degree relative, the risk of neural tube defect is elevated 10-fold.
- MSAFP is used to screen for neural tube defects, with the most accurate sampling being done between 16 and 18 weeks gestation.
- Three to 4% of the population will have an elevated MSAFP that may or may not be associated with neural tube defect. If the elevation is less than 3.0 multiples of the median and the gestational age is less than18 weeks, the sample is repeated. If the elevation is at least 3.0 multiples of the median, gestational age more than 18 weeks, or the second sample is elevated, the patient is referred for ultrasound.
- A low MSAFP is associated with an increased risk of Down's syndrome. A low MSAFP should *not* be repeated; the patient should be referred for counseling if the patient's risk of Down's syndrome (based on the MSAFP) is the same or greater than that of a 35-year-old woman.

- Three markers have been used to enhance the ability to screen for Down's syndrome, neural tube defect, and trisomy 18 in women under 35 years. Women over 35 should be offered amniocentesis.
- Pregnant women of Asian or Mediterranean descent with microcytic, hypochromic anemia in the presence of normal iron stores should undergo hemoglobin electrophoresis to rule out hemoglobinopathy. Pregnant women of African descent should undergo hemoglobin electrophoresis to rule out hemoglobinopathy.
- In the nonpregnant state, screening for Tay-Sachs disease is performed on serum. If the woman is using oral contraceptives or is pregnant, screening is performed using leukocytes.

Amniocentesis

- The safest gestational age for amniocentesis is 15 to 17 weeks and a 20- to 22-gauge needle is optimal. Approximately 1% of women experience temporary bleeding, leakage of amniotic fluid, or cramping after amniocentesis. Infection rates are less than 1%.
- Early amniocentesis (i.e., between 11 and 14 weeks gestation) is associated with a pregnancy loss rate of 1.5 to 3.3%.

Chorionic Villus Sampling

- The pregnancy loss rate after chorionic villus sampling is not statistically significantly higher than that seen with midtrimester amniocentesis. Cramping and spotting after chorionic villus sampling are common, and infection is rare.
- ACOG views chorionic villus sampling as a relatively safe and accurate procedure but recommends it not be done before 10 weeks gestation because there may be risk of transverse digital deficiency.

Known or Suspected Human Teratogens (Pregnancy Category D or X)

DRUGS

Acne preparations
Etretinate
Isotretinoin

Amebicidal
Carbarsone

Antibacterial
Kanamycin
Streptomycin
Sulfonamides
Tetracyclines
Tobramycin

Anticoagulants
Anisindione
Coumarin derivatives
Diphenadione
Ethyl biscoumacetate
Nicoumalone
Phenindione
Phenprocoumon
Warfarin

Anticonvulsants
Aminoglutethimide
Bromides
Ethotoin
Mephobarbital
Paramethadione
Phenobarbital
Phensuximide
Phenytoin
Primidone
Trimethadione
Valproic acid

Antidepressants
Amitriptyline
Butriptyline
Clomipramine
Dibenzepin
Dothiepin
Imipramine
Iprindole
Nortriptyline
Opipramol

Antidiabetic agents
Acetohexamide
Chlorpropamide
Tolazamide
Tolbutamide

Antihypertensives
ACE inhibitors
Reserpine

Antimalarial
Quinine

Antimanics (bimodal)
Lithium

Antineoplastics
Aminopterin
Azathioprine
Bleomycin
Busulfan
Chlorambucil
Cisplatin
Cyclophosphamide
Cytarabine
Daunorubicin
Doxorubicin
Fluorouracil
Mechlorethamine
Melphalan
Mercaptopurine
Methotrexate
Mithramycin
Procarbazine
Teniposide
Thioguanine
Thiotepa
Vinblastine
Vincristine

Antithyroid agents
Carbimazole
I[131]
Methimazole
Propylthiouracil

Autonomic, sympathomimetics (adrenergic)
Levarterenol
Metaraminol

Methoxamine

Diagnostic agents
Diatrizoate
Ethiodized oil
[125]I
[131]I
Iocetamic acid
Iodamide
Iodipamide
Iodoxamate
Iopanoic acid
Iothalamate
Ipodate
Metrizamide
Tyropanoate

Diuretics
Benzthiazide
Chlorothiazide
Chlorthalidone
Cyclopenthiazide
Cyclothiazide
Ethacrynic acid
Hydrochlorothiazide
Hydroflumethiazide
Methyclothiazide
Metolazone
Polythiazide
Quinethazone
Spironolactone
Triamterene
Trichlormethiazide

Expectorants
Hydriodic acid
Potassium iodide
Sodium iodide

Heavy metal antagonists
Penicillamine

Hormones
Chlorotrianisene
Clomiphene
Cortisone
Danazol
Dienestrol

Diethylstilbestrol
Ethisterone
Ethynodiol
Hydroxyprogesterone
Lynestrenol
Medroxyprogesterone
Norethindrone
Norethynodrel
Norgestrel

Narcotic antagonists
Cyclazocine
Levallorphan
Nalorphine

Sedative/hypnotics
Chlordiazepoxide
Diazepam

Ethanol
Mephobarbital
Meprobamate
Methaqualone
Metharbital
Pentobarbital
Phenobarbital
Secobarbital

Stimulants
Dextroamphetamine

Vaccines
Measles
Mumps
Rubella
Smallpox
Yellow fever

**CHEMICALS AND
OCCUPATIONAL
COMPOUNDS**
Anesthetic gases
Arsenic
Lead
Organic mercury
  compounds
Organic solvents
Polybrominated biphenyls
  (PBBs)
Polychlorinated biphenyls
  (PCBs)
Ionizing radiation

References

1. Cragin E. Conservatism in obstetrics. N Y Med J 1916;104:1.
2. Hook EB. Rates of chromosome abnormalities at different maternal ages. Obstet Gynecol 1981;58:282–285.
3. Friedman JM. Genetic disease in the offspring of older fathers. Obstet Gynecol 1981;57:745–749.
4. Brock DJ, Sutcliffe RG. Alpha-fetoprotein in the antenatal diagnosis of anencephaly and spina bifida. Lancet 1972;2:197–199.
5. Milunsky A, Alpert F, Neff RK, et al. Prenatal diagnosis of neural tube defects. Obstet Gynecol 1980;55:61–66.
6. Wald NJ, Cuckle H, Brock DJ, et al. Maternal-serum-alpha-fetoprotein measurement in antenatal screening for anencephaly and spina bifida early in pregnancy. Report of U.K. collaborative study on alpha-fetoprotein in relation to neural-tube defects. Lancet 1977;1:1323–1332.
7. Merkatz I, Nitowsky HM, Marci JN, et al. An association between low maternal serum alpha-fetoprotein and fetal chromosomal abnormalities. Am J Obstet Gynecol 1984;148:886–894.
8. Adams MM, Erickson JD, Layde PM, et al. Down's syndrome. Recent trends in the United States. JAMA 1981;246:758–760.
9. Combining maternal serum alpha-fetoprotein measurements and age to screen for Down syndrome in pregnant women under age 35. New England Regional Genetics Group Prenatal Collaborative Study on Down Syndrome Screening. Am J Obstet Gynecol 1989;160:575–581.
10. Bogart MH, Pandian MR, Jones OW. Abnormal maternal serum chorionic gonadotropin levels in pregnancies with fetal chromosome abnormalities. Prenat Diagn 1987;7:623–630.
11. Canick JA, Knight GJ, Palomaki GE, et al. Low second trimester maternal serum unconjugated oestriol in pregnancies with Down's syndrome in early pregnancy. Br J Obstet Gynaecol 1988;95:330–333.
12. Wald NJ, Cuckle HS, Densem JW, et al. Maternal serum screening for Down's syndrome in early pregnancy. BMJ 1988;287:883–887.
13. Phillips OP, Elias S, Shulman LP, et al. Maternal serum screening for fetal Down syndrome in women less than 35 years of age using alpha-fetoprotein, hCG and unconjugated estriol: a prospective 2-year study. Obstet Gynecol 1992;80:353–358.
14. Haddow JE, Palomaki GE, Knight GJ, et al. Prenatal screening for Down's syndrome with the use of maternal serum markers. N Engl J Med 1992;327:588–593.
15. Cheng EY, Luthy DA, Zebelman AM, et al. A prospective evaluation of a second-trimester screening test for fetal Down syndrome using maternal serum alpha-fetoprotein, hCG, and unconjugated estriol. Obstet Gynecol 1993;81:72–77.
16. Canick JA, Palomaki GE, Osathanondh R. Prenatal screening for trisomy 18 in the second trimester. Prenat Diagn 1990;10:546–548.
17. Crandall BF, Robinson L, Grau P. Risk associated with an elevated maternal serum α-fetoprotein level. Am J Obstet Gynecol 1991;165:581–586.
18. Maternal serum screening. ACOG Educ Bull 1996;228.
19. Hemoglobinopathies in pregnancy. ACOG Tech Bull 1996;220.
20. Stein J, Berg C, Jones J, et al. A screening protocol for a prenatal population at risk for inherited hemoglobin disorders: results of its application to a group of southeast Asians and blacks. Am J Obstet Gynecol 1984;150:333–341.
21. Hechtman P, Kaplan F, Bayleran J, et al. More than one mutant allele causes infantile Tay-Sachs disease in French-Canadians. Am J Hum Genet 1990;47:815–822.
22. McDowell GA, Mules EH, Fabacher P, et al. The presence of two different infantile Tay-Sachs disease mutations in a Cajun population. Am J Hum Genet 1992;51:1071–1077.

23. American College of Obstetricians and Gynecologists. Screening for Tay-Sachs Disease. ACOG Committee Opinion 162. Washington, DC: ACOG, 1995.

24. Kaback M, Lim-Steele J, Dabholkar D, et al. Tay-Sachs disease—carrier screening, prenatal diagnosis, and the molecular era. An international perspective, 1970 to 1993. The International TSD Data Collection Network. JAMA 1993;270:2307–2315.

25. National Institute of Child Health and Human Development, National Registry of Amniocentesis Study Group. Mid-trimester amniocentesis for prenatal diagnosis: safety and accuracy. JAMA 1976;236:1471–1476.

26. Medical Research Council. Diagnosis of Genetic Disease by Amniocentesis During the Second Trimester of Pregnancy. Ottawa, Canada: Medical Research Council, 1977.

27. An assessment of the hazards of amniocentesis: report to the Medical Research Council by their Working Party on Amniocentesis. Br J Obstet Gynaecol 1978;85(suppl 2): 1–41.

28. Richards DS, Seeds JW, Katz VL, et al. Elevated maternal serum alpha-fetoprotein with normal ultrasound: is amniocentesis always appropriate? A review of 26,069 screened patients. Obstet Gynecol 1988;71:203–207.

29. Penso CA, Sandstrom MM, Garber MF, et al. Early amniocentesis: report of 407 cases with neonatal follow-up. Obstet Gynecol 1990;76:1032–1036.

30. Hanson PW, Happ RL, Tennant FR, et al. Ultrasonography-guided early amniocentesis in singleton pregnancies. Am J Obstet Gynecol 1990;162:1376–1383.

31. Nevin J, Nevin NC, Dorman JC, et al. Early amniocentesis: experience of 222 consecutive patients, 1987–88. Prenat Diagn 1990;10:79–83.

32. Hanson PW, Happ RL, Tennant FR, et al. Early amniocentesis: outcome, risk, and technical problems at ≤12.8 weeks. Am J Obstet Gynecol 1992;166:1707–1711.

33. Henry GP, Miller WA. Early amniocentesis. J Reprod Med 1992;37:396–402.

34. Assel BG, Lewis SM, Dickerman LH, et al. Single-operator comparison of early and mid-second-trimester amniocentesis. Obstet Gynecol 1992;79:940–944.

35. Canadian Collaborative CVS-Amniocentesis Clinical Trial Group. Multicenter, randomized trial of chorionic villus sampling and amniocentesis. Lancet 1989;1:1–16.

36. Rhoads CG, Jackson LG, Schlesselman, et al. The safety and efficacy of chorionic villus sampling for early prenatal diagnosis of cytogenetic abnormalities. N Engl J Med 1989; 340:609–617.

37. American College of Obstetricians and Gynecologists. Chorionic Villus Sampling. ACOG Committee Opinion 160. Washington, DC: ACOG, 1995.

38. Jackson LG, Zachary JM, Fowler SE, et al. A randomized comparison of transcervical and transabdominal chorionic-villus sampling. The U.S. National Institute of Child Health and Human Development Chorionic-Villus Sampling and Amniocentesis Study Group. N Engl J Med 1992;327:594–598.

39. Hallack M, Johnson MP, Pryde PG, et al. Chorionic villus sampling: transabdominal versus transcervical approach in more than 4000 cases. Obstet Gynecol 1992;80:349–352.

40. Deleted in proof.

41. Ledbetter DH, Maring AO, Verlinsky Y, et al. Cytogenetic results of chorionic villus sampling: high success rate and diagnostic accuracy in the United States Collaborative Study. Am J Obstet Gynecol 1990;162:495–501.

42. Firth HV, Boyd PA, Chamberlain P, et al. Severe limb abnormalities after chorion villus sampling at 56–66 days' gestation. Lancet 1991;337:762–763.

43. Burton BK, Schulz CJ, Burd LI. Limb anomalies associated with chorionic villus sampling. Obstet Gynecol 1992;79:726–730.

44. Brambsati B, Simoni G, Travi M, et al. Genetic diagnosis by chorionic villus sampling before 8 gestational weeks: efficiency, reliability, and risks on 317 completed pregnancies. Prenat Diagn 1992;12:789–799.

45. Holmes LB. Report of National Institute of Child Health and Human Development Workshop on Chorionic Villus Sampling and Limb and Other Defects, October 20, 1992. Teratology 1993;48:7–13.

46. Olney RS, Khoury MJ, Alo CJ, et al. Increased risk for transverse digital deficiency after

chorionic villus sampling. Results of the United States multistate case-control study, 1988–1992. Teratology 1995;51:20–29.

47. Kuliev A, Jackson L, Froster U, et al. Chorionic villus sampling safety. Report to the World Health Organization/Euro meeting in association with the Seventh International Conference on Early Prenatal Diagnosis of Genetic Diseases, Tel-Aviv, Israel, May 21, 1994. Am J Obstet Gynecol 1996;174:807–811.

48. Maddalena A, Hicks BD, Spence WC, et al. Prenatal diagnosis in known fragile X carriers. Am J Med Genet 1994;51:490–496.

49. Strain L, Porteous ME, Gosden CM, et al. Prenatal diagnosis of fragile X syndrome: management of the male fetus with a permutation. Prenat Diagn 1994;14:469–474.

50. Nicolaides KH. Cordocentesis. Clin Obstet Gynecol 1988;311:123–125.

51. Paidas MJ, Berkowitz RL, Lynch L, et al. Alloimmune thrombocytopenia: fetal and neonatal losses related to cordocentesis. Am J Obstet Gynecol 1995;172:475–479.

52. Nicolini U, Nicolaides P, Fisk NM, et al. Fetal blood sampling from the intrahepatic vein: analysis of safety and clinical experience with 214 procedures. Obstet Gynecol 1990;76:47–53.

53. Antaklis AI, Papantantoniou NE, Mesgitis SA, et al. Cardiocentesis: an alternative method of fetal blood sampling for the prenatal diagnosis of hemoglobinopathies. Obstet Gynecol 1992;79:630–633.

54. Elias S, Emerson D, Simpson JL, et al. Ultrasound-guided fetal skin sampling for prenatal diagnosis of genodermatoses. Obstet Gynecol 1994;83:337–341.

55. Watson WJ, Chescheir NC, Katz VL, et al. The role of ultrasound in evaluation of patients with elevated maternal serum alpha-fetoprotein: a review. Obstet Gynecol 1991;78:123–128.

56. Nicolaides KH, Campbell S, Gabbe SG, et al. Ultrasound screening for spina bifida: cranial and cerebellar signs. Lancet 1986;2:72–74.

57. Hegge FN, Prescott GH, Watson PT. Fetal facial abnormalities identified during obstetric sonography. J Ultrasound Med 1986;5:679–684.

58. Sipes SL, Weiner CP, Sipes DR, et al. Gastroschisis and omphalocele: does either antenatal diagnosis or route of delivery make a difference in prenatal outcome? Obstet Gynecol 1990;76:195–199.

59. Vergani P, Mariani S, Ghidini A, et al. Screening for congenital heart disease with the four-chamber view of the fetal heart. Am J Obstet Gynecol 1992;167:1000–1003.

60. Kirk JS, Riggs TW, Comstock CH, et al. Prenatal screening for cardiac anomalies: the value of routine addition of the aortic root to the four-chamber view. Obstet Gynecol 1994;84:427–431.

61. Smith RS, Comstock CH, Kirk J, et al. Ultrasonographic left cardiac axis deviation: a marker for fetal anomalies. Obstet Gynecol 1995;85:187–191

62. Comstock CH. The antenatal diagnosis of diaphragmatic anomalies. J Ultrasound Med 1986;5:391–396.

63. Corteville JE, Gray DL, Langer JC. Bowel abnormalities in the fetus: correlation of prenatal ultrasonographic findings with outcome. Am J Obstet Gynecol 1996;175:724–729.

64. Callan NA, Blakemore K, Park J, et al. Fetal genitourinary tract anomalies: evaluation, operative correction, and follow-up. Obstet Gynecol 1990;75:67–74.

65. Gunn TR, Mora JD, Pease P. Antenatal diagnosis of urinary tract abnormalities by ultrasonography after 28 weeks' gestation: incidence and outcome. Am J Obstet Gynecol 1995;172:479–486.

66. Sharony R, Browne C, Lachman RS, et al. Prenatal diagnosis of skeletal dysplasias. Am J Obstet Gynecol 1993;169:668–675.

67. Gonclaves LF, Jeanty P, Piper JM. The accuracy of prenatal ultrasonography in detecting congenital anomalies. Am J Obstet Gynecol 1994;171:1606–1612.

68. Crane JP, LeFevre ML, Winborn RC, et al. A randomized trial of prenatal ultrasonographic screening: impact on the detection, management, and outcome of anomalous fetuses. Am J Obstet Gynecol 1994;171:392–399.

69. Goldstein RB, Filly RA, Callen PW. Sonography of anencephaly: pitfalls in early diagnosis. J Clin Ultrasound 1989;17:397–402.

70. Goldstein RB, Filly RA. Prenatal diagnosis of anencephaly: spectrum of sonographic appearances and distinction from the amniotic band syndrome. Am J Roentgenol 1988; 151:547–550.

71. Vintzileos AM, Egan JF, Smulian JC, et al. Adjusting the risk for trisomy 21 by a simple ultrasound method using long fetal long bone biometry. Obstet Gynecol 1996;87: 53–58.

72. Nyberg, DA, Luthy DA, Cheng EY, et al. Role of ultrasonography in woman with positive screen for Down syndrome on the basis of maternal serum markers. Am J Obstet Gynecol 1995;173:1030–1035.

73. Vintzileos AM, Campbell WA, Rodis JF, et al. The use of second-trimester genetic sonogram in guiding clinical management of patients at increased risk for fetal trisomy 21. Obstet Gynecol 1996;87:48–52.

74. Lockwood CJ, Lynch L, Berkowitz RL. Ultrasonographic screening for the Down syndrome fetus. Am J Obstet Gynecol 1991;165:349–352.

75. De Venciana M, Major CA, Porto M. Prediction of an abnormal karyotype in fetuses with omphalocele. Prenat Diagn 1994;14:487–492

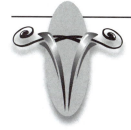

C H A P T E R 5

Early Pregnancy Monitoring

WILLIAM F. ZIEGLER
JOHN R. BRUMSTED

The objective of early pregnancy monitoring is to determine the implantation site and potential for normal development of a pregnancy as soon after conception as possible. This process begins with identifying risk factors that can affect normal embryo migration through the fallopian tube, implantation, and first-trimester development. Understanding the endocrinology of early pregnancy and the structural changes that occur over time is crucial if the practitioner is to differentiate a viable intrauterine pregnancy from an ectopic gestation or a conceptus destined to abort. With appropriate application, the increased sensitivity of hormonal assays and advances in transvaginal sonography enable the physician to make the timely diagnosis of first-trimester disorders, thus minimizing maternal morbidity. This chapter reviews the current use of hormonal assays and ultrasound in identifying early pregnancy disorders and provides treatment protocols in managing these clinical conditions.

EARLY PREGNANCY PHYSIOLOGY

Endocrinology of Early Pregnancy

Human Chorionic Gonadotropin

In early pregnancy, the trophoblastic cells excrete human chorionic gonadotropin (hCG). The hCG level is so specific and sensitive in pregnancy that it provides an excellent marker for the status of an early pregnancy. The primary function of hCG is to rescue the corpus luteum from atresia and prolong the secretion of progesterone, but this response is time limited. It is essential that by the time the corpus luteum ceases functioning, the fetal-placental unit should be established to support the pregnancy through the remainder of gestation.

hCG is a glycoprotein consisting of two noncovalently linked subunits. The α unit contains 92 amino acids that are common to other glycoprotein hormones: luteinizing hormone, follicle-stimulating hormone, and thyrotropin-stimulating hormone. The specificity of hCG is primarily due to its β subunit, which contains 145 amino acids with a unique terminal 24 amino acid sequence (1). The half-life of this hormone is relatively long (24 hours) because of its high sialic acid content. Immunohistochemical studies reported the cytotrophoblast is the major source of hCG before 6 weeks gestation and the syncytiotrophoblast the principle source thereafter (2).

In early pregnancy, the trophoblastic cells secrete predominately hCG in the form of an intact molecule containing both subunits (α-β dimer). There are small fractions (less than 1%) of free α and β subunits detectable in plasma. As the pregnancy progresses, the production of free α subunits increases. Other byproducts of the degradation of hCG are "nicked" hCG and β-core fragment, which are the major hCG-like materials in urine (3, 4). In the luteal phase of the menstrual cycle, hCG

115

can be detected in the maternal circulation within 9 to 11 days after conception (5). This is followed by a rapid rise in the serum concentration of hCG.

In determining the presence of a "normal" pregnancy, the rate of increase in the hCG concentration may be estimated by performing serial measurements. The time required for the hCG concentration to increase twofold is the doubling time. From the time of missed menses to 35 days after the last menstrual period, the doubling time is approximately 1.4 to 1.6 days and from 35 to 42 days gestation it is 2.0 to 2.7 days (6).

In many cases, the last menstrual period is unknown or uncertain, so sequential hCG measurements can be used to assess doubling time normalcy. For the purpose of early pregnancy monitoring, failure of the serum concentration of hCG to double over 48 hours indicates an abnormal gestation. In a normal pregnancy, for levels below 1200 mIU/mL, the doubling time is less than 1.9 days. This time interval increases to less than 2.3 days for values of 1200 to 6000 mIU/mL and less than 4.0 days for values above 6000 mIU/mL (7). At 10 weeks, the level peaks, reaching approximately 100,000 IU/L. This peak correlates with the rapid proliferation of the cytotrophoblast and syncytium of pregnancy, and hCG levels fall thereafter (8). In multiple gestations, the hCG levels 2 to 3 weeks after ovulation are over twofold higher than for a singleton pregnancy (9).

The two types of immunoassay currently used to measure hCG are competitive displacement and immunometric "sandwich" assays. Radioimmunoassay is a competitive assay that uses an antibody specific to the β subunit. There is competitive binding between endogenous hCG and added labeled β-hCG for the antibody. As the concentration of endogenous hCG increases, the antibody available to bind to the labeled β-hCG decreases. Therefore, measuring the amount of labeled β-hCG after separating the antibody-bound hCG from the free hCG allows quantitative measurements of the hCG concentration. Using radioactive I^{125} to tag the antibody-hCG complexes, fluorescence and luminescence are used to visually quantify the levels. These assays react differently with the free β-hCG subunit than with the intact α-β molecule, and this difference in immunoreactivity results in discrepant values obtained with various assays.

The immunometric or sandwich assay method is two-site specific, using two antibodies directed toward different parts of the hCG molecule. Endogenous hCG binds to an anti-hCG antibody, and this complex adheres to a solid phase of either plastic beads, test tubes, or microtiter plates. A second antibody carrying a radioactive, fluorescent, luminescent, or enzymatic signal is added and binds to the hCG on the solid phase. The endogenous hCG is the center of the sandwich assay. Several assays require addition of an appropriate substrate to yield a color reaction (10). Measuring the fluorescence intensity allows quantitative measurements of the hCG concentration. When one antibody is directed toward the α subunit and the other to the β subunit, then the assay measures only intact molecule. The use of polyclonal antibodies increases the sensitivity and specificity of the assay, resulting in detection of pregnancy before the time of expected menses. There are many procedural variations of this technique, and it is the basis of many commercially available home pregnancy tests.

Several international reference standards have been developed for calibrating hCG assays. Understanding the relationship between reference standards is essential to interpret any literature regarding pathologic pregnancy states and/or when monitoring an early pregnancy. Units of the International Reference Preparation are based on a preparation of highly purified hCG. The First International Reference Preparation (1st IRP-hCG) and most recently the third (3rd IRP-hCG) are provided by the World Health Organization and contain only the intact hCG molecule

(11). The Second International Standard (2nd IRP-hCG) was less pure and contained both intact and free β-hCG subunits. All three standards contain the same biological activity per international unit. One unit of 2nd IRP-hCG is approximately equivalent to two units of 1st or 3rd IRP-hCG (12).

The doubling time of hCG is influenced by gestational age and initial hCG concentration. As the pregnancy progresses, the clinical value of monitoring the hCG concentration decreases. After a gestational sac is visualized by ultrasound within the uterine cavity (approximately 25 to 35 days after ovulation), subsequent pregnancy monitoring should be continued with sonography (13).

Progesterone

Progesterone is the principle secretory product of the corpus luteum and essential for a successful pregnancy. Serum progesterone levels are used clinically to document ovulation, evaluate luteal phase defects, and assess fetal well-being during the first trimester. This hormone is best measured by a radioimmunoassay technique. In the luteal phase, progesterone production increases to approximately 10 ng/mL. In a normal pregnancy, the serum concentration of progesterone increases to about 25 ng/mL 2 weeks after ovulation (14). This level is approximately twice that of a nonpregnant cycle and remains constant until about 10 weeks gestation (15). Starting at the 12th week of gestation, plasma levels begin to gradually increase from a mean of 25 ng/mL to approximately 80 ng/mL by 28 weeks (16). After 28 weeks gestation, they increase steeply throughout the pregnancy until the last 4 to 6 weeks of gestation, reaching a mean concentration of 180 ng/mL. This level remains relatively constant until delivery.

A pregnancy is dependent on the corpus luteum for progesterone production until the seventh week of gestation. Removal of the corpus luteum before the seventh week of gestation results in a pregnancy loss. Ablation of the corpus luteum after 9 weeks gestation results in a *transient* decrease in progesterone without an abortion occurring (17, 18). From 7 to 10 weeks gestation, progesterone production shifts from the corpus luteum to the placenta, and the corpus luteum becomes dispensable at approximately 12 weeks gestation (19). As this shift from luteal to placental production occurs, there is a slight decline in the circulating progesterone level.

Serum progesterone concentration appears to be influenced by dietary intake because women on low-fat diets have been shown to exhibit a significantly lower luteal phase progesterone level compared with women on a standard meat-containing diet (20). A direct relationship has also been reported between caloric content and progesterone concentration. For each additional dietary increase of 239 kcal, the probability of a progesterone rise increased by 60% (21). Studies reported a decrease in progesterone after consumption of a meal. For example, a 34% reduction is observed with the nadir occurring 60 to 90 minutes after initiation of a meal in the nonpregnant state (22). During the first trimester, the postprandial decrease is still evident, along with significant variability in progesterone secretion over a 24-hour period. A diurnal variation has been suggested with the nadir occurring in the morning (23). Despite these variations, progesterone levels, compared with hCG, remain relatively static in the first trimester of pregnancy.

The major limitations in using serum progesterone for early pregnancy monitoring are

- Static levels during early pregnancy
- Overlap between normal and abnormal pregnancies
- Significant variation between individuals

Therefore, the clinical usefulness of progesterone measurements is limited. Several investigators described using a single progesterone value to diagnose pregnancy dysfunction in patients with natural conception. It appears that serum progesterone has three discriminatory zones. Less than 5 ng/mL is always associated with a nonviable gestation, greater than 25 ng/mL confirms a viable intrauterine pregnancy, and values of 5 to 25 ng/mL are indeterminate (24).

Estrogen

Because of wide variations in serum estrogen levels in the first trimester, measuring this hormone is not clinically useful in evaluating early pregnancy for location or viability. Estriol has, however, been used in association with maternal serum α fetal protein and hCG to assess fetal well-being and to screen for fetal aneuploidy in the second trimester.

Other Hormonal Markers

To enhance our ability to diagnose first-trimester disorders, many other potential endocrine markers of pregnancy viability have been examined. Several investigators reported use of serum inhibin, relaxin, and testosterone as possible indicators of pregnancy outcome (25–29). Compared with progesterone and hCG, these hormones exhibit a wide range of serum values with no discriminatory levels established. Many of these assays are difficult to perform, and the results may not differ from a normal viable first-trimester pregnancy (30). These recent findings do not improve patient care over the current recommendations for early pregnancy monitoring and should not be used until a benefit can be established.

Structural Development

The higher resolution of transvaginal ultrasound permits earlier identification of embryonic development. At 14 days after fertilization or 28 days gestation (based on a 28-day cycle), the gestational sac measures 2 mm in diameter. Rapid proliferation occurs during the following week, evident by visualization of the yolk sac and fetal pole. Cardiac activity can be documented in all viable pregnancies by 37 days (5 weeks, 2 days) gestation (31). By 39 days (5 weeks, 4 days) gestation, the embryo has reached a length of 2 to 4 mm, and at 7 weeks gestation, the crown-rump length is approximately 10 mm and the central nervous system begins to develop. Limb buds can be visualized by 8 weeks gestation when the crown-rump length is 20 mm. At 11 weeks gestation, the embryo measures 40 mm with all the major organs and structures of the body formed.

The sac diameter increases with advancing weeks, and structural changes within the sac correlate with gestational age, pregnancy viability, and eventual outcome. There appears to be a linear association between crown-rump length or mean gestational sac diameter and menstrual age (Tables 5.1 and 5.2) (32, 33).

Ultrasonography

Transvaginal ultrasonography has permitted detailed visualization of the developing conceptus in the first trimester. This allows early determination of gestational age, pregnancy location, viability, and number of gestational sacs. Serial examinations can assist in identifying pregnancy dysfunction and disorders of fetal growth. Transvaginal sonography is more useful than transabdominal ultrasound in early pregnancy monitoring because the vaginal technique allows visualization of an intrauterine pregnancy earlier in gestation.

Compared with transvaginal sonography, transabdominal ultrasound has sev-

TABLE 5.1. Estimated Gestational Age from Crown-Rump Measurements

Menstrual Maturity (wk + days)	Corrected "Regression Analysis" (mm)	Menstrual Maturity (wk + days)	Corrected "Regression Analysis" (mm)
6 + 2	5.5	10 + 2	33.2
6 + 3	6.1	10 + 3	34.6
6 + 4	6.8	10 + 4	36.0
6 + 5	7.5	10 + 5	37.4
6 + 6	8.1	10 + 6	38.9
7 + 0	8.9	11 + 0	40.4
7 + 1	9.6	11 + 1	41.9
7 + 2	10.4	11 + 2	43.5
7 + 3	11.2	11 + 3	45.1
7 + 4	12.0	11 + 4	46.7
7 + 5	12.9	11 + 5	48.3
7 + 6	13.8	11 + 6	50.0
8 + 0	14.7	12 + 0	51.7
8 + 1	15.7	12 + 1	53.4
8 + 2	16.6	12 + 2	55.2
8 + 3	17.6	12 + 3	57.0
8 + 4	18.7	12 + 4	58.8
8 + 5	19.7	12 + 5	60.6
8 + 6	20.8	12 + 6	62.5
9 + 0	21.9	13 + 0	64.3
9 + 1	23.1	13 + 1	66.3
9 + 2	24.2	13 + 2	68.2
9 + 3	25.4	13 + 3	70.2
9 + 4	26.7	13 + 4	72.2
9 + 5	27.9	13 + 5	74.3
9 + 6	29.2	13 + 6	76.3
10 + 0	30.5	14 + 0	78.3
10 + 1	31.8		

Reprinted with permission from Robinson HP, Fleming JE. A critical evaluation of sonar "crown-rump length" measurements. Br J Obstet Gynaecol 1975;82:702–710.

eral limitations in evaluating first-trimester pregnancies. The major consideration is decreased resolution, due primarily to the lower frequency of transabdominal transducers. Transvaginal transducer frequencies are 5 to 7.5 MHz compared with 3.5 to 5 MHz for transabdominal transducers. As the frequency increases, resolution of the image increases but the depth of penetration decreases. The transvaginal route only requires penetration of the vagina to view the uterus and adnexa, which may lie within 1 cm of the transducer. The pelvic structures rest at a much greater distance from the abdominal transducer, and this further decreases resolution. Visualization of the pelvic organs could be limited because of bowel interference or an empty bladder. In addition, transabdominal scanning requires the penetration of the abdominal wall, which can distort the image, especially in obese patients. An empty bladder alone does not compromise transvaginal sonography, but minimal distention may be useful with a severely anteverted uterus.

Because the high frequency of vaginal probes limits their penetration, large myomatous uteri or a fetuses greater than 14 to 16 weeks cannot be accurately scanned.

Because of the confines of the introitus, the transvaginal probe cannot be moved in all dimensions, and this may compromise visualization of pelvic and nonpelvic structures.

EARLY PREGNANCY MONITORING

The women who benefit most from early pregnancy monitoring are those at risk for pregnancy complications and those presenting with pelvic pain and/or vaginal bleeding. The risk factors for ectopic pregnancy are listed in Table 5.3. In many cases, screening for risk factors is as simple as taking a history, including a review of medical, surgical, and obstetric history. Therefore, it is the responsibility of the health care provider to identify those patients who would benefit from early evaluation.

Vaginal bleeding is the most common subjective complaint in the first trimester of pregnancy, affecting 15 to 20% of first-trimester pregnancies. This is the most common indication for first-trimester sonography, since an estimated 50% of these pregnancies end in fetal loss (34, 35). Approximately 18% of women experiencing vaginal bleeding in early pregnancy sonographically demonstrate a subchorionic hematoma (36). If a hematoma is documented in gestations less than 8 weeks, the spontaneous loss rate is approximately 10.5% when a viable fetus is noted. In those

TABLE 5.2. Estimated Gestational Age from Mean Gestational Chorionic Sac Diameter

Mean Gestational Sac Diameter (mm)	Gestational Age (wk)	Mean Gestational Sac Diameter (mm)	Gestational Age (wk)
10.0	5.0	36.0	8.8
11.0	5.2	37.0	8.9
12.0	5.3	38.0	9.0
13.0	5.5	39.0	9.2
14.0	5.6	40.0	9.3
15.0	5.8	41.0	9.5
16.0	5.9	42.0	9.6
17.0	6.0	43.0	9.7
18.0	6.2	44.0	9.9
19.0	6.3	45.0	10.0
20.0	6.5	46.0	10.2
21.0	6.6	47.0	10.3
22.0	6.8	48.0	10.5
23.0	6.9	49.0	10.6
24.0	7.0	50.0	10.7
25.0	7.2	51.0	10.9
26.0	7.3	52.0	11.0
27.0	7.5	53.0	11.2
28.0	7.6	54.0	11.3
29.0	7.8	55.0	11.5
30.0	7.9	56.0	11.6
31.0	8.0	57.0	11.7
32.0	8.2	58.0	11.9
33.0	8.3	59.0	12.0
34.0	8.5	60.0	12.2
35.0	8.6		

Modified from Hellman LM, Kobayashi M, Fillisti L, et al. Growth and development of the human fetus prior to the twentieth week of gestation. Am J Obstet Gynecol 1969;103:789–800.

TABLE 5.3. Risk Factors for Ectopic Pregnancies

Previous tubal or pelvic surgery
In utero diethylstilbestrol exposure
History of pelvic inflammatory disease or intrauterine device use
Previous ectopic pregnancy
Infertility
Ovulation-induction therapy
More than one lifetime sexual partner
Smoking
First-trimester bleeding

greater than 8 weeks, the loss rate decreases to 5% (37). When the hematoma is larger than two thirds of the chorionic sac diameter, fetal loss rate increases to 18.8% (37).

Early Monitoring for Detection of Ectopic Pregnancy or Potential for Abortion

The serum hCG level at which an intrauterine pregnancy should be visualized by ultrasound is described as the discriminatory zone. The 1st IRP-hCG discriminatory zone is 6500 IU/L for transabdominal ultrasound (38). Transvaginal ultrasound has increased the sensitivity of pregnancy detection, and it has been proposed that all normal intrauterine pregnancies should be visualized above an hCG concentration of 2000 IU/L (39). Recent studies proposed use of a higher level (3000 IU/L) to increase specificity for detection (39, 40). When the gestational age is known, a viable intrauterine pregnancy should be detected transvaginally in all cases at 35 days (5 weeks) gestation (41).

Important in performing transvaginal ultrasounds is the development of a strict scanning routine. At our institution, we begin with a bimanual examination to anticipate what may be seen on ultrasound. The probe is orientated in the sagittal plane during insertion and advanced slowly to visualize the cervix. After the probe is positioned in the posterior fornix, the uterus is evaluated for size, endometrial thickness, and the presence of an intrauterine gestation. The gestational sac should be measured in three planes followed by close inspection of its contents. Measurement of the fetal pole should be performed and the presence of heart motion documented. Each adnexa should be studied, looking for masses in the fallopian tube and/or ovary, followed by inspection of the posterior cul-de-sac for free fluid or blood. This technique can detect embryonic or fetal structures 1 to 2 weeks earlier than transabdominal sonography.

Appropriate diagnostic testing depends on the presence of symptoms and the ability to ascertain gestational age accurately. Figure 5.1 details the workup of an asymptomatic woman with risk factors for an ectopic or abortion, and Figure 5.2 details the workup of a high-risk patient with symptoms or a low-risk patient with bleeding or pain. For an asymptomatic patient known to be less than 6 weeks gestation (using date of last menstrual period) or with unknown dates, testing may begin with measuring the serum β-hCG concentration. When the hCG level is 2000 mIU/mL or greater, a transvaginal ultrasound can be performed because all normal intrauterine pregnancies will be visualized at that hCG level (39, 40). There is no benefit in measuring hCG after sonographic evidence of an intrauterine pregnancy, so subsequent monitoring should be via serial ultrasound examinations. If an intrauterine pregnancy is not documented, then ectopic gestation should be suspected and an ectopic protocol initiated (Fig. 5.3).

If the initial hCG concentration is less than 2000 mIU/mL, a repeat value should be obtained 48 hours later, when it should have doubled. Most abnormal pregnancies are associated with an increase of less than 66% in 48 hours (42). If the rise in hCG is normal and the patient is asymptomatic, then a transvaginal ultrasound can be performed once the hCG concentration is predicted to be greater than 2000 mIU/mL. Failure to visualize an intrauterine pregnancy when predicted by hCG levels or documentation of an abnormal rise in serum hCG concentration implies that an extrauterine gestation is present and the ectopic protocol must be initiated (Table 5.3).

Because twin gestations have higher hCG levels earlier, the correlation between a specific hCG level and expected state of physiologic growth (i.e., what one expects to see on an ultrasound at a given hCG level) does not correlate as well as it does in singleton pregnancies. In asymptomatic women with the potential for twins, intervention may be delayed by 48 hours to further clarify the location of the pregnancy.

Asymptomatic women who are at risk for ectopic or abortion and who are 6 weeks gestation or greater by reliable dates (Fig. 5.1) and all symptomatic women (Table 5.2) should have a transvaginal ultrasound performed initially. If an intrauterine pregnancy is not found, the asymptomatic woman should be evaluated with hCG measurements 48 hours apart as described above. If the symptomatic patient does not have an intrauterine pregnancy and has escalating pain, signs of peritoneal irritation, symptoms of hemodynamic instability, or a hemoperitoneum found on ultrasound, a laparoscopy should be performed at the earliest opportunity.

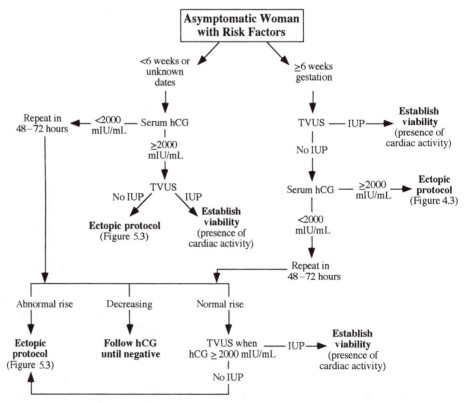

FIGURE 5.1. Early pregnancy monitoring for asymptomatic women with predisposing risk factors for an abnormal pregnancy. *IUP*, intrauterine pregnancy; *TVUS*, transvaginal ultrasound.

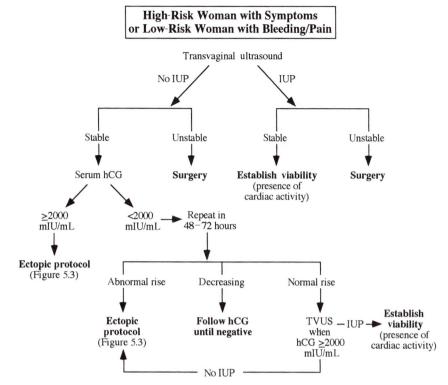

FIGURE 5.2. Early pregnancy monitoring in high-risk patients with symptoms and low-risk patients with vaginal bleeding or pain. *IUP,* intrauterine pregnancy; *TVUS,* transvaginal ultrasound.

In a clinically stable patient with a nonviable pregnancy (hCG levels have reached a plateau or are slowly falling) of unknown location, the ectopic protocol (Table 5.3) can be applied to ascertain location. An hCG level is obtained and an office curettage is performed using a vacuum aspiration syringe. If the hCG concentration 24 hours later has fallen or if chorionic villi are noted histologically in the uterine contents, then the patient is assumed to have a failed intrauterine pregnancy and the hCG concentration can be monitored weekly until undetectable. When the hCG level does not fall, it is assumed the pregnancy is extrauterine and medical treatment may be considered.

Imaging is most useful when an intrauterine pregnancy is seen, thus making the existence of an ectopic pregnancy unlikely. Using transvaginal sonography, the most reliable predictor of an ectopic pregnancy is the failure to visualize an intrauterine pregnancy at the appropriate gestational age and/or β-hCG level. Do not rely on seeing an ectopic pregnancy to establish the diagnosis. Findings that may suggest the presence of an extrauterine pregnancy are an endometrial thickness of greater than 10 mm and uterine area greater than 20 cm^2 but no intrauterine pregnancy (43). The presence of a complex pelvic mass and echogenic fluid in the posterior cul-de-sac can predict an extrauterine pregnancy with a specificity of 93.2% (44). Transabdominal ultrasound is not reliable in diagnosing an ectopic pregnancy unless an intact ectopic gestational sac containing a live fetus is seen.

Several studies implicated small sac size as predictive for impending pregnancy loss (45–47). In pregnancies less than 10 weeks gestation and a mean sac diameter

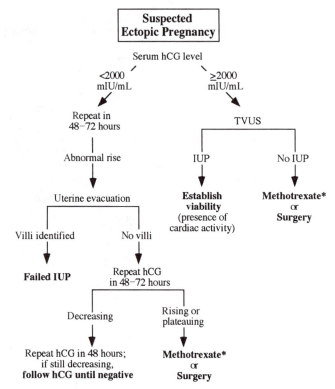

FIGURE 5.3. Ectopic protocol. *Asterisk* indicates if patient has no exclusion criteria for medical management (see Table 5.4). *IUP,* intrauterine pregnancy; *TVUS,* transvaginal ultrasound.

of greater than or equal to 8 mm, the absence of a yolk sac predicts a nonviable gestation with a sensitivity of 67% and specificity of 100%. In patients with a sac diameter of greater than 16 mm, absence of an embryo predicts nonviability with a sensitivity of 50% and specificity of 100% (48). The difference in gestational sac diameter and crown-rump length appears to correlate with an increased risk for fetal death, since a difference of less than 5 mm results in a demise rate of 80% compared with 10.8% when the difference is greater than or equal to 8 mm (49).

The documentation of fetal heart motion is pivotal in assessing pregnancy viability. Cardiac activity is visualized in 15% of viable gestations at 35 days (5 weeks) and increases to 100% by 37 days (5 weeks, 2 days) (31). The risk of fetal loss decreases to 7% after cardiac activity is visualized in pregnancies with a fetal pole greater than 5 mm or after 40 days gestation (50–52). As the embryo grows, the risk of fetal loss decreases to 3.3% with a crown-rump length of 6 to 10 mm and 0.5% if greater than 10 mm (52). Using a combination of gestational sac size, evidence of a yolk sac, embryo size, and presence or absence of cardiac pulsations enables early prediction of the viability of a pregnancy (48).

Doppler ultrasound has been used to increase the accuracy of distinguishing an ectopic pregnancy from an intrauterine gestation. A characteristic peritrophoblastic waveform has been reported with intrauterine pregnancies. This distinctive flow pattern exhibits low impedance and a peak systolic velocity higher than that seen in endometrial radial arteries. As the chorionic sac increases in size, the peak systolic velocity rises from 8 to 30 cm/sec with no intrauterine sac identified to 10 to 60 cm/sec with a 6- to 10-mm sac (53). An adnexal mass with increased vascularity but without a chorionic sac is highly suggestive of an ectopic pregnancy. In one study, the sensitivity of detecting an ectopic pregnancy by endovaginal ultrasound increased from 71% without Doppler to 87% with Doppler, providing a specificity of 99% (53). In 20% of ectopic pregnancies, a pseudogestational sac is seen within the uterine cavity. Ultrasound alone may not provide sufficient information to differentiate this from an early or abnormal intrauterine pregnancy. Doppler sonography can differentiate an intrauterine sac from a pseudosac by failing to detect peritrophoblastic flow. This modality may also provide additional information in diagnosing abnormal placentation early in the first trimester before the appearance of a yolk sac or fetal pole (Fig. 5.4).

The yolk sac diameter has been shown to correlate with gestational sac size and gestational age. The yolk sac grows 0.1 mm for every millimeter of growth of the gestational sac when the gestational sac diameter is less than 15 mm, slowing to 0.03 mm for every millimeter of growth when the sac diameter is over 15 mm (54). Abnormal pregnancies have been reported when the yolk sac diameter is two standard deviations below or above the mean, with positive predictive values of 60% and 44.4%, respectively. A large yolk sac (greater than 5.6 mm) in pregnancies less than 10 weeks is associated with poor outcomes (54). This is an area of controversy, however, because of reports failing to show any significant correlation between yolk sac size and pregnancy outcome (55, 56).

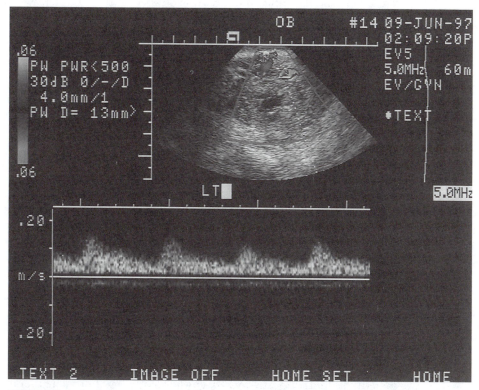

FIGURE 5.4. Endovaginal sonography demonstrated a left adnexa mass with an irregular hypoechoic area in this patient with an ectopic pregnancy. Color sonography (not shown) demonstrated increased vascularity to this area. Use of endovaginal pulse Doppler sonography demonstrates high diastolic blood flow with a low-impedance waveform, consistent with increased blood flow to the ectopic pregnancy.

Assessing the growth of early embryonic structures can facilitate detection of pregnancy dysfunction and provide information with regard to outcome. In summary, an abnormal pregnancy should be suspected if any of the following are noted:

- Chorionic sac with mean diameter greater than mm and without the presence of a yolk sac
- 6.5 week gestation without cardiac activity
- β-hCG level at least 10,800 mIU/mL without fetal cardiac activity (57)

Ectopic Pregnancy

The incidence of ectopic pregnancies has increased over the past two decades. It affects 2% of all gestations and is the leading cause of pregnancy-related maternal deaths in the first trimester (58, 59). Risk factors for ectopic pregnancy are listed in Table 5.3. The most common predisposing factor is a history of pelvic inflammatory disease. A history of this condition increases the risk for an ectopic pregnancy 10-fold compared with the general population. Approximately 11% of American women of reproductive age received treatment for pelvic inflammatory disease during the 1980s, with the highest average rate occurring in the 20- to 24-year age group (60, 61). After one ectopic pregnancy, there is a 15% increased risk for subsequent extrauterine gestation. Using transvaginal sonography along with hormonal monitoring in women at risk for ectopic pregnancy provides the best chance for early detection and treatment (62).

The diagnostic algorithms outlined in Tables 5.1, 5.2, and 5.3 identify women with an ectopic pregnancy with 100% sensitivity and without the use of laparoscopy (63). These algorithms rely on hCG determinations and transvaginal ultrasound. An alternative approach uses a single serum progesterone value to segregate patients into the three discriminatory zones, discussed in the earlier section entitled Progesterone:

- Greater than 25 ng/mL—viable pregnancy
- 5.0 ng/mL—nonviable pregnancy
- Greater than 5.0 but less than 25 ng/mL—pregnancy of undetermined viability

When the progesterone value is less than 5.0 ng/mL, an office curettage is performed and subsequent hCG values obtained. Failure of the hCG to fall is followed by methotrexate treatment. When the progesterone concentration is indeterminate, sequential hCG values and transvaginal ultrasound are required to finalize the diagnosis (64). In our institution, we found the use of progesterone concentrations to be of little additional value and do not use this information in the nonsurgical diagnosis of ectopic pregnancy.

Nonsurgical Treatment of Ectopic Pregnancy.   Women who should be considered for methotrexate therapy are divided into three groups:

- hCG level greater than 2000 mIU/mL and rising with no intrauterine pregnancy on vaginal sonogram
- hCG rising abnormally and associated with a negative uterine evacuation
- Unruptured ectopic pregnancy less than 3.5 cm in diameter noted on transvaginal ultrasound

Patients treated surgically and not considered for methotrexate therapy include those with an adnexal mass greater than 3.5 cm in diameter, free fluid in the cul-de-sac associated with pelvic pain, cardiac activity noted in an extrauterine gestational sac, hemodynamic instability, active pulmonary disease, or excess risk for complications from medical treatment (Table 5.4). All women treated with methotrexate must agree to comply with scheduled follow-up visits and blood tests (65).

TABLE 5.4. Exclusion Criteria for Medical Management of Ectopic Pregnancy

Extrauterine gestation with cardiac activity
Adnexal mass > 3.5 cm
Pelvic pain with free fluid
Hemodynamic instability
AST > 50 IU/L
Serum creatinine > 1.3 mg/dL
White blood cell count < 3000 mm^3
Active pulmonary disease
Patient noncompliance

Our treatment protocol includes a determination of the complete blood count (CBC), serum creatinine, aspartate aminotransferase (AST), blood type and Rh, and hCG concentration on the day of methotrexate administration. hCG levels are repeated on days 4 and 7 after treatment, with both samples saved and processed in the same assay to eliminate interassay variability. The hCG concentration should fall by at least 15% between days 4 and 7, and when these criteria are met, subsequent levels may be obtained at 1-week intervals until undetectable. When the hCG concentration fails to fall by at least 15% either initially or weekly, a repeat dose of methotrexate should be administered. Serum creatinine, CBC, and AST are repeated on day 7 to determine the potential for toxicity. Rh immunoglobulin is given routinely to women who are Rh negative (65, 66).

The dose of methotrexate given is 50 mg/m^2 intramuscularly in divided doses. It should be noted the calculation of the appropriate dose depends on determining the patient's surface area (m^2). This is done routinely by oncologists and pharmacists using nomograms that include patient height and weight. Repeat doses of methotrexate, when required, are identical to the initial amount. The indications for abandoning methotrexate treatment and resorting to surgery include evidence of hemodynamic instability, worsening pain with sonographic evidence of hemoperitoneum, or a persistent rise in hCG titer. An increase in pelvic pain is experienced by 20 to 34.3% of women treated medically (65, 66). These patients require prompt evaluation with physical examination, CBC, and transvaginal ultrasound to rule out tubal rupture and hemodynamic instability. In most cases, the pain subsides promptly without further treatment, but admission to the hospital with close observation may be required in selected cases.

With application of the diagnostic algorithms outlined, slightly more than 40% of patients can avoid initial surgical intervention. At least 85% of appropriately selected candidates successfully complete therapy, although up to 6% may require a second dose of methotrexate. The treatment protocol outlined is very well tolerated with less than one third of women experiencing the usually mild side effects. Data regarding reproductive performance after systemic methotrexate treatment indicate that posttreatment tubal patency and conception rates are comparable with those achieved with conservative laparoscopic management. However, methotrexate appears to have a significantly lower recurrent ectopic rate compared with salpingostomy (8% compared with 15.4%) (62).

Alternatives to the systemic methotrexate protocol described have been examined. The direct injection of a very low dose of methotrexate into the ectopic pregnancy under ultrasound guidance has a greater failure rate and is technically more cumbersome than systemic administration (67). Direct transvaginal injection of other substances, including prostaglandin and hyperosmolar glucose, has also been found to be inferior to systemic methotrexate. A trial of the antiprogestin mifepristone (RU-486) failed to demonstrate adequate efficacy. In summary, when medical therapy is appropriate, the systemic administration of methotrexate, 50 mg/m^2 intramuscularly in divided doses, should be considered the treatment of choice.

One other approach to the nonsurgical treatment of ectopic pregnancy deserves mention: expectant management. A criticism of the diagnostic algorithms cited is that many of the abnormal pregnancies identified would, in the past, have resolved spontaneously before detection. In fact, one study found that when the initial hCG concentration was less than 1000 mIU/mL, the ectopic pregnancy resolved spontaneously in 88% of cases (68). Unfortunately, our ability to predict individuals who will experience tubal rupture and hemoperitoneum during expectant management remains limited. Further investigation is needed before expectant management can be incorporated safely into modern treatment protocols.

Nonviable Intrauterine Pregnancy

The ability to discriminate between a dysfunctional intrauterine or an extrauterine pregnancy is at times difficult. Both clinical situations can present with pelvic pain and vaginal bleeding. To establish the diagnosis of a complete spontaneous abortion, one of two requirements must be fulfilled: villi are obtained from the expelled conception or a gestational sac with a fetal pole is seen on ultrasound before the pregnancy loss. A pseudosac can be seen in 14% of patients with an ectopic pregnancy, and therefore the presence of an intrauterine sac does not rule out the possibility of an ectopic pregnancy (69). An asymptomatic patient with minimal bleeding requires two hCG levels performed 48 hours apart. If the clinical situation is suspicious for an incomplete abortion with evidence of active vaginal bleeding or the cervical os is open and the patient complains of significant discomfort, then an office uterine evacuation can be performed with a vacuum aspiration syringe. This technique does not require analgesia, and the reevacuation rate is similar to sharp curettage without the morbidity of surgery (70). If trophoblastic villi are present on frozen-section examination of this tissue, then the diagnosis is an incomplete abortion and no further monitoring is needed. The absence of villi warrants an hCG determination on the procedure day and again 24 hours later. If a decline is noted, then either a complete spontaneous abortion has occurred or an extrauterine pregnancy is spontaneously resolving.

Follow-up of a complete abortion or resolving ectopic pregnancy should include monitoring the hCG titer until negative. Symptoms of an ectopic pregnancy should be reviewed with the patient, since the location of the pregnancy has not been confirmed. If at any point the titer plateaus or increases, then the ectopic protocol is followed.

The absence of fetal cardiac activity with any of the following findings confirms fetal demise or a missed abortion:

- Fetal pole or crown-rump length greater than 5 mm
- Gestational age greater than 46 days
- Gestational sac diameter greater than 20 mm (71–74)

A gestational sac that measures greater than 25 mm without a fetal pole (at least 7.5 weeks gestation) or greater than 20 mm without a yolk sac confirms the diagnosis of a blighted ovum (75). Two treatment options are available for these conditions, either expectant or active management. There are no hormonal or sonographic data to help predict when spontaneous passage of the products of conception will occur. A surgical procedure may be indicated during expectant management if hemorrhage occurs.

Those patients requesting active management can be offered either medical or surgical therapy. In pregnancies where the mean gestational sac diameter is 25 mm or less, an office early uterine evacuation could be performed using vacuum aspiration. Medical therapy involves inducing an abortion with any combination of mifepristone (RU-486), methotrexate, and/or prostaglandins. These medications have been used in the medical management of failing pregnancies and in the nonsurgical management of elective terminations.

Medically Induced Abortion.   Over the past few years the issue of medically induced abortion has received a great deal of public attention. The protocols for failing pregnancies include the use of single or combination therapy to expel the pregnancy. The first medication introduced in France in 1990 for this purpose was mifepristone (RU-486), a potent antiprogestin. Mifepristone has been shown to increase uterine activity and dilate the pregnant cervix. For pregnancies between 6.6 and 11 weeks, mifepristone has shown a spontaneous abortion rate of 82% when given as single-agent therapy, with expulsion of the pregnancy 2 to 5 days after ingestion of the medication (76). The success rate is enhanced with the administration of misoprostol, a synthetic prostaglandin E_1 (Cytotec). Patients receive a 600-mg oral dose of mifepristone followed 36 to 48 hours later by 600 μg of misoprostol orally. Using this protocol, 95% of missed or anembryonic pregnancies 13 weeks of gestation or less abort in a median time of 4 hours after ingestion of the misoprostol. Studies in the early 1990s on the effectiveness of combination therapy reported a 93% abortion rate with pregnancies less than 56 days (8 weeks) using a combination of 600 mg mifepristone and 400 μg misoprostol. Most women aborted within 4 hours after the administration of misoprostol (77). A more recent study confirmed the success rate for pregnancies at 7 weeks gestation or earlier (94.8%) but showed the efficacy slightly decreased between 49 and 56 days (7 to 8 weeks) (93.4%) and further decline at greater than 63 days (9 weeks) (83.3%). The two latter groups experienced an increase in vaginal bleeding that warranted an additional procedure in some cases (78). Vacuum aspiration because of medical failure or persistent pregnancy after expulsion occurs in 3% of pregnancies (77, 79, 80). The major side effects of this combination therapy are nausea, vomiting, and diarrhea (81). Patient's perception of this method are positive with regards to the level of psychological stress and the possibility of reduced physical trauma compared with vacuum aspiration (82).

To decrease the rate of side effects and the complication of persistent pregnancy, oral versus vaginal administration of misoprostol was examined. Pregnancies with a mean duration of amenorrhea of 51 days (7 weeks, 1 day) were administered a single oral dose of 600 mg mifepristone with 800 μg misoprostol vaginally 36 to 48 hours later. Pregnancies were expelled in 99% of the cases within 4 hours of administration of the misoprostol. One percent required additional treatment for hemorrhage but responded to medical management (83). The gastrointestinal side effects were also significantly reduced using the vaginal route.

Before receiving this therapy, all patients should be screened with documentation of a viable pregnancy on transvaginal sonogram and baseline blood work (including CBC, platelet count, AST, serum creatinine, blood type/Rh status, and serum β-hCG). If the patient is Rh negative, Rh immunoglobulin is administered intramuscularly before receiving any medication. It appears the best results are seen in pregnancies less than 50 days (7 weeks, 1 day) of amenorrhea, and side effects are reduced by using vaginal misoprostol administration. Mifepristone has recently received approval from the U.S. Food and Drug Administration for use in medically induced elective pregnancy terminations.

Methotrexate has been used for ectopic pregnancies and when combined with misoprostol has also been very effective for elective terminations. The protocol consists of methotrexate 50 mg/m² intramuscularly and misoprostol 800 μg vaginally 3 to 7 days later. This results in pregnancy expulsion in 90 to 100% of cases at 8 weeks gestation or earlier (84–86). This also appears to be affective for inducing abortion in 60% of pregnancies between 57 and 63 days gestation (8 to 9 weeks) (87). Patients with uterine or cervical anomalies and desirous of pregnancy termination could be at great risk if a suction curettage or a vacuum aspiration is performed. The use of medical therapy in these patients has been very effective and may decrease the morbidity risk compared with a surgical procedure (88).

FOLLOW-UP COUNSELING

Counseling a women about future reproductive potential and the recurrence of a pregnancy disorder is imperative for well-being. Putting the issue in perspective establishes a stable psychological foundation for her to either attempt conception again or seek further therapy. Concerns regarding secondary infertility, fetal anomalies in a subsequent pregnancy, and recurrent pregnancy loss are often raised. Spontaneous loss in the general population before 20 weeks gestation is reported to occur in 15 to 20% of recognized pregnancies. After one spontaneous abortion, the risk for a consecutive loss may be slightly increased (89). This does not reach statistical significance until after three or more consecutive losses.

The chance for a normal pregnancy outcome after three consecutive abortions without a prior live birth is only 50%; one previous live birth increases the chance of normal pregnancy to 63 to 70% (90–92). Women with this condition are termed habitual aborters and comprise approximately 1% of women (92). These patients require an evaluation for possible etiologies that could result in pregnancy loss, including anatomic causes, chronic disease states, immunologic problems, environmental factors, and genetic factors.

Patients undergoing an induced abortion often have concerns regarding fertility and possible complications with subsequent pregnancies. The risk of secondary infertility after surgical intervention is not consistent in the literature. Some investigators noted a slight increased risk of secondary infertility after a single abortion, whereas others fail to find an association (93–95). One study reported a direct correlation between secondary infertility and increasing number of induced abortions (95). The etiology is presumed secondary to postabortal intrauterine adhesion formation. Several studies evaluated the uterine cavity by hysteroscopy and reported uterine synechiae to occur in 16.7 to 19% of first-trimester surgical terminations. Adhesions have been reported to be as high as 50% after a first-trimester curettage. Even after a spontaneous abortion, intracavity adhesions were observed in 6.4% of the cases (96–98).

The role adhesions play in the development of secondary infertility is not well documented because infertility rates do not appear to be significantly different between surgical versus conservative management of abnormal pregnancies (25% and 22.9%, respectively) (94). One study evaluated the ability to conceive after a single spontaneous loss. After 18 months, 92% achieved conception versus 26% for those patients with greater than or equal to two losses (89). These results raise the possibility that early induced or spontaneous abortions may have the potential to promote uterine cavity pathology, which may affect fertility.

The influence of interpregnancy interval on pregnancy outcome has been investigated. There does not appear to be a pattern in the time interval from pregnancy loss to subsequent conception. The endocrine profile of the first menstrual cycle compared with the second after a spontaneous abortion reveals a lower level of estrone in the late luteal phase and a lower peak level of luteinizing hormone. This has been shown to result in a shorter luteal phase length (99). Similar endocrine abnormalities have been reported after termination of pregnancy (100, 101). This may predispose the pregnancy to an increased incidence of loss if conception occurs in the first cycle.

Even if the endocrine axis is reestablished, the endometrium may not be receptive. Endometrial biopsies were examined in women after a spontaneous abortion over two cycles. Both cycles revealed significant abnormalities, with the first being more abnormal than the second (102). Administering hormonal supplementation in the first cycle after surgical termination improves the endometrial thickness over no treatment and may enhance the reparative process within the endometrium (103). There are no data to support the idea that exogenous hormone supplementation improves pregnancy outcome over no therapy.

PRECONCEPTUAL COUNSELING

Preconceptual counseling is beneficial not only for women with medical problems but for all women who are attempting conception. Because more than 50% of pregnancies in the United States are unplanned, it is appropriate to discuss preventative care issues during the fertile period (104). The most crucial time in pregnancy is during organogenesis, which occurs between 17 and 56 days (2 to 8 weeks) after conception (105). Because some women do not realize they are pregnant until after this period, addressing preconception issues during a yearly office visit is appropriate for any women or couple contemplating pregnancy. Issues of nutrition, exercise, social activities, and immunization status should be addressed.

Evaluation of dietary habits are important for fetal development. Eating habits such as vegetarianism, fasting, eating disorders (anorexia and/or bulimia), and the use of vitamin supplements should be identified. Behavioral modifications are recommended in women who smoke, use recreational drugs, or consume alcohol. Abstention from these substances is always recommended, but in the first few weeks of gestation, pregnancy may not be suspected. Fetal alcohol syndrome occurs with chronic consumption, but the occasional drink during pregnancy has not been associated with a measurable risk of birth defects. Therefore, women who consume small amounts of alcohol on occasion in the first trimester may be put at ease.

Periconceptional intake of folic acid appears to reduce the risk of neural tube defects in all patients, not just high-risk pregnancies. Using folate-containing vitamins during the first 6 weeks of gestation results in a reduction in risk for neural tube defects of 73%. There is no reduction seen in those who begin folate supplementation after 6 weeks gestation (106). The U.S. Public Health Service recommends daily supplementation with 0.4 mg of folic acid for all U.S. women capable of becoming pregnant; this is twice the current average dietary intake of 0.2 mg (107). If the woman has previously had a child with a neural tube defect, she should be offered preventive treatment with 4.0 mg of folic acid daily starting 1 month before conception is planned and continuing through the first 3 months of pregnancy (108). This recommendation is supported by the Committee on Obstetrics: Maternal and Fetal Medicine of the American College of Obstetricians and Gynecologists, Washington, DC, and the Centers for Disease Control and Prevention (109, 110).

The preconceptual period is an appropriate time to discuss the impact of physical exercise and social activities on early pregnancy. Mild to moderate exercise appears to be beneficial and safe in early pregnancy. Strenuous exercise has been associated with smaller infants, which has been speculated to be secondary to hyperthermia

(111). The American College of Obstetricians and Gynecologists established guidelines for health care professionals to provide a safe exercise regime (112). Contraindications to exercise in the first trimester include a history of incompetent cervix, cervical cerclage, or persistent vaginal bleeding.

Neural tube defects have been associated with heat exposure from hot tubs, saunas, or a high fever in the first trimester. The length, frequency, and duration of exposure necessary to cause these effects have not been determined (113). Therefore, because no specific guidelines can be given, women should be advised to avoid unnecessary heat exposure if possible.

Contracting rubella in the first trimester can result in many birth defects, including congenital heart disease, microcephaly, mental retardation, cataracts, and deafness. Because the rubella vaccine is a live attenuated virus, it is contraindicated during pregnancy. Conception should be postponed and birth control recommended for 3 months after vaccination. If rubella infection is acquired within the first 8 weeks of pregnancy, the fetal infection rate reaches 50% and can result in spontaneous abortion and stillbirth (114).

CLINICAL NOTES

Early Pregnancy Monitoring

- Indicated for women at risk for ectopic pregnancy or abortion and women presenting with pelvic pain or vaginal bleeding.
- Failure of serum hCG to double over 48 hours indicates an abnormal pregnancy.
- Until 8 to 10 weeks gestation, transvaginal sonography is superior to transabdominal sonography to evaluate a pregnancy for viability and/or location.
- A consistent evaluation with transvaginal sonography should be done and include an evaluation of uterine size, endometrial thickness, and verification of the presence or absence of an intrauterine pregnancy. Measure gestational sac in three planes. Measure fetal pole. Document heart motion if present. Examine adnexa and posterior cul-de-sac.
- An abnormal pregnancy should be suspected if chorionic sac diameter is greater than 10 mm without presence of yolk sac, 6.5 weeks gestation without cardiac activity, or β-hCG at least 10,800 mIU/mL without cardiac activity.

Ectopic Pregnancy

- The most reliable predictor of ectopic pregnancy is failure to visualize (with transvaginal ultrasound) an intrauterine pregnancy at appropriate gestational age and/or hCG level.
- When medical therapy is appropriate, the systemic administration of methotrexate at 50 mg/m^2 intramuscularly in divided doses should be considered the treatment of choice.

Nonviable Intrauterine Pregnancy

- The absence of cardiac activity with any of the following confirms fetal demise or missed abortion: fetal pole or crown-rump length greater than 5 mm, gestational age greater than 46 days, or gestational sac diameter greater than 20 mm.
- Medically induced abortion can be performed by administering mifepristone 600 mg orally, followed 36 to 48 hours later by misoprostol 600 μg orally. Other regimens are also effective.

References

1. Bahl OP, Carlsen RB, Bellisario R. Human chorionic gonadotropin: amino acid sequence of the alpha and beta subunits. Biochem Biophys Res Commun 1972;48:416–422.

2. Maruo T, Ladines-Llave CA, Matsuo H, et al. A novel change in cytologic localization of human chorionic gonadotropin and human placental lactogen in first-trimester placenta in the course of gestation. Am J Obstet Gynecol 1992;167:217–222.

3. Ozturk M, Bellet D, Manil L, et al. Physiological studies of human chorionic gonadotropin (hCG), alpha hCG, and beta hCG as measured by specific monoclonal immunoradiometric assays. Endocrinology 1987;120:549–558.

4. Kato Y, Braunstein GD. Beta-core fragment is a major form of immunoreactive urinary chorionic gonadotropin in human pregnancy. J Clin Endocrinol Metab 1988;66: 1197–1201.

5. Lenton EA, Neal LM, Sulaiman R. Plasma concentrations of human chorionic gonadotropin from the time of implantation until the second week of pregnancy. Fertil Steril 1982;37:773–778.

6. Pittaway DE, Reish RL, Wentz AC. Doubling times of human chorionic gonadotropin increase in early viable intrauterine pregnancies. Am J Obstet Gynecol 1985;152: 299–302.

7. Pittaway DE, Wentz AC. Evaluation of early pregnancy by serial chorionic gonadotropin determinations: a comparison of methods by receiver operating characteristic curve analysis. Fertil Steril 1985;43:529–533.

8. Hay DL. Placental histology and the production of human choriogonadotrophin and its subunits in pregnancy. Br J Obstet Gynaecol 1988;95:1268–1275.

9. Jovanovic L, Landesman R, Saxena BB. Screening for twin pregnancy. Science 1977; 198:738.

10. Norman RJ, Menabawey M, Lowings C, et al. Relationship between blood and urine concentrations of intact human chorionic gonadotropin and its free subunits in early pregnancy. Obstet Gynecol 1987;69:590–593.

11. Storring PL, Gaines-Das RE, Bangham DR. International Reference Preparation of Human Chorionic Gonadotrophin for Immunoassay: potency estimates in various bioassay and protein binding assay systems; and International Reference Preparations of the alpha and beta subunits of human chorionic gonadotrophin for immunoassay. J Endocrinol 1980;84:295–310.

12. Ooi DS, Perkins SL, Claman P, et al. Serum human chorionic gonadotrophin levels in early pregnancy. Clin Chim Acta 1989;181:281–292.

13. Batzer FR, Weiner S, Corson SL, et al. Landmarks during the first forty-two days of gestation demonstrated by the beta-subunit of human chorionic gonadotropin and ultrasound. Am J Obstet Gynecol 1983;146:973–979.

14. Henzl MR, Segre EJ. Physiology of human menstrual cycle and early pregnancy: a review of recent investigations. Contraception 1970;1:315–338.

15. Lin TJ, Lin SC, Erlenmeyer F, et al. Progesterone production rates during the third trimester of pregnancy in normal women, diabetic women, and women with abnormal glucose tolerance. J Clin Endocrinol Metab 1972;34:287–297.

16. Tulchinsky D, Hobel CJ, Yeager E, et al. Plasma estrone, estradiol, estriol, progesterone, and 17-hydroxyprogesterone in human pregnancy. I. Normal pregnancy. Am J Obstet Gynecol 1972;112:1095–1100.

17. Csapo AI, Pulkkinen MO, Ruttner B, et al. The significance of the human corpus luteum in pregnancy maintenance. I. Preliminary studies. Am J Obstet Gynecol 1972; 112:1061–1067.

18. Csapo AI, Pulkkinen MO, Wiest WG. Effects of luteectomy and progesterone replacement therapy in early pregnant patients. Am J Obstet Gynecol 1973;115:759–765.

19. Batzer FR. Hormonal evaluation of early pregnancy. Fertil Steril 1980;34:1–13.

20. Bennett FC, Ingram DM. Diet and female sex hormone concentrations: an intervention study for the type of fat consumed. Am J Clin Nutr 1990;52:808–812.

21. Dorgan JF, Reichman ME, Judd JT, et al. Relation of energy, fat, and fiber intakes to plasma concentrations of estrogens and androgens in premenopausal women. Am J Clin Nutr 1996;64:25–31.

22. Nakajima ST, Gibson M. The effect of a meal on circulating steady-state progesterone levels. J Clin Endocrinol Metab 1989;69:917–919.

23. Nakajima ST, McAuliffe T, Gibson M. The 24-hour pattern of the levels of serum progesterone and immunoreactive human chorionic gonadotropin in normal early pregnancy. J Clin Endocrinol Metab 1990;71:345–353.

24. Stovall TG, Ling FW, Carson SA, et al. Serum progesterone and uterine curettage in differential diagnosis of ectopic pregnancy. Fertil Steril 1992; 57:452–458.

25. Tovanabutra S, Illingworth PJ, Ledger WL, et al. The relationship between peripheral immunoactive inhibin, human chorionic gonadotrophin, oestradiol and progesterone during human pregnancy. Clin Endocrinol 1993;38:101–107.

26. Illingworth PJ, Groome NP, Duncan WC, et al. Measurement of circulating inhibin forms during the establishment of pregnancy. J Clin Endocrinol Metab 1996;81:1471–1475.

27. Takeuchi T, Nishii O, Okamura T, et al. Free testosterone and abortion in early pregnancy. Int J Gynecol Obstet 1993;43:151–156.

28. Weiss G, Goldsmith LT, Sachdev R, et al. Elevated first-trimester serum relaxin concentrations in pregnant women following ovarian stimulation predict prematurity risk and preterm delivery. Obstet Gynecol 1993;82:821–828.

29. Aksoy S, Celikkanat H, Senoz S, et al. The prognostic value of serum estradiol, progesterone, testosterone and free testosterone levels in detecting early abortions. Eur J Obstet Gynecol Reprod Biol 1996;67:5–8.

30. Stewart DR, Overstreet JW, Celniker AC, et al. The relationship between hCG and relaxin secretion in normal pregnancies vs peri-implantation spontaneous abortions. Clin Endocrinol 1993;38:379–385.

31. Britten S, Soenksen DM, Bustillo M, et al. Very early (24–56 days from last menstrual period) embryonic heart rate in normal pregnancies. Hum Reprod 1994;9:2424–2426.

32. Robinson HP, Fleming JE. A critical evaluation of sonar "crown-rump length" measurements. Br J Obstet Gynaecol 1975;82:702–710.

33. Hellman LM, Kobayashi M, Fillisti L, et al. Growth and development of the human fetus prior to the twentieth week of gestation. Am J Obstet Gynecol 1969;103:789–800.

34. Jouppila P. Clinical consequences after ultrasonic diagnosis of intrauterine hematoma in threatened abortion. J Clin Ultrasound 1985;13:107–111.

35. Strobino BA, Pantel-Silverman J. First-trimester vaginal bleeding and the loss of chromosomally normal and abnormal conceptions. Am J Obstet Gynecol 1987;157:1150–1154.

36. Pedersen JF, Mantoni M. Prevalence and significance of subchorionic hemorrhage in threatened abortion: a sonographic study. Am J Radiol 1990;154:535–537.

37. Bennett GL, Bromley B, Lieberman E, et al. Subchorionic hemorrhage in first-trimester pregnancies: prediction of pregnancy outcome with sonography. Radiology 1996;200:803–806.

38. Kadar N, DeVore G, Romero R. Discriminatory hCG zone: its use in the sonographic evaluation for ectopic pregnancy. Obstet Gynecol 1981;58:156–161.

39. Kadar N, Bohrer M, Kemmann E, et al. The discriminatory human chorionic gonadotropin zone for endovaginal sonography: a prospective, randomized study. Fertil Steril 1994;61:1016–1020.

40. Shapiro BS, Escobar M, Makuch R, et al. A model-based prediction for transvaginal ultrasonographic identification of early intrauterine pregnancy. Am J Obstet Gynecol 1992;166:1495–1500.

41. Steinkampf MP, Guzick DS, Hammond KR, et al. Identification of early pregnancy landmarks by transvaginal sonography: analysis by logistic regression. Fertil Steril 1997;68:168–170.

42. Kadar N, Romero R. The timing of a repeat ultrasound examination in the evaluation for ectopic pregnancy. J Clin Ultrasound 1982;10:211–214.

43. Stabile I, Campbell S, Grudzinskas JG. Can ultrasound reliably diagnose ectopic pregnancy? Br J Obstet Gynaecol 1988;95:1247–1252.

44. Tongsong T, Pongsatha S. Transvaginal sonographic features in diagnosis of ectopic pregnancy. Int J Gynaecol Obstet 1993;43:277–283.

45. Bromley B, Harlow BL, Laboda LA, et al. Small sac size in the first trimester: a predictor of poor fetal outcome. Radiology 1991;178:375–377.

46. Nazari A, Check JH, Epstein RH, et al. Relationship of small-for-dates sac size to crown-

rump length and spontaneous abortion in patients with a known date of ovulation. Obstet Gynecol 1991;78:369–373.

47. Dickey RP, Olar TT, Taylor SN, et al. Relationship of small gestational sac-crown-rump length differences to abortion and abortus karyotypes. Obstet Gynecol 1992;79: 554–557.

48. Levi CS, Lyons EA, Lindsay DJ. Early diagnosis of nonviable pregnancy with endovaginal US. Radiology 1988;167:383–385.

49. Dickey RP, Olar TT, Taylor SN, et al. Relationship of small gestational sac-crown-rump length differences to abortion and abortus karyotypes. Obstet Gynecol 1992;79: 554–557.

50. Howe RS, Isaacson KJ, Albert JL, et al. Embryonic heart rate in human pregnancy. J Ultrasound Med 1991;10:367–371.

51. Levi CS, Lyons EA, Zheng XH, et al. Endovaginal US: demonstration of cardiac activity in embryos of less than 5.0 mm in crown-rump length. Radiology 1990;176:71–74.

52. Goldstein SR. Embryonic death in early pregnancy: a new look at the first trimester. Obstet Gynecol 1994;84:294–297.

53. Emerson DS, Cartier MS, Altieri LA, et al. Diagnostic efficacy of endovaginal color Doppler flow imaging in an ectopic pregnancy screening program. Radiology 1992;183: 413–420.

54. Lindsay DJ, Lovett IS, Lyons EA, et al. Yolk sac diameter and shape at endovaginal US: predictors of pregnancy outcome in the first trimester. Radiology 1992;183:115–118.

55. Kurtz AB, Needleman L, Pennell RG, et al. Can detection of the yolk sac in the first trimester be used to predict the outcome of pregnancy? A prospective sonographic study. Am J Radiol 1992;158:843–847.

56. Reece EA, Scioscia AL, Pinter E, et al. Prognostic significance of the human yolk sac assessed by ultrasonography. Am J Obstet Gynecol 1988;159:1191–1194.

57. Timor-Tritsch IE, Farine D, Rosen MG. A close look at early embryonic development with the high-frequency transvaginal transducer. Am J Obstet Gynecol 1988;159: 676–681.

58. Centers for Disease Control. Ectopic Pregnancy—United States, 1990–1992. MMWR Morb Mortal Wkly Rep 1995;44:46–48.

59. Centers for Disease Control. Ectopic Pregnancy—United States, 1988–1989. MMWR Morb Mortal Wkly Rep 1992;55:591–594.

60. Aral SO, Mosher WD, Cates W Jr. Self-reported pelvic inflammatory disease in the United States, 1988. JAMA 1991;266:2570–2573.

61. Westrom L, Joesoef R, Reynolds G, et al. Pelvic inflammatory disease and fertility: a cohort study of 1,844 women with laparoscopically verified disease and 657 control women with normal laparoscopic results. Sex Transm Dis 1992;19:185–192.

62. Yao M, Tulandi T. Current status of surgical and nonsurgical management of ectopic pregnancy. Fertil Steril 1997;67:421–433.

63. Stovall TG, Ling FW, Carson SA, et al. Nonsurgical diagnosis and treatment of tubal pregnancy. Fertil Steril 1990;54:537–538.

64. Stovall TG, Ling FW, Carson SA, et al. Serum progesterone and uterine curettage in differential diagnosis of ectopic pregnancy. Fertil Steril 1992;57:456–458.

65. Glock JL, Johnson JV, Brumsted JR. Efficacy and safety of single-dose systemic methotrexate in the treatment of ectopic pregnancy. Fertil Steril 1994;62:716–721.

66. Stovall TG, Ling FW, Gray LA. Single-dose methotrexate for treatment of ectopic pregnancy. Obstet Gynecol 1991;77:754–757.

67. Tulandi T, Atri M, Bret P, et al. Transvaginal intratubal methotrexate treatment of ectopic pregnancy. Fertil Steril 1992;58:98–100.

68. Trio D, Strobelt N, Picciolo C, et al. Prognostic factors for successful expectant management of ectopic pregnancy. Fertil Steril 1995;63:469–472.

69. Ackerman TE, Levi CS, Lyons E, et al. Decidual cyst: endovaginal sonographic sign of ectopic pregnancy. Radiology 1993;189:727–731.

70. Kizza AP, Rogo KO. Assessment of the manual vacuum aspiration (MVA) equipment in the management of incomplete abortion. East Afr Med J 1990;67:812–822.

71. Goldstein SR. Significance of cardiac activity on endovaginal ultrasound in very early embryos. Obstet Gynecol 1992;80:670–672.

72. Dickey RP, Olar TT, Taylor SN, et al. Relationship of small gestational sac-crown-rump length differences to abortion and abortus karyotypes. Obstet Gynecol 1992;79: 554–557.

73. Warren WB, Timor-Tritsch I, Peisner DB, et al. Dating the early pregnancy by sequential appearance of embryonic structures. Am J Obstet Gynecol 1989;161:747–753.

74. Goldstein I, Zimmer EA, Tamir A, et al. Evaluation of normal gestational sac growth: appearance of embryonic heartbeat and embryo body movements using the transvaginal technique. Obstet Gynecol 1991;77:885–888.

75. Nyberg DA, Laing FC, Filly RA. Threatened abortion: sonographic distinction of normal and abnormal gestation sacs. Radiology 1986;158:397–400.

76. Lelaidier C, Baton-Saint-Mleux C, Fernandez H, et al. Mifepristone (RU 486) induces embryo expulsion in first trimester non-developing pregnancies: a prospective randomized trial. Hum Reprod 1993;8:492–495.

77. Thong KJ, Baird DT. Induction of abortion with mifepristone and misoprostol in early pregnancy. Br J Obstet Gynaecol 1992;99:1004–1007.

78. Aubeny E, Peyron R, Turpin CL, et al. Termination of early pregnancy (up to and after 63 days of amenorrhea) with mifepristone (RU486) and increasing doses of misoprostol. Int J Fertil 1995;40:85–91.

79. McKinley C, Thong KJ, Baird DT. The effect of dose of mifepristone and gestation on the efficacy of medical abortion with mifepristone and misoprostol. Hum Reprod 1993;8:1502–1505.

80. World Health Organization. Termination of pregnancy with reduced doses of mifepristone. BMJ 1993;307:532–537.

81. El-Refaey H, Hinshaw K, Henshaw R, et al. Medical management of missed abortion and anembryonic pregnancy. BMJ 1992;305:1399.

82. Henshaw R, Naji S, Russell I, et al. Psychological responses following medical abortion (using mifepristone and gemeprost) and surgical vacuum aspiration. A patient-centered, partially randomised prospective study. Acta Obstet Gynecol Scand 1994; 73: 812–818.

83. El-Refaey H, Templeton A. Early induction of abortion by a combination of oral mifepristone and misoprostol administered by the vaginal route. Contraception 1994; 49:111–114.

84. Hausknecht RU. Methotrexate and misoprostol to terminate early pregnancy. N Engl J Med 1995;333:537–540.

85. Creinin MD, Darney PD. Methotrexate and misoprostol for early abortion. Contraception 1993;48:339–348.

86. Creinin MD, Vittinghoff E. Methotrexate and misoprostol vs misoprostol alone for early abortion: a randomized controlled trial. JAMA 1994;272:1190–1195.

87. Creinin MD. Methotrexate and misoprostol for abortion at 57–63 days gestation. Contraception 1994;50:511–515.

88. Schaff EA, Wortman M, Eisinger SH, et al. Methotrexate and misoprostol when surgical abortion fails. Obstet Gynecol 1996;87:450–452.

89. Kaplan B, Pardo J, Rabinerson D, et al. Future fertility following conservative management of complete abortion. Hum Reprod 1996;11:92–94.

90. Poland BJ, Miller JR, Jones DC, et al. Reproductive counseling in patients who have had a spontaneous abortion. Am J Obstet Gynecol 1977;127:685–691.

91. Thom DH, Nelson LM, Vaughan TL. Spontaneous abortion and subsequent adverse birth outcomes. Am J Obstet Gynecol 1992;166:111–116.

92. Warburton D, Fraser FC. Spontaneous abortion risks in man: data from reproductive histories. Collected in a medical genetics unit. Am J Hum Genet 1964;16:1–25.

93. Daling JR, Spadoni LR, Emanuel I. Role of induced abortion in secondary infertility. Obstet Gynecol 1981;57:59–61.

94. Ben-Baruch G, Schiff E, Moran O, et al. Curettage vs. nonsurgical management in women with early spontaneous abortions. J Reprod Med 1991;36:644–646.

95. Tzonou A, Hsieh CC, Trichopoulos D, et al. Induced abortions, miscarriages, and to-

bacco smoking as risk factors for secondary infertility. J Epidemiol Commun Health 1993;47:36–39.

96. Valle RF, Sciarra JJ. Intrauterine adhesions: hysteroscopic diagnosis, classification, treatment, and reproductive outcome. Am J Obstet Gynecol 1988;158:1459–1470.

97. Golan A, Schneider D, Avrech O, et al. Hysteroscopic findings after missed abortion. Fertil Steril 1992;58:508–510.

98. Friedler S, Margalioth EJ, Kafka I, et al. Incidence of post-abortion intra-uterine adhesions evaluated by hysteroscopy—a prospective study. Hum Reprod 1993;8:442–444.

99. Donnet ML, Howie PW, Marnie M, et al. Return of ovarian function following spontaneous abortion. Clin Endocrinol 1990;33:13–20.

100. Landgren BM, Unden AL, Diczfalusy E. Hormonal profile of the cycle in 68 normally menstruating women. Acta Endocrinol 1980;94:89–98.

101. Blazar AS, Harlin J, Zaidi AA, et al. Differences in hormonal patterns during the first postabortion menstrual cycle after two techniques of termination of pregnancy. Fertil Steril 1980;33:493–500.

102. Nakajima ST, Brumsted JR, Deaton JL, et al. Endometrial histology after first trimester spontaneous abortion. Fertil Steril 1991;55:32–35.

103. Farhi J, Bar-Hava I, Homburg R, et al. Induced regeneration of endometrium following curettage for abortion: a comparative study. Hum Reprod 1993;8:1143–1144.

104. Jones EF, Forrest JD, Henshaw SK, et al. Unintended pregnancy, contraceptive practice and family planning services in developed countries. Fam Plann Perspect 1988;20: 53–67.

105. Levitt C. Preconception health promotion. Prim Care 1993;20:537–549.

106. Milunsky A, Jick H, Jick SS, et al. Multivitamin/folic acid supplementation in early pregnancy reduces the prevalence of neural tube defects. JAMA 1989;262:2847–2852.

107. Centers for Disease Control and Prevention. Recommendations for the use of folic acid to reduce the number of cases of spina bifida and other neural tube defects. MMWR Morb Mortal Wkly Rep 1992;41:1–7.

108. Centers for Disease Control and Prevention. Use of folic acid for prevention for spina bifida and other neural tube defects 1983–1991. MMWR Morb Mortal Wkly Rep 1991;40:513–516.

109. Committee on Obstetrics Maternal and Fetal Medicine. Folic acid for the prevention of recurrent neural tube defects. Am Coll Obstet Gynecol 1993;120:1–3.

110. Centers for Disease Control and Prevention. Recommendations for use of folic acid to reduce number of spina bifida cases and other neural tube defects. JAMA 1993;269: 1233–1238.

111. Clapp JF III, Capeless EL. Neonatal morphometrics after endurance exercise during pregnancy. Am J Obstet Gynecol 1990;163:1805–1811.

112. Exercise during pregnancy and the postpartum period. ACOG Tech Bull 1994;189.

113. Milunsky A, Ulcickas M, Rothman KJ, et al. Maternal heat exposure and neural tube defects. JAMA 1992;268:882–885.

114. Rubella and pregnancy. ACOG Tech Bull 1992;171.

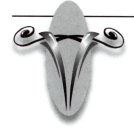

C H A P T E R   6

Vulvovaginitis

TRACEY A. BANKS

Vulvovaginitis is one of the most common reasons for a woman to visit her obstetrician/gynecologist. Vaginal discharge is among the top 25 reasons for a physician consultation by a patient (1). As commonplace as this diagnosis is, misdiagnosis can occur and lead to wrong treatment unless careful attentions to specific criteria are followed.

Most vaginal symptoms are caused by one of three types of vulvovaginitis: bacterial vaginosis, candida vulvovaginitis, and trichomoniasis. Other less common etiologies include contact vaginitis and desquamative exudative vaginitis. This chapter discusses the evaluation and treatment of vulvovaginitis with special emphasis on the pregnant and adolescent patient.

NORMAL VAGINAL FLORA AND DISCHARGE

The vagina is an ecosystem where the vaginal epithelium serves as the habitat for microbial flora, composed primarily of Gram-negative, Gram-positive, anaerobic, and facultatively anaerobic species (2). The predominant normal vaginal flora consists of facultative *Lactobacillus* species. These are long Gram-positive rods that exert protective effects in the vagina by the production of hydrogen peroxide, bacteriocins, and/or a lower pH that inhibits the colonization or overgrowth of potential pathogens. Physiologic or normal discharge is usually clear or white, viscous, and pools in the fornices of the vagina. It contains sloughed vaginal and cervical epithelial cells, mucoid endocervical secretions, and bacteria. The normal vaginal pH is usually less than 4.5. Minimal odor may be present. Normal vaginal discharge does not cause symptoms of burning or itching. The phase of the menstrual cycle influences the quantity and quality of normal discharge. During the follicular phase, there is a steady increase in vaginal liquid discharge, up to the point of ovulation. In the luteal phase, after ovulation, the discharge becomes more viscous and thick. Diet, medications, or over-the-counter dietary supplements affect the odor of the normal vaginal discharge. There may be excessive, but normal, vaginal discharge from cervical mucorrhea if there is a large cervical ectropion. In this case, no therapy is indicated, but if it is too bothersome to the patient, cryotherapy or CO_2 laser has been used and is occasionally helpful.

Mechanism of Infection

For the most part, there is remarkable stability of the vaginal endogenous flora even in the face of aggressive douching and short-term parenteral antibiotics. Estrogen and pH exert a strong influence on this stability. A complex interaction exists between the vaginal epithelium and both the endogenous and exogenous floras. A change in the existing conditions of the vaginal tissue may alter the flora in terms of numbers and species. Thus, benign normal vaginal flora can become pathologic and assume a different relationship to the host.

Diagnosis

The evaluation of women with vaginal symptoms requires a directed history, a physical examination, and in-office laboratory testing in all cases. Symptoms alone are insufficient as a basis for diagnosis and treatment plans (Table 6.1).

History

Vaginal discharge is the most common complaint in women with vaginitis. A thorough history should include the color, consistency, and volume of the vaginal discharge and the presence or absence of odor. It should include the onset, type, duration, and extent of symptoms. Other symptoms such as itching, vulvar pain, abdominal pain, and/or dysuria should be noted. Information regarding sexual history, previous sexually transmitted diseases, contraceptive methods, and dyspareunia is contributory. A list of current medications, including over-the-counter drugs, is included in the history. Often disregarded, but equally important, are the patient's concern or opinion about the diagnosis, remedies the patient has already tried, and, finally, the patient's response to past treatments.

Physical Examination

The physical examination should be deferred if vaginal creams were used in the past 72 hours, because they may obscure the diagnosis. The vulvar and vaginal vestibules,

TABLE 6.1. Diagnostic Features of Vulvovaginitis

Feature	Normal	Bacterial Vaginosis	Candida Vaginitis	Trichomonas Vaginitis
Symptoms	None or physiologic discharge	Thin, malodorous, white/gray discharge	Pruritus, white thick or watery discharge, vulva soreness	Profuse, offensive discharge, dyspareunia
Discharge	White or clear, variable minimal to no odor	Moderate, adherent, white to gray, homogenous	White, scant to moderate, varying from milky to cottage cheese-like	Profuse, yellowish, homogenous, frothy
Examination	Normal	No inflammation	Introital, vaginal, and vulvar erythema; exfoliations from scratching	Erythema and swelling of vulvar and vaginal wall; "strawberry" cervix
pH of vaginal fluid	<4.5	>4.5	<4.5	5–6.0
Amine (whiff) test	Negative	Positive	Negative	Occasionally positive
Saline microscopy	Normal epithelial cells and lactobacilli (long rods)	Clue cells, absence of leukocytes, decreased lactobacilli	Normal flora	Increased leukocytes, motile trichomonads, no clue cells or abnormal flora
10% KOH microscopy	Negative	Negative	Hyphae and budding yeast	Negative

including the vaginal introitus, are inspected and palpated for any erythema, swelling, lesions, or tenderness. Vaginal speculum examinations, with only water as a lubricant, are mandatory for the diagnosis and treatment of vulvovaginitis. Inspect the vaginal walls carefully for any evidence of vaginal ulcers secondary to improper tampon use or prolonged use of diaphragms or a pessary. Scrutinize the cervix for lesions, friability, or purulent material that may indicate cervicitis. The color, amount, texture, and odor of the vaginal and/or cervical discharge are noted. A bimanual examination is necessary to assess the size and tenderness of the uterus and adnexa.

Office Analysis

Simple office analysis provides the backbone for diagnosing the etiology of vulvovaginitis. This assessment includes the following tests:

1. pH of vaginal secretions—a drop of vaginal discharge is placed on litmus paper and color change is noted. The normal vaginal pH is 3.5 to 4.0.
2. Amine (Whiff) test—a positive test constitutes a "fishy" odor after 10% potassium hydroxide is added to vaginal secretions on the speculum or glass slide. This odor is caused by volatilization of amines in the discharge.
3. Microscopy (wet mount)—small amounts of vaginal discharge are placed on a plain unfrosted slide and mixed with one to two drops of normal saline at one end and one to two drops of 10% KOH at the other. The specimens are then covered with coverslips and examined microscopically.

Examination of the normal saline preparation includes assessment of the background flora where normal includes lactobacilli with long rods and abnormal reveals a predominance of short rods, cocci, and curved motile rods. A search for the presence of white blood cells, trichomonads, and/or clue cells (squamous epithelial cells studded with bacteria causing obscured borders) is also made. The potassium hydroxide preparation is examined for the presence of hyphae or budding yeast. Misdiagnosis occurs when slides are not systematically examined and carefully scrutinized for each type of vaginitis. Mixed infections can, and do, occur (3). An accurate diagnosis is subject to many variables. Despite this, the aforementioned laboratory tests, coupled with a thorough history and careful physical examination, provide an immediate and reliable clinical diagnosis.

At times, other diagnostic evaluations such as cultures for *Trichomonas vaginalis* and *Candida* species, using modified Diamond media in addition to Sabouraud's or Nickerson's agar (for *Candida* species), are required. Gram stain of vaginal secretions may be used to diagnose bacterial vaginosis and candidal vulvovaginitis. However, because nonmotile trichomonads are difficult to distinguish from leukocytes, the Gram stain is not useful in diagnosing this entity. If clinically indicated, urinalysis, pregnancy testing, or serum and/or cervical testing for concomitant sexually transmitted diseases, such as syphilis, human immunodeficiency virus (HIV), gonorrhea, or chlamydia, is performed.

If a microscope is not available, hydrogen peroxide may be able to differentiate yeast and bacterial vaginosis infections from those caused by trichomonas or desquamative inflammatory vaginitis. If the vaginal secretions contain white blood cells, the mixture of hydrogen peroxide and the vaginal discharge produces foaming bubbles. Leukocytes are present in cases of vulvovaginitis due to trichomonas or in desquamative vaginitis. In cases of vulvovaginitis caused by yeast or bacterial vaginosis, there are no white blood cells in the vaginal secretions; the mixture of vaginal secretions and hydrogen peroxide does not produce a foamy response. This information, in addition to the results of pH testing and the whiff test, may guide the clinician's diagnosis and therapy. The problem with this method is that the results are unreliable in the presence of a mixed infection.

During the episode of vulvovaginitis, and until treatment is completed, either intercourse is avoided or condoms are used. It is important to keep the external genitalia dry and to avoid perfumed feminine hygiene products. The patient should wear loose-fitting clothing and use only all-cotton undergarments.

BACTERIAL VAGINOSIS

Bacterial vaginosis is the most common vaginal infection among reproductive-age women, accounting for 40 to 50% of all cases of vaginitis (4). It has had many names in the past, including nonspecific vaginitis, *Haemophilus vaginalis* vaginitis, *Corynebacterium vaginale* vaginitis, and *Gardnerella vaginalis* vaginitis (5). The confusion over its name parallels the confusion over the disease entity itself. Initially believed to be a benign condition, recent investigations demonstrated that bacterial vaginosis is associated with a variety of upper genital tract infections and complications. These include pelvic inflammatory disease, postcesarean endometritis, posthysterectomy pelvic infection, chorioamnionitis, premature rupture of membranes, and preterm labor and delivery (6).

Epidemiology

Bacteria vaginosis is a common disorder that occurs among 35 to 64% of women attending sexually transmitted disease clinics, 15 to 20% of pregnant women, and 10 to 26% of women attending gynecologic clinics (7). Typically, bacterial vaginosis affects women in reproductive age, indicating a possible role of sex hormones in its pathogenesis, but it may occur in prepubertal and menopausal women infrequently. It is found equally in pregnant and nonpregnant women. There has been an association between bacterial vaginosis and intrauterine devices, although the exact mechanism by which the intrauterine device increases the risk of bacterial vaginosis is unknown (8). Oral contraceptives might have a protective effect on the development by promoting lactobacilli-predominant vaginal flora. This disease can also occur in women who have had a hysterectomy.

Pathogenesis

Bacterial vaginosis is a polymicrobial condition where there is a decrease in vaginal acidity and the concentration of lactobacilli. There is also a 100-fold or more increase in the concentrations of other organisms. These organisms include *G. vaginalis,* which is isolated from 45 to 99% of women with bacterial vaginosis; *Mycoplasma hominis; Prevotella;* bacteroides; *Peptostreptococcus* species; *Ureaplasma urealyticum;* and other anaerobic flora. The natural history is poorly understood. Many investigators view bacterial vaginosis as an alteration in the microecology of the lower genital tract, where microorganisms generally present in very low concentrations in reproductive-age women attain predominance over the physiologically favored lactobacilli's microflora. The specific triggers for this change in the vaginal flora are unknown. Although data exist that suggest bacterial vaginosis is sexually transmitted, this is still controversial (9).

Clinical Manifestations

Women often complain of a thin increased vaginal discharge present at the introitus. The discharge may be sticky and have a disagreeable or fishy odor. This odor is more noticeable after unprotected sexual intercourse. The basic pH of seminal fluid causes a volatilization of amines and the production of a strong odor. Mild to moderate itching may also occur with the vaginal discharge. These symptoms, however, could be absent in approximately half of the women with bacterial vaginosis (4). On examination, a thin grayish-white homogeneous discharge that adheres to the vaginal wall may be noted (Fig. 6.1).

In some cases of bacterial vaginosis due predominately to *Gardnerella*, gas-filled cystic structures on the vaginal walls or cervix are seen. This is vaginitis emphysematosa and will clear with treatment of the bacterial vaginosis. Vaginitis emphysematosa may also be seen with infections due to trichomonas.

Diagnosis

Traditionally, the most widely accepted clinical criteria for diagnosis include three of the following four criteria (8):

1. Milky homogenous adherent discharge
2. Vaginal pH greater than 4.5
3. Presence of clue cells in the vaginal fluid on light microscopy
4. Positive whiff test

The presence of clue cells, vaginal epithelial cells with bacteria densely adherent to them and obscuring their borders, is the single most reliable predictor of bacterial vaginosis (10) (Fig. 6.2). Few inflammatory cells or lactobacilli are seen on the wet smear. The presence of leukocytes on the smear indicates a concurrent process, such as cervicitis, trichomonas, or atrophic vaginitis. To accurately diagnose bacterial vaginosis, at least 20% of the epithelial cells seen on the wet mount should be clue cells (11). Interpretation of these signs can be difficult. Vaginal pH is highly sensitive but

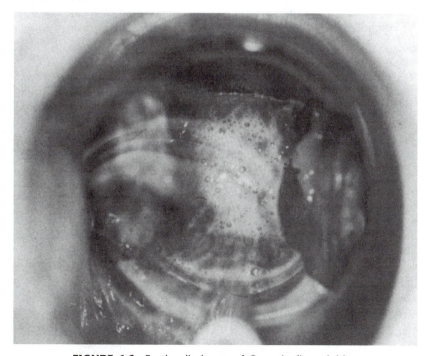

FIGURE 6.1. Frothy discharge of *G. vaginalis* vaginitis.

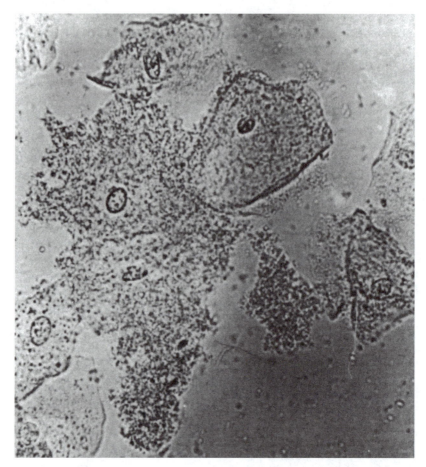

FIGURE 6.2. Stippled clue cell of *G. vaginalis* vaginitis.

not specific; it is influenced by vaginal bleeding, douching, and recent intercourse. Currently, the presence of clue cells and two of the other three signs are sufficient to confirm the diagnosis of bacterial vaginosis.

Clue cells and changes in bacterial flora may be detected on the Papanicolaou (Pap) smear. These are normally an incidental finding and have limited diagnostic significance in comparison with other methods. Gram stains are another means of diagnosing bacterial vaginosis that can be done in the office setting. A criteria for interpreting Gram stains was devised by Spiegal et al. (12). Bacterial vaginosis was diagnosed if the number of *Gardnerella* morphotypes and other bacteria (cocci, fusiforms, and curved rods) were increased and if there were fewer than five *Lactobacillus* morphotypes (large Gram-positive rods) per oil immersion field. Using these criteria, the Gram stain has a sensitivity of 93% and a specificity of 70% for diagnosing bacterial vaginosis.

Vaginal culture, which has a high degree of sensitivity, is not practical because these organisms are members of the normal flora. Unless clinical signs are present, the incidental finding of *G. vaginalis* in a vaginal culture is not used to diagnose bacterial vaginosis.

Oligonucleotide probe tests have the advantage of being specific and can be adjusted in sensitivity to detect either high or low concentrations of bacteria. A commercially available version of this test is reported to be 94% sensitive and 81% specific for the diagnosis of bacterial vaginosis in a population seeking treatment for sexually transmitted diseases (13). These types of tests are ideal in offices where microscopy is not available or is unsatisfactory. They are objective and do not require microscopy skills. Other tests available only in research laboratories look for the metabolic products of microorganisms unique to the vaginal fluid of women with bacterial vaginosis.

Sequelae

Several researchers established a correlation between abnormal bacterial flora of the genital tract and upper genital tract infections. Bacterial vaginosis may contribute significantly to the development of these upper tract infections (4). Almost 67% of the time, the anaerobes and facultative bacteria responsible for bacterial vaginosis are recovered from the upper genital tracts of women with pelvic inflammatory disease. These studies provide strong evidence for the important role that anaerobic bacteria play in the etiology and pathogenesis of acute pelvic inflammatory disease.

The development of postoperative infection depends on a complex interaction between host defense mechanisms and the bacterial inoculum. Most postoperative pelvic infections involve an ascending route of bacterial spread from the vagina and cervix. Similarities between the bacteria associated with bacterial vaginosis and those of postpartum and postsurgical infections suggest that bacterial vaginosis may play a role in the origin of these infections (14). Preliminary data suggest that bacterial vaginosis increases the risk of postoperative infections in both the postpartum and postsurgical settings. However, few prospective studies are able to confirm this suspicion. If this is true, it may be prudent to consider treatment of bacterial vaginosis (symptomatic or asymptomatic) before performing surgical or invasive procedures. To clarify this relationship, additional prospective studies must be done.

Considerable information shows that bacterial vaginosis is associated with a two- to threefold increased risk of preterm premature rupture of the membranes, preterm labor and birth, and infectious maternal morbidity (15). Hillier et al. (16) demonstrated that women with bacterial vaginosis during the second trimester were 40% more likely to give birth to premature low-birth-weight infants than women without bacterial vaginosis. This relationship remained unchanged after adjustment for confounding variables. The causative mechanism(s) for these adverse outcomes is unknown. One line of thinking is that microorganisms of bacterial vaginosis produce factors, including proteases, that can facilitate transport of bacteria to fetal membranes and impair fetal membrane integrity. Prospective investigations to determine if treatment of bacterial vaginosis reduces the incidence of premature rupture of the membranes and preterm births are currently lacking. Currently, pregnant women with asymptomatic bacterial vaginosis are not routinely screened or treated for this syndrome. Some advocate the screening of all gravidas with a history of preterm labor or rupture of membranes, although this is controversial.

Treatment

Asymptomatic Patients

Approximately 50% of women with microbiologic findings suggestive of bacterial vaginosis are asymptomatic. Studies suggest that spontaneous resolution of laboratory-proven bacterial vaginosis occurs in most asymptomatic women (17). Currently, treatment of asymptomatic patients is not recommended. It has been recommended that patients with bacterial vaginosis scheduled to undergo endometrial biopsy, hysteroscopy, hysterosalpingography, intrauterine device insertion, or hysterectomy receive a full course of therapy before the procedure. Although bacterial vaginosis has been associated with premature rupture of membranes, preterm labor, chorioam-nionitis, and postpartum endometritis, routine treatment of asymptomatic pregnant patients has not been recommended universally or accepted.

Systemic Therapy

A multitude of antimicrobial agents has been used for the treatment of bacterial vaginosis, including sulfa vaginal creams, ampicillin, and doxycycline (Table 6.2). Metronidazole is currently the treatment of choice with reported cure rates of 72 to 100% (18). Metronidazole is inactive against facultative lactobacilli and therefore helps the recolonization of this organism and thus the restoration of the normal flora after successful therapy. Various treatment regimens with metronidazole exist. The two most common dosages are 500 mg orally, twice daily for 5 to 7 days, and 2 g as a single dose. The 7-day course achieves higher cure rates compared with the single 2-g dose. The single-dose regimen increases compliance and has fewer side ef-fects and a lower cost. These factors may render its clinical effectiveness equal to that of the 7-day regimen, but there are no firm data to support this argument.

The common side effects of metronidazole are nausea, vomiting, anorexia, metal-lic taste in the mouth, secondary yeast infections, headache, dizziness, and darkening of the urine. Skin rashes are less common. The patient should not drink alcoholic bev-erages while taking metronidazole because it may produce a disulfiram-like effect.

There is some concern about the use of systemic metronidazole in pregnancy be-cause of potential teratogenicity. A recent analysis of seven studies suggests no increase in birth defects among infants exposed in the first trimester, but currently there are no prospective studies that address this issue (19). Metronidazole should be used with caution in patients with central nervous system diseases or blood dyscrasias.

Oral clindamycin has a significant cure rate against anaerobic bacteria and *G. vaginalis*. A dose of 300 mg twice daily for 7 days produced a 94% cure rate that is comparable with metronidazole (20). It is particularly useful in pregnancy, metronidazole treatment failure, and where patients cannot tolerate metronidazole. Adverse reactions include gastrointestinal complaints (nausea, loose stool) and, on rare occasions, skin rash. It is safe to use in pregnancy, regardless of trimester.

Intravaginal Therapy

Metronidazole vaginal gel 0.75% (MetroGel-vaginal) is an effective alternative to oral metronidazole (21). It provides cure rates similar to those for oral metronidazole, de-

TABLE 6.2. Treatment Options for Bacterial Vaginosis

Drug	Formulation	Cost[a] ($)
ORAL THERAPY		
Metronidazole (Flagyl, Protostat)	500 mg twice daily for 5–7 days	13.39
	2 g as a single dose	6.49
Clindamycin	300 mg twice daily for 7 days (comes in 375-mg tablets)	37.79
INTRAVAGINAL THERAPY		
Metronidazole gel (MetroGel 0.75%)	One applicator (5 g) twice daily for 5 days	39.29
Clindamycin cream (Cleocin 2%)	One applicator (5 g) at bedtime for 7 days	39.49

[a]Prices were based on a local major pharmacy in the Chicago area (1997).

creases bacterial vaginosis associated microorganisms, and is safe. The currently recommended dosage is one applicator (5 g) intravaginally twice a day for 5 days.

Clindamycin (Cleocin) is another vaginal preparation found to be effective in limited clinical trials. The currently recommended regimen is clindamycin cream 2%, one applicator (5 g) intravaginally at bedtime for 7 days. This regimen appears to be safe and well tolerated in nonpregnant women. The major side effect is vaginal candidiasis, which occurs in up to 10% of patients with bacterial vaginosis treated with clindamycin cream.

Sexual Partners

The role of sexual transmission of microorganisms in bacterial vaginosis is controversial. Randomized, double-blinded studies show no improvement in cure rates when sexual partners were also treated (22, 23). Therefore, the data indicate no benefit in treating the sexual partners of women with bacterial vaginosis. However, some clinicians favor doing so in women who have intractable or recurrent disease.

Recurrence

The treatment of recurrences can be difficult. Although many women have isolated recurrences that respond to single repeated courses of therapy, some women have continuing recurrences. This latter group has been the subject of few studies, and the most appropriate way to manage them is unclear. This group is difficult to treat. Options that can be tried include longer antibiotic usage, prophylactic antibiotic usage at the time of exposure (if known), or long-term (14 days) Betadine douching.

CANDIDA VULVOVAGINITIS

Epidemiology

Candida vulvovaginitis is the second most common diagnosis in women with vaginal symptoms. Approximately 75% of women have at least one episode of candida vulvovaginitis during their reproductive years, with 40 to 50% of these women experiencing a second attack (24). Fortunately, fewer than 5% of women suffer repeated recalcitrant infections.

Pathogenesis

Twenty-five to 40% of women who have positive vaginal cultures for candida are asymptomatic. This suggests a colonization of *Candida* species (similar to that of many bacterial vaginosis-associated organisms) in low numbers that may increase when faced with an altered vaginal environment. Thus, asymptomatic colonization may progress to symptomatic candida vulvovaginitis when changes occur in the host vaginal environment. The natural vaginal flora, predominated by lactobacilli, provides a colonization-resistant mechanism to prevent candida germination and superficial mucosal invasion. Approximately 85 to 90% of yeast isolated from the vagina are *Candida albicans* strains. The remainder are due to nonalbicans *Candida* species, the most common of which are *Torulopsis glabrata*, *Candida parapsilosis*, and *Candida tropicalis*. These nonalbicans species can induce vaginitis and are often more resistant to conventional therapy (25).

Predisposing Factors

Multiple factors such as pregnancy, high-dose oral contraceptives, diabetes mellitus, broad-spectrum antibiotics, tight and poorly ventilated clothing, perfumed toilet paper, douches, and feminine hygiene sprays increase the rate of asymptomatic vaginal colonization with candida. In only some cases, however, is the precipitating factor identified to explain the transformation from asymptomatic carrier to symptomatic vaginitis.

Clinical Manifestations

The most common symptom is vulvar pruritus, which occurs in virtually all symptomatic patients and is usually more severe at night. Patients may also complain of a burning sensation after urination. This is intensified in the presence of excoriation from scratching or extensive maceration of the vulva. Vaginal discharge is typically white and cottage cheese-like in consistency but may vary from watery to homogeneously thick. Other symptoms include vaginal irritation, soreness, burning, dyspareunia, and external dysuria. Odor is rarely present and not offensive. The symptoms are usually exacerbated in the week preceding the onset of menses. There is some relief after the onset of menstrual flow.

Physical examination of the labia and vulva often reveals erythema and swelling with discrete pustulopapular peripheral lesions. A spectrum of manifestations occurs. At one end, there is an exudative syndrome of copious discharge and white plaques on the vaginal walls. At the other end, there is minimal discharge and severe erythema with extensive vulvar involvement (26). Male counterparts frequently experience a transient rash, erythema and pruritus, or a burning sensation of the penis that occurs minutes or hours after unprotected intercourse.

Diagnosis

The diagnosis of candida vulvovaginitis is not made on the basis of clinical manifestations alone. By the same token, positive vaginal cultures may reflect colonization and are not used as the sole basis of diagnosis either. One makes the diagnosis by identifying the presence of hyphae or budding yeast in vaginal secretions mixed with 10% potassium hydroxide preparation. Microscopic examination of a saline preparation of vaginal secretions to exclude the presence of clue cells or trichomonads is necessary as well. Large numbers of leukocytes are invariably absent and, if present, suggest a mixed infection. The vaginal pH is normal (4.0 to 4.5), and a pH in excess of 4.7 indicates bacterial vaginosis, trichomoniasis, or a mixed infection. The Pap smear is unreliable as a diagnostic test for candidal vulvovaginitis. As with cultures, the presence of yeast may represent colonization and not infection.

Cultures using Nickerson's media and Sabouraud dextrose agar plates are indicated in the presence of negative microscopy. Some candida species, like *T. glabrata*, may not have typical hyphae or spores and may be difficult to identify on microscopy. There is no reliable serologic technique for the diagnosis of symptomatic candidal vaginitis. A latex agglutination slide technique, using polyclonal antibodies, is available commercially. Its sensitivity is moderately good, but this test provides no advantage over the standard microscopic examination (24).

The diagnosis of candidal vulvovaginitis in postmenopausal women, women who are breast-feeding, or prepubertal children should raise the possibility of underlying diabetes mellitus.

Recurrent Candida Vulvovaginitis

Recurrent candida vulvovaginitis is the occurrence of at least four mycologically proven symptomatic episodes of candidal vaginitis within a 12-month period, with the exclusion of other vaginal pathogens (25). Up to one third of patients with chronic fungal vaginitis may have a nonalbicans species present. Fungal cultures may aid in confirming the diagnosis and selecting appropriate therapy. Most patients have chronic or recurrent episodes of fungal vaginitis despite the absence of underlying medical illnesses or predisposing factors. Risk factors include uncontrolled diabetes, exogenous hormone therapy, positive HIV serology, repeated courses of broad-spectrum antibiotics, tight-fitting clothing, and local hypersensitivity to the candida antigen. Theories to explain the pathogeneses of recurrent candida vulvovaginitis include reinfection from exogenous sources such as sexual partners, oral-genital sex, the intestinal reservoir, or vaginal relapse. The hypothesis for vaginal relapse is that recurrent infections are due to the same infecting organism, declining in numbers only to subsequently increase again and result in a recurrence.

Treatment

Antifungal agents are available topically as creams, lotions, vaginal tablets, and suppositories (Table 6.3). There is no evidence to suggest that the vehicle influences efficacy. The patient's preference should guide the choice of therapeutic vehicles. Extensive vulvar inflammation dictates local vulvar applications of cream.

Topical Agents

The various imidazole and triazole vaginal preparations are broad-spectrum antimycotics and have superior efficacy compared with polyene preparations (Nystatin). The efficacy and dosing regimens of the various azole derivatives are all comparable. Terconazole, a triazole, is more effective against the nonalbicans *Candida* species than the imidazoles and is equally as effective against *C. albicans*. There is a major trend toward shorter courses and single-dose regimens. These have demonstrated effectiveness in several clinical trials. These trials, however, did not include patients with severe and more intractable infections. This has led some authors to advocate single-dose therapy in patients with infrequent episodes of mild to moderate severity (26). Side effects may include local irritation or discomfort.

Oral Agents

Ketoconazole (400 mg daily for 5 days), itraconazole (200 mg daily for 3 days or 400 mg for 1 day), and fluconazole (150 mg for 1 day) are all highly effective in achieving clinical and mycologic cures in acute candida vaginitis (27). Only fluconazole (Diflucan) has U.S. Food and Drug Administration approval for this indication. Compared with conventional topical therapy, oral therapy demonstrates equal, if not slightly superior, efficacy. Most women, given the choice, prefer oral therapy, although it is more expensive.

The potential side effects of oral therapy are important to remember. Ketoconazole incurs gastrointestinal upset up to 10% of the time and, rarely, anaphylaxis. The major concern is the risk of hepatotoxicity, which occurs in 1 of 10,000 to 15,000 women treated. Similar side effects are less frequent with itraconazole and fluconazole.

Pregnancy

The incidence of candida vulvovaginitis during pregnancy is 2- to 20-fold higher than that in nonpregnant women. The altered hormonal milieu of pregnancy makes reinfection more common and definitive cure more difficult. Most topical antifungal agents are effective, especially when prescribed for longer periods of 1 to 2 weeks. Nevertheless, single-dose therapy with clotrimazole also has been efficacious in pregnant women. Vaginal antifungal therapy is safe in pregnancy, and there is minimal systemic absorption. Oral antifungal agents are not recommended for use during pregnancy. Because oral triazoles (and possibly ketoconazole) are excreted in breast milk, these drugs should not be used in women who are breast-feeding.

TABLE 6.3. Treatment Options for Candida Vulvovaginitis

Drug	Formulation	Rx	Cost[a] ($)
ACUTE CASES			
Miconazole			
200-mg suppository (Monistat-3)	1 suppository intravaginally at bedtime for 3 nights	No	14.89
2% vaginal cream (Monistat 7)	1 applicator intravaginally at bedtime for 7 nights	No	14.99
100-mg vaginal tablet (Monistat)	1 vaginal tablet at bedtime for 7 nights	No	14.99
Clotrimazole			
Gyne-Lotrimin, Mycelex G			
100-mg vaginal tablet	1 tablet intravaginally at bedtime for 7 nights	No	10.99
1% vaginal cream	1 applicator intravaginally at bedtime for 7 nights	No	10.99
Mycelex 500-mg vaginal tablet	1 tablet intravaginally one time	No	16.39
Butoconazole			
Femstat 2% cream	1 applicator intravaginally at bedtime for 3 nights	No	15.99
Terconazole			
Terazol 3 80-mg suppository or 0.8% vaginal cream	1 suppository or 1 applicator intravaginally at bedtime for 3 nights	Yes	32.69
Terazol 7 0.4% vaginal cream	1 applicator intravaginally at bedtime for 7 days	Yes	32.69
Tioconazole			
Vagistat 6.5% ointment	1 applicator intravaginally at bedtime one time	No	17.99
Ketoconazole			
Nizoral 400 mg	1 tablet daily for 5 days	Yes	34.29
Fluconazole			
Diflucan 150 mg	1 tablet orally one time	Yes	17.39
Itraconazole			
Sporanox			
200 mg	1 tablet orally daily for 3 days	Yes	34.49
400 mg	1 tablet one time	Yes	27.71
PROPHYLATIC REGIMENS			
Ketoconazole 100 mg	1 tablet daily for 6–12 months	Yes	51.19/mo
Clotrimazole 500 mg	1 tablet vaginally weekly or monthly for 6–12 months	No	24.09
Fluconazole 150 mg	1 tablet orally each month for 6–12 months	Yes	17.39
RESISTANT CASES			
Any of the above drugs at dosage levels used for 7-day regimens for a 14–21 day course			
Boric acid 600-mg capsule	600-mg capsule daily intravaginally for 14 days (requires suppository formulation by pharmacist)	Yes	
Gentian violet	Apply to vagina, once or twice in 1 week	Yes	

[a]Prices were based on a local major pharmacy in the Chicago area (1997).

Recurrence

In recurrent candidal vulvovaginitis, management aims for control rather than cure. The first step is to confirm the diagnosis, preferably with vaginal cultures. Next, any predisposing factors are identified and eradicated. Patients using oral contraceptives are more susceptible to recurrent yeast infections, but others do not feel it is necessary to discontinue low-dose estrogen contraceptives when long-term antimycotic agents are prescribed. Similarly, the yield of doing a glucose tolerance test on asymptomatic, healthy, premenopausal women to diagnose latent or chemical diabetes is extremely low and is not worthwhile. To avoid recurrences, patients are counseled to avoid tight-fitting clothing and synthetic underwear. Douching is not useful and should be discouraged. Dietary alteration is also ineffective. Unfortunately, in most women with recurrent or chronic candida vulvovaginitis, no underlying or predisposing factor(s) can be identified. In women, recurrent candida vulvovaginitis may be a marker of HIV infection. Testing for the virus is warranted in at-risk patients with a recent onset of recurrent recalcitrant candidal vaginitis. Testing for the virus in all women with recurrent candida vulvovaginitis is not indicated.

Most women with recalcitrant infection require long-term suppressive therapy. The best suppressive prophylaxis is with daily low doses of ketoconazole (100 mg daily for 6 to 12 months). Low doses of ketoconazole have fewer side effects but can cause idiosyncratic reactions such as hepatitis (incidence of 1 in 5,000 to 1 in 10,000). Therefore, liver enzymes should be periodically monitored. Cessation of antifungal therapy leads to a resurgence of symptoms in more than 50% of the women troubled by recurrent candida vulvovaginitis. There are modest reductions in recurrent candida vulvovaginitis with monthly and weekly clotrimazole, 500-mg suppositories, and monthly fluconazole, 150-mg, for one year.

Recurrent candida vulvovaginitis does not appear to be due to resistant yeast. Long-term ketoconazole therapy does not induce the emergence of resistant strains. These patients usually respond to oral azoles or topical flucytosine therapy. Other modalities, less commonly used, include intravaginal boric acid gelatin capsules, 600 mg each, twice a day for 14 days or gentian violet painted on the vaginal walls. Treating the sexual partner does not cause a significant reduction in the recurrence rate. For most women, the use of antibiotic therapy does not mandate the use of prophylactic antifungal medication. However, in women with recurrent candida vulvovaginitis, it may be prudent to administer topical antimycotic therapy together with antibiotics. The consumption of yogurt containing *Lactobacillus acidophilus* as prophylaxis may reduce vaginal colonization and candidal vaginitis in women with recurrent infections. More confirmatory studies are needed.

Women who suffer from recurrent candida vulvovaginitis may experience physical and psychological sequelae. Symptoms of chronic dyspareunia may cause sexual and marital relations to suffer. These patients need support, counseling, and reassurance that virtually all cases of recurrent candida vulvovaginitis can be controlled.

TRICHOMONAS VAGINALIS INFECTION

Epidemiology

Trichomonas vaginalis infection is the most prevalent nonviral sexually transmitted disease in the United States; it accounts for 15 to 20% of vulvovaginitis cases. In asymptomatic patients attending family planning clinics, 5% of women had the disease. It was found in 13 to 25% of asymptomatic women attending gynecology clinics and in 50 to 75% of asymptomatic prostitutes (28). The normally acidic environment in the vagina discourages the growth of *Trichomonas*. Menstruation, semen, or the presence of other pathogens that render the vaginal fluid more basic favor the growth of these protozoans. Other known risk factors for trichomonas infection include multiple sexual partners, black race, previous history of sexually transmitted diseases, coexistent infection with *Neisseria gonorrhoeae*, and nonuse of either barrier or hormonal contraceptives.

Pathogenesis

Trichomonas infection is predominately sexually transmitted. The etiologic agent, *T. vaginalis*, is a flagellated anaerobic protozoan. Transmission appears to be higher from men to women, because 70% of men have disease within 48 hours of exposure compared with 85% of exposed women (29, 30). Perinatal transmission occasionally occurs and is detected in about 5% of newborn girls born to infected mothers. This is the only documented nonvenereal transmission, and the infection was confined to the genital tract. Although there is no prolonged evaluation on infant carriage, it is presumed that the infection clears in these female infants as the effects of the maternal hormonal milieu dissipates (31). Although *Trichomonas* will survive for short periods on moist objects or exposed bodily fluids, there are no documented cases of transmission by indirect or fomite exposure.

Clinical Manifestations

Trichomonas infection ranges from an asymptomatic carrier state to severe acute inflammatory disease. It is asymptomatic in 50% of women and 90% of men (30). In some studies, one third of asymptomatic infected women became symptomatic within 6 months (32). The incubation period of symptomatic trichomonal infection, although controversial, ranges from 3 to 28 days.

The most common complaint is vaginal discharge, described as malodorous by 10% of patients. Other symptoms include vulvar irritation, dyspareunia, dysuria, and/or pruritus. These symptoms can be severe. Lower abdominal pain may also be present, but its presence should raise the possibility of concomitant salpingitis. Symptoms tend to appear or worsen during or immediately after menstruation or during pregnancy.

On examination, excessive vaginal discharge is present in 50 to 75% of patients. The classically described frothy or bubbly yellow-green discharge is present in less than one half of these patients. The discharge is gray in 75% of patients. Vulvar finding may be absent, or in severe cases, diffuse vulvar erythema may be evident. Vulvar and vaginal erythema and edema is typical. In less than 10% of women, capillary dilatation and punctate hemorrhages of the cervix result in the characteristic "strawberry cervix." There should be no mucopurulent endocervical discharge unless *C. trachomatis* or *N. gonorrhoeae* is also present.

Diagnosis

Similar to bacterial vaginosis and candida vaginitis, the diagnosis of trichomonas is not made based on clinical features alone. Definitive diagnosis requires the demonstration of the organism. The teardrop-shaped parasite is slightly larger than a leukocyte and is mobile (Fig. 6.3). If the slide is too cold, the solution too hypertonic, or too many leukocytes surround the organisms in solution, the parasite may not be very mobile and may be rounder in shape. The vaginal pH is almost always above 5.0. Gram stains are of little value because of the inability to differentiate trichomonas from leukocytes. The use of Giemsa, acridine orange, and other stains has no advantage over saline preparation. The Pap smear lacks adequate sensitivity and does not offer advantage over saline preparation microscopy. Diamond's media culture

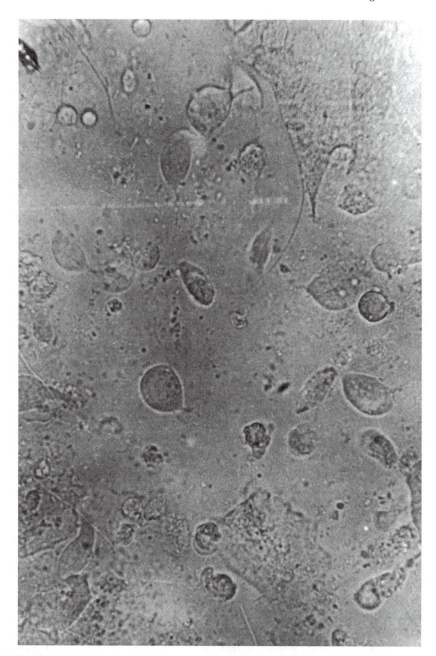

FIGURE 6.3. Trichomoniasis: high-power microscopic view of secretions showing multiple trichomonads.

has a sensitivity of 95% and remains the gold standard in the diagnosis of trichomonas. Cultures are incubated anaerobically, and growth is usually detected within 48 hours. Culture is indicated in patients with an elevated pH, excessive leukocytes, and the absence of motile trichomonads and clue cells. Newer methods of identification based on demonstration of a trichomonal antigen or nucleic acids are being developed.

Pregnancy

Recent studies suggest that infection with *T. vaginalis* is associated with premature delivery, low birth weight, and postpartum endometritis (33). The role of *Trichomonas* in contributing to adverse pregnancy outcome(s) is controversial. Although some reports found an association between *T. vaginalis* with prematurity, there is little evidence that the microorganism ascends into the uterus, placenta, or to the neonate.

Treatment

Because trichomonas is highly infectious, all patients and their recent sexual contacts require therapy (Table 6.4). The mainstay of therapy for trichomonas infection continues to be the 5-nitroimidazoles; only metronidazole (Flagyl) is available in the United States. Systemic therapy is required to fully treat this infection because organisms may be present in the urinary and genital tracts. Treatment consists of the following options (34):

TABLE 6.4. Therapeutic Options for Trichomonas Vaginitis

Drug	Formulation	Cost[a] ($)
STANDARD TREATMENT		
Metronidazole (Flagyl, Protostat)		
500 mg	2 g (four tablets) orally in a single dose	6.49
500 mg (should treat partner as well)	500 mg orally twice daily for 7 days	13.39
PERSISTENT OR RECURRENT CASES		
Metronidazole	500 mg orally twice daily for 14 days or repeat 2 g orally	23.80
Clotrimazole (Gyne-Lotrimin, Mycelex-G) 100-mg tablet	1 tablet vaginally at bedtime for 7 nights	10.99
ADJUNCTIVE THERAPY		
Povidone-iodine suppositories (Betadine)	1 suppository intravaginally twice daily for 14–28 days	
Metronidazole gel (MetroGel)	5 g intravaginally twice daily for 5 days	39.29
PREGNANCY		
Metronidazole	2 g orally one time after first trimester	6.49
Clotrimazole 100-mg tablet	1 tablet intravaginally at bedtime for 7 nights	10.99
LACTATION		
Metronidazole	2 g orally one time, with discontinuation of breast-feeding for 24 hr	6.49

[a]Prices were based on a local major pharmacy in the Chicago area (1997).

1. 2 g of metronidazole as a single oral dose for both men and women, achieving cure rates of 82 to 88%, which increases to 95% when partners are simultaneously treated
2. 250 mg orally three times daily for 7 days, with a cure rate of 95%
3. 500 mg twice daily for 7 days

Disadvantages to the prolonged dosages include decreased compliance, greater vaginal flora disruption, and a longer period of alcohol abstinence. Intrauterine devices may be left in place except in those with severe (upper reproductive tract) infections. Patients on medications that activate the liver enzymes, such as phenobarbitol or dilantin, may require either higher doses or longer periods of therapy to effect a cure.

For those patients who cannot take oral therapy, vaginal treatments with either metronidazole or Vagisec Plus are therapeutic options, although complete eradication of the organism is not usually achieved.

Also of concern is the potential teratogenicity of metronidazole in pregnancy. As mentioned earlier, use of metronidazole in the first trimester requires caution. A single 2-g oral dose is best for lactating women. Breast feeding should be discontinued for 24 hours after treatment.

Recurrence

When initial therapy is unsuccessful, the most common reasons are noncompliance and reinfection. If single-dose therapy is ineffective, a repeated 2-g dose is given to both the patient and her sexual contacts. This is successful in 85% of cases (34). Other possibilities to consider include misdiagnosis or infection with multiple sexually transmitted diseases. If compliance is assured and sexual partners have been treated, continued infection is most likely due to resistance. Fortunately, metronidazole resistance remains rare and does respond to higher doses and prolonged treatment with metronidazole. The patient takes 1 to 2 g of daily oral metronidazole for 10 to 14 days. Sexual partners also require re-treatment. Many practitioners augment a high daily oral dose (1 to 2 g) with the use of topical intravaginal agents to increase the concentrations in the vaginal fluids. Such regimens include 0.75% metronidazole gel or a 500-mg gelatin capsule of metronidazole placed in the vagina twice daily. For those patients unable to tolerate the oral preparation because of vomiting, intravenous administration of 2 to 4 g daily is an option. In rare cases of metronidazole allergy, an intravenous incremental dosing protocol has been used with good results (35).

Alternative treatments to the 5-nitroimidazoles, like metronidazole, are considered palliative. These are the only drugs with documented efficacy. Topical clotrimazole intravaginally for 7 days has variable low cure rates. Other options of vinegar douches, hypertonic (20%) saline douches, sitz baths, and povidone-iodine douches or suppositories offer questionable benefit.

ATROPHIC VAGINITIS

Atrophic vaginitis is a symptomatic vaginal inflammatory condition caused by estrogen-deficient vaginal epithelium. It is important to distinguish it from simple vaginal atrophy. Decreased endogenous estrogen results in thinned epithelium and decreased glycogen content, all of which contribute to a reduction in vaginal pH. These changes in the vaginal environment promote an overgrowth in coliform organisms and the disappearance of *Lactobacillus*.

Most women are asymptomatic, especially in the absence of coitus. Symptoms include vaginal spotting and soreness, external dysuria, pruritus, and dyspareunia. Burning is a frequent complaint, and intercourse often exacerbates this symptom. On examination, the vaginal surface appears thin, smooth, pale pink, without rugae, and with a predominance of parabasal cells on vaginal smear. The discharge is minimal and may be blood-like, thick, or watery. The vaginal pH is greater than 5. Microscopy reveals the absence of organisms, increased leukocytes, and small round epithelial cells. The normal *Lactobacillus*-dominated flora is replaced by a mixed flora of Gram-negative rods. Treatment consists primarily of intravaginal estrogen cream inserted into the vagina once daily or every other day for 2 weeks. In patients unwilling or unable to use estrogen, topical vaginal lubricants are an option. A long-lasting lubricant, such as Replens, is preferable to KY jelly.

DESQUAMATIVE INFLAMMATORY VAGINITIS

This is a rare disorder characterized by a diffuse exudative vaginitis, epithelial cell exfoliation (increased parabasal cells), and a profuse purulent vaginal discharge in the absence of an identifiable cause. Unlike patients with atrophic vaginitis, estrogen does not induce a therapeutic response. Patients complain of a purulent vaginal discharge, dyspareunia, and burning sensations in the vulva. On examination, the vagina is intensely reddened with acute inflammation of the upper half or all of the vagina. There may be denuded areas in the vagina, especially in the fornices. The vaginal walls are extremely friable and easily traumatized. Occasionally, areas of epithelium exhibit a grayish pseudomembrane that peels or becomes desquamated. The pH is usually greater than 5.0. There is a marked increase in leukocytes and basal and parabasal epithelial cells. *Lactobacilli* are minimally present. In up to two thirds of patients with the vulvovaginal disease, there are concurrent oral lesions. The cause of this entity is unknown. Evidence suggests a microbial possibly Gram-positive coccal cause. As a result, management is controversial. One therapeutic option that can be offered is the use of 2% topical clindamycin intravaginally nightly for 2 weeks (36).

ACUTE DERMATITIS

Acute dermatitis is a common affliction with a myriad of sources. In contact dermatitis, the vulva becomes erythematous, pruritic, and often exfoliated from scratching. Common offenders are vaginal hygienic products, laundry detergents, perfumed soaps or toilet paper, tight-fitting and/or synthetic undergarments, and local anesthetic medications. Therapy involves removing the offending agent and administering topical corticosteroids for a short course of 7 to 10 days.

PEDIATRIC VULVOVAGINITIS

The most common causes of vulvovaginitis in the pediatric population include poor hygiene and threadworms. Poor hygiene is frequently the cause of vaginal contamination from fecal material; bubble baths, soaps, shampoos, sand, and tight clothing may also cause irritation. Other causes of vulvovaginitis include β-hemolytic streptococci, shigella, sexually transmitted diseases, foreign bodies, inflammatory dermatoses, and desquamative vulvovaginitis.

Diagnosis, as with an adult, includes a full history and physical examination. Common complaints include pruritus, irritation, pain, dysuria, and discharge. Depending on the severity of the symptoms, examination can be in the frog-leg position, which will often show a scanty discharge traced to poor hygiene. If discharge is persistent, purulent, or recurrent or if there is a concern about sexual abuse, examination in the knee-chest position is preferable. An otoscope may be helpful to visualize the vagina and cervix. Often, the child is too uncomfortable for a pelvic examination, and examination under general anesthesia is required.

Treatment of vulvovaginitis in the child and/or adolescent depends on the cause. The use of cotton underpants, avoidance of nylon tights or tightly fitting clothing, frequent handwashing, and "front to back" wiping after urination or defecation may address those cases precipitated by poor hygiene.

Further discussion of problems encountered in prepubertal and adolescent girls is available in Chapter 1.

CLINICAL NOTES

Normal Vaginal Flora and Discharge

- The normal vaginal pH is less than 4.5, there is minimal odor, and the phase of the menstrual cycle influences the quantity of normal discharge.
- All women with complaints of vulvovaginitis should have a directed history, physical examination, and in-office laboratory testing because symptoms alone are an insufficient basis for diagnosis and treatment.
- Office analysis of a woman with symptoms of vulvovaginitis includes a pH of vaginal secretions, an amine or whiff test, and wet mount using both saline and 10% KOH.

Bacterial Vaginosis

- Bacterial vaginosis accounts for 40 to 50% of all cases of vaginitis among reproductive-age women. It has been implicated as an etiologic agent in pelvic inflammatory disease, postcesarean endometritis, postoperative vaginal cuff cellulitis, premature rupture of the membranes, and preterm labor.
- Bacterial vaginosis can occur in women who have had a hysterectomy.
- There are four clinical criteria for diagnosis of bacterial vaginosis: milky homogenous discharge, vaginal pH greater than 4.5, at least 20% of epithelial cells on wet mount are clue, and a positive whiff test.
- Approximately 50% of women with microbiologic evidence of bacterial vaginosis are asymptomatic. Currently, treatment of asymptomatic patients is not universally recommended.
- The therapy of choice for bacterial vaginosis is metronidazole (Flagyl), 500 mg orally twice daily for 5 to 7 days or 2 g orally as a single dose. Alternative therapies includes clindamycin, 300 mg orally twice daily for 7 days. Intravaginal therapy with metronidazole gel 0.75%, 5 g intravaginally bid for 5 days, or clindamycin cream 2%, 5 g intravaginally for 7 nights, are also effective.
- It is not currently recommended that sexual partners of women with bacterial vaginosis undergo therapy, although some recommend this for women with intractable or recurrent disease.

Candida Vulvovaginitis

- Twenty-five to 40% of women with positive vaginal cultures for candida are asymptomatic. About 85 to 90% of yeast isolated from the vagina are *Candida albicans* strains.
- Diagnosis of vaginal yeast infection is made by identification of hyphae or budding yeast in vaginal secretions mixed with 10% KOH solution and a normal vaginal pH.
- The presence of candidal vulvovaginitis in women who are menopausal or breast-feeding or in prepubertal children should raise suspicions of underlying diabetes mellitus.

- Up to 33% of patients with recurrent candida vulvovaginitis (at least four mycologically proven symptomatic episodes of candidal vaginitis in a 12-month period with the exclusion of other pathogens) have a nonalbicans species present.
- Of the topical agents, the imidazole and triazole vaginal preparations are the best broad-spectrum antimycotics.
- Oral agents used for candida vulvovaginitis include ketoconazole, 400 mg/day for 5 days, itraconazole 200 mg/day for 3 days, or 400 mg as a single dose, or fluconazole, 150 mg as a single dose, are all highly effective.
- The incidence of candida vulvovaginitis is markedly increased in pregnant women. Vaginal therapy is recommended during pregnancy, not oral therapy.
- In women, recurrent candida vulvovaginitis may be a marker of HIV infection.
- Women with recalcitrant candidal infection require long-term suppressive therapy, e.g., ketoconazole, 100 mg/day for 6 to 12 months with monitoring of liver enzymes periodically. Treatment of the sexual partner does not seem to significantly reduce the recurrence rate.

Trichomonas vaginalis Infection

- *Trichomonas vaginalis* infection is the most prevalent nonviral sexually transmitted disease in the United States and accounts for 15 to 20% of the cases of vulvovaginitis.
- Transmission of trichomonas is higher from men to women, and it may be detected in about 5% of newborn girls born to infected mothers.
- Trichomonas infection is asymptomatic in 50% of women and in 90% of men.
- Definitive diagnosis of trichomonas infection requires demonstration of the organism. The vaginal pH is usually greater than 5, and a gray or yellow-green malodorous discharge may be present.
- All patients with trichomonas infection and their recent sexual contacts require therapy, with metronidazole (Flagyl) being the drug of choice. Treatment with vaginal preparations may not result in complete eradication of the organism.
- For (rare) metronidazole resistance, the use of metronidazole, 1 to 2 g/day for 10 to 14 days, usually results in eradication of the organism.

Other Causes of Vulvovaginitis

- Atrophic vaginitis is usually asymptomatic but may cause vaginal spotting, dysuria, pruritus, and/or dyspareunia. The vaginal pH is greater than 5. Treatment is with intravaginal estrogen cream or topical lubrication.
- Desquamative inflammatory vaginitis is rare but causes a diffuse exudative vaginitis, epithelial exfoliation, and profuse purulent vaginal discharge. The cause is unknown, and treatment is controversial. One therapeutic option is the use of 2% topical clindamycin intravaginally for 2 weeks.
- The most common causes of vulvovaginitis in the pediatric population are poor hygiene, threadworms, and foreign body.

References

1. Kent HL. Epidemiology of vaginitis. Am J Obstet Gynecol 1991;165:1168–1176.
2. Larsen B. Vaginal flora in health and disease. Clin Obstet Gynecol 1993;36:107–121.
3. Ferris DG, Hendrich J, Payne PM, et al. Office laboratory diagnosis of vaginitis. J Fam Pract 1995;41:575–581.
4. Biswas MK. Bacterial vaginosis. Clin Obstet Gynecol 1993;36:166–176.
5. Eschenbach DA. History and review of bacterial vaginosis. Am J Obstet Gynecol 1993;169:441–445.
6. McCoy MC, Katz VL, Kuller JA, et al. Bacterial vaginosis in pregnancy: an approach for the 1990s. Obstet Gynecol Surv 1995;50:482–488.
7. Mead PB. Epidemiology of bacterial vaginosis. Am J Obstet Gynecol 1993;169:446–449.
8. Amsel R, Totten PA, Spiegal CA, et al. Nonspecific vaginitis. Diagnostic criteria and microbial and epidemiologic associations. Am J Med 1983;74:14–22.

9. Gardner HL. *Haemophilus vaginalis* vaginitis after twenty-five years. Am J Obstet Gynecol 1980;137:385–391.

10. Eschenbach DA, Critchlow CW, Watkins H, et al. A dose duration study of metronidazole for the treatment of nonspecific vaginosis. Scand J Infect Dis Suppl 1993;40:73.

11. Sobel JD. Vulvovaginitis. Dermatol Clin 1992;10:339–358.

12. Spiegal CA, Amsel R, Holmes KK, et al: Diagnosis of *Haemophilus vaginalis* by direct Gram stain of vaginal fluid. J Clin Microbiol 1983;18:170.

13. Hillier SH. Diagnostic microbiology of bacterial vaginosis. Am J Obstet Gynecol 1993; 169:455–459.

14. Soper DE. Bacterial vaginosis and postoperative infection. Am J Obstet Gynecol 1993;160:467–469.

15. Gravett MG, Hummel D, Eschenbach DA, et al. Preterm labor associations with subclinical amniotic fluid infection and with bacterial vaginosis. Obstet Gynecol 1986; 67:229.

16. Hillier SL, Nugent RP, Eschenbach DA, et al. Association between bacterial vaginosis and preterm delivery of a low birth weight infant. N Engl J Med 1995;333:1737–1742.

17. Bump RC, Zuspan FP, Buerschig WJ, et al. The prevalence, six month persistence, and predictive values of laboratory indicators of bacterial vaginosis (nonspecific vaginitis) in asymptomatic women. M J Obstet Gynecol 1984;150:917–924.

18. Joesoef MR, Schmid GP. Bacterial vaginosis: review of treatment options and potential clinical indication for therapy. Clin Infect Dis 1995;20:s72–s79.

19. Piper JM, Mitchel EF, Ray WA. Prenatal use of metronidazole and birth defects: no association. Obstet Gynecol 1993;82:348–352.

20. Greaves WL, Chungafung J, Morris B, et al. Clindamycin versus metronidazole in the treatment of bacterial vaginosis. Obstet Gynecol 1988;72:799–802.

21. Hillier SL, Lipinski C, Briselden AM, et al. Efficacy of intravaginal 0.75% metronidazole gel for treatment of bacterial vaginosis. Obstet Gynecol 1993;81:963–967.

22. Vejtorp M, Bollerup AC, Vejtorp L, et al. Bacterial vaginosis: a double-blind randomized trial of the effect of treatment of the sexual partner. Br J Obstet Gynaecol 1988;95:920–926.

23. Moi H, Erkkola R, Jerve F, et al. Should male consorts of women with bacterial vaginosis be treated? Genitourin Med 1989;65:263–268.

24. Hurley R. Recurrent *Candida* infection. Clin Obstet Gynecol 1981;8:209.

25. Sobel JD. Pathogenesis and treatment of recurrent vulvovaginal candidiasis. Clin Infect Dis 1992;14(suppl 1):S80–90.

26. Sobel JD. Candidal vulvovaginitis. Clin Obstet Gynecol 1993;36:153–165.

27. Reef SE, Levine WC, McNeil MM, et al. Treatment options of vulvovaginal candidiasis, 1993. Clin Infect Dis 1995;20(suppl 1):S80–90.

28. Rein MF, Muller M. *Trichomonas vaginalis* and trichomoniasis. In: Holmes KK, Mardt PA, Sparling AF, et al., eds. Sexually Transmitted Disease. New York: McGraw-Hill, 1989: 481–492.

29. Hasseltine HC, Wolters SL, Campbell A. Experimental human vaginal trichomoniasis. J Infect Dis 1942;71:127–130.

30. Weston TET, Nico CS. Natural history of trichomonal infection in males. Br J Vener Dis 1963;39:251–257.

31. Bramley M. Study of female babies of women entering confinement with vaginal trichomoniasis. Br J Vener Dis 1976;52:58–62.

32. Wolner-Hanssen P, Krieger JN, Stevens CE, et al. Clinical manifestations of vaginal trichomoniasis. JAMA 1989;261:571–576.

33. Heine P, McGregor JA. *Trichomonas vaginalis:* a reemerging pathogen. Clin Obstet Gynecol 1993;36:137–143.

34. Lossick JG. Treatment of *Trichomonas vaginalis* infections. Rev Infect Dis 1990;12(suppl 6): S665–S681.

35. Pearlman MD, Yashar C, Ernst S, et al. An incremental dosing protocol for women with severe vaginal trichomoniasis and adverse reaction to metronidazole. Am J Obstet Gynecol 1996;174:934–936.

36. Sobel JD. Desquamative inflammatory vaginitis: a new subgroup of purulent vaginitis responsive to topical 2% clindamycin therapy. Am J Obstet Gynecol 1994;171: 1215–1220.

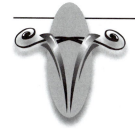

C H A P T E R 7

Sexually Transmitted Diseases

HUNTER HAMMILL

Sexually transmitted diseases are commonly encountered in the office setting. Occasionally, patients present with significant concern about their contacts and request screening for sexually transmitted disease(s). Patients also commonly present with either no symptoms or with symptoms related to genital sores, ulcers, growths, or discharges. It is important to ask the patient if any lesions are present. The lesion should be examined and cultured or biopsied if needed. It is paramount to remember that if one sexually transmitted disease is detected, other pathology or diseases may coexist.

HERPES SIMPLEX

Herpes simplex virus (HSV) is a common infection and can be divided into two types: HSV type 1, usually associated with lesions above the umbilicus or oral/facial lesions, and HSV type 2, associated with genital and neonatal infections. Although type-specific serologic testing is available, its use is normally limited to research settings. Culture does permit viral typing and may be helpful in counseling patients about frequency of recurrences. Both HSV-1 and -2 can be transmitted to other sites by direct contact with infected secretions or autoinoculation. Asymptomatic shedding is very common, especially in the first year after a primary episode. This probably represents a major source of sexual transmission. Recurrences are more common in men than in women, and HSV-2 genital lesions recur more frequently than genital lesions caused by HSV-1 (1, 2).

Symptoms

In the primary infection of genital herpes, the lesions are often severely painful. In more than two thirds of women, a flu-like syndrome and burning, dysuria, and an exquisitely tender vulva may be present. Acute urinary retention may occur. In 10 to 20% of patients, extragenital lesions are present in the primary outbreak (3). Symptoms usually appear within 3 to 7 days of contact. Not all cases of primary herpes are dramatic; mild or even asymptomatic initial infections do occur. The length of time for viral shedding averages 7 to 10 days for primary infection. Primary lesions may involve any area of the female genitalia. They are initially vesicles that go on to ulcerate and may coalesce, covering most of the vulvar area. The inflammatory response results in vulvar edema, and bilateral inguinal adenopathy is also present. Although the nodes may be mild or moderately tender, they are not fluctuant. The lesions in primary herpes may require 2 to 6 weeks to resolve completely. After the primary infection, the virus becomes latent in sensory nerve ganglion (4, 5).

Approximately 50% of patients develop recurrent infection within 6 months of outbreak. Trigger factors for recurrent outbreak vary from person to person but can include sunlight, fever, menses, emotional stress, or local trauma. For recurrent infections, the lesions are not as severely painful but still may be quite uncomfortable. Recurrences appear at the sites of the primary lesions. The symptoms are quite localized to the genital lesions and systemic symptoms are uncommon. A prodromal sensation of burning, tingling, itching, or hypersensitivity may be present for several hours before the appearance of lesions. The length of viral shedding is shortened in recurrent infections, usually lasting 3 to 6 days. By the seventh to ninth day, most lesions are healed. Recurrences tend to be more severe in women than in men (3).

Diagnosis

Definitive diagnosis is by culture. The specimen should be obtained at the base of an open vesicle. Vesicles contain their highest viral levels in the first 24 to 48 hours of appearance, so cultures are best obtained early in the course of infection (6). If there will be a delay in transport to the laboratory, the specimen should be stored at 4 to 9°C; for longer delays, it should be stored at −70°C. The virus usually grows rapidly so cultures may be positive in 2 to 3 days, although occasionally it may be several weeks before a final report is available. Serologic testing may be helpful in diagnosing primary infection but is of no clinical value for recurrent infections.

Treatment

The acute outbreak of primary herpes may require hospitalization for pain control and possible catheterization. The use of oral or intravenous narcotics and topical anesthetics for the lesions is recommended. Topical acyclovir will decrease viral shedding time, pain, and facilitate healing of lesions in primary outbreaks but does neither of these for recurrent infections (7). It is not as effective, however, as the oral agents. Intravenous antiviral medications (e.g., acyclovir [Zovirax]) are indicated in severe primary outbreaks or disseminated herpetic infections.

For recurrent outbreaks, oral analgesics are recommended. If the patient becomes aware of prodromal symptoms, oral acyclovir, famciclovir, or valacyclovir may be started. This will decrease viral shedding and may circumvent a symptomatic recurrence. For patients suffering more than six outbreaks per year or in whom medical or personal circumstances would benefit from suppression, strong consideration should be given to the use of prophylactic oral antiviral therapy. Acyclovir has been shown to be efficacious in decreasing the frequency and number of recurrences with minimal side effects (8). Famciclovir (Famvir) is also approved by the Food and Drug Administration for suppression of recurrent genital herpes. Patients must be counseled that although recurrences are less frequent, viral shedding still occurs, so they are still capable of transmitting the disease.

The following is the recommended regimen for primary outbreak:

- Topical acyclovir: apply every 3 hours, six times daily for 7 to 10 days. Use gloves to avoid inoculation of fingers; do not use intravaginally *and*
- Acyclovir 200 mg orally five times a day for 7 to 10 days, *or*
- Acyclovir 400 mg three times a day, *or*
- Valacyclovir 1000 mg twice daily, *or*
- Famciclovir 250 mg orally every 8 hours for 5 days.

The following is the recommended regimen for recurrent episodes:

- Acyclovir 200 mg orally 5 times a day for 5 days, *or*
- Acyclovir 400 mg orally three times a day for 5 days, *or*
- Acyclovir 800 mg orally twice daily for 5 days, *or*
- Famciclovir 125 mg orally twice daily for 5 days, *or*
- Valacyclovir 1000 mg orally twice daily.

The following is the recommended regimen for suppression of recurrent outbreaks:

- Acyclovir (Zovirax) 400 mg orally twice daily every day, *or*
- Famciclovir (Famvir) 250 mg orally twice daily every day.

For severe primary infection or disseminated infection, acyclovir, intravenous 5 mg/kg every 8 hours for 5 days, is used.

Special Considerations

Pregnancy

In pregnancy, the recurrence rate of herpes is high (9). Herpes infection in pregnancy is clinically significant because of the potential for harm, even death, to the neonate. The incidence of neonatal infection is approximately 12 per 100,000 live births (10). There are three forms of neonatal infection: disseminated (with the highest morbidity and mortality even with treatment), central nervous system only (high morbidity, some mortality even with treatment), and skin/eye/mouth involvement only (low morbidity and mortality with treatment). About half of all infected neonates who do not receive prompt therapy die. Of the neonates who survive herpetic infection, many suffer profound neurologic sequelae. Preventing neonatal infection is difficult because 70 to 80% of afflicted newborns are born to mothers with no history of prior infection or signs or symptoms at or around the time of delivery.

For a primary outbreak (at the time of delivery) in the mother, the risk to the infant is large, with 50% of neonates developing infection. The risk of neonatal transmission at the time of delivery is highest with a primary maternal infection, particularly if this occurs in the third trimester because there are no developed maternal antibodies. A primary outbreak in the first trimester of pregnancy can cause spontaneous abortion, preterm labor, chorioretinitis, microcephaly, intrauterine growth retardation, or skin lesions (11). Ultrasound follow-up at 18 weeks gestation and again in the third trimester should be done. There is less likelihood of adverse fetal effects for primary infections in the early second trimester, and beyond 20 weeks gestation, no adverse fetopathy has been reported. In recurrent infections (at the time of delivery), only 4% of infants ultimately become infected.

In the absence of lesions or prodromal symptoms, vaginal delivery should be expected, excluding other obstetric indications for cesarean section. Patients with active disease in labor should be delivered by cesarean section to decrease the risk of vertical transmission. Although cesarean section markedly decreases the risk, it does not negate it altogether. Ideally, cesarean section would be performed within 4 to 6 hours of rupture of membranes (at term) in a patient with lesions or prodrome, but regardless of duration of ruptured membranes, it is of benefit.

A clinical dilemma that arises is what to do with the patient with lesions or prodromal symptoms and preterm premature rupture of the membranes. Most agree that in a pregnancy with a high likelihood of neonatal survival and acceptable morbidity risk, one should proceed with cesarean section. For pregnancies under 31 to 32 weeks gestation, there are case reports of expectant management, with delivery occurring 1 to 5 weeks later and none of the infants suffered HSV infection (12, 13).

CONDYLOMATA ACUMINATA (VENEREAL WARTS)

Condyloma acuminatum, or human papilloma virus (HPV), presents in many forms in the gynecologist's office. Epidemiologic studies suggested that condyloma may occur in 0.1% of all age groups. However, this may increase with adolescence. There has also been much concern about the various types of the papilloma virus. There is some concern that HPV types 16, 18, 31, 33, 35, and 39 are more frequently associated with genital cancer (14).

HPV is seen most frequently in women of reproductive age and is acquired most commonly through sexual contact. Poor personal hygiene, vaginitis, or an altered immune state are predisposing factors to the growth of the warts. Condylomata tend to flourish during pregnancy but usually regress postpartum. The incubation time from exposure to outbreak is approximately 3 to 6 months. Patients may complain of pruritus or may be asymptomatic. Untreated, the warts may increase in size and proliferate or regress spontaneously. In women, warts are most frequently noted in the vulva, perineal body, perianal region, introitus, and lower third of the vagina. It is less common to see warts in the upper vaginal area and cervix, although it does occur. For discussion of the effects of HPV infection on cervical cytology, see Chapter 9.

Diagnosis

Diagnosis is most often made by visualization of the lesions. If doubt exists, a biopsy should be taken. Because of variations in inter- and intraobserver interpretation, Papanicolaou smears are not a reliable method for diagnosis. Although there are genetic probes available to identify HPV and some subtypes, the clinical utility of these tests has not been determined, and they should be viewed as research tools only.

Treatment

The indications for treatment of genital warts include cosmesis, relief of local symptoms, and/or relief of psychological stress caused by the presence of the lesions. In pregnancy, it is done to relieve significant obstruction of the birth canal that may preclude or significantly complicate vaginal delivery. The risk of neonatal transmission, particularly to the larynx, is quite small. Approximately 10 to 20% of patients have spontaneous resolution of the lesions. Any associated infection(s) should be eradicated before treating the warts. It is important to counsel patients that although the warts may be eradicated, the virus, once present, will never be lost from the genital tract. As a result, recurrences of warts are common.

Podophyllin (Podocon-25, Podofin) is a cytotoxic agent that is contraindicated during pregnancy. Podophyllin can be used in a 10% solution once or twice a week. Because there is transmucosal systemic absorption, it should not be used intravaginally. It is most effective when used on lesions under 2 cm in size. Podophyllin causes blanching of the warts shortly after application, and patients may complain of a burning sensation. Chemical burns may be seen in as many as 30 to 50% of patients. They may wash the area within 2 to 4 hours to avoid the severe irritation of the skin that may occur with prolonged exposure. If the warts fail to regress after four applications, an alternative therapy may be needed. Neurologic, hematologic, and febrile complications, including death, have been seen as complications associated with topical podophyllin. Podophyllin should not be used in children.

A purified podophyllin resin, podofilox, is also available as a prescription ointment, Condylox 0.5%, that patients may apply twice daily for 3 consecutive days per week but for no more than 3 weeks. This ointment does not need to be washed off, is less toxic, and is more efficacious than podophyllin 20% (15). It is category C for pregnancy.

Bichloracetic acid and trichloroacetic acid in up to 85% solution in alcohol is an effective treatment for small lesions as well. Solution can be applied with a swab daily for up to 4 weeks. Because this is a more liquid solution than podophyllin, some recommend applying petrolatum ointment to the skin around the wart and on the corresponding area contralaterally to avoid extensive irritation. Alternatively, talcum powder or bicarbonate soda may be used to protect the opposing skin or to remove any acid that has not reacted. The patient may wash the solution off after 6 to 8 hours and may find a sitz bath with baking soda effective in relieving any discomfort. There are fewer side effects with this regimen than with podophyllin, and this treatment may be used safely in pregnancy. Neither compound appears to be effective in treating vaginal or cervical warts.

5-Fluorouracil (Efudex), 5% cream, may eliminate lesions in 3 to 7 days but is associated with severe side effects, including erythema, edema, and shallow ulcerations of the skin. It should not be used in pregnant women and is not considered a first-line therapy in the treatment of genital warts.

Iquimod (Aldara) cream, 5%, a newly released agent, can be used topically three times a week for up to 8 weeks. Patients apply this themselves at home. It should be used at bedtime and washed off in 6 to 10 hours. It is rated category B in pregnancy. It may elicit a strong local response with erythema, but this usually looks worse than it feels.

Interferon alfa 2b (Intron A) is an effective therapy given by local injection. It is usually reserved for recurrent and/or resistant genital warts. The maximum dose to be used at any one time is 3 million units. Treatment is usually given three times per week for approximately 3 weeks. When this treatment is offered, patients may have a flu- or viral-like syndrome within the first 24 hours (16). With repeated injections, this side effect often subsides. Systemic use of interferon for the treatment of genital warts is not recommended because of the immunosuppression that occurs.

Cryotherapy is another modality used in treating genital warts. Lesions are frozen every 1 to 2 weeks, and it is important to freeze just the lesion and not the surrounding skin. Its most common clinical role in HPV is in the treatment of multiple cervical warts. It is safe for use in pregnancy. Burning and ulceration may follow therapy, although it usually resolves in 7 to 10 days with little or no scarring.

Surgical excision via loop electrosurgical excision procedure (LEEP), scalpel excision, scissor excision, punch biopsy, or CO_2 laser is another method that can be used, particularly when large lesions or perianal lesions are present. Large lesions may obliterate the entire perineum. If CO_2 laser is used for surgical ablation, the lesions must be destroyed down to the base or the incidence of recurrence will be higher.

MOLLUSCUM CONTAGIOSUM

Molluscum contagiosum is a dome-shaped lesion with central umbilication. These lesion are found on epithelial surfaces but not on mucosal membranes. Sometimes a curd-like milky core can be expressed. Lesions are slow growing and usually multiple. It is a member of the pox virus, and infection is usually self-limiting, lasting 6 to 9 months on average. There are two forms of infection. One is seen in young children, resulting from skin to skin contact or fomite transmission, and the other occurs in adolescents and adults and results from sexual transmission (17).

Diagnosis

Diagnosis of this lesion is primarily made by gross appearance, or a skin biopsy may be performed. Skin biopsy is usually performed when the diagnosis is in question.

Treatment

Effective treatment can be achieved with skin curettage, cryotherapy, expression of the umbilicated core, or excision. The latter causes scarring, so it is not routinely recommended. The use of podophyllin or trichloroacetic acid is also effective. Podophyllin should not be used in children.

LYMPHOGRANULOMA VENEREUM

Lymphogranuloma venereum (LGV) is a sexually transmitted disease caused by chlamydia trachomatous serotypes L1, L2, and L3 (not to be confused with the chlamydia serotypes D through K of pelvic inflammatory disease [PID]) (18). LGV has a low incidence in the United States, with most cases occurring in men. In third world countries, it is more common, with some areas reporting an incidence of up to 11% (19).

Clinical Manifestations

The incubation period from exposure to appearance of a painless lesion is 4 to 21 days. The patient may have a primary chancre, although this is often not noticed because it is transient and painless. If it is intraurethral, it may cause symptomatic urethritis. In women, the primary lesion occurs most commonly on the posterior area of the vulva. The lesion usually heals without scarring in several days. Approximately 1 to 4 weeks later, the secondary stage begins. The patient notes tender inguinal lymphadenopathy, which is unilateral in two thirds of patients. The lymph nodes involved are those that drain the primary lesion. In men, the lesion usually is on the penis or in the urethra, so the inguinal nodes are involved. In women, if the lesion is on the vulva, the inguinal and femoral nodes are involved. If the lesion is rectal, the deep iliac nodes are affected; if it is in the upper vagina or cervix, the obturator and iliac nodes are infected. The adenopathy progresses to extensive adenitis and, ultimately, suppuration with multiple draining sinuses. Rupture of the infected node relieves pain and fever, but drainage of thick purulent material may continue for weeks or months. Only about one third of buboes rupture; the remainder harden and slowly diminish in size. If involvement of the femoral nodes occurs, the inguinal ligament dividing them may produce a "groove" sign This is only seen in 10 to 20% of patients (20). Systemic symptoms of myalgia, arthritis, and/or fever may be present. Patients may also complain of symptoms consistent with lower abdominal and/or back pain secondary to deep pelvic and lumbar lymph node involvement.

Left untreated, the infection progresses to a tertiary stage with continued tissue destruction and scarring. As a result, sinuses, fistulas, and strictures involving the vulva, perineum, and rectum may develop. Ultimately, elephantiasis and hypertrophic ulceration results. Women most frequently present in either the secondary or tertiary stage.

Diagnosis

A diagnosis based on clinical or historical grounds is hard to make. Diagnosis can be made on the basis of positive chlamydial serology for acute infection, isolation of chlamydia from infected tissue, and occasionally on histopathology. Aspirate with culture from a bubo or genital or rectal tissue yields chlamydial organism(s) in only about 30% of cases (21). The complement fixation test for chlamydial antibodies may be used and is considered diagnostic if titers are greater than 1:64. (Mucosal infections with chlamydia are usually associated with lower titer levels.)

Treatment

Treatment for LGV is doxycycline 100 mg twice daily for 21 days. Alternative regimens include erythromycin 500 mg orally four times a day for 21 days, sulfamethoxazole 1000 mg orally twice daily for 21 days, or tetracycline 500 mg four times a day for 21 days.

Aspiration of fluctuant nodes through adjacent healthy skin should be done to prevent sinus tract formation. Surgical excision of affected nodes, however, will only serve to further impair already compromised lymphatic drainage and is not recommended. Antibiotics will help with constitutional symptoms but will only have a limited effect in resolution of buboes.

CHANCROID

Chancroid is caused by *Haemophilus ducreyi.* Worldwide it is a very common infection. Although considered rare in the United States, major outbreaks have been reported recently (22, 23). It is most commonly reported in men, particularly young men with recent contact with prostitutes (24). The incubation time varies from 1 day to several weeks, with a median of 5 to 7 days. Lesions usually begin as small papules and progress over 2 to 3 days to an ulcerated state. Extragenital chancroid is rare. The lesion is painful, tender, and not usually indurated, and there may be multiple lesions. Men often have single ulcers, whereas women typically have multiple lesions. The ulcer diameter ranges from 1 to 20 mm. The ulcers can include the entire vagina and fourchette and the anal area (25). Unilateral, tender, inguinal adenopathy is common and present in about 50% of patients. Approximately 25% of cases may develop a bubo 7 to 10 days after the appearance of the lesion. Left untreated, the bubo will rupture, with resultant development of an inguinal ulcer.

Diagnosis

Diagnosis of these painful genital ulcers based on clinical findings is difficult and often inaccurate. Other sexually transmitted diseases causing genital ulcers such as syphilis, herpes, and LGV must be excluded and may even be concurrent with chancroid. Culture of material from the base of an ulcer or aspiration of a bubo should be done. Isolation of *H. ducreyi* is technically difficult but definitive. Diagnosis can be confirmed by Gram stain of the exudate where a "school of fish" pattern of the Gram-negative coccobacilli may be seen. The most reliable material to use for Gram stain in an attempt to diagnose chancroid is pus aspirated from a bubo. The sensitivity of Gram stain, however, is low.

Treatment

First-line treatment involves erythromycin ethinyl succinate, erythromycin base (Eryc, E-Mycin), ceftriaxone (Rocephin), or azithromycin (Zithromax) (26). Partners should also receive treatment, regardless of symptomatology, and should abstain from any sexual contact until the treatment is completed. Fluctuant nodes should be aspirated through adjacent healthy skin.

The following are the recommended regimens:

- Erythromycin base (Eryc, E-Mycin) 500 mg orally four times a day for 7 days, *or*
- Erythromycin ethinyl succinate 1 g orally in a single dose, *or*
- Ceftriaxone (Rocephin) 250 mg intramuscularly in a single dose, *or*
- Azithromycin (Zithromax) 1 g orally in a single dose.

Alternative regimens are as follows:

- Amoxicillin (Amoxil) 500 mg plus clavulanic acid 125 mg orally three times a day for 7 days, *or*
- Ciprofloxacin (Cipro) 500 mg orally twice daily for 3 days, *or*
- Azithromycin (Zithromax) 1 g orally in a single dose.

CHLAMYDIA

Chlamydia trachomatis is the most common sexually transmitted disease in the world. Serotypes D through K are the ones associated with PID. *C. trachomatis* is an intracellular parasite that infects women most commonly at the transformation zone of the cervix. Most female patients with chlamydia are asymptomatic, although some may complain of a mucopurulent cervical discharge. The incubation time is 1 to 3 weeks, although many infections remain asymptomatic. Chlamydia has been associated with PID, mucopurulent cervicitis, a pneumonia-like syndrome in neonates, and a conjunctivitis syndrome in the infant (27).

Diagnosis

The diagnosis is currently made either by culture or rapid diagnostic tests. Although tissue culture is the gold standard in identifying *C. trachomatis,* rapid diagnostic tests using DNA probes are readily available, accurate, and recommended. To test sites other than the cervix, polymerase chain reaction (PCR) or ligase chain reaction tests or culture should be used. It is important to remember that the discharge from the cervical os is not where the parasite resides. Although a proper specimen for gonorrhea is obtained by placing the swab in the endocervical discharge, this is not true for chlamydia. The chlamydia collection swab should be rubbed against the endocervical canal so that infected endocervical cells are included in the sample. Chlamydia can also be isolated from the urethra, although the yield is higher from the cervix. Because there is a high rate of concurrent infection, any woman being tested for chlamydia should be screened for gonorrhea as well.

Cytology and serology are not used for the diagnosis of chlamydial infection. The sensitivity of cytologic tests is quite low. Serologically, there is a high prevalence of antichlamydial antibodies in the population, making it impossible to distinguish between acute or ongoing infections.

Treatment

The treatments of choice are tetracycline (Achromycin) or doxycycline (Vibramycin, Doryx) (28). Newer agents, such as azithromycin (Zithromax), are also available. During pregnancy, erythromycin base or ethinyl succinate or amoxicillin are treatments of choice. Partners in the past 1 to 2 months should be tested for chlamydia, gonorrhea, and other sexually transmitted diseases. If this is not done, the partner will serve as a source of reinfection.

The recommended regimens are

- Doxycycline (Vibramycin, Doryx) 100 mg orally two times a day for 7 days, *or*
- Azithromycin (Zithromax) 1 g orally in a single dose.

The alternative regimens are

- Ofloxacin (Floxin) 300 mg orally two times a day for 7 days, *or*
- Erythromycin base (Eryc, E-Mycin) 500 mg orally four times a day for 7 days, *or*
- Erythromycin ethyl succinate 800 mg orally four times a day for 7 days.

Special Considerations

Follow-up Test of Cure
Chlamydial infection with serotypes D through K, although often asymptomatic, may be quite insidious because of its silent nature and is associated with tubal damage, infertility, and chronic pain. Patients treated for a positive chlamydia culture should

have a test of cure after the full course of therapy has been completed. At least 2 weeks should elapse, particularly if one is using rapid diagnostic tests, before a test of cure is done because dead particles of the organism could give a false-positive result.

NEISSERIA GONORRHOEAE

Neisseria gonorrhoeae is still a major cause of infectious cervicitis and PID. Although men are usually symptomatic, up to 90% of women are asymptomatic (29). When women are symptomatic, the most common complaints are a mucopurulent discharge, dysuria, and/or abnormal vaginal bleeding. Mucopurulent discharge is present in about 25% of symptomatic women. Infection of the female genital tract is primarily seen in the endocervix, although the urethra, Skene's glands, Bartholin's glands, and anus may also be involved. Approximately 10% of infected women also have a pharyngeal infection with gonococcus (30). For almost half of patients with pharyngeal infections, cultures done at other sites are negative. Risk of transmission from a male to a female after one exposure is high, about 80 to 90% (31). The incubation period after exposure is 3 to 5 days. In 15 to 20% of women with pelvic site infection, acute PID develops. The patients present with fever and lower abdominal tenderness. They most commonly present at the end of, or shortly after, their menstrual cycle. Untreated, gonorrhea is associated with severe sequelae such as infertility, increased incidence of ectopic pregnancy, and chronic pelvic pain. Infertility may occur in as high as 20% of patients without early treatment of *N. gonorrhoeae* (32).

Diagnosis

The diagnosis of gonorrhea is made either with culture or with a rapid diagnostic test such as a DNA gene probe or PCR test. Rapid diagnostic tests have a high sensitivity rate up to 98% (33, 34). If culture is done, modified Thayer-Martin media is used and the specimen must be placed in either a CO_2 incubator or in a covered bottle where oxygen has been removed (usually by placing a lighted tea candle in the bottle and then putting the lid on). The specimen should not be refrigerated.

For either culture or rapid testing, the specimen should be obtained from the discharge in the endocervix. A single endocervical swab detects up to 90% of infections with gonorrhea, whereas two consecutive endocervical swabs or an endocervical and separate anal swab increase the detection rate to 99%.

The rapid tests are unable to determine if the organism present is a resistant one. To detect a penicillinase-producing strain, culture is required. Up to 30% of gonococcal isolates are resistant to penicillin and tetracycline.

Gram stain of an endocervical discharge may reveal polymorphonuclear neutrophils with intracellular Gram-negative diplococci. Although reliable for diagnosis in symptomatic urethritis, it detects cervical, rectal, or asymptomatic urethral infections only 50% of the time. It is not a useful diagnostic test for pharyngeal infection.

Treatment

The treatment of choice for gonorrhea is ceftriaxone (Rocephin), 125 mg intramuscularly, although alternative agents such as single-dose ciprofloxacin (Cipro) 500 mg are also effective. Approximately 30 to 50% of women with genital gonorrhea have coexisting chlamydial infection. Therefore, the treatment regimen should provide coverage for both organisms. Partners of infected women should be screened and treated to prevent reinfection. Patients with persistent symptoms after treatment should have a repeat culture performed (35). Treatment of gonorrhea with currently recommended regimens is probably sufficient to address any early incubating syphilis, with the exception of spectinomycin (Trobicin).

The recommended regimens are

- Ceftriaxone (Rocephin) 125 mg intramuscularly in a single dose, *or*
- Cefixime (Suprax) 400 mg orally in a single dose, *or*
- Ciprofloxacin (Cipro) 500 mg orally in a single dose, *or*
- Azithromycin (Zithromax) 1 g orally in a single dose, *or*
- Ofloxacin (Floxin) 400 mg orally in a single dose, *plus*
- A regimen effective against possible coinfection with *C. trachomatis,* such as doxycycline 100 mg orally twice daily for 7 days, given concurrently.

SYPHILIS

Syphilis still remains a significant sexually transmitted disease in the United States, particularly in pregnancy. Most cases occur in persons 15 to 30 years of age. In 1993, 3000 cases of congenital syphilis were reported (36). Between 1985 and 1990, there was a 75% increase in the incidence of the disease. Although rates are highest in the urban southeastern United States and Texas, changes have occurred nationwide, including areas of the United States where it was once uncommon (37). The current increase in syphilis is thought to be related to the recent epidemic of drug use, particularly cocaine, because there is often an exchange of sex for drugs.

Syphilis is caused by a spirochete, *Treponema pallidum,* and, aside from congenital infection, is primarily acquired through sexual contact. It may be transmitted through kissing active lesions, transfusion of fresh blood, or direct inoculation. The risk of infection to a partner of an infected person is approximately 30% (38).

Clinical Symptoms

Syphilis has been called "the great imitator." It can present in any stage and with almost any symptoms. Primary syphilis is associated with the chancre lesion, a painless ulceration that occurs at the site of entry of the spirochete. It is indurated with a smooth base and raised firm borders. There is no exudate unless secondary infection occurs. There is little pain or bleeding if the lesion is scraped for a dark-field examination. The chancre may occur in the cervix, vagina, vulva, or at a nongenital site like the oropharynx. Multiple chancres can occur, and this is particularly true in patients infected with human immunodeficiency virus (HIV) (39). Its location is dependent on the site of inoculation. Because it is usually not noticed by the patient, most women are unaware of being infected until serologic testing is done. After exposure to syphilis, a 10- to 90-day incubation period precedes the appearance of the chancre. The incubation period depends on the initial inoculum size (40). If untreated, the primary chancre resolves spontaneously within 3 to 6 weeks. Patients with a history of previous syphilis and who are reexposed will either not develop a lesion or will develop only a small papule.

From 6 weeks to 6 months later, the patient then develops the secondary stage of syphilis. This is when the highest number of treponemes are in the body, especially the blood. The primary chancre may still be present during this stage. This presents as low-grade fever, malaise, and lymphadenopathy. Epitrochlear adenopathy, a rare occurrence, should strongly raise suspicions for the diagnosis of syphilis. In addition, there is a rash that may involve mucous membranes and/or cutaneous sites, including the palms of the hands and soles of the feet. If hair follicles are involved, a temporary localized alopecia may develop. The nature of the rash is variable. It may be macular, maculopapular, papular, pustular, or any variation thereof. With the exception of congenital syphilis, it is never vesicular. It may be quite pronounced or rather unimpressive. In warm moist areas of the body, gray plaques, called condylomata lata, may develop, which are highly infectious. Lesions of mucous membranes, or mucous patches, may also develop. These are a silvery-gray shallow ulceration with a raised red border, also highly infectious. During the secondary stage, there is hematogenous and lymphatic dissemination of the spirochete.

Involvement of the central nervous system is present in up to 40% of patients with secondary syphilis. Headaches and meningismus are common, and changes in the cerebrospinal fluid may be noted (41). Involvement of cranial nerves II to VIII may also be seen. These are manifestations of the secondary stage of syphilis and should not be confused with the tertiary complication of neurosyphilis (42). It is important to realize that virtually any organ of the body may be involved. If untreated, the symptoms of secondary syphilis resolve spontaneously.

What follows the second stage is an asymptomatic latent phase that is quite variable in duration. The Center for Disease Control and Prevention (CDC) defines early latent phase as less than 1 year's duration of infection and in approximately 25% of patients, the symptoms of secondary stage may recur. The World Health Organization (WHO) defines early latent phase as infection of less than 2 years' duration. Seventy-five percent of relapses occur in the first year after infection. Although the skin lesions in relapses are not as copious, condylomata lata are quite common. Syphilis is sexually communicable by patients in primary, secondary, or early latent stages. The late latent stage is not sexually contagious but can be transmitted to a fetus transplacentally. The CDC defines late latent stage as more than 1 year's duration of infection, whereas the WHO defines it as more than 2 years' duration.

If latent syphilis is untreated, about 33% of patients go on to develop tertiary syphilis with involvement and progressive destruction of the central nervous system and/or ascending aorta, although almost any organ may be involved. Another expression of tertiary syphilis is gummas, a lesion with a coagulated necrotic center and evidence of small-vessel obliterative endarteritis. These principally appear in the skin, liver, bones, and spleen.

Diagnosis

Diagnostic testing involves the use of nontreponemal specific screening tests like the Venereal Disease Research Laboratory (VDRL), rapid plasma reagin (RPR), or automated reagin test (ART). If positive, these tests are confirmed by treponemal specific tests like the fluorescent treponemal antibody absorption test (FTA-ABS) or the microhemagglutination assay test (MHA-TP). The nonspecific tests detect the presence of nontreponemal antibodies, and their sensitivity and specificity vary. The RPR has greater than 90% sensitivity and 98% specificity. In about 2% of patients, a prozone phenomenon occurs, especially in secondary syphilis when the antigenic load is at its highest. Therefore, when the index of suspicion is high but the test is reported as negative, it may be useful to contact the laboratory and request a repeat test with higher than normal dilutions. Clinicians must realize, however, that other disease states and/or physiologic states (e.g., pregnancy) can yield false-positive results. Any strong immunologic stimulus (vaccination, acute viral or bacterial infections) may cause a transient false-positive reaction. Persistent false positives may be seen with drug abuse, connective tissue diseases, or a state of hypergammaglobulinemia.

Confirmatory testing is done in the presence of a positive screening test. Treponemal tests specifically detect the treponemal antigen. The MHA-TP test is cheaper and simpler so is more commonly used than the FTA-ABS examination. If a specific treponemal test is positive, antibody titers should be obtained. For patients with a history of treated syphilis, a fourfold rise in the antibody titer signifies recurrent infection, and appropriate re-treatment is necessary. In primary syphilis, the treponemal specific tests become positive before the nontreponemal or reaginic tests. However, the MHA-TP test is not as sensitive as the FTA-ABS test for primary syphilis. This is important to remember in instances where suspicion is high for primary syphilis but the reaginic test is negative. Other disease caused by spirochetes (e.g., Lyme disease) will give positive nontreponemal and/or treponemal test results.

Dark-field examination can be done on specimens obtained directly from syphilitic lesions. This may be the diagnostic method of choice for patients with a chancre because the nonspecific and specific serologic tests may be nonreactive when the chancre first appears.

Testing during pregnancy is recommended at the first prenatal visit and again at term, particularly in high-risk populations.

If a patient has any neurologic symptoms, a lumbar puncture to look for neurosyphilis is recommended. Lumbar puncture is also recommended in HIV-positive patients where asymptomatic neurosyphilis may occur or in cases where inadequate treatment (including benzathine penicillin) was given. More detailed discussion of HIV-infected patients and syphilis is found in Chapter 8.

Treatment

Penicillin G, in benzathine, aqueous procaine, or aqueous crystalline form, is the drug of choice for treatment of all stages of syphilis. Because of the high rate of failure of other treatment modalities, patients with known penicillin allergy should undergo desensitization with subsequent administration of penicillin. An oral desensitization protocol can be safely done in the labor and delivery area or in the office where emergency facilities are immediately available. For one oral desensitization protocol, see Table 7.1.

Treatment should include antibody titer checks every 3 months for 1 year. Titers decrease more quickly in earlier stages of disease, when titers are low, and in patients without a previous history of syphilis. Successful treatment of primary and secondary syphilis causes a fourfold decrease in titers at 6 months and an eightfold decrease at 12 months. Successful treatment of early latent disease causes a fourfold decrease in titer at 12 months posttherapy. If the infection had been present for more than 1 year, antibody titers should also be drawn again at 18 and 24 months posttherapy.

With treatment, the nonspecific tests do revert to negative. A positive RPR after 1 year in a patient treated for primary syphilis or after 2 years in a patient treated for secondary syphilis indicate either persistent infection, reinfection, or a false-positive reaction. In most patients, once a specific treponemal test is positive, it stays positive for life. However, after treatment with benzathine penicillin G, up to 24% of those with a positive FTA-ABS and up to 13% of those with a positive MHA-TP test may revert to negative (43).

One to 2 hours after treatment, patients can develop an acute febrile reaction related to breakdown of the spirochetes called the Jarisch-Herxheimer reaction. Symptoms include fever, chills, myalgias, headache, tachycardia, hyperventilation, vasodilation, and mild hypotension. This occurs in 10 to 25% of patients overall but is most common in the treatment of secondary syphilis, where the incidence is 70 to 90%. It lasts for 12 to 24 hours, has varying degrees of severity, and is usually self-limiting. Treatment is with two aspirin every 4 hours for 24 to 48 hours. Pretreatment with prednisone serves as prophylaxis and is recommended when treating either cardiovascular or symptomatic neurosyphilis. In pregnant patients, this reaction has

TABLE 7.1. Oral Penicillin Desensitization Protocol of Wendel[a]

Dose[b]	Penicillin V Suspension (units/mL)	Amount[c] mL	Amount[c] Units	Cumulative Dose (Units)
1	1,000	0.1	100	100
2	1,000	0.2	200	300
3	1,000	0.4	400	700
4	1,000	0.8	800	1,500
5	1,000	1.6	1,600	3,100
6	1,000	3.2	3,200	6,300
7	1,000	6.4	6,400	12,700
8	10,000	1.2	12,000	24,700
9	10,000	2.4	24,700	48,700
10	10,000	4.8	48,000	96,700
11	80,000	1.0	80,000	176,000
12	80,000	2.4	164,000	336,700
13	80,000	4.8	320,000	656,700
14	80,000	8.0	640,000	1,296,700

Adapted from MMWR Morb Mortal Wkly Rep. 1998;47(RR-1):47.
[a]Patients are desensitized as above. After desensitization, patients are observed for 30 minutes before parenteral injection of benzathine penicillin. Patients who have been desensitized previously, have received their benzathine penicillin intramuscularly, and are returning for their second shot will not require additional desensitization. Although desensitization is usually lost within 2 days of terminating the penicillin therapy, long-acting benzathine penicillin will sustain the sensitized state for periods up to 3 weeks.
[b]Interval between doses, 15 min; elapsed time, 3 hr and 45 min; cumulative dose, 1.3 million units.
[c]The specific amount of drug is diluted in approximately 30 mL of water and then given orally.

been associated with increased uterine activity and preterm delivery. All patients receiving initial treatment should be counseled regarding this reaction and instructed to report any symptoms they may develop.

Special Considerations

Syphilis in Pregnancy

The highest congenital infection rate is seen with recent maternal or current disseminated secondary infections in the mother. Fetal infection before the 16th week of gestation is rare, so treatment of the mother during the first 16 weeks of pregnancy almost ensures the fetus will not be infected. Fifty percent of infants of women with untreated primary or secondary syphilis are affected at birth, and the remainder develop neonatal infection. The risk of congenital infection for early latent infection is 40% and 6 to 14% for late latent infection (44). In summary then, the shorter the duration of the mother's infection, the higher the likelihood of fetal transmission.

In the perinatal time period, the mucocutaneous tissues and bones are most commonly affected (i.e., the saddle nose or saber shins). The earliest sign of congenital syphilis is a rhinitis ("snuffles"). Necrotizing funisitis is almost pathognomonic for syphilis. A rash may develop, and, as in adults, any organ of the body may be involved. Neonatal death is usually a result of liver failure, pneumonia, or pulmonary hemorrhage. If the child is untreated and lives beyond the first 6 to 12 months, they enter a latent period. Over the ensuing years, interstitial keratitis, eighth nerve deafness, and other signs and symptoms develop. Penicillin treatment for all neonates born to syphilitic mothers is warranted given the profound morbidity and potential for mortality that exists. Quantitative antibody titers should be repeated at 3, 6, and 12 months posttherapy.

Syphilis and HIV

Given the strong association between HIV and genital ulcer disease, concurrent infection with HIV and syphilis is common. It is thought by some, but not all, that the HIV-infected patient with syphilis may present with greater constitutional symptoms; organ involvement, particularly uveitis; and a significant predisposition to neurosyphilis (45, 46). For most patients with HIV, serologic testing provides accurate information. It has been suggested that patients with HIV and syphilis should be treated more aggressively than patients without HIV. A further discussion of syphilis in HIV-positive patients is found in Chapter 8.

Cerebrospinal Fluid Examination

Controversy surrounds who among asymptomatic patients should undergo lumbar puncture for the detection of neurosyphilis. This is further compounded by the lack of agreement regarding the specific laboratory criteria that must be met for the diagnosis of asymptomatic neurosyphilis. Ideally, all patients with disease of greater than 1 year's duration should undergo lumbar puncture. Clinically, it is uniformly thought that all patients with syphilis and neurologic or ophthalmologic symptoms require examination of the cerebrospinal fluid. In addition, most would agree that failure of initial therapy, an antibody titer of greater than or equal to 1:32 in infection known to be more than 1 year in duration, and history of nonpenicillin therapy in infection known to be more than 1 year in duration are sufficient grounds for a spinal tap. Discussion regarding the use of lumbar puncture in syphilis for patients who are HIV positive is found in Chapter 8.

There is no single test that can diagnose neurosyphilis. Combinations of reactive serology, specific abnormalities on examination of the cerebrospinal fluid (e.g., elevated protein and cell count), and/or a reactive VDRL or PCR on cerebrospinal fluid are used. The RPR should not be done on cerebrospinal fluid for the diagnosis of neurosyphilis.

For asymptomatic neurosyphilis, treatment prevents destruction of the nervous system and the development of symptoms. For symptomatic neurosyphilis, treatment prevents further destruction but will not reverse the damage that has been done.

The recommended regimen for adults (nonpenicillin allergic or after desensitization) is as follows:

- Primary, secondary, or early latent stage: benzathine penicillin G, 2.4 million units intramuscularly in a single dose
- Late latent stage or syphilis of unknown duration: benzathine penicillin, 2.4 million units intramuscularly once a week for 3 consecutive weeks
- Neurosyphilis: penicillin G procaine 2 to 4 million units every 4 hours intravenously for 10 to 14 days *or* penicillin G procaine 2 to 4 million units intramuscularly once a week for 3 consecutive weeks

GRANULOMA INGUINALE

Granuloma inguinale is a chronic, progressive, ulcerative disease caused by *Calymmatobacterium granulomatis* and usually found in the genitalia. There are fewer than 100 cases per year in the United States, but it is more frequent worldwide. Although it is primarily a sexually transmitted disease, extragenital lesions do suggest alternative modes of spread.

Symptoms

The incubation time is between 8 and 80 days. The initial lesion is a small painless papule or nodule that soon ulcerates and becomes beefy-red, with exuberant granulomatous changes. It is almost "velvety" in its appearance. The ulcer bleeds easily and, unless secondary infection occurs, is painless. In women, the most common sites involved are the labia and fourchette, although the vaginal walls or cervix may also be involved. It is frequently diagnosed in pregnancy, and it is suspected that pregnancy intensifies the disease (47). Inguinal groin swellings, called "pseudobuboes," result from the subcutaneous spread of granulomas into the inguinal region. It is not a true adenitis. Lymphedema and subsequent elephantiasis of the external genitalia may result in severe cases. Healing is accompanied by scarring. Systemic disease, although rare, does occur and is more common in women with primary lesions of the cervix. In cases of concurrent infection with another sexually transmitted disease, secondary bacterial infection of lesions, or extensive spread of lesions, constitutional symptoms may also be noted.

Diagnosis

The diagnosis is usually made on clinical grounds but can be confirmed with histologic examination of a biopsy or scrapings taken from the edges of a lesion. Active lesions should be cleaned with saline before biopsy. The gold standard for diagnosis is the presence of intracellular Donovan bodies.

Treatment

There is no real consensus regarding the ideal form of therapy. Larger lesions seem to require longer periods of treatment. Lesions tend to heal from the edges inward, and most recommend continued therapy until complete epithelialization occurs to avoid relapse.

Recommended treatment regimens are tetracycline 500 mg four times a day, doxycycline (Vibramycin, Doryx) 100 mg twice daily, or trimethoprim-sulfamethoxazole (800 mg/160 mg) (Bactrim) two tablets twice daily.

PELVIC INFLAMMATORY DISEASE

PID, also called acute salpingitis, is the most frequent acute infection in reproductive-age nonpregnant women. It is estimated that one million women a year are treated for PID in the United States. An estimated 150,000 surgical procedures are performed each year specifically addressing complications of PID. In 1990, the direct costs for PID, such as ectopic pregnancy and infertility, were estimated to be 2.7 billion dollars (48–51). Among sexually active females, the highest rate of infection occurs in those 15 to 19 years of age.

Approximately 25% of women who suffer from PID also experience one or more long-term complications, the most common of which is infertility. Other morbidities include chronic pelvic pain, dyspareunia, increased risk for ectopic pregnancy, and/or tubo-ovarian abscesses.

Symptoms

PID is polymicrobial in nature, although the most frequently associated organisms are *N. gonorrhoeae* and *C. trachomatis*. It most commonly presents during or shortly after menstruation. The patient presents with fever, lower abdominal/pelvic pain, and a mucopurulent discharge. On examination, cervical motion tenderness and adnexal tenderness are present. On laboratory studies, a leukocytosis may be present.

Diagnosis

The most commonly used method of diagnosing PID is on the basis of clinical history and physical findings. Making a clinical diagnosis is not the most accurate method and is difficult because of the wide variety of signs and symptoms that may be present (52). Laparoscopy is currently the gold standard for diagnosis, although it is neither economically feasible nor practical for all patients with the suspected diagnosis of PID to undergo this procedure. The criteria accepted for the diagnosis of PID are listed in Table 7.2.

Treatment

The goal of treatment is to prevent infertility, ectopic pregnancy, and other long-term sequelae associated with PID. Although the general population has a 3% rate of infertility, in women who have had at least one episode of treated PID, the average infertility rate is 21% (53). The likelihood of infertility is directly related to the number of episodes of PID a woman suffers. With one episode, her risk is 11%; after two, it rises to 34%; and with three or more episodes, it rises to 54% (54). The effectiveness of therapy in preventing subsequent infertility is also related to the time between onset of symptoms and treatment of disease. The less time that elapses between the two, the lower the woman's risk of infertility (55).

Of patients treated in the United States, only 20 to 25% are hospitalized. The remainder are treated as outpatients. The CDC published guidelines for the treatment of PID on an outpatient or hospitalized basis. Indications for acceptable reasons to hospitalize a patient are listed in Table 7.3. If a patient is being treated as an outpatient, a repeat physical examination within 24 to 48 hours is warranted to verify response to therapy. Presence of a tubo-ovarian abscess, either noted on examination or confirmed by imaging study, warrants hospitalization.

TABLE 7.2. Diagnostic Criteria for PID

ALL THREE ARE REQUIRED FOR DIAGNOSIS
Lower abdominal tenderness
Adnexal tenderness
Cervical motion tenderness

ONE OR MORE INCREASES THE SPECIFICITY OF THE DIAGNOSIS
Fever (oral temperature >38.3°C [>101.8°F])
Abnormal cervical or vaginal discharge
Elevated erythrocyte sedimentation rate
Elevated C-reactive protein level
Laboratory proven infection with *N. gonorrhoeae* or *C. trachomatis*

DEFINITIVE CRITERIA FOR DIAGNOSING PID INCLUDE
Histopathologic evidence of endometritis on endometrial biopsy
Transvaginal sonography or other imaging techniques showing thickened fluid-filled
    tubes with or without free pelvic fluid or tubo-ovarian complex
Laparoscopic abnormalities consistent with PID

Adapted from MMWR Morb Mortal Wkly Rep 1998;47(RR-1):80

TABLE 7.3. Recommendations for Hospitalization of Patients with PID

Diagnosis is uncertain, and surgical emergencies such as appendicitis cannot be excluded.

Patient is pregnant.

Patient does not respond clinically to oral antimicrobial therapy.

Patient is unable to follow or tolerate an outpatient oral regimen.

Patient has severe illness, nausea and vomiting, or high fever.

Patient has a tubo-ovarian abscess.

Patient is immunodeficient (i.e., has HIV infection with low CD4 counts, is taking immunosuppressive therapy, or has another disease).

Adapted from MMWR Morb Mortal Wkly Rep 1998; 47(RR-1):82.

TABLE 7.4. Outpatient Treatment of PID

REGIMEN A

Ofloxacin (Floxin) 400 mg orally bid for 14 days + metronidazole (Flagyl) 500 mg orally BID for 14 days

REGIMEN B

Ceftriaxone (Rocephin) 250 mg IM once, *or*

Cefoxitin (Mefoxin) 2 g IM plus probenecid 1 g orally in a single dose concurrently once, *or*

Other parenteral third-generation cephalosporin (e.g., ceftizoxime [Cefizox] or cefotaxime [Claforan]), *plus*

Doxycycline (Vibramycin, Doryx) 100 mg orally BID for 14 days, *plus*

Clindamycin (Cleocin) 450 mg orally QID, *or*

Metronidazole (Flagyl) 500 mg orally BID for 14 days

Adapted from MMWR Morb Mortal Wkly Rep 1998;47(RR-1):84.

TABLE 7.5. Inpatient Treatment of PID[a]

REGIMEN A

Cefoxitin (Mefoxin) 2 g IV q 6 hr *or* cefotetan (Cefotan) 2 g IV q 12 hr, *plus*

Doxycycline (Vibramycin) 100 mg IV or orally q 12 hr

REGIMEN B

Clindamycin (Cleocin) 900 mg IV q 8 hrs, *plus*

Gentamicin (Garamycin) loading dose IV or IM (2 mg/kg of body weight), followed by a maintenance dose (1.5 mg/kg) q 8 hr. Single daily dosing may be substituted.

ALTERNATIVE PARENTERAL REGIMENS

Ofloxacin (Floxin) 400 mg IV q 12 hr *plus* metronidazole (Flagyl) 500 mg IV q 8 hr, *or*

Ampicillin/sulbactam (Unasyn) 3 g IV q 6 hr *plus* doxycyline (Vibramycin, Doryx) 100 mg IV or po q 12 hr, *or*

Ciprofloxacin (Cipro) 200 mg IV q 12 hr *plus* doxycycline 100 mg IV or orally q 12 hr *plus* metronidazole 500 mg IV q 8 hr

Adapted from MMWR Morb Mortal Wkly Rep 1998;47(RR-1):82–83

[a]These regimens should be used untill at least 48 hours after the patient demonstrates substantial clinical improvement. They may then be changed to doxycycline (Vibramycin) 100 mg orally BID for a total of 14 days of treatment. If tubo-ovarian abscess is present, many health care providers use clindamycin (Cleocin) 900 mg orally TID for continued therapy instead of doxycycline.

Sexual partners should also be examined and treated with a regimen appropriate for uncomplicated gonorrhea and chlamydia.

For outpatient therapy options, see Table 7.4. For inpatient treatment, see Table 7.5. This regimen is given for at least 48 hours after the patient clinically improves. After discharge, the patient continues doxycycline 100 mg twice daily for a total of 14 days *or* clindamycin (Cleocin) 900 mg intravenously every 8 hours *plus* a gentamycin (Garamycin) loading dose of 2 mg/kg, followed by maintenance dose of 1.5 mg/kg every 8 hours. This regimen is given for at least 48 hours after the patient clinically improves. After discharge, the patient continues doxycycline 100 mg twice daily for a total of 14 days or clindamycin 450 mg orally five times a day for 10 to 14 days.

SCABIES

Scabies is a highly contagious infection caused by *Sarcoptes scabiei,* also known as the itch mite. It is an obligate parasite that burrows into, resides in, and reproduces in human skin. It is worldwide in its distribution and occurs in all races and socioeconomic classes. It is not a vector for other infectious disease. It is transmitted by intimate contact, often sexual, but casual contact may incur transmission as well. Fomites may also be an important means of transmission.

Symptoms

Most persons with scabies complain of intense pruritus that is worse at night. Areas prone to infection include interdigital spaces, wrists, axillary folds, the periumbilical area, pelvic area, penis, and ankles. In infants or toddlers, the head, neck, palms, and soles may be involved. Infection is usually erythematous, and papules or vesicles may be present. Excoriations are often seen. Chronic infection may lead to pruritic reddish-brown nodules, especially in children. They may not disappear for weeks or months after therapy is completed.

Diagnosis

The classic linear burrows (short wavy lines that cross skin lines) should be sought to assist in the diagnosis. Formal diagnosis is made by microscopically examining skin scrapings of suspected sites for the organism, eggs, or feces. Skin samples are obtained by either scraping or shaving the superficial layers of skin over a burrow. This is done to a depth sufficient to cause a very small amount of bleeding.

Treatment

The drug of choice for treatment is permethrin (Nix 1% or Elimite 5%) cream, which has a higher cure rate than lindane (Kwell) (56). Permethrin is safe for use in pregnancy, it is category B, but should not be used in infants less than 2 months old. Household contacts should also be treated, and recently worn clothes and linens should be washed in hot soapy water and placed in a hot dryer. Dry cleaning is also sufficient to kill the mite(s). Fingernails should also be trimmed as part of the treatment, and patients should be counseled that the itching may persist for up to 2 weeks after therapy.

The treatment regimens are as follows:

- Permethrin (Nix 1% or Elimite 5% cream): apply head to toe, avoiding mouth, nose, and eyes, and wash off after 8 to 10 hours.
- Crotamiton (Eurax) 10% cream or lotion: apply from chin to feet for two consecutive nights and wash off 24 hours after second application. Pregnancy category C, but less topical absorption than lindane (Kwell).

- Lindane (Kwell) 1%: apply from head to toe, avoiding mouth, nose, and eyes, and wash off after 8 to 12 hours. Pregnancy category B. In children, wash off after 6 to 8 hours. Do not apply immediately after a bath or shower because this will increase the amount of topical absorption. It may cause seizures if overused or misused in children.

PEDICULOSIS PUBIS

Pediculosis pubis is also known as the crab louse. An estimated 3 million cases occur each year in the United States. It may be spread through fomites, although the usual acquisition is through sexual contact. The chance of contracting this with a single sexual encounter is 95%—making this the most contagious sexually transmitted disease known. It is more common in women than in men up to age 19, after which it is more common in men. Incubation time is 30 days.

Symptoms

Most patients complain of intense pruritus or irritation in the pubic hair area. If there are a large number of lice and, hence, lots of bites, there may be systemic complaints of low-grade fever and malaise.

Diagnosis

The diagnosis is made by visualizing the lice, larvae, and/or nits with a magnifying glass.

Treatment

All sexual contacts, family members, and close contacts should be treated, even if they are asymptomatic. Recently worn clothing or linens should be washed in hot soapy water and dried in a hot dryer. Dry cleaning is also acceptable. Petrolatum jelly should be applied to infested eyelashes. After therapy, a fine tooth comb should be used to remove any remaining lice and/or nits. If lice or eggs are found 5 to 7 days after therapy, repeat the treatment.

The treatment regimens are as follows:

- Permethrin (Nix 1% rinse or Elimite 5% cream): apply to affected areas and wash off after 10 minutes.
- Pyrethrin with piperonyl butoxide (Rid): apply as for permethrin.
- Lindane (Kwell 1% shampoo): apply for 4 minutes and wash off.

CLINICAL NOTES

- Primary outbreaks of herpes are more severe than recurrences and may require hospitalization. Urinary retention may be present. Eighty percent of patients will suffer a recurrent outbreak the year after the primary outbreak.
- Not all patients are aware of the primary outbreak of herpes or exposure to the virus.
- Cultures for herpes should be taken from the base of the lesion.
- Acyclovir may be used for prophylaxis in patients with frequent recurrences.
- The risk of neonatal infection with herpes is highest in those mothers suffering from a primary outbreak at or around the time of delivery. For recurrent maternal infections, the risk of fetal transmission is much lower.
- Condylomata acuminata are common, up to 20% of patients will have spontaneous resolution of the warts, and there are both medical and surgical modalities to treat it.

- LGV is caused by chlamydia and is a painless ulcer in the early stages. If untreated it results in fistulas, strictures, and elephantiasis.
- Chancroid causes a painful ulcer and subsequent bubo formation. It is caused by *H. ducreyi.*
- *C. trachomatis* infects most women at the transformation zone of the cervix. Adequate detection depends on obtaining the culture or specimen from the sidewall(s) of the endocervical canal.
- Asymptomatic chlamydial infection is associated with tubal damage, infertility, and chronic pain. A test of cure should be done in all treated patients.
- Gonorrhea is readily transmitted from a male to a female. In 15 to 20% of women, acute PID results.
- When treating gonorrhea, a regimen effective against *C. trachomatis* should also be given. These two infections are often concurrent.
- Syphilis may present in any fashion and in any organ system. The primary ulcer is painless.
- Syphilis is sexually contagious in the primary, secondary, and early latent phases.
- After treatment for syphilis, titers should be periodically checked to ensure adequate therapy and/or detect reinfection.
- Syphilis is most easily transmitted to the fetus in the primary or secondary stages, although it is also transmissible in the latent phase. The shorter the duration of the maternal infection, the higher the likelihood of fetal transmission.
- Granuloma inguinale, also called Donovanosis, presents as a nontender ulcer. It causes the formation of pseudobuboes.
- PID is a major cause of hospitalization in reproductive-age women in the United States. It is also a significant cause of infertility, chronic pelvic pain, and increased risk of ectopic pregnancy.
- Scabies is caused by a mite and is highly contagious. It does not act as a vector for other infectious diseases.
- Pediculosis pubis, or crabs, is the most contagious sexually transmitted disease known.

Characteristics of the Ulcerative Sexually Transmitted Diseases

	Incubation Time (days)	Adenopathy		Bubo Formation		Ulcer		Ulcer		Bleeds Easily[a]		Scarring	
		Bilateral	Unilateral	Yes	No	Single	Multiple	Tender	Non-tender	Yes	No	Yes	No
LGV	4–21		X (2/3)	X		X			X				X
Chancroid	5–7		X	X		Men	Women	X		X?		?	
Herpes	3–7	X			X		X	X			X		X
Primary syphilis	10–90	X			X	X			X		X		X
Granuloma inguinale	8–80	X			X	X			X	X		X	

[a]In the absence of secondary infection.

Sexually Transmitted Diseases: Should the Partner(s) Be Treated?

	Average Incubation	Treat Partners?		Which Partners?
		Yes	No	
Herpes	3–7 days		X	
Venereal warts	3–6 mo	X	X	Treatment of partners is controversial; unless symptomatic, most do not
Molluscum contagiosum	2–7 wk	X		Partners in last 1–2 mo; examine and treat if affected
Lymphogranuloma venereum	4–21 days	X		Last 30 days
Chancroid	5–7 days	X		Immediate
Chlamydia	1 day–several weeks	X		Last 1–2 mo
Gonorrhea	3–5 days	X		Immediate
Syphilis	10–90 days (primary)	X		All contacts in primary, secondary, and early latent; late latent and tertiary not sexually communicable
Granuloma inguinale	8–80 days		X	
Pelvic inflammatory disease	Varies by organism	X		Immediate
Crabs	30 days	X		Contacts in last month
Scabies	4–6 wk	X		Contacts in last 4–6 wk

Treatment Regimens for Sexually Transmitted Diseases

HERPES

Primary outbreak	*Recurrence*	*Severe disease*	*Prophylaxis*
Acyclovir	Acyclovir	Acyclovir, intravenous	Acyclovir
Valacyclovir	Famciclovir		Famciclovir
Famciclovir	Valacyclovir		

HUMAN PAPILLOMA VIRUS

Medical options	*Surgical options*
Podophyllin 10% solution	Cryotherapy
Condylox 0.5%	LEEP
Bichloracetic or Trichloroacetic acid, up to 85%	CO_2 laser ablation
	Scalpel excision
5-FU, 5% cream	
Iquimod 5%	
Interferon alfa 2b	

MOLLUSCUM CONTAGIOSUM

Options
Podophyllin
Trichloroacetic acid
Skin curettage
Cryotherapy
Expresssion of umbilicated core
Excision

LYMPHOGRANULOMA VENEREUM

Recommended	*Alternative*
Doxycycline	Erythromycin
	Sulfisoxazole
	Tetracycline

CHANCROID

Recommended	*Alternative*	*Comments*
Ceftriaxone	Amoxicillin	Drain buboes
Erythromycin	Ciprofloxacin	Do not excise nodes
	Azithromycin	

CHLAMYDIA

Recommended	*Alternative*
Doxycycline	Ofloxacin
Azithromycin	Erythromycin

GONORRHEA

Recommended	*Concurrent*
Ceftriaxone	See regimen for chlamydia
Cefixime	
Ciprofloxacin	
Azithromycin	
Ofloxacin	

Continued

Treatment Regimens for Sexually Transmitted Diseases

SYPHILIS

Primary	*Secondary*	*Early latent*	*Late latent*	*Neurosyphilis*
Benzathine penicillin	Benzathine penicillin	Benzathine penicillin	Benzathine penicillin	Penicillin G procaine

GRANULOMA INGUINALE
Options
Tetracycline
Doxycycline
Trimethoprim-sulfamethoxazole

SCABIES

Recommended	*Children, pregnant, women*	*Infants*
Permethrin	Permethrin	Pyrethrins/piperonyl butoxide
Crotamiton	Lindane	
Lindane		

CRABS
Options
Permethrin
Pyrethrin with piperonyl butoxide
Lindane

References

1. Koelle DM, Benedetti J, Langenberg A, et al. Asymptomatic reactivation of herpes simplex virus in women after the first episode of genital herpes. Ann Intern Med 1992;116:433.
2. Koutsky LA, Stevens CE, Holmes KK, et al. Underdiagnosis of genital herpes by current clinical and viral-isolation procedures. N Engl J Med 1992;326:1533
3. Corey L, Adams H, Brown Z, et al. Genital herpes simplex viral infection: clinical manifestations, course, and complications. Ann Intern Med 1983;98:958.
4. Baringer JR, Swoveland P. Recovery of herpes simplex virus from human trigeminal ganglion. N Engl J Med 1973;288:648.
5. Baringer JR. Recovery of herpes simplex virus from human sacral ganglion. N Engl J Med 1974;291:828.
6. Spruance SL, Overall JC Jr, Kern ER, et al. The natural history of recurrent herpes simplex labialis: implications for antiviral therapy. N Engl J Med 1977;297:69.
7. Corey L, Nahmias AJ, Guinan EM, et al. A trial of topical acyclovir in genital herpes simplex virus infections. N Engl J Med 1982;306:133.
8. Goldberg LH, Kaufman R, Kurtz TO, et al. Long-term suppression of recurrent genital herpes with acyclovir. Arch Dermatol 1993;129:582–587.
9. Maccato M. Herpes in pregnancy. Clin Obstet Gynecol 1993;36:869
10. Sullivan-Bolyai J, Hull HF, Wilson C, et al. Neonatal herpes simplex infection in King County, Washington. Increasing incidence and epidemiological correlates. JAMA 1983;250:3059.
11. Hulto C, Arvin A, Jacobs R, et al. Intrauterine herpes simplex virus infections. J Pediatr 1987;110:97.
12. Ray DA, Evans AT, Elliott JP, et al. Maternal herpes infection complicated by prolonged preterm premature rupture of the membranes. Am J Perinatol 1985;2:96.
13. Utley K, Bromberger P, Wagner L, et al. Management of primary herpes in pregnancy complicated by ruptured membranes and extreme prematurity: a case report. Obstet Gynecol 1987;69:471.
14. Chuang TY. Condylomata acuminata (genital warts). An epidemiologic view. J Am Acad Dermatol 1987;16:376–384.
15. Edwards A, Atma-Ram A, Thin RN. Podophyllotoxin 0.5% v podophyllin 20% to treat penile warts. Genitourin Med 1988;64:263–265.
16. Clark DP. Condyloma acuminatum. Dermatol Clin 1987;4:779–788.
17. Felman YM, Nikitas JA. Sexually transmitted molluscum contagiosum. Derm Clin 1983;1:103.
18. Borchardt KA, Neves S. Lymphogranuloma venereum. In: Borchardt KA, ed. Sexually Transmitted Diseases: Epidemiology, Pathology, Diagnosis, and Treatment. 1st ed. Boca Raton, FL: CRC Press, 1997:117.
19. Sischy A. Syphilis serology in patients with primary syphilis and non-sexually transmitted diseases in Southern Africa. Genitour Med 1991;67:129.
20. Hayes LJ. Evidence for naturally occurring recombination gene encoding of LGV isolates. Infect Immun 1994;62:56.
21. Perine PL, Osoba AO. Lymphogranuloma venereum. In: Holmes KK, Mardh PA, Sparling PF, et al., eds. Sexually Transmitted Diseases. 2nd ed. New York: McGraw-Hill, 1990:195.
22. Schmid GP, Sanders LL Jr, Blount JH, et al. Chancroid in the United States: reestablishment of an old disease. JAMA 1987;258:3265.
23. Flood JM, Sarafian SK, Bolan GA, et al. Multistrain outbreak of chancroid in San Francisco, 1989–1991. J Infect Dis 1993;167:1106–1111.
24. Centers for Disease Control. Chancroid—California. MMWR Morb Mortal Wkly Rep 1982;31:173–175.
25. Albritton WL. Biology of *Haemophilus ducreyi*. Microbiol Rev 1989;53:377–389.
26. Drugs for sexually transmitted diseases. Med Lett Drugs Ther 1995;37:117–122.

27. Barns R. Laboratory diagnosis of human chlamydial infections. Clin Microbiol Rev 1989;2:119.

28. Recommendations for the prevention and management of *Chlamydia trachomatis* infections, 1993. Centers for Disease Contol and Prevention. MMWR Morb Mortal Wkly Rep 1993;42:1–39.

29. Handsfeld HH, Sparling PF. *Neisseria* gonorrhea. In: Mandell GL, Bennett JE, Dolin R, eds. Principles and Practices of Infectious Diseases. 4th ed. New York: Churchill Livingstone, 1995:1909–1925.

30. Bro-Jornensen A, Jensen T. Gonococcal pharyngeal infections. Report of 110 cases. Br J Vener Dis 1973;49:491.

31. Dans PE. Gonococcal anogenital infection. Clin Obstet Gynecol 1975;18:103.

32. Division of STD Prevention, Sexually Transmitted Disease Surveillance, 1994. Washington, DC: U.S. Department of Health and Human Services, CDC, September 1995.

33. Judson FN. Gonorrhea. Med Clin North Am 1990;74:1353.

34. Ho BS, Feng WG, et al. Polymerase chain reaction for the detection of *Neisseria gonorrhoeae* in clinical samples. J Clin Pathol 1992;45:439–442.

35. MMWR treatment guidelines: sexually transmitted diseases. MMWR Morbid Mortal Wkly Rep 1998;47:62.

36. Domingue G. Syphilis. In: Borchardt KA, ed. Sexually Transmitted Diseases: Epidemiology, Pathology, Diagnosis, and Treatment. Boca Raton, FL: CRC Press, 1997:130.

37. Centers for Disease Control. Primary and secondary syphilis—United States, 1981–1990. MMWR Morb Mortal Wkly Rep 1991;40:314.

38. Sparling PF. Natural history of syphilis. In: Holmes KK, Mardh PA, Sparling PF, et al., eds. Sexually Transmitted Diseases. New York: McGraw-Hill, 1984:298.

39. Chapel TA. The variability of syphilitic chancres. Sex Transm Dis 1978;5:68.

40. Magnuson HJ, Thomas EW, Olansky S, et al. Inoculation of syphilis in human volunteers. Medicine 1956;35:33.

41. Lukehart S, Hook FW, Baker-Zander SH, et al. Invasion of the central nervous system by *Treponema pallidum*. Implications for diagnosis and therapy. Ann Intern Med 1988;109:855.

42. Slatiel P, Melmed CA, Portnoy D. Sensorineural deafness in early acquired syphilis. Can J Neurol Sci 1988;10:114.

43. Romanowski B, Sutherland R, Fick GH, et al. Serologic response to treatment of infectious syphilis. Ann Intern Med 1991;114:1005.

44. Fiumara NF, Fleming WL, Downing JG, et al. The incidence of prenatal syphilis at the Boston City Hospital. N Engl J Med 1952;247:48.

45. Hutchinson CM, Rompalo AM, Reichart CA. Characteristics of patients with syphilis attending Baltimore STD clinics: multiple high risk subgroups and interactions with human immunodeficiency virus. Arch Intern Med 1991;151:511.

46. Musher DM, Hamill RJ, Baughn RE. Effect of human immunodeficiency virus (HIV) infection on the course of syphilis and the response to treatment. Ann Intern Med 1990;113:872–881.

47. O'Farrell N. Donovanosis (granuloma inguinale) in pregnancy. Int J STD AIDS 1991;2:447–448.

48. Curran JW. Economic consequences of pelvic inflammatory disease in the United States. Am J Obstet Gynecol 1980;138:848.

49. Jones OG, Saida AA, St. John RK. Frequency and distribution of salpingitis and pelvic inflammatory disease in short stay in hospitals in the United States. Am J Obstet Gynecol 1980;138:905.

50. Washington AE, Cates W, Zadi AA. Hospitalizations for pelvic inflammatory disease. Epidemiology and trends in the United States, 1975–1981. JAMA 1984;251:2529.

51. Washington AE, Katz P. Cost of and payment source for pelvic inflammatory disease. Trends and projections, 1983 through 2000. JAMA 1991;266:2565.

52. Chaparro MV, Ghosh S, Nashed A, et al. Laparoscopy for confirmation and prognostic evaluation of pelvic inflammatory disease. Int J Gynecol Obstet 1978;15:307.

53. Westrom L. Effect of acute pelvic inflammatory disease on fertility. Am J Obstet Gynecol 1975;122:876.
54. Westrom L. Incidence, prevalence, and trends of acute pelvic inflammatory disease and its consequences in industrialized countries. Am J Obstet Gynecol 1980;138:880.
55. Viberg L. Acute inflammatory conditions of the uterine adnexa. Acta Obstet Gynecol Scand 1964;43:5.
56. Amer M, El-Garib I. Permethrin vs crotamiton and lindane in the treatment of scabies. Int J Dermatol 1992;31:357.

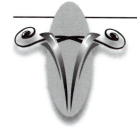

CHAPTER 8

Gynecologic Manifestations of Human Immunodeficiency Virus Infection

ANDREW W. HELFGOTT

As the number of people infected with human immunodeficiency virus (HIV) and afflicted with acquired immunodeficiency syndrome (AIDS) continues to grow worldwide, so too does the impact of these disease entities on health care systems. Current World Health Organization statistics estimate 30.7 million people to be affected by HIV or AIDS, with 1.8 million reported AIDS cases worldwide (1). From 1981 through June 1996, 612,078 cases of AIDS in patients older than 13 years were reported to the U.S. Centers for Disease Control and Prevention (CDC). Of these cases, 84% were adolescent and adult males, whereas 15% were adolescent and adult females. Thirty-six percent of these patients were Caucasian, 43% were African-American, and 20% were Hispanic. The year 1996 was a dubious milestone for African-Americans, since they became the leading race afflicted by the AIDS epidemic in the United States (2).

The CDC has received reports of 92,242 cases of AIDS in women since reporting first began (2). From 1991 to 1995, the number of women diagnosed with AIDS increased by 63%. This increase was greater than that seen with any other group of persons with AIDS (3). Although estimating the number of persons living with HIV infection or AIDS is difficult because of the differences in populations, estimates range from 650,000 to 900,000 for U.S. men, women, and children. Among women, the prevalence is thought to be 1 in 1000 (0.1%), and this is estimated to be a three-fold increase over the past 5 years (4). In 1996, women comprised 20% of adult cases of AIDS, with women 15 to 24 years old accounting for 7% of these and 25 to 44 years old accounting for 77%. In both age groups, the AIDS incidence rates increased faster through heterosexual contact than through intravenous drug abuse.

The incidence of AIDS cases reported to the CDC between 1991 and 1995 increased most rapidly in women infected through heterosexual contact. Heterosexual transmission accounted for 46% of cases in women in the Northeast, 52% in the Midwest, 58% in the South, and 50% in the West. This represents a change in the geographic distribution of HIV/AIDS, which initially affected the Northeastern states most severely (3).

AIDS has become a leading contributor to morbidity and mortality for women and is the third leading cause of death in women aged 25 to 44 years (5). When analyzed by race, HIV was the leading cause of death in African-American women aged 25 to 44 years in the United States in 1991 (6). African-American and Hispanic women continue to be significantly overrepresented in terms of AIDS cases. The HIV prevalence within the cultural and social networks combined with partner selection plays a role in the demographics of the HIV/AIDS epidemic. AIDS cases contracted through intravenous drug abuse are more common in men of African-American and Hispanic descent; thus, the sexual partners of these infected men are predicted to contract the virus at greater rates.

CLINICAL COURSE OF HIV/AIDS IN WOMEN

Little information exists in the literature to describe the complications of HIV infection or the disease course of HIV/AIDS in women. Small series of patients from metropolitan centers with high prevalence rates have been reported, but well-designed prospective studies have not as of yet. From the information currently available, it appears that the course of HIV infection in women mirrors that of men (7, 8). Overall, *Pneumocystis* pneumonia is the most common AIDS-defining illness for both men and women (9). Carpenter et al. (10) reported esophageal candidiasis as the most common AIDS-defining illness in his cohort of 200 women, but other larger studies did not support these findings (11, 12).

Regarding survival after an AIDS-defining illness, once again the data available are limited. Earlier studies reported survival advantages for men that ranged from slight (13, 14) to significant (15–17). More recently, reports of the opposite have been published (18–20). Unfortunately, there are many confounders that have an impact on the outcome of these studies, necessitating careful study. It is well known that women with HIV infection are diagnosed later in the course of their disease (21). Furthermore, HIV-infected women tend to access medical care less readily than HIV-infected men and thus do not receive standard antiretroviral therapy and antibiotic prophylaxis (17). These factors could significantly affect the survival rates of women, and if health care improves in these women, there may be no real difference in survival rates between the sexes. We await results from large multicenter studies on the course of HIV/AIDS.

In addition to the well-known morbidities associated with HIV infection and AIDS, women suffer the burden of gynecologic manifestations of the disease. These include abnormal cervical cytology, vaginal infections, pelvic inflammatory disease (PID), genital ulcer disease, and menstrual irregularities.

Clark et al. (11) reported on the clinical manifestations of HIV/AIDS in a cohort of women in Louisiana. The investigators retrospectively reviewed the charts of women followed at their center; the median duration of follow-up was 18 months. Of the 224 women evaluated, 17.5% had abnormal cervical cytology (cervical intraepithelial neoplasia [CIN]). Thirty-five percent had clinical evidence of a vulvovaginal candida infection or colonization with yeast. The occurrence of sexually transmitted diseases (STDs) was relatively impressive as well, with high infection rates for syphilis (22.2%), gonorrhea (7.2%), and chlamydia (12.3%). Evidence of PID was present in 5.3% of these women. Sixteen percent of the women had clinical evidence of genital infection with human papilloma virus (HPV), and 26.9% had trichomonal infections of the vagina (11). These authors also examined the occurrence of nongynecologic opportunistic infections in their cohort of women. *Pneumocystis carinii* pneumonia was the most common opportunistic infection in this group, followed by esophageal candidiasis and wasting syndrome. These findings were similar to that of men.

In a more recent study, women admitted to an AIDS inpatient medical service were offered a comprehensive gynecologic examination. Although very few women were admitted for gynecologic disease, 51% had vaginitis and 45% had cervical dysplasia. Twenty-three percent had evidence of genital HPV infection, and 20% had evidence of genital herpes. A diagnosis of PID was made in 5% of the women examined. Furthermore, the investigators found that the standardized checklist of gynecologic symptoms did not effectively predict gynecologic disease (22).

The authors concluded that although most women infected with HIV seek medical care for HIV-related illnesses, a very high percentage (80% in this study) of such women also require treatment for a concomitant gynecologic condition. The authors stressed that a thorough gynecologic examination should be performed in all HIV-infected women, because an absence of symptoms in the history is inadequate for ruling out gynecologic manifestations of HIV (22).

Given the growing impact of HIV infection and AIDS on women's health care, the primary care provider clearly needs to know when to screen for HIV infection. For patients who present to the clinic with a previously diagnosed HIV infection, the provider needs to have knowledge of an appropriate women's health maintenance schedule and the gynecologic conditions associated with HIV infection and AIDS.

SCREENING FOR HIV INFECTION

Although a great deal of information is available regarding the rationale for testing during pregnancy, no consensus exists regarding the recommendations for when to offer testing to the woman presenting for gynecologic care. Only offering HIV testing to patients with risk factors has, however, been notoriously inadequate. Routine testing in a low-risk population, however, is a potentially expensive and low-yield endeavor.

Women who present to their care provider for entities such as STDs, abnormal cervical cytology, substance abuse, or domestic violence are at substantial risk for HIV infection. Some advocate offering HIV testing to STD clinic patients because of the high comorbidity rate of HIV and other STDs (23). Others recommend offering testing to women with abnormal cervical cytology for the same reasons (24).

The screening and early identification of HIV-infected women is important because HIV infection is now considered a chronic illness with infected individuals doing well on combination antiretroviral therapy. Advances in therapeutic regimens have significantly increased the length of time that infected individuals survive. Early aggressive treatment for HIV-infected patients is justified by the scientific literature (25).

CARE OF THE HIV-INFECTED WOMAN

Unfortunately, the first reaction by health care providers to a woman with HIV infection is to refer her to an infectious disease specialist. Although the expertise of the infectious disease specialist in managing antiretroviral therapy combinations is invaluable, many gynecologic manifestations of AIDS are best managed by a primary care provider. Although becoming more rare, it is still not uncommon to see HIV-infected women receiving antiretroviral therapy but without adequate gynecologic care.

A description of the initial evaluation of a woman infected with HIV is shown in Table 8.1. A comprehensive patient history includes information about previous STD infections and abnormal cervical cytology smears. A full physical examination, including pelvic examination with samples for cytology and STD screening, is also necessary, and laboratory tests for indicators of disease progression and nutritional status are warranted. Social services should be consulted, and the physician should initiate a thorough patient education conversation about safer sexual practices, attempting to reduce the likelihood of further virus transmission.

TABLE 8.1. Initial Evaluation of the HIV-Infected Woman

Routine history, including history of other sexually transmitted diseases
Routine physical examination, including baseline Mini-Mental State Examination
Baseline laboratory evaluation
    Complete blood count with platelets
    Biochemistry screening profile (Chem-20)
    Urinalysis
    Tuberculin skin test without anergy panel
    T-lymphocyte subset analysis (CD4, CD8 counts)
    Toxoplasmosis serology (IgG, IgM)
    Hepatitis A, B, C serologies
    Quantitative polymerase chain reaction for HIV RNA (to measure viral load)
Patient education
    Evaluate baseline knowledge of disease
    Discuss management plan
    Educate regarding prevention of disease transmission
Social services referral
Infectious disease specialist referral

Physical Examination

Because there are many different manifestations of HIV infection, all organ systems need to be examined closely. The following review, although thorough, should not dictate the degree to which the provider may individualize the examination for each patient. Although the essential components of a comprehensive examination are described below, the recommended frequency of examinations is much more controversial.

The examination should begin with the patient's general appearance. Wasting syndrome is now considered a major sign of advanced disease and can be treated with combinations of nutritional supplements and pharmacologic treatment. Next, the physician should carefully examine the woman's skin for dermatoses that may be related to HIV infection or AIDS. Kaposi's sarcoma is rare in women but has been reported (26). The fundus of the eye should be examined for lesions associated with cytomegalovirus and toxoplasmosis. The throat and oral cavity can be the site of oral candidiasis, Kaposi's sarcoma, aphthous ulcers, and other oral manifestations of HIV, with subsequent referral to the dentist or other oral health care provider for appropriate management of any lesions found. The neck should be palpated for lymphadenopathy. Careful auscultation of the heart and lungs for evidence of cardiac or pulmonary manifestations of HIV is important. *P. carinii* pneumonia is the most common opportunistic infection in both men and women, and the incidence of tuberculosis has risen during the HIV epidemic. The breasts should be examined in the usual manner and the patient instructed on breast self-examinations. The abdomen should be examined for signs of HIV-related disease, including organomegaly. A cursory psychological/neurologic examination includes checking orientation (to time, person, and place), deep tendon reflexes, muscle tone and strength, and motor skills.

An approach to the yearly gynecologic examination of an HIV-infected woman is detailed in Table 8.2. The pelvic examination should include careful inspection of the external genitalia and perineum for lesions. Genital ulcer disease, HPV, her-

TABLE 8.2. Annual Gynecologic Examination for the HIV-Infected Woman

Breast examination	STD screens
Mammography (starting at age 40)	Gonorrhea
Pelvic examination	Chlamydia
Bimanual	Syphilis
Pap smear[a]	Wet mount of vaginal swab
	Candidiasis
	Bacterial vaginosis
	Trichomoniasis

[a]Some authorities believe a Pap smear should be done every 6 months in more severely immunocompromised women (CD4 < 200/mm³). See Table 8.3 for an approach to the HIV-infected woman with an abnormal Pap smear.

pes simplex virus, and other lesions have all been described in this patient population. Next, a speculum examination is performed, again with careful inspection of the vagina (including the vaginal walls) for the presence of any lesions. The entire vaginal vault and cervix needs to be examined for any evidence of herpes, HPV, candida, or other infection. The Papanicolaou (Pap) smear should be performed, and specimens for gonorrhea and chlamydia collected. If symptoms warrant, wet prep and potassium hydroxide specimens should also be collected for identifying bacterial vaginosis, trichomoniasis, and vaginal candidiasis. The bimanual examination should pay special attention to cervical motion tenderness and masses, because PID and tubo-ovarian abscesses are commonly seen in HIV-infected women (27, 28). A thorough discussion of the diagnosis and management of gynecologic manifestations of HIV/AIDS appears in a section below.

Laboratory Testing

Although most providers of women's health care do not usually evaluate the immunologic status of their patients, some baseline laboratory tests should nonetheless be ordered and the results shared with the AIDS or infectious disease specialist. The advantages to ordering these tests early in the primary care evaluation include convenience to the patient and more timely information for the infectious disease consultant. In the instance of severe immunocompromise, earlier diagnosis may shorten the delay to starting antiretrovirals and prophylactic antibiotics.

A routine complete blood count with platelet count is in order. Specific evaluation of the immune system is accomplished with T-lymphocyte subset analysis. A quantitative analysis of HIV RNA by polymerase chain reaction provides assessment of the degree of HIV infection. This may significantly influence the initiation of anti-HIV therapy. Serologies for toxoplasmosis and hepatitis viruses (A, B, and C) are warranted, whereas cytomegalovirus and herpes simplex virus antibody testing is of little value. A routine urinalysis should be performed. The association of HIV infection with tuberculosis infection warrants placement of a tuberculin skin test (preferably a purified protein derivative or Mantoux test). The placement of an anergy panel with the tuberculin test is no longer recommended by the CDC (29).

On pelvic examination, patients should be tested for gonorrhea and chlamydia, and any abnormal lesions should be cultured for herpes simplex virus or other pathogens. There is no clear consensus on the schedule for obtaining the Pap smear in HIV-infected women. The 1993 CDC guidelines recommended an initial Pap should be done upon the diagnosis of HIV (30). If that test is normal, another Pap should be repeated within 6 months. If that test is normal, the woman can revert to yearly Pap smears, although some experts advocate follow-up every 6 months. Table 8.3 reviews an approach to the abnormal Pap smear result in this patient population. A smear that reveals inflammation or reactive atypia should be treated and repeated in 3 months. Any patient with atypical specimen cells of uncertain significance or squamous intraepithelial lesions (low or high grade) should undergo colposcopy.

Unfortunately, the 1993 CDC guidelines regarding Pap smears overlook many important issues (e.g., poor patient compliance and problems with Pap smears predicting cervical lesions in this patient population). Presently, a multitude of different protocols are followed for frequency of Pap smears and initiation of colposcopic evaluation in HIV-infected women. A safe, although perhaps overly cautious, approach is baseline colposcopic evaluation for all HIV-infected women and appropriate follow-up based on findings (31) *or* routine twice-annual Pap smear screening (32).

Patient Counseling

At the conclusion of the physical examination, it is important to spend time educating the patient. There are three main issues on which to focus. First, the importance of seeking health care and continuing gynecologic follow-up should be stressed. Part of this process includes explaining the plan of management for her HIV, including referral to an HIV specialist in addition to regular gynecologic visits.

The next goal is to improve the patient's knowledge of HIV and its transmission. This should lead to a discussion about methods to reduce spread to an uninfected partner(s). Safer sexual practice methods must be discussed in detail with extensive questioning and role playing to ensure patient comprehension and hopefully improve compliance.

Finally, the patient must be made aware of the enormous psychosocial implications of HIV/AIDS. Information about resources such as social workers, support groups, and health care providers specializing in HIV care must be made available to the patient at that first visit to facilitate her receiving adequate long-term care for her disease. These resources are discussed further in the next section.

Social Work Referral

A referral to a social service agency to access optimal care is imperative. In caring for women who are HIV infected, there are a number of socioeconomic issues that must be considered and addressed to provide optimal care. Case management, health education, substance abuse services, child care, support groups, and legal services are just some of the important resources to which HIV-infected women need ready access.

Most HIV-infected women are of African-American or Hispanic descent. Most live in the large metropolitan areas in households with low incomes (33). A significant number report drug use, although not necessarily intravenous. Many of these women rely on public assistance and may lack acceptable housing for their families (34, 35). The public health care system itself can contribute to the isolation and

TABLE 8.3. Approach to Abnormal Pap Smear Findings in HIV-Infected Women

Infection or inflammation	Treat; repeat Pap smear in 3 mo
Atypical squamous cells of undetermined significance	Colposcopy
Squamous intraepithelial lesions (low or high grade)	Colposcopy

alienation that HIV-infected women experience. Because the early years of the AIDS epidemic predominantly affected gay men, the original HIV/AIDS organizations and care facilities were oriented toward providing service to that population. These clinics are often inadequately prepared to deal with the health problems of women and children (36).

The diagnosis of HIV infection is itself stigmatizing, further isolating the patient. This isolation and fear of loss of autonomy with increased dependence on a social services system that may have failed them in the past are some reasons that women refuse to divulge their HIV status and seek care for their HIV infection (34, 37, 38). If a partner or her children are also infected, the emotional toll on the patient is obviously compounded. Given these circumstances, it becomes apparent why some women consider their HIV infection the least of their problems (34, 37–39).

GYNECOLOGIC HEALTH ISSUES IN THE HIV-INFECTED WOMAN

In 1993, the CDC revised the definition and surveillance criteria for HIV and AIDS to include certain gynecologic manifestations as markers for the progression of women from HIV infection to full-blown AIDS (40). Table 8.4 details the CDC clas-

TABLE 8.4. Classification System of HIV Disease

CD4 Count	A	B	C
>500	A1	B1	C1
200–500	A2	B2	C2
<200	A3	B3	C3

CATEGORY A
Asymptomatic HIV infection
Persistent generalized lymphadenopathy
Acute retroviral syndrome

CATEGORY B (FORMERLY "ARC")

Bacillary angiomatosis	Hairy leukoplakia (oral)
Candidiasis	Herpes zoster
(oral or recurrent vaginal)	Idiopathic thrombocytopenic purpura
Cervical dysplasia	Listeriosis
Constitutional symptoms	Pelvic inflammatory disease
(e.g., fever or diarrhea) for >1 mo	Peripheral neuropathy

CATEGORY C (AIDS-DEFINING CONDITIONS)

CD4 count	Cytomegalovirus	*Mycobacterium avium*
< 200 cells/mm³	Encephalopathy (HIV)	*Mycobacterium kansasii*
Candidiasis (pulmonary	Herpes simplex	*Mycobacterium*
or esophageal)	(chronic or	*tuberculosis*
Cervical cancer	esophageal)	*Pneumocystis carinii*
Coccidioidomycosis	Histoplasmosis	Pneumonia (recurrent)
Cryptococcosis	Isosporiasis	Progressive multifocal
(extrapulmonary)	Kaposi's sarcoma	leukemia
Cryptosporidiosis	Lymphoma	Salmonellosis

From Centers for Disease Control and Prevention. 1993 Revised classification systems for HIV infection and expanded surveillance case definitions for AIDS among adolescents and adults. MMWR Morb Mortal Wkly Rep 1993;41(RR-17):1–19.

sification system. Women presenting with diseases such as recurrent or difficult-to-treat vulvovaginal candidiasis, abnormal cervical cytology such as CIN, and multiple episodes of PID are now classified as CDC class B. Furthermore, invasive cervical cancer (ICC) was included in the CDC stage C list of AIDS-defining illnesses. These changes in CDC classifications acknowledge the impact of gynecologic manifestations on AIDS progression.

Contraception and Prevention of Disease Transmission

Current literature supports the idea that the risk of acquiring HIV infection through heterosexual transmission is greater for women than men (41). Multiple factors support this, including the larger surface area of vaginal mucosa exposed to viral secretions and the greater time of exposure to infectious fluids both during and after the sexual act (42). Physiologic factors may play a role in the heterosexual transmission of HIV as well. It is thought that the acidic pH of the vagina may be virucidal, decreasing the risk of transmission from women to men (43). Although vaginal mucosal trauma is often quoted as another factor that enhances transmission from men to women, this microtrauma is not a prerequisite because there are reports of transmission of HIV-1 virus to women artificially inseminated by infected semen donors (44).

Unprotected intercourse not only places women at risk for HIV infection but has the additional risks of unplanned pregnancies and infection with other STDs. Thus, for the physician providing care to HIV-infected women and women at risk for HIV infection, contraception for family planning and prevention of STDs is of paramount importance. Unfortunately, what prevents conception may not necessarily prevent HIV transmission, and the most effective means of preventing HIV infection is not necessarily the ideal contraceptive method. Any discussion of contraception must take into account the duality of the issue: prevention of conception and prevention of HIV and other STD transmission.

In evaluating and prescribing a contraceptive method, the care provider must consider its effectiveness, side effects, contraindications, convenience of use, and cost. These issues are of importance regardless of the woman's HIV status and are discussed further in Chapter 3. With the HIV-infected woman, potential for preventing HIV transmission, impact on disease progression, and drug interactions with anti-HIV therapies must also be considered.

Barrier Methods

Condoms have become a mainstay in preventing the heterosexual transmission of HIV and other STDs. Latex condoms must be used because animal skin condoms do not provide adequate protection from HIV transmission. Condoms act as a physical barrier in protecting the vagina and anus from infectious secretions. Despite highly publicized efforts to promote condoms for prevention of transmission of HIV and other STDs, women continue to be unaware of these benefits or, in some cases, choose to not use them. Condoms have been shown to effectively prevent the spread of many STDs, including herpes, hepatitis B, chlamydia, gonorrhea, and cytomegalovirus (45–47) and have been proven effective against transmission of HIV-1 in vitro (48, 49). Other investigators showed the efficacy of condoms in the prevention of HIV in vivo as well. Data from the European Study Group (and other published studies) reveal no seroconversion to HIV-1 among couples who report using condoms on a consistent basis (50). Study patients who used condoms on a less consistent basis had seroconversion rates of 10 to 18% (50–53). There was significant reduction in the risk of HIV-1 seroconversion (up to 90%) when condoms were used consistently and correctly.

Kamenga et al. (54), reporting from Zaire, demonstrated an HIV-1 transmission rate of only 4% in a cohort of prostitutes with consistent condom use. In the control group, where condom use was less consistent, the transmission rate approached 20%. Among women in the cohort who did seroconvert despite condom use, cases of pregnancy, urethritis, and instances of condom breakage were reported. In 1995, Kissinger et al. (55) reported that despite intensive educational efforts in a cohort of HIV-infected women, there was a low rate of condom usage and a high incidence of STDs. Among those women reporting regular condom use, 21% had an episode of STD infection. It is thought that even with attempts at consistent use, mechanical, educational, and behavioral factors have a significant impact on use of the condom to prevent HIV transmission.

Despite these potential shortcomings, the consistent and correct use of latex condoms is effective in the prevention of HIV transmission. Inconsistent condom use results in unwanted pregnancies, acquisition of STDs, and heterosexual transmission of HIV. Younger minority women of poor socioeconomic status tend to experience more failures when using condoms. This is, unfortunately, the same population at highest risk for HIV infection.

Barrier methods other than condoms, including the diaphragm, vaginal contraceptive sponge, and female condom, have also been recommended for women. Although both the vaginal sponge and diaphragm are effective in providing contraception and protection against STDs, concerns exist regarding their ability to prevent heterosexual transmission of HIV. The diaphragm provides poor protection from HIV-1 infection because it only covers the cervix, leaving the lower vagina exposed to potentially contaminated semen and other secretions. Seroconversion after only vaginal exposure to infectious secretions has been demonstrated in laboratory animals and in humans. Cervical ascension of the virus into the endometrium is thus *not* essential for HIV-1 transmission and infection (56). Other concerns exist regarding the sponge and diaphragm methods as effective agents in HIV prevention. Both require significant effort on the part of the user for each sexual act, and abrasions caused by their placement may cause disruption in the vaginal epithelium and may serve to enhance susceptibility to HIV.

The female, or vaginal, condom is a relatively new development in the efforts to prevent transmission of STDs. There are significant concerns regarding its potential for improper insertion and use. In addition, they are expensive, and this makes them relatively inaccessible to the population most at risk. The female condom has been shown to be effective in preventing pregnancy and STDs (57).

The female condom has been shown to prevent the transmission of HIV-1 and other viruses in vitro (57, 58), but its ability to prevent HIV-1 transmission in vivo has not been evaluated. Because of this uncertainty, the female condom alone should not be actively promoted for prevention of HIV transmission. Also, its efficacy in preventing other STDs and pregnancy is, as with traditional latex condoms, directly related to the consistency of proper use.

In summary, couples who use latex condoms consistently and correctly can expect significant protection from the transmission of HIV-1 and other STDs. The lack of information about other barrier methods for the prevention of HIV-1 transmission makes the diaphragm and female condom less preferable.

Oral Contraceptive Pills

Oral contraceptive pills (OCPs) have been proven effective for both prevention of pregnancy and reduction of severity of PID (59). OCPs are the most commonly used means of contraception, and major side effects are rare. There are three major concerns about the use of OCPs in HIV-infected women: impact on the immune system, effect on HIV transmission, and interactions with anti-HIV medications.

There is significant evidence that the sex steroids in contraceptive pills can alter both systemic and local (mucosal) immunity. Estrogen can inhibit cell-mediated responses to various stimuli. It has been shown to decrease levels of immunoglobulins in cervical and vaginal secretions by direct suppression of mucosal plasma cell immunoglobulin production (60). Progesterone also has an inhibitory effect on the immune system, suppressing antibody production. In the pregnant state, with significantly elevated progesterone levels, women have a decreased immune response to various pathogens as well (61).

Measurements of cervical mucus immunoglobulin concentrations have been demonstrated to be lowest at time of ovulation, measuring at levels less than 10% of those before ovulation; they elevate soon after ovulation (62). Women using OCPs have antibody concentrations in cervical mucus that remain lower throughout the menstrual cycle than those not using OCPs. A rise in the antibody concentrations tends to occur during the 7 days of the cycle not influenced by oral contraceptives (i.e., when the patient either takes no pill or placebos).

The local absorption of antigens is also influenced by sex steroid hormones. Studies in mice reveal that the permeability of the vagina to antigens is significantly affected by changes in serum concentrations of estrogen and progesterone (63). This is manifested by a decrease in cellular immunity, specifically a decrease in T-lymphocyte and macrophage activity.

Given the above information, it is possible that the use of OCPs may affect susceptibility to HIV infection and progression of disease in infected women. Unfortunately, there are no data to address this question, and investigation is warranted. These theoretic concerns, however, do not preclude use of OCPs in HIV-infected women.

The data regarding the impact of oral contraceptive use on HIV transmission are mixed. Most studies that address this issue are retrospective and cross-sectional in design, limiting their usefulness. Studies that found an association between OCP use and HIV transmission are confounded by patients' high-risk sexual activity and study design (64, 65).

There are physiologic adaptations that occur with OCP use, including cervical ectopy and changes in the amounts of cervical mucus. Theoretically, the decrease in menstrual flow usually seen with OCP use lessens the exposure of denuded endometrium to infectious fluids during and after a sexual act. For the male partner of an HIV-infected women, decreased menstrual flow should decrease their exposure to infectious fluids. Thus, oral contraceptive use might decrease the risk of transmission of HIV, but this remains to be proven.

Finally, there is significant concern about the interaction of OCPs with drugs commonly used in HIV-infected women. Use of some antiseizure medications or antibiotics decreases efficacy of OCPs in preventing contraception (66). This may also be true of antiretroviral medications, which are metabolized in the liver. The effect of protease inhibitors on the pharmacokinetics of oral contraceptive or vice versa warrants careful investigation. It appears that protease inhibitors, specifically ritonavir (Norvir), decreases estradiol levels in women taking OCPs (67).

Spermicides and Microbicides
During the past 15 years, use of spermicides and other microbicides has been advocated for prevention of HIV and other STD transmission. Spermicides consist of two

components: the actual spermicide agent and the base or carrier in which the agent is carried. The only agents available in the United States are nonoxynol-9 and octoxynol. These are surfactants that destroy the sperm cell membrane.

Spermicides are relatively easy to use and require little planning before use. Free from systemic side effects, they are available without a prescription and are relatively inexpensive. Evidence for an in vitro effect of nonoxynol-9 on gonorrhea and other bacterial infections of the vagina exists in the literature, but it has a lesser effect on preventing chlamydia infection (68) and has been found ineffective in preventing vaginal candidiasis (69).

By preventing the spread of STDs, nonoxynol-9 can indirectly affect HIV transmission. A 0.05% concentration has also been shown to inactivate the HIV-1 virus directly within 60 seconds of contact in vivo (70, 71).

Miller et al. (72) used nonoxynol-9 in six macaques that were subsequently exposed to simian immunodeficiency virus. Spermicide use prevented seroconversion in three animals exposed. Zekeng et al. (73) examined the relationship between condom and spermicide use and HIV-1 transmission in female sex workers in Cameroon. The HIV transmission rate was 0.1 (95% confidence interval [CI], 0.1 to 0.6). This report was actually the first epidemiologic evidence to support the use of nonoxynol-9 to reduce HIV transmission.

Unfortunately, the relationship between nonoxynol-9 and prevention of HIV-1 is not without controversy. Kreiss et al. (74) examined prostitutes in Nairobi who reported spermicide use. In this study, 45% (27/60) of the participants who reported using a contraceptive sponge permeated with nonoxynol-9 seroconverted to HIV-positive status. The seroconversion rate in the placebo group was only 3.6% (20/56). Confounders to the association between HIV transmission and spermicide use include significantly higher exposure rates to the nonoxynol-9 (with some participants using 14 sponges per day) and lack of means to quantify the epithelial trauma caused by frequent sponge changing. Kreiss et al.'s results thus might not be applicable to persons using the sponge less frequently.

Reports of colposcopically visible epithelial disruption of the vaginas of nonoxynol-9 users have been present in the literature for some time (75). Nonoxynol-9 contains high levels of peroxides, and it is postulated that when the spermicide is used frequently, these compounds cause vaginal tissue irritation and epithelial damage. Such damage to the vaginal epithelium may be a factor in increasing susceptibility to HIV-1 (75–77).

Currently, most lubricated condoms have nonoxynol-9 as the active spermicidal ingredient, although there is no evidence suggesting the nonoxynol-9 prevents HIV transmission better than condoms alone. There are also no scientific data to support the routine use of additional spermicide for the prevention of HIV, but use of additional spermicide (or some other contraceptive method) is warranted for improving efficacy in prevention of pregnancy and STDs. The current CDC recommendations for prevention of HIV-1 transmission are for consistent and correct use of latex condoms with or without a spermicide (57).

Intrauterine Device

The intrauterine device (IUD) has long been associated with PID and its attendant complications. Although it is an effective contraceptive agent with excellent compliance, the IUD is probably not an ideal contraceptive agent for HIV-infected women because it is thought to be associated with endometrial trauma at the time of insertion (78). The heavier menstrual flow seen with copper IUDs may increase the risk of transmitting HIV to the woman's partner.

Progestational Agents

Progestin implants for contraception have been available for some time. Levonorgestrel is the progestational agent in silastic capsules that are implanted in the woman's arm (Norplant). Generally well tolerated, the implants are left in place and remain as active contraceptive agents for up to 5 years.

In addition to the fact that the implants provide little protection from STDs, Norplant has been associated with heavy and prolonged menstrual bleeding. This bleeding has also been described as irregular. Although these complications are usually self-limiting and easily treated, they cause concerns in the HIV-infected woman.

Progesterone has been shown to induce changes in vaginal pH. It also has been associated with changes in the vaginal epithelium itself, indirectly causing a thinning of the epithelium. Finally, it has been demonstrated that progesterone has a role in changing the consistency of the cervical mucus (79). These physiologic effects of progesterone on the vagina cause further concern about use of a progestational agent and risk of enhanced transmission of HIV. These concerns are for both the uninfected woman who may be more susceptible to HIV from an infected partner and for the sexual partner of an infected woman who may be at increased transmission risk from prolonged and irregular menstrual bleeding.

Up until recently many of these concerns were theoretic, based more on supposition than scientific fact. Marx et al. (80) recently reported their experience with progesterone implants and simian immunodeficiency virus in macaques. Eighteen animals had the progesterone implants inserted, and the 10 controls received placebo implants. Both groups were inoculated intravaginally with simian immunodeficiency virus. The investigators found that the macaques with the progesterone implants had thinning of the vaginal epithelium and an increased rate of simian immunodeficiency virus transmission compared with the placebo group, and the treatment group tended to have significantly higher plasma levels of viral DNA compared with the infected placebo animals. Finally, several of the simian immunodeficiency virus-infected macaques in the progesterone group experienced more rapid progression of their disease.

Despite this study, very little is actually known about the impact of this commonly used method of contraception on the transmission or disease course of HIV in women. The work of Marx et al. is preliminary and involves monkeys and simian immunodeficiency virus. Furthermore, preliminary investigations in humans do not reveal similar findings (81). Additional research is required before definitive statements can be made on the use of progestational agents in HIV-infected women.

Abnormal Cervical Cytology

Among the criteria specific to women addressed in the 1993 CDC HIV classification revisions were the additions of CIN and cervical dysplasia (both moderate and severe) to category B (diseases caused by or complicated by HIV infection). ICC was classified as category C (an AIDS-defining illness; Table 8.4) (40).

The high prevalence of CIN in HIV-positive women makes it an extremely important issue when considering the medical management of HIV-infected women. Unfortunately, not enough is known about the epidemiology or etiology of CIN in this population. A lack of consensus on the optimal screening schedule in this population and methods of screening and follow-up have contributed to the debate.

An association between immunosuppression and abnormal cervical cytology was established by Sillman and Sedlis (82), who identified an increased prevalence of HPV-related lesions and abnormal cervical dysplasia in a cohort of women who were immunosuppressed from long-term steroid therapy or transplant rejection prophylaxis. Since then, many authors described an association between HIV infection and increased prevalence of CIN. Maiman et al. (24) reported in 1990 that up to 10% of the women in his colposcopy clinic were HIV positive, and Shafer et al. (83) reported that HIV-infected women had a 4- to 10-fold increased risk for CIN compared with HIV-negative control subjects. Several other authors corroborated the association of HIV infection with a higher prevalence of CIN and an increased rate of HPV infection (84).

Many early studies describing the association of the development of CIN in HIV-infected women were dismissed summarily for lack of control groups, problems with study design, and failure to control confounding variables (85). Subsequently, many better-designed studies managed to meet some of the control standards and did corroborate the earlier reports of an association between HIV infection and the development of CIN (86–88). In a widely accepted publication, Wright et al. (88) reported on 303 HIV-infected women with a prevalence of CIN of 21%. In their cohort, as the women became increasingly immunosuppressed, the prevalence of CIN increased to 29% in women with CD4 cell counts less than $200/mm^3$ (compared with 17% in women with CD4 counts greater than $500/mm^3$; $P < .05$). The author concluded that HIV infection itself (odds ratio, 3.5) and CD4 counts (odds ratio, 2.7) were independently associated with the development of CIN.

Although an association between HIV infection and cervical neoplasia certainly exists, the actual relationship is difficult to describe. There is no single agent or behavior associated with the development of CIN; its etiology is multifactorial. Many risk factors for HIV infection, such as early intercourse, multiple partners, HPV infection, and substance abuse, are also associated with the development of CIN. The increased prevalence of HPV combined with the risk-taking behaviors seen in HIV-infected populations seem to account, at least in part, for the increased prevalence of CIN in HIV-infected women.

It appears that other factors are involved as well. The association of prevalence and severity of CIN with the individual degree to which patients are immunosuppressed (as manifested by declining CD4 counts) has been well documented (83, 89). Local changes in the immune response of the cervix in the presence of HIV infection also appear to play a role. The depletion of Langerhans cells in the cervical mucus of HIV-infected women has been documented (90), and it has been hypothesized that in the presence of HPV infection, depletion of Langerhans cells may facilitate the development of CIN. This relationship between decreased Langerhans cells in the cervical mucus and the demonstration of an abnormality in the CD4:CD8 ratio of cervical lymphocytes before the development of systemic immunosuppression supports the theory of a local immunosuppressive effect of HIV as a major role player in the development of CIN in this patient population (91).

Factors other than immunosuppression have also been implicated in the development of CIN in HIV-infected women. Reports of higher rates of CIN in HIV-infected intravenous drug abusers compared with women contracting HIV by heterosexual transmission (58% versus 23%; odds ratio, 2.2; 95% CI, 1.2 to 3.8) indicate that intravenous drug abuse may compound the immunosuppressed state. Furthermore, the lifestyle of drug-abusing women (e.g., multiple sex partners, smoking, HPV infection) may progressively increase their risk for development of CIN (92, 93).

Screening

A great deal of the debate regarding CIN in the presence of HIV infection revolves around screening methods, screening intervals, and management of screening results. The issue first came to the forefront when Maiman et al. (94) reported on the poor correlation of cervical cytology obtained by Pap smear with histology obtained by colposcopic biopsy. In this report, 32 HIV-infected women underwent Pap smear examinations and colposcopy with biopsies taken. Thirteen (41%) of the patients had evidence of CIN on the colposcopic biopsy, yet only one of the cytology smears revealed CIN. The sensitivity was unacceptably low (8%), leading the authors to conclude that there was a high rate of false-negative Pap smears among HIV-infected women. The investigators cautioned health care providers about the need for colposcopic biopsy of suspicious lesions for all HIV-infected women. The authors strongly believed that routine colposcopic examination done in conjunction with Pap smears should be the primary screening method for CIN among this patient population.

This report was soundly criticized because it had no HIV-negative control group and the degree of immunosuppression was not measured. It nevertheless provoked a great deal of debate. Many authors subsequently examined the sensitivity of Pap smears compared with colposcopic biopsy (88, 95). In the largest of these, Wright et al. (88) performed a cross-sectional study of 398 HIV-infected women and 352 HIV-negative control subjects. The sensitivity of the Pap smear was 81%, with a specificity of 87%. The authors concluded that Pap smear screening alone *is* sufficient to detect CIN in HIV-infected women.

Unfortunately, this did not resolve this troublesome issue. Multiple authors found problems with the use of Pap smear screening alone for the detection of CIN in this population. Olaitan et al. (96) found a false-negative rate of 14% using cervical cytology alone to detect CIN. Fink et al. (97) also determined that cervical screening by cytology was limited by a high false-negative rate. Both authors supported the use of annual cervical cytology and colposcopic screening with biopsy of any suspicious lesions.

There are many factors that must be evaluated in examining the issue and making a decision between Pap smear and colposcopic examination in this patient population. The population of women in the studies, operator training and skill in obtaining the Pap smear, and level of expertise of cytopathologists all may have an impact on the results. Although some would argue that colposcopy is invasive and too costly to do routinely on HIV-infected women, others would contend that, in the appropriate hands, the procedure causes minimal discomfort and should be used routinely. Given the high prevalence of cervical and vulvar dysplasias in HIV-infected women and major problems with compliance, some experts argue that colposcopy as a screening tool can indeed be justified.

Unfortunately, no clear consensus on screening is available. The CDC guidelines recommend annual screening for CIN using Pap smears (40). Individualization of the screening protocol for the patient population served may be best. It is easy to recommend colposcopy for all HIV-infected women, but if equipment or training are lacking, these recommendations are not realistic.

Treatment

Many current standard therapies for the treatment of CIN have been used in the treatment of HIV-positive women. It appears that regardless of the method used, the outcomes are less than satisfactory. Of all treatment modalities, cryotherapy is the least desirable because it could potentially obscure a lesion. Maiman et al. (98) demonstrated that using cryotherapy as a primary treatment plan resulted in a 48% recurrence rate in the HIV-positive population, compared with only 1% in HIV-negative women. The loop electrosurgical excision procedure (LEEP) also had a high failure rate. Wright et al. (99) found that loop excision failed in 60% of HIV-infected women, compared with 13% in the control group (odds ratio, 10.5; $P < .0001$).

Cuthill et al. (100) examined the complications encountered in treating CIN in HIV-infected women. Fifteen HIV-infected women with CIN treated by laser, cone biopsy, or cryotherapy were compared with 44 HIV-negative control subjects. Eleven percent of the HIV-infected women had excessive bleeding compared with only 1% of the HIV-negative women (odds ratio, 11.3; $P = .02$). After treatment, 53% of the HIV-positive group developed an infectious complication (versus 18% in control subjects; $P < 0.002$). The authors concluded that HIV-infected women were more vulnerable to complications after treatment for CIN and should be monitored closely.

No consensus for the best method for treating CIN in HIV-infected women exists. Maiman (31) recommends close surveillance and repetitive treatment when and where needed. Among the recommendations made are

- Excisional therapy (cone biopsy, laser cone, or LEEP cone) instead of ablative therapy (cryotherapy), so that the biopsy specimen can be reviewed for margins
- Diagnostic procedures for the usual indications, for example, diagnostic cone biopsy for failure to visualize the transformation zone completely
- Diligent and conscientious follow-up with colposcopy as required after definitive therapeutic measures have been taken
- Aggressive treatment of recurrences or persistent lesions as needed to eradicate the disease

Follow-up

The course of CIN in HIV-infected women has been described as more aggressive, with more rapid progression of disease and frequent recurrence. Fruchter et al. (101) reported a 39% recurrence rate of CIN after appropriate therapy, compared with 9% in HIV-negative control subjects. In this cohort, patients who were more immunosuppressed suffered more frequent recurrence (18% with CD4 greater than $500/mm^3$, 45% with CD4 less than $500/mm^3$). This group also described multiple recurrences of CIN in HIV-positive women; 62% of patients developed recurrent CIN by 36 months follow-up compared with only 18% in the HIV-negative control group. These recurrences were predicted by low CD4 counts. The authors caution care providers of the multiple recurrences of CIN—up to three recurrences despite acceptable therapies.

One suggested protocol follows women who have atypical squamous cells of undetermined significance or low-grade squamous intraepithelial lesions with colposcopy at the time of cytologic diagnosis and again in 6 months. Treatment is warranted for any evidence of disease progression. Higher grade squamous intraepithelial lesions or carcinoma in situ are treated immediately upon diagnosis and receive frequent follow-up for recurrence or progression. The authors proposing this protocol believe that once a tissue diagnosis is obtained on biopsy, expectant management with follow-up is acceptable (91). Of course, this type of approach requires patient compliance with follow-up appointments.

In following the HIV-infected woman for HPV-associated lesions, the entire lower genital tract needs to be evaluated for the presence of suspicious lesions, specifically intraepithelial neoplasias. Among the lesions that have to be ruled out are vaginal intraepithelial neoplasia, vulvar intraepithelial neoplasia, and anal intraepithelial neoplasia. These lesions have all been described in this patient population. Korn et al. (102) reported 15% of women with CIN had concomitant vulvar intraepithelial neoplasia. Williams et al. (103) described anal intraepithelial neoplasia in 14% of the 144 women in the cohort examined. Of the patients with CIN, 44% had evidence of abnormal anal cytology. Thus, it is important to pay close attention to the entire lower genital tract when performing a pelvic examination or colposcopy on the HIV-infected woman. If any lesions or suspicious areas are found, colposcopy and/or colposcopic biopsies must be performed, and consequent treatment should be aggressive with diligent follow-up.

Invasive Cervical Cancer

With the increasing prevalence of HIV/AIDS in women and the common occurrence of CIN in that patient population, one would expect the incidence of invasive cervical cancer (ICC) to increase as well. This trend has not been seen to date. Many factors may account for this: limited access of HIV-infected women to health care, lack of gynecologic care providers to women at many HIV care sites, and sensitivity limitation of Pap smears. Because of delay in seeking health care, it is not uncommon for the presenting illness of women to be an opportunistic infection. Failure to provide a thorough gynecologic examination at the time of presentation would lead to an underdiagnosis of ICC in this population.

Klevens et al. (104) examined 16,794 women diagnosed with AIDS in 1993 and examined the characteristics of the 217 (1.3%) who were diagnosed with ICC. The women with ICC were younger, more likely to be African-American, and more likely to live in the southern states. They were also more likely to be intravenous drug abusers. Overall, Hispanics were 0.6 times less likely to be reported with ICC ($P <$ .01). Of the intravenous drug-abusing patients, African-Americans were 0.5 times less likely to be diagnosed with ICC ($P < .001$). These findings were attributed to the many factors that limit access to care for minority patient populations.

Although abnormal cervical cytology remains a problem requiring a great deal of follow-up, it does not appear to contribute significantly to mortality in HIV-infected women. This is not true of ICC in this population. It appears that cervical cancer is much more aggressive in the HIV-infected woman, and patients tend to present with more advanced and metastatic disease. Maiman et al.'s (105) report of an HIV-infected 16-year-old with stage IIIB cervical cancer who expired from her cancer shortly after her 17th birthday attests to the aggressive nature of the disease in this patient population. Another study from the same group compared 16 HIV-positive women with ICC with 68 HIV-negative women with ICC. The HIV-positive group had more advanced disease (stages III and IV) compared with the seronegative group (50% versus 18%). The tumors tended to be of a higher grade and had more lymph node involvement in the HIV-positive group. Most patients had squamous cell cancer and tended to expire from cancer-related entities rather than HIV/AIDS. As with CIN, there appears to be a relationship between the degree of immunosuppression and the course of disease, with more severely immunocompromised women doing more poorly.

The methods for treating the HIV-infected patient with ICC are beyond the scope of this review. Patients should not have their ICC neglected simply because they are HIV positive. The prognosis is significantly influenced by immune function, and most of these women succumb to ICC before other HIV/AIDS-related illness.

Vaginal Infections

Vulvovaginitis in the nonimmunocompromised patient is reviewed in Chapter 6. Cases of recurrent recalcitrant vulvovaginal candidiasis in women subsequently found to be HIV infected have been reported. In 1987, Rhoades et al. (106) described chronic vulvovaginal candidiasis as a presenting complaint prompting investigation of HIV status. The patients were severely immunocompromised and had concomitant oral candidiasis at diagnosis. The authors concluded that chronic vulvovaginal candidiasis is an important marker for HIV infection.

Iman et al. (107) examined the hierarchical patterns of mucosal candidiasis infection in HIV-seropositive women. Their report described an increased incidence and prevalence of vaginal candidiasis in HIV-positive women, even before reduction in CD4 counts. The likelihood of oral and esophageal candidiasis occurring increased as the immune system became progressively more compromised.

It would make sense that immunocompromised women would have a weakened cellular and mucosal immunity, thus placing them at risk for vaginal infection. In 1993, the CDC revised its classifications to include recurrent vulvovaginitis as an opportunistic infection (Table 8.4) (40). The original articles describing recurrent vulvovaginal candidiasis were, unfortunately, fraught with problems and have been roundly criticized (108). Strict definition of recurrent vulvovaginal candidiasis requires at least four microbiologically proven episodes of acute vulvovaginal candidiasis within a 12-month period in the absence of any other courses of vaginal symptomatology, including bacterial vaginosis, trichomoniasis, and other entities (109), and none of the early studies established the diagnosis of recurrent vulvovaginal candidiasis using these definitions. Concerns regarding these findings stimulated well-designed, prospective, controlled trials to examine vulvovaginal candidiasis in HIV-infected women.

LeRoy et al. (110) examined the prevalence and evidence of genital infections and their association with HIV-1 infection in third-trimester pregnant women compared with noninfected control subjects in Kigali, Rwanda. The HIV-infected group had a significantly higher incidence of *Trichomonas* vaginitis (20.2% versus 10.9%, $P = .007$) but only a slightly higher incidence of candida vaginitis (22.3% versus 20.1%).

Spinillo et al. (111) collected vaginal, rectal, and oral cultures for *Candida* species from 84 HIV-positive and 384 HIV-negative women attending an STD clinic in Italy. Overall, the prevalence of vaginal candidiasis was increased in the HIV-positive group (62% versus 32%, $P < .001$). The interval to recurrent vulvovaginal fungal infection was shorter in the HIV-infected group. Patients with full-blown AIDS and/or symptomatic HIV infection tended to have a higher prevalence of candida vaginal infection than women with asymptomatic disease, although the results were not statistically significant.

In a follow-up report, the various species of yeast were identified. There was a much higher incidence of *Torulopsis glabrata* in the HIV-infected group, and patients with this species more commonly reported recurrent vulvovaginitis with multiple treatments before participation in the protocol. Most *Candida albicans* species were found to be sensitive for all the antifungal drugs tested, but many isolates of *Torulopsis* were resistant to the azole antifungals tested (112).

Duerr et al. (113) examined the rate of colonization by CD4 counts. Patients with a CD4 count of 500 mm^3 or greater had yeast colonization rates similar to patients in the HIV-negative control group. When CD4 counts were below 200 cells/mm^3, the risk for colonization and symptomatic vulvovaginitis was three times greater than in HIV-positive women with CD4 counts above 500 cells/mm^3 and four times greater than in HIV-negative women.

As with many gynecologic manifestations of disease, there is no consensus regarding vulvovaginal candidiasis. Women should be examined when complaining of a vaginal discharge and treated aggressively if yeast is found. It would appear that recurrent difficult to treat cases, when they occur, are in the more severely immunocompromised women.

Pelvic Inflammatory Disease

The seroprevalence of HIV among women diagnosed with PID can be quite high, ranging from 4.2 to 21.3% (27, 28, 114, 115). It is important for health care providers who treat women with STDs to understand the impact of HIV on the course of PID. STDs and PID in nonimmunocompromised women are reviewed in Chapter 7.

Hoegsberg et al. (114) reported the prevalence of HIV among women hospitalized with PID. Of the 110 patients included in the report, 15 were HIV positive (13.6% seroprevalence). Among the HIV-infected patients, 40% had a white blood cell count of less than 10,000/mm^3 at admission. HIV infection was not associated with a higher frequency of other STDs, although there was a trend toward more cases of syphilis among the HIV-infected women. The trend in the rate of surgical intervention between the HIV-infected group (26.6%) and the HIV-negative group (8.4%) was not statistically significant ($P = .058$).

In 1993, Korn et al. (115) looked at the clinical course of PID in 23 HIV-infected women compared with 108 seronegative control subjects. The HIV-infected women had significantly lower abdominal tenderness scores ($P < .05$) and a trend toward lower white blood cell counts at admission and discharge. They more often required surgical intervention than the negative control subjects ($P < .05$). The authors believed that HIV-infected women may have an altered immune response to PID, preventing optimal response to therapy, and may require additional surgical procedures. No differences were seen in duration of treatment, length of hospitalization, or incidence of tubo-ovarian abscesses.

Kamenga et al. (116) studied 57 HIV-positive and 113 HIV-negative women with PID in Abidjan, Ivory Coast. The HIV-infected women statistically had more genital ulcers and were more likely to require hospitalization and to require subsequent surgical intervention (odds ratio, 6.5; 95% CI, 1.1 to 67.5). There were no differences among the microorganisms identified as the causative agents. Both groups reported similar response to treatment rates (95% versus 93%).

This group also examined the influence of the percentage of CD4 cells on the characteristics of PID. The authors identified an inverse linear association between the percentage of CD4 cells and a temperature of at least 38°C. The women with lower CD4 counts also tended to have a higher frequency of genital ulcers and adnexal masses, but no statistical significance was achieved. No association between CD4 percentages and the need for hospitalization, surgical intervention or clinical severity was seen (116).

Barbosa et al. (117) reported the effects of HIV infection on the clinical course of acute PID among women admitted as inpatients in Brooklyn, New York. The seroprevalence of HIV in this cohort was 8.3%. The HIV-infected women were more likely to have a previous STD and a previous diagnosis of PID than the HIV-negative women. The HIV-positive women had significantly lower white blood cell counts at both admission and discharge and lower lymphocyte counts on discharge than the negative control subjects. The HIV-infected group had higher temperatures on admission and were more likely to still be febrile 48 hours after the initiation of therapy (54% versus 28%, $P < .01$) These differences between the groups disappeared after the fifth hospital day. The authors also reported that the HIV-infected women with PID required changes in their therapeutic regimens more frequently than the HIV-negative cohort (41% versus 13%, $P < .01$). After excluding patients who required surgery, the HIV-positive group had a longer duration of hospital stay (10.6 versus 6.4 days, $P < .01$). Although the severity of disease appeared greater in the HIV-positive group, no differences were seen in frequency of tubo-ovarian abscesses or the need for surgical intervention. In terms of etiologic agents, there was no difference in the number of cases of gonorrhea or chlamydia between the two groups.

At the 1997 National Conference on Women and HIV, Moorman et al. (118), of the Multicenter PID/HIV Study conducted by the CDC and various clinical care sites, presented results on the association of HIV infection with various endometrial pathogens in women with acute PID. The HIV-infected group was more likely to have had genital mycoplasma, streptococcal species, and cytomegalovirus than the HIV-negative control subjects. The HIV-infected women were also much more likely to show signs of chronic infection, whereas the HIV-negative women more commonly showed signs of acute infection.

In summary, the data regarding the effect of HIV infection on etiologic agents causing PID, course of disease, and complications of PID are confusing at best. Currently, it is considered prudent to hospitalize any HIV-infected woman suspected of having PID for intravenous antibiotics. It appears that conventional therapeutic regimens (see Chapter 7) are also effective in the HIV-infected group, but careful attention to febrile morbidity, response to therapy, and disease resolution is warranted in this patient population. Women who are on anti-HIV therapy or who are severely immunocompromised merit special surveillance for treatment response, drug interactions, and other complications.

Genital Ulcer Disease

A number of reports describe the occurrence of aphthous ulcers in immunocompromised patients. These ulcers generally affect the mucosal surfaces of the gastrointestinal tract, from the oropharynx to the anus. They are single or multiple lesions caused predominately by viruses, usually herpes simplex virus or cytomegalovirus. *Treponema pallidum* and *Haemophilus ducreyi* have also been identified as causative agents responsible for this type of ulceration. Zalcitabine (Hivid, ddC) has been implicated in causing esophageal ulcerations (119), and foscarnet (Foscavir) has also been associated with mucosal ulceration formation (120, 121). Nongenital mucosal ulcers tend to have dramatic improvement and healing with the use of steroid therapy. Thalidomide has also proven useful therapy for these lesions (122).

More recently, reports have surfaced on the emergence of large, painful, necrotic lesions in the genital area of HIV-infected women. Termed genital ulcer disease, these lesions have proven difficult to treat because of the difficulty in identifying the etiologic agent(s) responsible for the lesions.

Covina and McCormack (123) described a vulvar ulcer of unknown etiology in an HIV-infected woman. This patient had a history of genital warts that were ablated with laser therapy. She subsequently developed a right vestibular ulcer that continued to expand despite treatment with erythromycin, ceftriaxone (Rocephin), acyclovir (Zovirax), and doxycycline (Vibramycin, Doryx). In addition to the genital ulcer, the patient described multiple painful ulcerations of her lips and oropharynx that healed spontaneously but recurred. Despite multiple cultures of the genital and oral ulcers, no etiologic agent was identified. Biopsies of the vulvar lesions revealed acute and chronic inflammation with granulation tissue, dysplasia, and condyloma formation. The patient was subsequently found to be HIV infected and started on zidovudine (Retrovir, azidothymidine). Shortly after the zidovudine was initiated, the vestibular ulcer reepithelialized, and the patient subsequently remained ulcer free. This interesting case report of aphthous ulcerations of both the oropharyngeal cavity and the vulvar indicates the difficulty of determining the etiologic agent and appropriate treatment for such lesions.

La Guardia et al. (124) retrospectively examined the frequency of genital ulcers in 307 HIV-positive women. They also looked at the microbiologic and histopathologic characteristics of the genital ulcers in this population. There were 43 genital ulcers in 36 women, with 7 of the women (19%) experiencing recurrent ulcers. The overall prevalence of genital ulcer disease in these patients was 11.7%. The patients had extensive evaluations of the lesions, with testing for chlamydia, gonorrhea, herpes simplex virus, cytomegalovirus, and fungi. Cultures for bacterial organisms, acid-fast bacilli, and other species were performed as well. Six of 43 cases of ulcer disease had a biopsy performed, with the specimens undergoing special staining for cytomegalovirus, herpes, acid-fast bacilli, and fungi. Sixty percent of the cases were negative for all organisms, 28% were positive for herpes simplex virus on culture, and 12% were infected with bacteria. In five cases, mixed infections, including *Gardnerella vaginalis, Chlamydia trachomatis, Staphylococcus aureus,* and/or cytomegalovirus were identified. Four patients with genital ulcer disease (9%) had known positive serology for syphilis before the occurrence of any ulcers.

The women with genital ulcer disease were relatively immunocompromised, with a mean CD4 count of 210 cells/mm^3. The six cases that obtained a biopsy were found to have a variety of organisms present, including herpes simplex virus, cytomegalovirus, C. *trachomatis,* and *G. vaginalis.* This report by La Guardia et al. (124) was the first to provide descriptive data of the prevalence of genital ulcer disease in a cohort of HIV-infected women.

La Guardia et al.'s report was informative but troubling. It called to attention the significant lack of information available regarding genital ulcer disease in women in the United States. This may be a result of underreporting of these ulcers by women and their health care providers. The authors were unable to identify the etiologic agent involved in the ulcers in 60% of the cases. This may be a function of the retrospective nature of the report, lack of specific isolation techniques, or other problems. For example, there were no attempts to identify *H. ducreyi* as an etiologic agent. This organism, which causes chancroid, has been identified as a common cause of similar types of ulcerative lesions in men and women in Africa (125, 126). Syphilis has also been identified as a common cause of genital ulcerative lesions in Africa (125, 126), and no dark-field examinations for *Treponemes* were performed in La Guardia's cohort either.

Finally, many organisms were identified that are not usually associated with genital ulcers: C. *trachomatis,* S. *aureus,* and *G. vaginalis.* These agents may have been causative or may have represented concomitant infections, colonization, or contamination by vaginal fluid. Vaginal discharge on the perineum can cause a local irritation and inflammation. Combined with physical trauma associated with pruritus and chafing, this can cause tissue breakdown and small excoriated areas. A severely immunocompromised state and subsequent local infection can then cause further tissue breakdown, necrosis, secondary infection, and the development of a large necrotic lesion. This is a plausible theory to explain the presence of these unexpected organisms in the ulcers described in La Guardia et al.'s report.

The authors reiterated the serious lack of knowledge about genital ulcer disease in women and encouraged further investigation into this devastating disease. The authors specifically recommended investigation of pathogenesis, response to therapy, and the role of HIV in causing the ulcers (124).

Anderson et al. (127) also retrospectively reviewed HIV-infected women suspected of having genital ulcer disease. They questioned investigators from various AIDS Clinical Trials Group sites about clinical characteristics, diagnostic testing, and management of genital ulcer disease. The authors reported data from 29 women who were diagnosed with genital ulcerations. Sixty-eight percent of the women described in the report had AIDS based on the 1993 CDC revised classification system

(40). The median CD4 count of all 29 patients was 50 cells/mm^3. Thirty-seven percent of the women had concomitant oropharyngeal ulcerations, and 19% had progression of their genital ulcers to fistula formation.

Those women who were antiretroviral naive responded to initiation of zidovudine (Retrovir, azidothymidine) with resolution of their genital ulcerations. Most women (86%) receiving antiherpetic therapies such as acyclovir (Zovirax) had no response to therapy. The authors also examined the use of steroids (topical, intralesional, and systemic), and for the most part, all modes of delivery were associated with marginal to good results. Finally, the use of broad-spectrum intravenous antibiotic therapy was successful in 12 of 19 cases (63%) in which they were used (127).

These investigators concluded that the clinical presentation and causes of genital ulcers were similar to that of oropharyngeal ulcers and likely shared the same pathophysiologic mechanism. Most women in their cohort were severely immunocompromised. The genital ulcer disease was generally extensive, progressed to fistula formation in 19% of the cases, and often recurred. Healing and ulcer resolution often took a long time. The authors called for further research into the pathophysiology and therapeutic regimens to treat this disease.

Some would suggest that HIV infection itself can cause the development of the genital ulcers. Unfortunately, the large percentage of severely immunocompromised women in the studies reviewed also indicates that declining immunofunction also plays a role in the development of genital ulcers. The actual etiology of genital ulcer disease remains unknown in most cases. The response of patients to treatment also varied, and empiric antiviral therapy and systemic antibiotic therapy seemed to not be of any benefit when the etiologic agent had not been identified. Treatment with antiretrovirals did, however, appear to help. Steroid therapy was beneficial in healing lesions. All pharmacologic therapy should be withheld until sufficient specimens have been collected in search of an etiologic agent.

Although the physician's first reaction to genital ulcer disease may be to take the patient to the operating room for extensive debridement, this would devascularize the area and further compromise the healing process. Biopsies must be obtained with specimens sent for special staining procedures and cytology and homogenization with testing for all the above-mentioned infectious entities. Because these lesions are exquisitely tender, adequate anesthesia is required for obtaining the biopsies. The comprehensive investigation of a woman with what appears to be genital ulcer disease should include serologic tests for syphilis, cultures for herpes, cytomegalovirus, acid-fast bacilli, bacteria (anaerobic and aerobic), and fungi.

While the patient is anesthetized, it is prudent to clean the lesions, vigorously removing exudate and necrotic tissue. This can be achieved with the use of gauze sponges and a solution of warm saline, Betadine, and hydrogen peroxide. Subsequent perineal hygiene with a perineal care bottle and a warm dilute solution of saline, Betadine, and hydrogen peroxide is essential. Sitz baths are helpful as well. Because these lesions are exquisitely tender, the patient should have ample pain medications ordered.

Therapeutic regimens such as broad-spectrum antibiotics (usually administered intravenously) and antiherpetic medications (acyclovir [Zovirax] or valacyclovir [Valtrex]) with a short course of systemic corticosteroids can be initiated, although it is preferable to await the culture and biopsy results. The true dilemma arises when no etiologic agent is identified. At that time, the above-mentioned therapies and the anti-HIV therapies should be continued in an attempt to achieve a response. We have had success using topical silver sulfadiazine (Silvadene) cream applied to the area in selected cases of extensive ulcerations that were especially slow to heal.

It is imperative for the care provider and patient to understand the chronic course and recurrent nature of genital ulcer disease. Patients should see their health care provider for any ulcerative lesions in the genital or perennial area, no matter how trivial it may seem. It may not take long before such a small ulceration can become full-blown genital ulcer disease.

Menstrual Irregularities

Theories regarding menstrual irregularities in women who are HIV infected are based on current information regarding metabolic abnormalities in HIV-positive men. Gonadal failure, low testosterone, impotence, and other testicular abnormalities in men with HIV are reported in the literature (128–130). Croxson et al. (129) go to great lengths to describe the abnormalities in the hypothalamic-pituitary-gonadal axis, causing abnormalities in hormonal levels and the male reproductive tract in HIV-infected men.

There are several reports examining menstrual irregularities among women infected with HIV. Most are cross-sectional studies and have small numbers of patients. A possible increase in the rates of amenorrhea and oligomenorrhea has been reported, but most studies had significant problems in design. Most had substance abusers in their cohorts yet did not control for this factor, and some did not have a control group at all.

Because of the paucity of data, little is known about the impact of HIV infection on the menstrual cycle, abnormal bleeding patterns, and/or amenorrhea. There are plausible explanations for why menstrual abnormalities might occur. The impact of substance abuse on the hypothalamic-pituitary-gonadal axes is well known, and many HIV-infected patients have a history of substance abuse. Many women infected with HIV/AIDS experience wasting syndrome, with significant weight loss. As is seen in women with eating disorders, low weight or excessive weight loss can alter hormone production and create menstrual irregularities and amenorrhea.

The immune suppression associated with HIV may also cause menstrual irregularities. This has been seen in patients immunosuppressed for medical or transplant reasons. Specific effects of HIV infection alone on the hypothalamic-pituitary-gonadal axis could potentially account for menstrual irregularities (131). Opportunistic infection(s) of the female reproductive organs may contribute to menstrual irregularities (132).

There are two studies that prospectively examined the impact of HIV infection on the menstrual cycle. Shah et al. (133) attempted to determine if a higher prevalence of menstrual symptoms was present in women infected with HIV compared with an HIV-negative control group. This cross-sectional study examined 55 HIV-infected women and 55 control subjects and attempted to classify abnormalities of the menstrual cycle, such as oligomenorrhea, amenorrhea, and menorrhagia. The authors also attempted to establish an association between menstrual irregularities and immunologic status as measured by CD4 counts. No significant differences were found in the prevalence of menstrual irregularities between the two groups. The HIV-infected cohort was then subdivided for analysis into a symptomatic group (based on CDC staging) and an asymptomatic group. No significant differences in menstrual irregularities were seen between these two groups. This report, then, did not support previous reports of menstrual irregularities in HIV-infected women. Although the study attempted to control for substance abuse as a confounder and did contain a control group, it was nonetheless flawed. The sample size was small and had insufficient power to exclude the effect of HIV and immunosuppression on menstrual irregularities. Furthermore, of the women classified as HIV negative, the true HIV status in 47 of the 55 women was unknown.

Ellerbrock et al. (134) also examined the menstrual characteristics of women who were HIV positive. In their cross-sectional study, 197 HIV-infected women and 189 HIV-negative control subjects were examined and interviewed extensively regarding menstrual irregularities. Information about immune status was also obtained. In the 12-month duration of the study, the number of menstrual periods, duration, and quantity of blood flow in the HIV-infected group was no different from the control group. The information in this study regarding menstrual problems in the HIV-infected group was then stratified by CD4 counts. The numbers of women with abnormal bleeding patterns were similar in each category. Even women who were significantly immunocompromised (CD4 count less than 50 cells/mm^3) had no differences in the number of menstrual periods, duration of menstrual flow, or abnormal patterns. The authors concluded that HIV infection and immunosuppression did not have a significant impact on the menstrual cycle or cause abnormal bleeding patterns in this cohort.

The population infected with HIV are difficult to follow long term, making information regarding menstrual irregularities and abnormal bleeding difficult to gather. None of the reports cited examined measurements of body mass index or bioimpedance analysis nor have they established quantitative measures of nutritional status. These types of studies would indicate when HIV-infected women develop wasting syndrome and start losing significant body mass. In theory, this is when abnormalities in the hypothalamic-pituitary-gonadal axis resulting in menstrual irregularities would be expected to develop.

Overall, the few well-designed studies with large cohorts of HIV-infected women matched with negative control subjects do not support the association of menstrual irregularities and HIV infection. Because of the problems inherent to these studies, more work remains to be done before this question can be satisfactorily answered.

CLINICAL NOTES

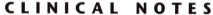

Screening for HIV Infection

- The primary care physician must maintain a high level of clinical suspicion for HIV infection.
- Patients with STDs, abnormal cervical cytology, substance abuse, domestic violence, and other associated social circumstances should be offered testing.

Care of the HIV-Infected Woman

- The history should include prior STDs, abnormal Pap smears, and other related conditions. Although gynecologic symptoms should always be addressed, women with HIV and concomitant gynecologic problems may not display the usual symptoms.
- The physical examination must include a thorough gynecologic examination with Pap smear and cultures (Table 8.2). KOH and wet prep should be done if indicated.
- Preliminary laboratory tests should be ordered (Table 8.2), including assessments of immune system and nutritional status.
- The patient should be referred to an infectious disease or AIDS specialist for initiation of anti-HIV therapies.
- The patient should be referred to a broad spectrum of social services.
- Extensive counseling on anticipated disease course and means to reduce transmission to others is imperative.

Gynecologic Health Issues in the HIV-Infected Woman

- The CDC guidelines for classification of HIV/AIDS were revised in 1993 to include more gynecologic conditions (Table 8.4).
- Contraception and prevention of transmission of HIV or infection with other STDs must be addressed. Condoms are the best method, with nonoxynol-9 spermicide to improve the prophylaxis against pregnancy and STDs.
- Abnormal cervical cytology requires aggressive treatment and follow-up (Table 8.3). Patients found to have ICC deserve definitive treatment, because they are more likely to die of cancer than HIV/AIDS.
- Vaginal infections may frequently recur or be resistant to treatment, especially as the degree of immunocompromise worsens.
- Patients found to have PID likely need hospital admission for intravenous antibiotics.
- It can be difficult to find the cause in a case of genital ulcer disease. These patients should *not* be taken for surgical debridement. Rather, specimens should be taken under anesthesia before scrubbing of necrotic tissue with a solution of saline, Betadine, and hydrogen peroxide. Empiric therapy may then be started, although only antiretrovirals have been found helpful.
- It is not clear whether women who are infected with HIV have more menstrual irregularity problems than HIV-negative women. Confounders include drug abuse and generalized wasting syndrome.

References

1. World Health Organization. Report on the Global HIV/AIDS Epidemic. New York: United Nations, 1997.
2. HIV/AIDS Surveillance Report. Centers for Disease Control and Prevention. 1997; 9:1–37.
3. Wortley PM, Fleming PL. AIDS in women in the United States. JAMA 1997;278:911–916.
4. Karon JM, Rosenberg PS, McQuillan G, et al. Prevalence of HIV infection in the United States, 1984 to 1992. JAMA 1996;276:126–131.
5. Centers for Disease Control and Prevention. National Vital Statistics. Atlanta, GA: CDC, 1996.
6. Centers for Disease Control and Prevention. National Vital Statistics. Atlanta, GA: CDC, 1994.
7. Anastos K, Denenberg RN, Solomon L. Human immunodeficiency virus infection in women. Med Clin North Am 1997;8:533–553.
8. Sha BE, Benson CA, Pottage JC, et al. HIV infection in women: an observational study of clinical characteristics, disease progression and survival for a cohort of women in Chicago. J Acquir Immune Defic Syndr Hum Retrovirol 1995;8:486–495.
9. Fleming PL, Ciesielski CA, Byers RH, et al. Gender differences in reported AIDS-indicative diagnoses. J Infect Dis 1993:168:61–67.
10. Carpenter CJC, Mayer K, Stein MD, et al. Human immunodeficiency virus infection in North American women: experience with 200 women and a review of the literature. Medicine 1991;70:307–325.
11. Clark RA, Brandon W, Dumestre J, et al. Clinical manifestation of infection with the human immunodeficiency virus in women in Louisiana. Clin Infect Dis 1993;17:165–172.
12. Greenberg AE, Thomas PA Landesman SH, et al. The spectrum of HIV-1 related disease in New York City. AIDS 1992:6:849–859.
13. Friedland GH, Saltzman B, Vileno J, et al. Survival differences in patients with AIDS. J Acquir Immune Defic Syndr 1991;4:144–153.
14. Rothenberg RM, Woelfel R, Stoneburner J, et al. Survival with the acquired immunodeficiency syndrome: experience with 5,833 cases in New York City. N Engl J Med 1991;317:1217–1302.
15. Whyle BC, Swanson C, Cooper D. Survival of patients with the acquired immunodeficiency virus in Australia. Med J Aust 1987;150:358–362.

16. Lemp G, Payne S, Neal D, et al. Survival trends for patients with AIDS. JAMA 1990; 263:402–406.

17. Lemp GF, Hirozawa AM, Cohen JB, et al. Survival for women and men with AIDS. J Infect Dis 1992;166:74–79.

18. Chiasson R, Keruly J, Moore R. Race, sex, drug use, and progression of human immuno-deficiency virus disease. N Engl J Med 1995;333:751–756.

19. Cozz-Lepri A, Pezzotti P, Dorructi M, et al. HIV disease progression in 854 women and men infected through injecting drug use and heterosexual sex and followed for up to 9 years from seroconversion. The Italian Seroconversion Study. BMJ 1994;309: 1573–1542.

20. Turner B, Markson L, McKee L, et al. Health care delivery, Zidovudine use and survival of women and men with AIDS. J Acquir Immune Defic Syndr 1994;7:1250–1262.

21. Scheonbaum EE, Webber MP. The underrecognition of HIV infection in an inner city emergency room. Am J Publ Health 1993;83:363–368.

22. Frankel RE, Selwyn P, Mezger J, et al. High prevalence of gynecologic disease among hospitalized women with HIV infection. Clin Infect Dis 1997;25:706–712.

23. McCombs SB, McCray E, Frey RL, et al. Behaviors of heterosexual sexually transmitted disease clinic patients with sex partners at risk for human immunodeficiency virus in-fection. Sex Transm Dis 1997;24:461–468.

24. Maiman M, Fruchter RG, Serur E, et al. Human immunodeficiency virus and cervical neoplasia. Gynecol Oncol 1990;38:377–382.

25. Panel on Clinical Practices for Treatment of HIV Infection. Convened by the Depart-ment of Health and Human Services (DHHS) and the Henry J. Kaiser Family Founda-tion. Guidelines for the Use of Antiretroviral Agents in HIV-Infected Adults and Ado-lescents. Washington, DC: U.S. Public Health Service, 1997.

26. Kloser PC. Primary care of women with HIV disease. In: Cotton D, Watts DH, eds. The Medical Management of AIDS in Women. New York: Wiley-Liss, 1997:189.

27. Sperling RS, Friedman F Jr, Joyner M, et al. Seroprevalence of the human immunode-ficiency virus in women admitted to the hospital with pelvic inflammatory disease. J Re-prod Med 1991;36:122–124.

28. Safrin S, Dattel BJ, Hauer L, et al. Seroprevalence of epidemiologic correlation of hu-man immunodeficiency virus infection in women with acute pelvic inflammatory dis-ease. Obstet Gynecol 1990;75:666–670.

29. Centers for Disease Control and Prevention. Anergy skin testing and prevention ther-apy for HIV infected persons: review and recommendations. MMWR Morb Mortal Wkly Rep 1997;46:RR-15.

30. Centers for Disease Control and Prevention. 1993 STD treatment guidelines. MMWR Morb Mortal Wkly Rep 1993;42:RR-14.

31. Maiman M. Management of cervical neoplasia in HIV positive women. In: Cotton D, Watts DH, eds. The Medical Management of AIDS in Women. New York: Wiley-Liss, 1997:221–234.

32. Minkoff HL, DeHovitz JA. Care of women infected with the human immunodeficiency virus. JAMA 1991;266:2253–2258.

33. Kneisil CR. Psychosocial and economic concerns of women affected by HIV infection. In: Cohen FL, Durham, JD, eds. Women, Children and HIV/AIDS. New York: Springer, 1993:241–250.

34. Shayne VT, Kaplan BJ. Double victims: poor women and AIDS. Women Health 1991;17:21–37.

35. Buckingham SL, Rehm SJ. AIDS and women at risk. Health Soc Work 1987;12:5–11.

36. Stuntzner-Gibson D. Women and HIV disease: an emerging social crisis. Soc Work 1991;36:375–378.

37. Woodruff G. Women and children and HIV. Readings J Rev Comment Mental Health 1993;8:18–22.

38. Ybarra S. Women and AIDS: implications for counseling. J Counsel Dev 1991;69,285–287.

39. Gillman R, Newman B. Psychosocial concerns and strengths of women with HIV infec-tion: an empirical study. Families Soc J Contemp Hum Serv 1996:131–141.

40. Centers for Disease Control and Prevention. 1993 Revised classification systems for HIV infection and expanded surveillance case definitions for AIDS among adolescents and adults. MMWR Morb Mortal Wkly Rep 1993;41(RR-17):1–19.

41. Peterman TA, Stoneburner RL, Allen JR, et al. Risk of human immunodeficiency transmission from heterosexual adults with transfusion associated infections. JAMA 1988; 259:55–58.

42. European Study Group. Risk factors for male to female transmission of HIV. BMJ 1989; 298:411–415.

43. Klebanoff SJ, Coombs RW. Viricidal effect of *Lactobacillus acidophilus* on human immunodeficiency virus type 1: possible role in heterosexual transmission. J Exp Med 1991;174:289–292.

44. Stewart GL, Tyler JPP, Cunningham AL, et al. Transmission of human T-cell lymphotropic virus type III (HTLV-III) by artificial insemination by donor. Lancet 1985;1: 581–584.

45. Judson FN, Ehret JM, Bodin GF, et al. In vitro evaluations of condoms with and without nonoxynol-9 as physical and chemical barriers against *Chlamydia trachomatis,* herpes simplex virus type 2, and human immunodeficiency virus. Sex Transm Dis 1989;16:51–56.

46. Katznelson S, Drew WL, Mintz L. Efficacy of the condom as a barrier to the transmission of cytomegalovirus. J Infect Dis 1984;150:155–157.

47. Minuk GY, Bohme CE, Bowen TJ. Condoms and hepatitis B virus infection (letter). Ann Intern Med 1986140:584.

48. Rietmeijer CA, Krebs JW, Feorino PM, et al. Condoms as physical and chemical barriers against human immunodeficiency virus. JAMA 1988;259:1851–1853.

49. Conant M, Hardy D, Sernatinger T, et al. Condoms prevent transmission of AIDS-associated retrovirus. JAMA 1986;255:1706.

50. European Study Group. Comparison of female to male and male to female transmission of HIV in 563 stable couples. BMJ 1992;302:809–813.

51. Fischl MA, Dickinson GM, Scott GB, et al. Evaluation of heterosexual partners, children and household contacts of adults with AIDS. JAMA 1987;257:640–644.

52. DeVincenzi I. Heterosexual transmission of HIV in a European cohort of couples. Ninth International Conference on AIDS, Berlin, 1993. Abstract WSC-21.

53. Saracco A, Musicco M, Nicolosi A, et al. Man to woman sexual transmission of HIV: longitudinal study of 343 steady partners of infected men. J Acquir Immune Defic Syndr 1993;6:497–502.

54. Kamenga M, Ryder RW, Jingu M, et al. Evidence of marked sexual behavior changes associated with low HIV-1 seroconversion rate in 149 married couples with discordant HIV-1 serostatus. AIDS 1991;5:61–67.

55. Kissinger P, Clark R, Dumestre J, et al. High incidence of sexually transmitted disease and low prevalence of condom use as a primary method of contraception among HIV infected women attending public inner city HIV outpatient clinics. Presented at the HIV Infected Women Conference, February 1995.

56. Kell PD, Barton SE. Unrevealing the mysteries of vulval ulceration in human immunodeficiency virus-seropositive women. Am J Obstet Gynecol 1991;164:935–936.

57. Centers for Disease Control and Prevention. Update: barrier and protection against HIV infection and other sexually transmitted diseases. MMWR Morb Mortal Wkly Rep 1993;42:589–597.

58. Drew WL, Blair M, Miner RC, et al. Evaluation of the virus permeability of a new condom for women. Sex Transm Dis 1990;17:110–112.

59. Wolner-Hanssen P, Svensson L, Mardh PA, et al. Laparoscopic findings and contraceptive use in women with signs and symptoms suggestive of acute salpingitis. Obstet Gynecol 1985;66:233–238.

60. Schumacher GF. Immunology of spermatozoa and cervical mucus. Hum Reprod 1998; 3:289–300.

61. Grossman CJ. Interactions between the gonadal steroids and the immune system. Science 1985;227:257–261.

62. Forrest B. Women, HIV, and mucosal immunity. Lancet 1991;337:835–836.
63. Apr MB, Apr EL. Antigen recognition in the female reproductive tract. I. Update of intraluminal protein traces in the mouse vagina. In: MacDonald TC, Challacombe SJ, Bland PW, et al., eds. Advances in Mucosal Immunology. Norwell, MA: Kluwer Academic Publishers, 1990:608–609.
64. Hitti J, Walker CK, Nsubuga PSJ, et al. Oral contraceptive use and HIV infection. Eighth International Conference on AIDS, Amsterdam, 1992. Abstract POC 4309.
65. Plourde PJ, Plummer FA, Pepin J, et al. HIV type 1 infection in women attending a sexually transmitted disease clinic in Kenya. J Infect Dis 1992;166:86–92.
66. Physician's Desk Reference. Montvale, NJ: Medical Economics, 1996:1872.
67. Quellet D, Hsu A, Qian J, et al. Effect of ritonavir on the pharmacokinetics of ethinyl estradiol I healthy female volunteers. Presented at the International Conference on AIDS, 1996. Abstract Mo.B.1198.
68. Kappus EW, Quinn TD. The spermicide nonoxynol 9 does not inhibit *Chlamydia trachomatis* in vitro. Sex Transm Dis 1986;13:134–137.
69. Rosenberg MJ, Rojanapithayakorn W, Feldblum PH, et al. Effect of the contraceptive sponge on chlamydia infection, gonorrhea and candidiasis. A comparative clinical trial. JAMA 1987;257:2308–2312.
70. Hicks DR, Martin LS. Getchell JP, et al. Inactivation of HTLV-III/LAV infected cultures of normal human lymphocytes by nonoxynol-9 in vitro. Lancet 1985;2:1422–1423.
71. Polsky B, Baron PA, Gold WM, et al. In vitro inactivation of HIV-1 by contraceptive sponge containing nonoxynol-9 (letter). Lancet 1988;1:1456.
72. Miller CJ, Alexander NJ, Gettie A, et al. The effect of contraception containing nonoxynol 9 on the genital transmission of simian immunodeficiency virus in *Rhesus Macaques*. Fertil Steril 1992;57:1126–1128.
73. Zekeng L, Feldblum PJ, Oliver R, et al. Barrier contraceptive use and HIV infection among high-risk women in Cameroon. AIDS 1993;7:725–731.
74. Kreiss J, Ngugi E, Holmes K, et al. Efficacy of nonoxynol-9 contraceptive sponge in preventing heterosexual acquisition of HIV in Nairobi prostitutes. JAMA 1992;268:477–482.
75. Niruthisard S, Roddy RE, Chutiuongse S. The effects of frequent nonoxynol-9 use on the vaginal and cervical mucosa. Sex Transm Dis 1991;18:176–179.
76. Roddy RE, Cordero M, Cordero C, et al. A dosing study of nonoxynols and genital irritation. Int J STD AIDS 1993;4:165–170.
77. Chrepil M, Droegmueller W, Owen JA, et al. Studies of nonoxynol-9: its effect on the vagina of rabbits and rats. Fertil Steril 1980;33:445–450.
78. Fathall MF. Relationship between contraceptive technology and HIV transmission: an overview. In: Alexander N, Gabelnick H, Spieler J, eds. Heterosexual Transmission of AIDS. New York: Wiley, 1990:225–237.
79. Stratton P, Alexander NJ. Heterosexual spread of HIV infection. Reprod Med Rev 1994;3:113–136.
80. Marx P, Spira A, Gettie A, et al. Progesterone implants enhance SIV vaginal transmission and early virus load. Nat Med 1996;2:1084–1089.
81. Patton DL, Thwin SS, Agnew KJ, et al. Influence of the normal menstrual cycle and combination of oral contraceptives on vaginal epithelium and flora. Infect Dis Obstet Gynecol 1997;4:348–364.
82. Sillman FH, Sedlis R. Anogenital papilloma virus and neoplasia in immunodeficient women: an update. Dermatol Clin 1991;9:353–369.
83. Shafer A, Friedman W, Mielka, et al. Frequency of cervical neoplasia in women with HIV is related to degree of immunosuppression. Am J Obstet Gynecol 1991;164:593–599.
84. Vermund SH, Kelley K, Klein RS, et al. High risk of human papilloma virus infection and cervical squamous intraepithelial lesions among women with symptomatic human immunodeficiency virus infection. Am J Obstet Gynecol 1991;165:392–400.
85. Centers for Disease Control. Risk for cervical disease in HIV infected women—New York City. MMWR Morb Mortal Wkly Rep 1990;39:846–849.

86. Mandelblatt JS, Fahs M, Garibaldi K, et al. Associations between HIV infection and cervical neoplasia: implications for clinical care of women at risk for both conditions. AIDS 1992;6:173–178.

87. Adachi A, Fleming I, Burk RD, et al. Women and human immunodeficiency virus infections and abnormal pap smears: a prospective study of colposcopy and clinical outcome. Obstet Gynecol 1993;81:372–377.

88. Wright TC, Ellerbrock TV, Chiasson MA, et al. Cervical intraepithelial neoplasia in women infected with human immunodeficiency virus: prevalence, risk factors, and validity of Papanicolaou smears. Obstet Gynecol 1994;84:591–597.

89. Conti M, Agarossi A, Muggiesen MA, et al. High progression rate of HPV and CIN in HIV infected women. Eighth International Conference on AIDS, 1990. Abstract PO-B-3050.

90. Barton S, Maddox D, Smith J, et al. A study of Langerhans cells in the cervical epithelium in women with HIV infection. Sixth International Conference on AIDS, 1990. Abstract 2013.

91. Olaitan A, Johnson MA. Cervical intraepithelial neoplasia in women with HIV. J Int Assoc Phys AIDS Care 1997;3:15–17.

92. Bradbeer C. Is infection with HIV a risk factor for cervical intraepithelial neoplasia? Lancet 1987;2:1277–1278.

93. Crocchiolo P, Lizioli A, Guisis F, et al. Cervical dysplasia and HIV infection. Lancet 1988;1:238–239.

94. Maiman M, Tarricone N, Vieira J, et al. Colposcopic evaluation of human immunodeficiency virus seropositive women. Obstet Gynecol 1991;78:84–88.

95. Johnson JC, Burnett AF, Willet GD, et al. High frequency of maternal and clinical human papilloma virus infections in immunocompromised human immunodeficiency virus-infected women. Obstet Gynecol 1992;79:321–327.

96. Olaitan A, Mocroft A, McCarthy K, et al. Cervical abnormality and sexually transmitted disease screening in human immunodeficiency virus-positive women. Obstet Gynecol 1997;89:71–75.

97. Fink MJ, Fruchter RG, Maiman M, et al. The adequacy of cytology and colposcopy in diagnosing cervical neoplasia in HIV seropositive women. Gynecol Oncol 1994;55:133–117.

98. Maiman M, Fruchter RG, Serur E, et al. Recurrent cervical intraepithelial neoplasia in human immunodeficiency seropositive women. Obstet Gynecol 1993;82:170–174.

99. Wright TC, Koulous J, Schnoll F, et al. Cervical intraepithelial neoplasia in women infected with the human immunodeficiency virus: outcome after loop electrosurgical excision. Gynecol Oncol 1994;52:105.

100. Cuthill S, Maiman M, Fruchter RG, et al. Complications after treatment of cervical intraepithelial neoplasia in women infected with the human immunodeficiency virus. J Reprod Med 1996;40:823–829.

101. Fruchter RG, Maiman M, Sedlis A, et al. Multiple recurrences of cervical intraepithelial neoplasia in women with the human immunodeficiency virus. Obstet Gynecol 1996;87:336–344.

102. Korn AP, Autry M, DeRemer PA, et al. Sensitivity of the Papanicolaou smear in human immunodeficiency virus-infected women. Obstet Gynecol 1994;83:401–404.

103. Williams A, Darragh T, Vranizan K, et al. Anal and cervical human papillomavirus infection and risk of anal and cervical epithelial abnormalities in human immunodeficiency virus-infected women. Obstet Gynecol 1994;83:205–211.

104. Klevens RM, Fleming P, Mays M, et al. Characteristics of women with AIDS and invasive cervical cancer. Obstet Gynecol 1996;88:269–273.

105. Maiman M, Fruchter RG, Serur E, et al. Human immunodeficiency virus infection and invasive cervical carcinoma. Cancer 1993;71:402–406.

106. Rhoades JL, Wright C, Redfield RR, et al. Chronic vaginal candidiasis in women with human immunodeficiency virus infection. JAMA 1987;257:3105–3107.

107. Iman N, Carpenter CJ, Mayer KH, et al. Hierarchical patterns of mucosal candidiasis infection in HIV-seropositive women. Am J Med 1990;89:142–146.

108. White MH. Is vulvovaginal candidiasis an AIDS-related illness? Clin Infect Dis 1996;22(suppl 2):S124–S122.

109. Sobel JD. Pathogenesis and treatment of recurrent vulvovaginal candidiasis. Clin Infect Dis 1992;14(suppl 1):S148–S153.

110. LeRoy U, DeClercy A, Ladner J, et al. Should screening of genital infections be part of antenatal care in areas of high HIV prevalence? A prospective cohort study from Kigali, Rwanda. 1992–1993. The Pregnancy and HIV (EGE) Group. Genitourin Med 1995;71:207–211.

111. Spinillo A, Micheleone G, Cavanna C, et al. Clinical and microbiological characteristics of symptomatic vulvovaginal candidiasis in HIV seropositive women. Genitourin Med 1994;70:268–272.

112. Spinillo A, Nicola S, Colonna L, et al. Frequency and significance of drug resistance in vulvovaginal candidiasis. Gynecol Obstet Invest 1994;38:130–133.

113. Duerr A, Sierra MF, Feldman J, et al. Immune compromise and prevalence of *Candida* vulvovaginitis in human immunodeficiency virus infected women. Obstet Gynecol 1997;90:252–256.

114. Hoegsberg B, Abulafia O, Sedlis A, et al. Sexually transmitted diseases and human immunodeficiency virus infection among women with pelvic inflammatory disease. Am J Obstet Gynecol 1990;163:1135–1139.

115. Korn AP, Landers DV, Green JR, et al. Pelvic inflammatory disease in human immunodeficiency virus infected women. Obstet Gynecol 1993;82:765–768.

116. Kamenga MC, DeCock KM, St Louis ME, et al. The impact of human immunodeficiency virus infection on pelvic inflammatory disease: a case-control study in Abidjan, Ivory Coast. Am J Obstet Gynecol 1995;172:919–925.

117. Barbosa C, Macasaet M, Brockmann S, et al. Pelvic inflammatory disease and human immunodeficiency virus infection. Obstet Gynecol 1997;89:65–70.

118. Moorman A, Schwartz, Irwin K, et al. Influence of HIV infection on the relationship of endometritis and endometrial pathogens among women with acute pelvic inflammatory disease. National Conference on Women and HIV, Pasadena, 1997:108. Abstract 103.6.

119. Indorf AS, Pegram PS. Esophageal ulceration related to zalcitabine (ddC). Ann Intern Med 1992;117:133–134.

120. Caumes E, Gatineau M, Bricaire F, et al. Foscarnet-induced vulvar erosion (letter). J Am Acad Derm 1993;28:799.

121. Saint-Marc T, Fournier F, Touraine JL, et al. Uvula and oesophageal ulcerations with foscarnet (letter). Lancet 1992;340:970–971.

122. Paterson Dl, Georghiov PR, Allworth AM, et al. Thalidomide as treatment of refractory aphthous ulceration related to human immunodeficiency therapy. Clin Infect Dis 1995;20:250–254.

123. Covino JM, McCormack WM. Vulval ulcer of unknown etiology in a human immunodeficiency virus-infected woman: response to treatment with zidovudine. Am J Obstet Gynecol 1990;163:116–118.

124. La Guardia KD, White M, Saigo PE, et al. Genital ulcer disease in women infected with human immunodeficiency virus. Am J Obstet Gynecol 1995;172:553–562.

125. Bogaerts J, Ricart CA, Van Dyck E, et al. The etiology of genital ulcerations in Rwanda. Sex Transm Dis 1989;16:123–126.

126. Plummer FA, D'Costa L, Nsanze H, et al. Clinical and microbiologic studies of genital ulcers in Kenyan women. Sex Transm Dis 1985;12:193–197.

127. Anderson J, Clark R, Watts DH, et al. Idiopathic genital ulcers in women infected with human immunodeficiency virus. J Acquir Immune Defic Syndr 1996;13:343–347.

128. McCutchen A, Slahian B, Jacobson D, et al. Evaluation of pituitary-testicular axis dysfunction in HIV/AIDS. Ninth International Conference on AIDS. Berlin, June 1993. Abstract Po-B24–1951.

129. Croxson S, Chapman WE, Miller LK, et al. Changes in the hypothalamus pituitary gonadal axis in human immunodeficiency virus infected homosexual men. J Clin Endocrinol Med 1989;68:312–321.

130. Dobs AS, Dempsey NA, Ladenson PW, et al. Endocrine disorders in men infected with human immunodeficiency virus. Am J Med 1988;84:611–616.

131. Merenick JA, McDermott MJ, Asp AA, et al. Evidence of endocrine involvement early in the course of HIV infection. Clin Endocrinol Metab 1990;70:566–571.

132. Familari V, Larocca L, Tamburrini E, et al. Premenopausal cytomegalovirus oophoritis in a patient with AIDS (letter). AIDS 1991;5:458–459.

133. Shah PN, Smith JR, Wells C, et al. Menstrual symptoms in women infected by the human immunodeficiency virus. Obstet Gynecol 1994;83:392–400.

134. Ellerbrock TV, Wright TC, Bush TJ, et al. Characteristics of menstruation in women infected with human immunodeficiency virus. Obstet Gynecol 1996;87:1030–1034.

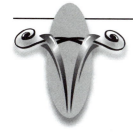

Abnormal Papanicolaou Smears and Human Papilloma Virus

MOLLY A. BREWER
ALMA SBACH
JUDY SANDELLA

The incidence of cervical cancer has significantly decreased over the past 40 years because of the use of the Papanicolaou (Pap) smear for screening, yet cervical cancer is the second most common malignancy of women in the world. Cervical cancer is a major health problem, particularly in underdeveloped countries where preventive health care is the exception rather than the rule. It is estimated that in the United States in 1997, there will be 14,500 new cases of cervical cancer and 4800 deaths from this malignancy (1). Worldwide, the incidence of cervical cancer is much higher; there is a sevenfold difference between rates among Caucasians in the United States and native Peruvians, who have the highest incidence.

Within the United States, racial and regional differences in incidence are attributed to varying exposures to risk factors and barriers to access for preventive health care. According to Surveillance, Epidemiology, and End Results data from the National Cancer Institute, Vietnamese women in the United States have the highest incidence with rates of 43 in 100,000 annually from 1988 to1992. In comparison, Japanese women in the United States had an incidence of 5.8 in 100,000 (2).

THE PAP SMEAR

George Papanicolaou first observed that cancer cells could be observed in smears taken from the cervix. This led to the development of a cytologic test named after Dr. Papanicolaou, the Pap smear. Neoplastic changes confined to the cervix were also found to be assessable by the Pap smear, and these changes were presumed to precede invasive cancer (3). By enabling preinvasive lesions to be identified and then treated, the Pap smear became the standard of care for prevention of cervical cancer, although its efficacy was never tested. Since that time, it has been further refined and subjected to closer scrutiny.

Several parts of the collection and preparation process of the cervical Pap smear are potentially fraught with error. The sample must be collected from the uterine cervix, which may be difficult to visualize (3). Once obtained, the smear must *immediately* be sprayed with fixative to avoid drying artifacts. Finally, the smear must be read by a trained cytotechnologist. Much controversy has arisen in the past 10 years regarding the number of smears that can be accurately screened by one person per day. Laboratories must provide quality control, and the Centers for Disease Control and Prevention (CDC) currently requires that 10% of all negative smears are routinely rescreened. This is a poor method of ensuring that smears are read correctly because it depends on the laboratory to decide which 10% will be rescreened. Interpretation of cytology is one of the more difficult areas of microscopy, as no underlying stroma is present to use as a point of reference (3). In addition, there is usually minimal clinical history, and this may affect the cytologic interpretation, as the history is one aspect of making a correct diagnosis.

The Pap smear may exhibit cells from the entire reproductive tract, depending on the hormonal status of the woman. Abnormal smears can result from abnormalities of the ectocervix, endocervix, vagina, vulva, distal urethra, endometrium, and even the fallopian tube and ovary if the tubes are patent. So although an abnormal Pap smear most likely represents abnormal cytology of the uterine cervix, an abnormal smear in the presence of a normal ectocervical and endocervical examination and sampling requires investigation of the remaining components of the genital tract.

CLASSIFICATION OF THE PAP SMEAR

Dr. Papanicolaou described smears as classes I to V, with class I being normal and classes IV and V being invasive cancer. A class II smear was thought to represent either an infectious etiology or benign atypia, and class III indicated a suspicion of cancer. In 1988, the National Cancer Institute reclassified the Pap smear cytologic interpretations for several reasons (4–9):

1. The Papanicolaou system did not reflect an understanding of vaginal or cervical neoplasia.
2. The Papanicolaou system lacked histopathologic terminology and did not provide a diagnosis for the preinvasive disorders.
3. The old system did not reflect diagnostic interpretations adequately.

The new classification, the Bethesda system, addressed the issue of inadequate specimens by requiring a commentary that the smear was either adequate for interpretation, less than optimal, or unsatisfactory with an explanation for the last two categories. The new system placed the smear in a general category of "within normal limits" or "other," which included a descriptive diagnosis. The descriptive diagnoses listed were of infection (with a description of type), reactive or reparative changes, epithelial cell abnormalities, and nonepithelial malignant neoplasms. For vaginal smears, a category of hormonal status was added. If there were epithelial abnormalities, the new system distinguished between squamous and glandular components and had several descriptions for the abnormalities, including abnormal squamous or glandular cells of undetermined significance (ASCUS or AGUS), low-grade squamous intraepithelial neoplasia (LGSIL, favor human papilloma virus [HPV] or cervical intraepithelial neoplasia [CIN]), or high-grade squamous intraepithelial neoplasia (HGSIL). This new system was an attempt to aid in specifying the abnormality and guiding further diagnostic workup. In 1991, after 3 years of experience with the Bethesda system, it was modified to clarify the necessity for further workup (7, 10, 11). Infection and reparative/reactive changes were reclassified into a new category, benign cellular changes. The atypical category for both squamous and glandular cells was retained but was qualified by a descriptive of the process (i.e., whether it was reactive or neoplastic) (12). The updated system is shown in Table 9.1. The Bethesda system classifies cytologic interpretations, whereas the pathologic definitions still include CIN or dysplasia. CIN was first described cytologically by Richart in 1964; subsequently, Richart et al. (13) described its colposcopic appearance in their classic paper on CIN. The term CIN was used to describe a spectrum

TABLE 9.1. The 1991 Bethesda System

ADEQUACY OF THE SPECIMEN
Satisfactory for evaluation
Satisfactory for evaluation but limited by . . . (specify reason)
Unsatisfactory for evaluation . . . (specify reason)

GENERAL CATERGORIZATION (OPTIONAL)
Within normal limits
Benign cellular changes: See descriptive diagnoses
Epithelial cell abnormalities: See descriptive diagnoses

DESCRIPTIVE DIAGNOSES
Benign cellular changes
Infection
    Trichomonas vaginalis
    Fungal organisms morphologically consistent with *Candida* species
    Predominance of coccobacilli
    Bacteria morphologically consistent with *Actinomyces* species
    Cellular changes associated with herpes simplex virus
    Other[a]

Reactive changes
Reactive cellular changes associated with
    Inflammation (includes typical repair)
    Atrophy with inflammation ("atrophic vaginitis")
    Radiation
    Intrauterine contraceptive device
    Other

Epithelial cell abnormalities
Squamous cell
    Atypical squamous cells of undetermined significance: qualify[b]
        Low-grade squamous intraepithelial lesion encompassing HPV[a]; mild
            dysplasia/CIN 1
        High-grade squamous intraepithelial lesion encompassing moderate and severe
            dysplasia, CIS/CIN 2, and CIN 3
    Squamous cell carcinoma
Glandular cell
    Endometrial cells, cytologically benign, in a postmenopausal woman
    Atypical glandular cells of undetermined significance: qualify[b]
    Endocervical adenocarcinoma
    Endometrial adenocarcinoma
    Extrauterine adenocarcinoma
    Adenocarcinoma, NOS
Other malignant neoplasms: specify

Hormonal evaluation (applies to vaginal smears only)
Hormonal pattern compatible with age and history
Hormonal pattern incompatible with age and history: specify
Hormonal evaluation not possible due to: specify

NOS, non-organ-specific.
[a]Cellular changes of HPV previously termed koilocytosis, koilocytotic atypia, or condylomatous atypia are
included in the category of low-grade squamous intraepithelial lesion.
[b]Atypical squamous or glandular cells of undetermined significance should be further qualified, if possible, as
to whether a reactive or a premalignant/malignant process is favored.

of intraepithelial abnormalities that ranged from mild dysplasia to carcinoma in situ (CIS). CIN 1, or mild dysplasia, is now classified as LGSIL by the Bethesda system. Normal squamous epithelium has nuclei that are equidistance, uniform, and pyknotic, whereas CIN 1 is characterized by nuclear enlargement, hyperchromicity, chromatin clumping, and irregularity of the nuclear membrane with polynucleation. With CIN 1, cellular patterns change and there is crowding and disorganization of nuclei and an increase in nuclear concentration. This is primarily seen in the superficial cell layers and is described pathologically as extending less than one third the distance from the surface to the basal layer. Colposcopically, these are seen as a small focus of abnormality (HPV/CIN 1) (13) (Fig. 9.1).

The Bethesda system now classifies CIN 2 and 3 as HGSIL (4–6). CIN 2, or moderate dysplasia, is characterized by increased nuclear crowding and cellular uniformity in the deeper epithelial zones. It is usually described as extending two thirds of the way from the surface to the basal layer and is more frequently multifocal than mild dysplasia. There may be a sharp demarcation between areas of different cytologic abnormalities, and the cells may align in whorls. Colposcopically, areas of moderate and severe dysplasia are sharply demarcated from normal tissue (Fig. 9.2). CIN 3 (severe dysplasia or CIS) describes extension of abnormal cells two thirds of the distance between the surface and the basal layer. CIS is described pathologically as having tightly packed neoplastic nuclei extending from the surface to the basal layer without extension into the basement membrane. It differs in appearance colposcopically from CIN 1 and HPV by the increased thickness of the acetowhite epithelium, presence of punctation, and abnormal vessels (Fig. 9.3). On colposcopy, invasive cancer may mimic CIN 3 or may have exophytic areas (Fig. 9.4).

It is difficult to distinguish CIS from occult invasive carcinoma and microinvasion. As a result, invasion may be missed relatively frequently on colposcopy (14–16). At the other end of the spectrum, HPV is typically confused with low-grade dysplasia on colposcopy and is often overtreated with either the loop electrical excision procedure (LEEP) or multiple biopsies.

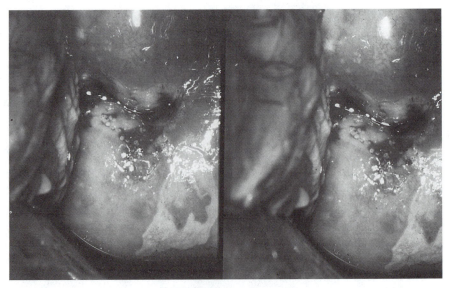

FIGURE 9.1. Condyloma.

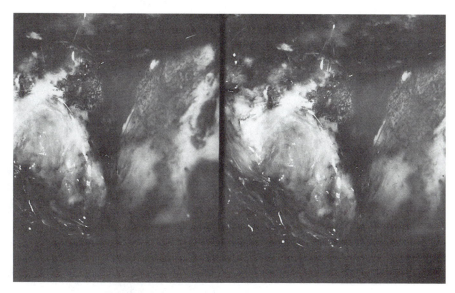

FIGURE 9.2. Cancer—squamous cell carcinoma.

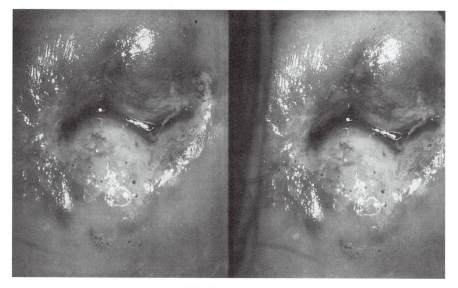

FIGURE 9.3. CIN 3.

Adenocarcinoma in situ (ACIS) was first described as a clinical entity in 1952 (17). ACIS is thought to be the preinvasive form of cervical adenocarcinoma just as CIS is thought to be the preinvasive component of cervical squamous cell carcinoma. It is characterized by morphologic features similar to invasive adenocarcinoma but without the invasive component. It is frequently found adjacent to invasive adeno-carcinoma. ACIS may be of the endocervical type (more common) or the en-dometrioid type (less common) (18). It is characterized by neoplastic glandular cells that coexist with normal columnar cells. The endocervical-type CIS originates in the more superficial portion of the gland, or "primary cleft" (18, 19).

ACIS occurs in women in their late 20s to mid-30s, an age group in which many women are nulliparous. The peak incidence for invasive adenocarcinoma occurs ap-

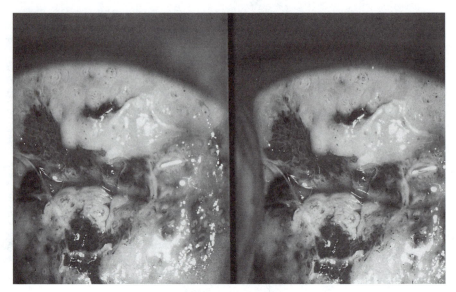

FIGURE 9.4. CIN 2.

proximately 5 to 7 years after the peak incidence for ACIS (20). There appears to be a strong link between adenocarcinoma and HPV 16/18 and, presumably, the same link exists for HPV and ACIS (21–23).

RISK FACTORS FOR DYSPLASIA

Multiple risk factors, including smoking, early age at first intercourse, multiple sexual partners, and HPV, may contribute to the development of CIN. Of these, HPV and smoking are the major risk factors. Studies show a relative risk of almost 3 (three times increased risk) for cervical dysplasia in smokers with HPV compared with non-smokers with HPV (24, 25). The risk factors of early age at first intercourse and multiple sexual partners are probably related to increased HPV exposure and infection.

Human Papilloma Virus

The strongest independent risk factor for cervical dysplasia is infection with HPV. HPV is a small oncogenic DNA virus that may induce neoplastic changes on mucosal and epidermal surfaces (26, 27). It is composed of eight early genes and two late genes, which refer to the portion of the cell cycle that the virus affects. The early genes are responsible for transforming properties and the late genes for structural proteins. HPV was initially discovered by the identification of koilocytosis on Pap smears in the 1970s (27). In the late 1970s, HPV infections began to be linked to CIN and invasive cervical neoplasms and subsequently has been shown to be associated with most cases of cervical neoplasia (24–33).

HPV is a sexually transmitted virus that has been extensively characterized. HPV may cause anogenital warts, with most occurring on the vulva, perineum, or in the perianal region. These warts may spontaneously regress or may persist. Pregnancy, human immunodeficiency virus (HIV), chronic renal failure, and other conditions associated with immunodeficiency may exacerbate HPV infections. Over 60 types have been identified, of which at least 8 are associated with cervical infections.

Different HPV types are associated with different clinical manifestations and are generally site specific, reflecting a specific interaction between viral and cellular gene expression (27). For example, types 6 and 11 are most commonly associated with HPV changes, CIN 1, and genital warts and types 16 and 18 are most commonly associated with CIN 3 and invasive cancer. HPV type has been strongly correlated with risk of invasive cancer, and types have been classified as low risk, intermediate risk, and/or high risk. Types 6, 11, and 42 to 44 are strongly linked to benign changes that seldom progress to invasion. Types 16, 18, 45, and 56, however, are strongly linked to the development of invasive cancer and are considered high risk. HPV types 31, 33, 35, 51, and 52 are considered intermediate risk because they have the highest association with high-grade dysplasia but a lower odds ratio for invasive cancer (34, 35). Adenocarcinoma is most commonly associated with HPV type 18 (22).

Once genes within the viral genome have been inserted into the host DNA, they become intimately associated with the transformation and regulatory activities within the cell. HPV structural proteins have been demonstrated in CIN lesions, CIS, and invasive carcinoma (32, 36). Progression to cancer is thought to occur when the host fails to control existing persistent viral genomes (30, 37). In benign lesions, viral DNA replicates in the host cell in an episomal form that is separate from the host genetic material (33). Malignant changes may occur when the viral genome is incorporated into the host genome, disrupts the host's intragenomic regulation, and maintains the cell in this transformed state (30, 37, 38). Viral genetic material may then change the host regulatory functions and hence initiate the first step in the development of neoplastic changes.

Evidence of HPV infections by colposcopy, Pap smear, and biopsy may regress, remain stable, or progress (32, 36, 38). Spontaneous regression is associated with low-grade lesions on biopsy and Pap smear, whereas high-grade lesions are frequently associated with progression. HPV types 16 and 18 are most commonly associated with high-grade dysplasia or carcinoma, and lesions caused by these types are less likely to regress spontaneously (39, 40).

Multiple studies demonstrate a strong association between HPV infections and CIN (32, 36, 40–48). High-risk HPV, particularly types 16 and 18, are associated with progression of CIN to high-grade dysplasia. Types 16 and 18 increase the risk by 11 times; 52% of all CIN is attributable to types 16 and 18 (46). Women infected with HPV have a significantly higher rate of CIN development than uninfected women (28% versus 3%) (46). Other studies found similar results with progression of CIN from low-grade to high-grade dysplasia associated predominantly with HPV types 16 and 18 (40, 46). Regression is more consistently seen in association with low-risk types (6 and 11) (40–42, 44, 45, 49, 50). Low-risk types can and do progress to higher grade dysplasia, although not as commonly as high-risk types (40–45, 50). Although smoking, intercourse at an early age, and multiple sexual partners are associated with progression of CIN in other studies, one prospective nonintervention study of 342 women found that HPV type was the major predictive variable in CIN progression, with other factors having little effect (24, 25, 39, 40, 51).

The initial discovery that HPV could subclinically infect the cervix without causing overt warty changes and the observation that koilocytosis on Pap smear was linked to HPV and dysplasia were the two factors linking HPV infection to cervical dysplasia/neoplasia. Subsequent studies strengthened that association considerably (24, 25, 30, 38–45, 52–54). HPV changes are frequently confused with CIN on colposcopy, especially by inexperienced colposcopists (13, 26, 27, 34). As a result, overtreatment is common. This was part of the rationale for adopting the Bethesda system of classification.

MANAGEMENT OF PATIENTS WITH AN ABNORMAL PAP SMEAR

Patients who present with abnormal Pap smear results fall into two groups: high risk and low risk. Risk is determined in two ways. The first is the differential diagnosis. The low-risk group includes LGSIL favoring HPV, LGSIL favoring dysplasia, ASCUS favoring reaction, and AGUS favoring reaction (55, 56). The high-risk group includes HGSIL, AGUS favoring dysplasia, squamous cell carcinoma, and adenocarcinoma. The second determination of risk lies in the patients' history of abnormal Pap smears. Patients with their first low-risk cytology after having yearly normal Pap smears fall into the low-risk group. Patients who have had multiple abnormal Pap smears, patients from sexually transmitted disease clinics, patients without frequent surveillance, patients who have been noncompliant with screening or treatment, and patients with HIV fall into a higher risk group (57).

It is important to understand that not all HPV/low-grade dysplasia progresses to cancer. Approximately 25% of HPV lesions regress, 55% persist, and 20% progress (13, 40, 49, 52). Patients in the low-risk category with HPV/LGSIL, ASCUS, or AGUS (favor reactive) can be followed with Pap smears every 6 months. By 9 months, 78% of patients with CIN 1 or LGSIL have regression and 7% have progression (58, 59). In contrast, moderate dysplasia, now classified as HGSIL, shows a regression rate of 54% and a progression rate of 30% (60). Patients in the high-risk category, by virtue of diagnosis or history, should be treated.

Colposcopy

Colposcopy has been the standard of care for an abnormal Pap smear. However, it lacks sensitivity for microinvasive carcinoma. In a retrospective review, 24 patients, which represented 0.06% of the population studied, developed invasive carcinoma within 14 months of treatment for microinvasive disease (61). This failure rate was largely attributable to failure to colposcopically diagnose or take a biopsy of the affected area at the time of original diagnosis. Retrospective review of Pap smears showed malignant cells on three Pap smears that were not documented with biopsy (61). In prospective studies, colposcopy had a sensitivity of 69 to 95% and specificity of 67 to 93% for diagnosing CIN (13, 14, 62–64). There were variable results in the diagnosis of invasion; sensitivity ranged from 0 to 78% in the colposcopic diagnosis of carcinoma. In these prospective studies, three diagnoses of microinvasion or invasion were made at the time of colposcopy despite a negative biopsy (13, 14, 62–64). The total number of invasive carcinomas was small. A larger retrospective study showed 10 to 15% incorrect diagnoses of microinvasive carcinoma (65).

Endocervical Curettage

Although some believe an endocervical curettage (ECC) is not necessary if the colposcopy is adequate, one large retrospective study found that ECC was the one test that consistently found an abnormality in patients with invasive cancers (66–69). Although ECC did not identify carcinoma, the abnormality was the impetus for further diagnostic procedures that identified the invasive component. Although ECC is painful for the patient and represents a superficial biopsy that does not sample the underlying stroma, it is a worthwhile and relatively easy diagnostic procedure to do.

Inadequate colposcopy, especially in older women, may be associated with a significant number of endocervical abnormalities, including microinvasion and invasion, that would be identified on the ECC (67). A positive ECC is usually associated with abnormalities within the canal and warrants further diagnostic procedures, such as cold knife conization (CKC) of the cervix or LEEP conization (70). There is enough evidence to show that a positive ECC has a high probability of representing an invasive or microinvasive cancer that ECC should be done with every colposcopy (71). The technique for colposcopy is described below.

Other Screening Modalities

Cervicography and cervicoscopy have been described as alternative methods to colposcopy or the Pap smear. Cervicography is performed by taking a color slide of the cervix with a 35-mm camera after acetic acid lavage. The resulting cervigrams are described as technically defective, negative, or suspicious. Cervicoscopy is performed by visualizing the cervix without magnification after lavage with acetic acid; the examination is classified as negative or positive depending on whether acetowhite epithelium is present. Although cervicoscopy appears to be slightly more accurate than cytology and cervicography, both cervicography and cervicoscopy lack sensitivity and specificity as screening tests (72).

ThinPrep (Cytyc Corp., Marlboro, MA) is a relatively new technique that varies from the traditional Pap smear in that it is liquid based. Instead of being smeared on a slide, the sample is rinsed in a vial of preservative solution. The vial is placed into a ThinPrep 2000 processor and a thin layer of cells is prepared, transferred to a glass slide, fixed, and stained. It is then read in the conventional manner. With this new technique, studies suggested less atypia, a lower rate of false-negative results, fewer fixation artifacts, and fewer unsatisfactory specimens; hence, fewer repeat specimens are required (73–77). None of these studies had adequate control subjects. All ThinPrep results were compared with those of the conventional Pap smear, which is well known to have relatively low sensitivity. Without biopsy specimens for controls, there is no way to estimate the incidence of overtreatment that might result with this technology. Further studies are needed before the Pap smear is replaced.

Currently, there is strong interest in developing an automated method for analyzing cervical cytology to lessen the reliance on cytotechnologists. Although these methods have not been perfected, they are promising. Automated screening would be particularly useful in developing countries where the major interest is on detection of significant lesions (77).

A screening modality that is better than the Pap smear would be of great benefit to patients and would help to avoid overtreatment and underdiagnosis. The ThinPrep has potential but lacks data. A very promising technique has been developed through MD Anderson Cancer Center and University of Texas Optics Division that has a superior sensitivity and specificity to Pap smear and colposcopy. Fluorescence spectroscopy is a new and exciting technique that is completely noninvasive and involves fluorescence light being applied to the surface of the cervix. This light excites naturally occurring fluorophores within the tissue, resulting in tissue emission of fluorescence of a different wavelength depending on the intrinsic fluorescence of the tissue, the scattering within the tissue, and the biochemical composition of the tissue. It is a real-time measurement that is fully automated and does not require the expertise needed for colposcopy. The higher the grade of the dysplasia, the more absorption and the less emitted fluorescence (78–83). Preliminary data and cost analysis of this technique show that fluorescence spectroscopy of the cervix has a higher sensitivity than the Pap smear and a higher specificity than colposcopy in differentiating squamous intraepithelial lesion(s) from no squamous intraepithelial lesion(s) and LGSIL from HGSIL. Spectroscopically directed biopsy is significantly less expensive than colposcopy with LEEP (Mitchell M, Zuluaga A, Richards-Kortum R, unpublished data, 1998).

TREATMENT OF PATIENTS WITH ABNORMAL PAP SMEARS

Observation

The natural history of CIN is variable and depends primarily on the HPV type involved. There has been a general reluctance to simply follow CIN without treatment because of the fear that dysplasia would progress to cancer. Many women received multiple procedures in an attempt to eradicate the virus and any CIN 1 present, an approach that is costly and results in excessive morbidity. In up to 62% of patients, CIN 1 completely regresses over 1 to 3 years (59). Again, observation is appropriate for patients with low-risk LGSIL, ASCUS (favor reactive), or AGUS (favor reactive).

Interventions

Multiple modalities have been used over the years to treat CIN. Laser ablation and cryotherapy have been used for the treatment of mild dysplasia and CKC or laser conization have been used to treat severe dysplasia (84, 85).

Cryotherapy

Cryotherapy has the lowest complication rate of all ablative therapies and the equipment is the least costly. Richart and colleagues (86, 87) prospectively evaluated 2839 women receiving cryotherapy for CIN 1 to 3 and found a very low incidence of recurrence of dysplasia over 14 years (0.41 to 0.44%). However, in patients with HGSIL, failure rates of cryotherapy range from 10 to 40%, depending on the size of the lesion (88). Because a large proportion of LGSIL and HPV lesions regress without treatment, cryotherapy has fewer indications at present. However, cryotherapy is a well-tested method and has a reasonable efficacy with persistent low-risk lesions; it remains one of the least invasive methods of treating dysplasia. A description of a cryotherapy technique is found in Appendix 9.1.

Laser Conization

Laser conization became popular with the increased use of the laser as an ablative and surgical tool. Laser conization has no advantage compared with CKC, is technically more difficult, and requires more costly equipment. For these reasons, this technique is less frequently used. Laser ablation is still used by some, but its primary use remains as ablation of vaginal and/or vulvar intraepithelial neoplasia.

Cold Knife Conization

CKC is used both for diagnostic and therapeutic purposes. Part of the efficacy of CKC in treating CIN may be due to elimination of HPV by removal of susceptible cells (89). It provides an excellent pathology specimen and may reveal invasion where none was suspected (90–92). Post-CKC hysterectomy has shown residual disease in 42 to 82% of patients who had positive margins and 18 to 23% of patients with negative margins (91, 93, 94). Some studies concluded that postconization cervical cytology is more useful than cone margins as a predictor of recurrent or persistent disease, although other studies concluded the opposite (91, 92, 94). Women with positive margins may be followed conservatively and thus avoid further surgery (95, 96).

In some institutions, CKC specimens can be evaluated as a frozen section before hysterectomy. Advantages of this approach include avoiding the need for two procedures, planning a surgical treatment with greater accuracy, and avoiding the delay associated with a two-step procedure. The diagnosis of invasion can be made using frozen sections with excellent sensitivity and specificity: 89 and 100%, respectively (97, 98). However, this technique is limited to institutions with experience with frozen cones and is not widely available because many pathologists are reluctant to use a frozen cone biopsy to guide treatment because of the potential of missing an invasive lesion.

Complications of CKC are well known; they include hemorrhage, pelvic cellulitis, cervical stenosis, and incompetent cervix (85). In addition, CKC requires general anesthesia, which adds significantly to the cost of the procedure.

Loop Electrosurgical Excision Procedure

There has been a change in treatment patterns in the past few years as a new technique has become more popular, LEEP. (A technique for LEEP is described in Appendix 9.2.) As data have accumulated, it is evident that this technique has complications similar to, but not the same as, those of CKC: infection, bleeding, burns to the vagina, cervical stenosis, cervical incompetence, and recurrence of dysplasia. Bleeding usually occurs between 5 and 10 days after the procedure as the eschar sloughs off the cervix. Bleeding can usually be controlled with Monsel's solution. Stenosis is rare (1%) and occurs primarily in the nulliparous, perimenopausal, or the postmenopausal patient. If stenosis occurs, dilation of the cervix should first be tried. If this does not allow sampling of the cervix, a repeat LEEP can be done of the stenotic os followed by dilatation and hormones for the menopausal patient (99). Cervical incompetence is usually a complication of multiple procedures.

Because general anesthesia is not required for LEEP, it is possible to perform colposcopy, biopsies, and LEEP in the same visit. This "see and treat" protocol has become increasingly more popular for convenience and cost effectiveness. There is, however, a relatively high rate of negative specimens (14 to 40%) with the see and treat approach with LEEP. These are attributable to thermal injury, incomplete tissue sampling, and false-positive colposcopy with biopsy having been therapeutic (100, 101). Even if colposcopy is done at the time of initial visit, there was still an overtreatment (LEEP with negative specimen) problem of 39% in one population (102). Although the see and treat approach may eliminate compliance problems and reduce the risk of missing an invasive cancer, it is also associated with excessive loss of cervical tissue and significant overtreatment (102). Patients with CIN 2 or 3 on outside Pap smears probably benefit from the see and treat strategy. Because of the possibility of overtreatment, the see and treat protocol is not recommended for younger patients or those with cytologic evidence of CIN 1; these patients benefit from having their biopsies reviewed before treatment.

Most patients with CIN 2 or 3 treated with LEEP are disease free at 6 months of follow-up (102). Pregnancy outcomes after LEEP are generally good. A 1995 study evaluated 574 women after LEEP and found an incidence of 8.5 pregnancies per 100 woman years compared with 7.4 per 100 woman years in women with CIN who did not receive LEEP. In women treated with LEEP, the pregnancy outcome was comparable with the untreated population (103).

A 1997 article comparing CKC, laser conization, and LEEP showed a decrease in complication with LEEP along with a decrease in operating time. Margins were equally assessable with LEEP and CKC. Laser cone showed the highest rate of complication. The only drawback for the LEEP procedure was the slightly shorter cone depth and a slightly higher risk of recurrence (104).

ADENOCARCINOMA IN SITU

There has been increasing interest in the management of ACIS as women delay their childbearing and opt for conservative management. Treatment of ACIS has traditionally been extrafascial hysterectomy because of the concern for disease further up the canal. Skip lesions have been described in which glands with CIS are found adjacent to normal glands. Three recent retrospective studies showed that even with negative margins on the cone specimen and a negative ECC, there may be residual disease further up the canal or in the endometrium; this may consist of ACIS or adenocarcinoma with invasion (105–107). CKC or LEEP specimens with negative margins and negative ECC are associated with a 30 to 50% risk of residual disease further up the canal and a 10 to 15% risk of invasive carcinoma. Patients with positive margins and/or positive ECC have a 75 to 80% probability of residual disease. These patients should have a repeat cone (LEEP or CKC) and endometrial biopsy because they have a high rate (10 to 20%) of invasive adenocarcinoma. These estimates for an invasive component may be somewhat high (erroneously) but are ominous nevertheless. Patients who wish to preserve their fertility must be carefully counseled about meticulous follow-up with Pap smears using the cytobrush, ECC, and endometrial biopsy every 3 months for the first 2 years. There is preliminary evidence that LEEP cone may be superior to CKC if done carefully enough to avoid cautery artifact. The LEEP cone with two endocervical specimens allows biopsy of the entire endocervical canal. This may provide a better pathologic specimen with less disruption of the endocervical canal because a thinner specimen may be obtained (Mitchell M, Brewer M, unpublished data, 1998).

DIAGNOSIS AND/OR TREATMENT FAILURE

Progression of dysplasia to carcinoma after treatment is considered a treatment failure. As discussed earlier, the most important predictive factor for progression, regardless of treatment, is HPV type. Types 16, 18, 31, and 33 are associated with a significantly higher rate of progression than nononcogenic HPV types (43). Infrequent or suboptimal Pap smears are another risk factor for progression. In 20 patients who developed CIN 3 or invasive carcinoma after three normal Pap smears, over half of them had a smear that was obscured by inflammation or a minimum 2-year lapse since their last Pap smear (108). After CKC for preinvasive disease, 1.4% of women may develop invasive cancer 1 to 16 years later. In one study, 25% of patients who subsequently developed invasion had carcinoma deep in the cervical stroma that was inaccessible to a subsequent CKC and was probably buried from the prior cone procedure (109).

One problem in evaluating risk of progression has been inadequate biopsy specimens. Dysplasia and CIS often coexist in the cervix. If the biopsy was taken from an area with CIS, then a true sample has been taken, and the diagnosis of progression from CIS to invasive cancer is accurate. However, if the biopsy was not taken from the most severe lesion, then what is called progression is actually failure to have originally diagnosed the more severe lesion (110).

Colposcopy by an inexperienced practitioner increases the risk for progression of dysplasia to invasive cancer (111). Webb (111) wrote the following: "Colposcopic triage of the abnormal Pap smear is increasingly undertaken by gynecologists who have only modest colposcopic experience. Ideally, colposcopy should only be performed by an expert colposcopist." Error rates due to inexperience in colposcopic diagnosis of microinvasive and occult carcinoma range from 10 to 15% (15, 62, 111). This is of particular concern today as more and more physicians with minimal colposcopic experience are performing colposcopy with directed biopsy. These practitioners lack the colposcopic expertise to determine the worst areas most suggestive of disease and some are unaware of the appropriate disposition for these patients. The most common cause of treatment failure is deviation from protocol and use of ablative treatment without adequate pathologic evaluation to rule out invasive cancer (61).

HIV AND ABNORMAL CERVICAL CYTOLOGY

Women with HIV or acquired immunodeficiency syndrome should be treated as high-risk patients and may be at risk for rapid progression of CIN to cervical cancer (112, 113). Some investigators found that routine screening with the Pap smear is adequate surveillance for HIV-positive women, whereas others believe colposcopy is a better screening method for this group (57, 114, 115). Some studies demonstrate that the rates of CIN are inversely proportional to CD4 counts in HIV-positive women (115). When cervical cancer is diagnosed in HIV-positive women, they usually have a more advanced state of disease and carry a poorer prognosis for their cancer than their non-HIV-infected counterparts. This delay in diagnosis may, in part, be due to socioeconomic factors and lack of compliance or access to health care (116). (Further discussion of gynecologic problems in HIV-infected women, including abnormal cervical cytology, can be found in Chap. 8.)

ABNORMAL PAP SMEAR IN PREGNANCY

The cytologic features associated with CIN in pregnancy do not differ from those seen in the nonpregnant state. With pregnancy, there is eversion of the endocervical canal and gaping of the external os. This is readily apparent by the latter first trimester in the primigravid woman and occurs even earlier in the multiparous woman. These physiologic changes help facilitate colposcopic evaluation of the squamocolumnar junction.

The indications for colposcopy in the pregnant woman are the same as those for the nonpregnant woman. On visualization of the cervix, the pregnant female may demonstrate an acetowhite change because of the active squamous metaplasia of pregnancy. In addition, cervical mucus is more copious, and the cervix is easily traumatized. Application of the speculum and acetic acid require a delicate touch to avoid bleeding.

If the colposcopic examination is visually consistent with CIN 1 or 2, no biopsy is necessary. Most would advocate repeat colposcopy and cytology in each of the remaining trimesters of pregnancy and 2 months postpartum. If the colposcopic impression changes or cytologic testing indicates progression during the pregnancy, biopsy of the most abnormal area is warranted.

Gravid patients with CIN 3 on the Pap smear should undergo careful colposcopic examination to rule out microinvasion. If signs of microinvasion are noted, such as abnormal vascular patterns with markedly dilated vessels, vessels running horizontally in the epithelium, "corkscrew" or "comma" vessels, or an increase in intercapillary distance, a biopsy or biopsies must be obtained. If none of these findings are noted, the patient may be followed with reexamination by colposcopy and cytology every 6 weeks for the remainder of the pregnancy. A repeat cytologic and colposcopic examination should be done 6 to 8 weeks postpartum.

It is important to remember that if, at any point of the pregnancy, there is colposcopic or cytologic suspicion of microinvasive disease or frank invasion, a biopsy is required for diagnosis. Small biopsies of the most abnormal areas on colposcopy are recommended to minimize bleeding. Cervical sites of biopsy bleed quite briskly during pregnancy, so preparations for this should be made before obtaining the specimen.

If the Pap smear demonstrates malignant cells but they cannot be seen on colposcopy and biopsy, a diagnostic conization may be necessary. If the Pap smear or biopsy indicates invasive cancer, a conization (either CKC or LEEP) should be done to evaluate the extent of invasion. This should be done in the operating room with the help of a perinatologist if the patient is greater than 24 weeks gestation. Preterm labor and bleeding are the most common complications; gestational age and extent of disease determine treatment.

The Pap smear is one of the oldest screening tests but is associated with significant error in technique and interpretation. These factors have a direct impact positively or negatively on a subsequent treatment plan(s).

It is anticipated that screening for dysplasia and cervical cancer will become fully automated with spectroscopic methods that are not subject to the same degree of error and the incidence of cervical cancer will decrease significantly in the screened population. Until that time, it is of critical importance that both underdiagnosis and overtreatment are avoided. In addition, with the development of HPV vaccines, there is a possibility that elimination of cervical dysplasia will be within our reach.

CLINICAL NOTES

- Cervical cancer is the second most common malignancy in the world. In the United States, Vietnamese women have the highest incidence (43/100,000).
- The cervical sample must be sprayed with fixative *immediately* after applying it to the slide to avoid drying artifacts.
- Although an abnormal Pap smear most likely represents abnormal cytology of the cervix, it may also reflect abnormal cytology of other genital tract structures.
- The Bethesda system classifies cytologic interpretations, whereas the pathologic definitions still include dysplasia. HPV changes or CIN 1 are categorized as LGSIL in the Bethesda system, whereas CIN 2, CIN 3, and CIS are categorized as HGSIL.
- The strongest independent risk factor for cervical dysplasia is infection with HPV. Although specific types of HPV are associated with risk of invasive cancer, HPV typing is still a research, and not a clinical, tool.
- Patients with an abnormal Pap with HPV/LGSIL, ASCUS, or AGUS (favor reactive) and no history of abnormal Pap smears may be followed with Pap smears every 6 months.
- Patients with an abnormal Pap with HGSIL; AGUS favoring dysplasia; squamous cell carcinoma; adenocarcinoma; history of abnormal Pap smears and/or referred from sexually transmitted disease clinics and/or history of noncompliance and/or HIV infection; or lack of frequent surveillance must be treated.
- Colposcopy lacks sensitivity for microinvasive carcinoma. Its sensitivity for CIN diagnosis is 69 to 95% and its specificity for diagnosing CIN is 67 to 93%.
- ECC is a worthwhile and easy diagnostic procedure to do that is particularly helpful in identifying endocervical abnormalities.
- Observation as therapy is appropriate in patients with low-risk abnormal cytology and histories.
- Cryotherapy is an acceptable method of treatment for CIN 1 to 3, although the risk of treatment failure increases in HGSIL, depending on the size of the lesion.
- LEEP is an acceptable mode of therapy for CIN and has a lower complication rate than CKC or laser.
- Patients with ACIS are traditionally treated with extrafascial hysterectomy. For women wishing to preserve fertility, follow-up with Pap smears (using the cytobrush), ECC, and endometrial biopsy every 3 months for 2 years may be done.

A Technique for Cryotherapy

Cryotherapy is done in the office without anesthesia, although pretreatment ingestion of a nonsteroidal drug, approximately 1 hour before the procedure, will help diminish the pain of uterine cramping the patient may experience. Cryotherapy is best done shortly after a completed menstrual cycle because this allows the most active phase of regeneration to occur before the next menses.

A speculum as large as the patient will tolerate is used. The abnormal location and topography of the abnormal epithelium is visualized with colposcopy. The probe that best matches the configuration of abnormality is attached to the cryotherapy unit and its surface is covered with a water-soluble lubricant (to ensure adequate heat transfer and to achieve a deeper level of cryonecrosis). If the lesion is more than one and one half times the probe's size, the lesion should be subdivided, with each segment frozen separately.

Still at room temperature, the tip of the probe is positioned onto the tissues, taking care the entire lesion is covered with the metal tip. The unit is activated to circulate the refrigerant. Crystallization of the back of the probe tip should be noted and within 10 to 15 seconds should spread from the edge of the probe onto the tissues. The amount of time spent in freezing is not important; ensuring that the edge of the ice ball extends at least 5 to 6 mm beyond the edge of the probe into normal appearing epithelium *is* important. With extension of the ice ball 5 to 6 mm laterally into normal tissue, there is adequate depth of tissue destruction to destroy all glands involved with CIN.

Once the entire area of abnormal tissue is frozen, the probe is removed. After a waiting period of 5 to 10 minutes to allow for thawing, the technique is repeated once more. Use of the "freeze-thaw-freeze" technique increases the reliability of cell death. This is important because cryonecrosis tends to be patchy and may be associated with a wide zone of sublethal injury in adjacent tissues.

The patient should be observed for 15 to 20 minutes after the procedure to ensure no vasomotor reaction (light-headedness, possible headache, and, rarely, loss of consciousness). The patient should refrain from intercourse, tampons, and douching for 3 weeks and should be seen for follow-up in 3 to 4 months. The patient should be counseled to expect a *profuse* watery discharge in the 2 to 3 weeks after the procedure.

LEEP Technique

Coloscopy is done before LEEP to fully visualize the lesion with acetic acid. Lugol's solution is then applied to the cervix, and the nonstaining areas and squamocolumnar junction are visualized. Benzocaine 20% gel or spray is used on the cervix in preparation for the lidocaine injection. The cervix is then injected with 10 to 20 mL of 2% lidocaine with epinephrine (1:50,000 or 1:100,000). This technique provides excellent analgesia. Using a Potocky needle (Fig. 9.5), which is more rigid than a spinal needle, the cervix is injected at the 12, 3, 6, and 9 o'clock positions. Occasionally, after the injection of lidocaine, some patients experience a rapid heart rate that may last for 2 to 3 minutes.

For LEEP, the Cabot system is favored, using the monopolar output and a blend of coagulation and cut. A 2.0 × 0.8 cm loop is used for the ectocervical specimen at a power of 7 W for the average, multiparous, premenopausal patient. However, with a small or low-grade lesion or in a nulliparous or postmenopausal patient in whom a conservative LEEP is indicated, a 15 × 10-mm or a 15 × 8-mm loop is used for the ectocervical specimen. The cervix should remain moist throughout the procedure. Starting at the 6 or 12 o'clock position, the ectocervical specimen is removed in an anterior-to-posterior direction or vice versa, rather than laterally, to avoid lateral vaginal wall damage. The electrode must be activated before actually touching the cervix to avoid cautery artifact to the specimen and avoid cautery damage to the cervical os. The loop is pushed perpendicularly to the surface of the cervix to a depth of 8 mm at the os, which is approximately up to the crossbar of the electrode, and an oblong specimen that is thinner on the edges and thicker in the middle is removed. The specimen is marked at the 12 o'clock position (usually with a stitch), and the margins are inked according to the recommendations of the pathology department. If at any time the

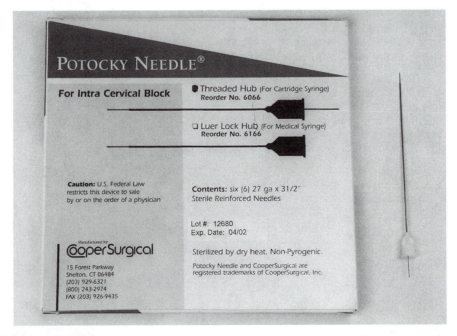

FIGURE 9.5. Potocky Needle used for intracervical block. (Reprinted with permission from CooperSurgical, Inc., Shelton, CT.)

loop stalls, the pressure is released, the power stopped, and the procedure restarted at the area that would have originally been the exit site.

If the procedure is a LEEP cone, a 1.0×1.0-cm loop is used, the power is reduced to 5 W, and either one or two specimens are removed. The direction of the endocervical canal is ascertained by inserting the end of a cotton tip applicator or uterine sound to ensure central placement of the specimen. It should be emphasized that the loop should never be advanced too slowly because cautery artifact results and the margins will not be interpretable. Nor should the loop be advanced too rapidly because the steam envelope that precedes the loop will not excise the tissue. To avoid stenosis, the external os is fulgurated for hemostasis but the internal os is not.

References

1. Wingo PA, Tong T, et al. Cancer statistics, 1995. CA Cancer J Clin 1995;45:8–30.
2. Miller et al., eds. Surveillance, epidemiology, and end results incidence rates among women, 1988–1992. Bethesda, MD: National Cancer Institute, SEER Program, 1997.
3. Koss LG. The Papanicolaou test for cervical cancer detection. JAMA 1989;261:737–743.
4. Lundberg GD. The 1988 Bethesda system for reporting cervical/vaginal cytological diagnoses. JAMA 1989;262:931–934.
5. Kurman RJ, Malkasian GD, Sedlis A, et al. From Papanicolaou to Bethesda: the rationale for a new cervical cytologic classification. Obstet Gynecol 1991;77:779–781.
6. Luff RD. The Bethesda system for reporting cervical/vaginal cytologic diagnosis: report of the 1991 Bethesda workshop. The Bethesda System Editorial Committee. Hum Pathol 1992;23:719–721.
7. Isacson C, Kurman RJ. The Bethesda system: a new classification for managing Pap smears. Contemp Obstet Gynecol 1995;40:67–74.
8. Tabbara S, Saleh ADM, Andersen WA, et al. The Bethesda classification for squamous intraepithelial lesions: histologic, cytologic, and viral correlates. Obstet Gynecol 1992;79:338–346.
9. Sherman ME, Schiffman MH, Erozan YS, et al. The Bethesda system: a proposal for reporting abnormal cervical smears based on the reproducibility of cytopathologic diagnosis. Arch Pathol Lab Med 1992;116:1155–1158.
10. Bottles K, Reiter RC, Steiner AL, et al. Problems encountered with the Bethesda system: the University of Iowa experience. Obstet Gynecol 1991;78:410–414.
11. Herbst AL. The Bethesda system for cervical/vaginal cytologic diagnosis: a note of caution. Obstet Gynecol 1990;76:449–450.
12. Widra EA, Dookhan D, Jordan A, et al. Evaluation of the atypical cytologic smear. J Reprod Med 1994;39:682–684.
13. Richart RM, Doyle GB, Ramsay GC. Colpomicroscopic studies of the distribution of dysplasia and carcinoma in situ on the exposed portion of the humane uterine cervix. Cancer 1965;18:950–954.
14. Edebiri AA. The relative significance of colposcopic descriptive appearances in the diagnosis of cervical intraepithelial neoplasia. Int J Gynecol Obstet 1990;33:23–29.
15. Benedet JL, Boyes DA, Nichols TM, et al. Colposcopic evaluation of patients with abnormal cervical cytology. Br J Obstet Gynaecol 1976;83:177–182.
16. Anderson MC, Jordan JA, Morse AR, et al. A Textbook and Atlas. New York: Thieme-Stratton, 1984:134–177.
17. Hepler TK, Dockerty MB, Randall LM. Primary adenocarcinoma of the cervix. Am J Obstet Gynecol 1952;63:800–808.
18. Noda K, Kimura K, Ikeda M, et al. Studies on the histogenesis of cervical adenocarcinoma. Int J Gynecol Path 1983;1:336–346.
19. Jaworski RC. Endocervical glandular dysplasia, adenocarcinoma in situ, and early invasive (microinvasive) adenocarcinoma of the uterine cervix. Semin Diagn Pathol 1990;7:190–204.
20. Kjaer SK, Brinton LA. Adenocarcinomas of the uterine cervix: the epidemiology of an increasing problem. Epidemiol Rev 1993;15:486–498.
21. Duggan MA, McGregor SE, Benoit JL, et al. The human papillomavirus status of invasive cervical adenocarcinoma. Hum Pathol 1995;26:319–325.
22. Leminen A, Paavonen J, Vesterinen E, et al. Human papillomavirus types 16 and 18 in adenocarcinoma of the uterine cervix. Am J Clin Pathol 1991;95:647–652.
23. Shingleton HM. Do squamous cell carcinomas and adenocarcinomas of the cervix have the same risk factors? Gynecol Oncol 1993;51:299–300.
24. Schiffman MH. Recent progress in defining the epidemiology of human papillomavirus infection and cervical neoplasia. J Natl Cancer Inst 1992;84:394–398.
25. Schiffman MH, Bauer HM, Hoover RN, et al. Epidemiologic evidence showing that human papillomavirus infection causes most cervical intraepithelial neoplasia. J Natl Cancer Inst 1993;85:958–964.

26. Cuzick J, Szarewski A, Terry G, et al. Human papillomavirus testing in primary cervical screening. Lancet 1995;345:1533–1536.

27. Howley PM, Schlegel R. The human papillomaviruses. Am J Med 1988;85:155–158.

28. Schneider A, Meinhardt G, Kirchmayr R, et al. Prevalence of human papillomavirus genomes in tissues from the lower genital tract as detected by molecular in situ hybridization. Int J Gynecol Pathol 1991;10:1–14.

29. Stewart AM, Eriksson AM, Manos MM, et al. Intratype variation in 12 human papillomavirus types: a worldwide perspective. J Virol 1996;70:3127–3136.

30. zur Hausen H, de Villiers EM. Human papillomaviruses. Annu Rev Microbiol 1994; 48: 427–447.

31. Bosch FX, Manos MM, Munoz N, et al. Prevalence of human papillomavirus in cervical cancer: a worldwide perspective. J Natl Cancer Inst 1995;87:796–802.

32. Kataja V, Syrjanen K, Mantyjarvi R, et al. Prospective follow-up of cervical HPV infections: life table analysis of histopathological, cytological and colposcopic data. Eur J Epidemiol 1989;5:1–7.

33. Shah KV. Genital warts, papillomaviruses, and genital malignancies. Annu Rev Med 1988;39:371–379.

34. Barrasso R, Coupez F, Ionesco M, et al. Human papilloma viruses and cervical intraepithelial neoplasia: the role of colposcopy. Gynecol Oncol 1987;27:197–207.

35. Lorincz AT, Reid R, Jenson AB, et al. Human papillomavirus infection of the cervix: relative risk associations of 15 common anogenital types. Obstet Gynecol 1992;79:328–337.

36. Kataja V, Syrjanen S, Mantyjarvi R, et al. Prognostic factors in cervical human papillomavirus infections. Sex Trans Dis 1992;19:154–160.

37. zur Hausen H. Papillomaviruses in human cancer. Cancer 1987;59:1692–1696.

38. zur Hausen H. Papillomaviruses in human genital cancer. Med Oncol Tumor Pharmacother 1987;4:187–192.

39. Ikenberg H, Sauerbrei W, Schottmuller U, et al. Human papillomavirus DNA in cervical carcinoma correlation with clinical data and influence on prognosis. Int J Cancer 1994;59:322–326.

40. Morrison EAB, Ho GYF, Vermund SH, et al. Human papillomavirus infection and other risk factors for cervical neoplasia: a case-control study. Int J Cancer 1991;49:6–13.

41. Syrjanen K, Mantyjarvi R, Vayrynen M, et al. Human papillomavirus (HPV) infections involved in the neoplastic process of the uterine cervix as established by prospective follow-up of 513 women for two years. Eur J Gynaecol Oncol 1987;8:5–16.

42. Syrjanen KJ. Current concepts of human papillomavirus infections in the genital tract and their relationship to intraepithelial neoplasia and squamous cell carcinoma. Obstet Gynecol Surv 1984;39:252–265.

43. Kenemans P. HPV genotype as a prognostic factor for progression to cervical carcinoma in young women. Eur J Obstet Gynecol 1994;55:24–25.

44. Syrjanen K, Hakama M, Saarikoski S, et al. Prevalence, incidence and estimated lifetime risk of cervical human papillomavirus infections in a non-selected Finnish female population. Sex Transm Dis 1990;17:15–19.

45. Syrjanen K, Mantyjarvi R, Vayrynen M, et al. Factors influencing the biological behavior of cervical human papillomavirus (HPV) infections in prospectively followed-up women. Arch Geschwulstforsch 1985;55:457–466.

46. Koutsky LA, Galloway DA, Holmes KK. Epidemiology of genital human papillomavirus infection. Epidemiol Rev 1988;10:122–163.

47. Ho GY, Burk RD, Klein S, et al. Persistent genital human papillomavirus infection as a risk factor for persistent cervical dysplasia. J Natl Cancer Inst 1995;87:1365–1371.

48. Mitchell MF, Hittleman WN, Hong WK, et al. The natural history of cervical intraepithelial neoplasia: an argument for intermediate endpoint biomarkers. Cancer Epidemiol Biomarkers Prev 1994;3:619–626.

49. Morrison EAB. Natural history of cervical infection with human papillomaviruses. Clin Infect Dis 1994;18:172–180.

50. Evander M, Edlund K, Gustafsson A, et al. Human papillomavirus infection is transient in young women: a population-based cohort study. J Infect Dis 1995;171:1026–1030.

51. Remmink AJ, Walboomers JMM, Helmerhorst TJM, et al. The presence of persistent high-risk HPV genotypes in dysplastic cervical lesions is associated with progressive disease: natural history up to 36 months. Int J Cancer 1995;61:306–311.

52. Lancaster WD, Jenson AB. Natural history of human papilloma virus infection of the anogenital tract. Cancer Metastasis Rev 1987;6:653–664.

53. Wright TC, Richart RM. Role of human papillomavirus in the pathogenesis of genital tract warts and cancer. Gynecol Oncol 1990;37:151–164.

54. Reeves WC, Brinton LA, Garcia M, et al. Human papillomavirus infection and cervical cancer in Latin America. N Engl J Med 1989;320:1437–1441.

55. Widra EA, Dookhan D, Jordan A, et al. Evaluation of the atypical cytologic smear. J Reprod Med 1994;39:682–684.

56. Richart RM, Wright TC Jr. Controversies in the management of low-grade cervical intraepithelial neoplasia. Cancer 1993;71:1413–1421.

57. Adachi A, Fleming I, Burk RD, et al. Women with human immunodeficiency virus infection and abnormal Papanicolaou smears: a prospective study of colposcopy and clinical outcome. Obstet Gynecol 1993;81:372–377.

58. Montz FJ, Monk BJ, Fowler JM, et al. Natural history of the minimally abnormal Papanicolaou smear. Obstet Gynecol 1992;80:385–388.

59. Nasiell K, Roger V, Nasiell M. Behavior of mild cervical dysplasia during long-term follow-up. Obstet Gynecol 1986;67:665–669.

60. Nasiell K, Nasiell M, Vaclavinkova V. Behavior of moderate cervical dysplasia during long-term follow-up. Obstet Gynecol 1983;61:609–614.

61. Shumsky AG, Stuart GCE, Nation J. Carcinoma of the cervix following conservative management of cervical intraepithelial neoplasia. Gynecol Oncol 1994;53:50–54.

62. Richart RM, Crum CP, Townsend DE. Workup of the patient with an abnormal Papanicolaou smear. Gynecol Oncol 1981:12:S265–S276.

63. Stafl A, Wilbanks GD. An international terminology of colposcopy: report of the nomenclature committee of the International Federation of Cervical Pathology and Colposcopy. Obstet Gynecol 1991;77:313–314.

64. Javaheri G, Fejgin MD. Diagnostic value of colposcopy in the investigation of cervical neoplasia. Am J Obstet Gynecol 1980;137:588–594.

65. Benedet JL, Anderson GH, Boyes DA. Colposcopic accuracy in the diagnosis of microinvasive and occult invasive carcinoma of the cervix. Obstet Gynecol 1985;65:557–562.

66. Swan RW. Evaluation of colposcopic accuracy without endocervical curettage. Obstet Gynecol 1979;53:680–684.

67. Dinh TA, Dinh TV, Hannigan EV, et al. Necessity for endocervical curettage in elderly women undergoing colposcopy. J Reprod Med 1989;34:621.

68. Urcuyo R, Rome RM, Nelson JH Jr. Some observations on the value of endocervical curettage performed as an integral part of colposcopic examination of patients with abnormal cervical cytology. Am J Obstet Gynecol 1977;128:787–792.

69. Drescher CW, Peters WA III, Roberts JA. Contribution of endocervical curettage in evaluating abnormal cervical cytology. Obstet Gynecol 1983;62:343.

70. Krebs HB, Wheelock, JB, Hurt WG. Positive endocervical curettage in patients with satisfactory and unsatisfactory colposcopy: clinical implications. Obstet Gynecol 1987;69:601–605.

71. El-Dabh A, Rogers RE, Davis TE, et al. The role of endocervical curettage in satisfactory colposcopy. Obstet Gynecol 1989;74:159–163.

72. Cecchini S, Bonardi R, Mazzotta A, et al. Testing cervicography and cervicoscopy as screening tests for cervical cancer. Tumori 1993;79:22–25.

73. McGoogan E, Reith A. Would monolayers provide more representative samples and improved preparations for cervical screening? Overview and evaluation of systems available. Acta Cytol 1996;40:107–119.

74. Hutchinson ML, Agarwal P, Denault T, et al. A new look at cervical cytology. Acta Cytol 1992;36:499–504.

75. Bur M, Knowles K, Pekow P, et al. Comparison of ThinPrep preparations with conventional cervicovaginal smears. Acta Cytol 1995;39:631–642.

76. Awen C, Hathway S, Eddy W, et al. Efficacy of ThinPrep preparation of cervical smears: a 1,000-case, investigator-sponsored study. Diagn Cytopathol 1994;11:33–37.

77. Richart RM, Patten SF Jr, Lee JS. Prospects for automated cytology. Obstet Gynecol Clin North Am 1996;23:853–859.

78. Ramanujam N, Mitchell MF, Mahadevan A, et al. Development of a multivariate statistical algorithm to analyze human cervical tissue fluorescence spectra acquired in vivo. Lasers Surg Med 1996;19:46–62.

79. Mahadevan A, Michell MF, Silva E, et al. Study of the fluorescence properties of normal and neoplastic human cervical tissues. Lasers Surg Med 1993;13:647–655.

80. Ramanujam N, Mitchell MF, Mahadevan A, et al. Fluorescence spectroscopy: a diagnostic tool for cervical intraepithelial neoplasia (CIN). Gynecol Oncol 1994;52:31–38.

81. Ramanujam N, Mitchell MF, Mahadevan A, et al. In vivo diagnosis of cervical intraepithelial neoplasia (CIN) using 337 nm laser induced fluorescence. Proc Natl Acad Sci USA 1994;91:10193–10197.

82. Ramanujam N, Mahadevan A, Mitchell MF, et al. Fluorescence spectroscopy of the cervix. Clin Consult Obstet Gynecol 1994;6:62–69.

83. Malpica A, Wright T, Atkinson N, et al. Spectroscopic diagnosis of cervical squamous intraepithelial neoplasia in vivo using laser induced fluorescence spectra at multiple excitation wavelengths. Lasers Surg Med 1996;19:63–74.

84. Ahlgren M, Ingemarsson I, Lindberg LG, et al. Conization as treatment of carcinoma in situ of the uterine cervix. Obstet Gynecol 1975;46:135–140.

85. Villasanta U, Durkan JP. Indications and complications of cold conization of the cervix. Obstet Gynecol 1966;27:717–723.

86. Richart RM, Townsend DE. Outpatient therapy of cervical intraepithelial neoplasia with cryotherapy or CO_2 laser. In: Osofsky HJ, ed. Advances in Clinical Obstetrics and Gynecology. Vol. 1. Baltimore: Williams & Wilkins, 1982:235–246.

87. Richart RM, Townsend DE, Crisp W, et al. An analysis of "long-term" follow-up results in patients with cervical intraepithelial neoplasia treated by cryotherapy. Am J Obstet Gynecol 1980;137:823–826.

88. Ferenczy A. Management of patients with high grade squamous intraepithelial lesions. Cancer 1995;76:1928–1933.

89. Elfgren K, Bistoletti P, Dillner L, et al. Conization for cervical intraepithelial neoplasia is followed by disappearance of human papillomavirus deoxyribonucleic acid and a decline in serum and cervical mucus antibodies against human papillomavirus antigens. Am J Obstet Gynecol 1996;174:937–942.

90. Killackey MA, Jones WB, Lewis JL Jr. Diagnostic conization of the cervix: review of 460 consecutive cases. Obstet Gynecol 1986;67:766.

91. Buxton EJ, Luesley DM, Wade-Evans T, et al. Residual disease after cone biopsy completeness of excision and follow-up cytology as predictive factors. Obstet Gynecol 1987; 70:529–532.

92. Paterson-Brown S, Chappatte OA, Clark SK, et al. The significance of cone biopsy resection margins. Gynecol Oncol 1992;46:182–185.

93. Phelps JY III, Ward JA, Szigetti J II, et al. Cervical cone margins as a predictor for residual dysplasia in post-cone hysterectomy specimens. Obstet Gynecol 1994;84: 128–130.

94. Abdul-Karim FW, Nunez C. Cervical intraepithelial neoplasia after conization: a study of 522 consecutive cervical cones. Obstet Gynecol 1985;65:77–81.

95. Monk A, Pushkin SF, Nelson AL, et al. Conservative management of options for patients with dysplasia involving endocervical margins of cervical cone biopsy specimens. Am J Obstet Gynecol 1996;174:1695–1700.

96. Lapaquette TK, Dinh TV, Hannigan EV, et al. Management of patients with positive margins after cervical conization. Obstet Gynecol 1993;82:440–443.

97. Neiger R, Bailey SA, Wall AM III, et al. Evaluating cervical cone biopsy specimens with frozen sections at hysterectomy. J Reprod Med 1991;36:103–107.

98. Hoffman MS, Collins E, Roberts WS, et al. Cervical conization with frozen section before planned hysterectomy. Obstet Gynecol 1993;82:394–398.

99. Curtis M. The use of the loop electrosurgical excision procedure (LEEP) in relieving stenosis of the external cervical os. J Gynecol Surg 1996;12:201–203.

100. Ferenczy A, Choukroun D, Arseneau J. Loop electrosurgical excision procedure for squamous intraepithelial lesions of the cervix: Advantages and potential pitfalls. Obstet Gynecol 1996;87:332–337.

101. Alvarez RD, Helm CW, Edwards RP, et al. Prospective randomized trial of LLETZ versus laser ablation in patients with cervical intraepithelial neoplasia. Gynecol Oncol 1994;52:175–179.

102. Brady JL, Fish ANJ, Woolas RP, et al. Large loop diathermy of the transformation zone: is "see and treat" an acceptable option for the management of women with abnormal cervical smears? J Obstet Gynecol 1994;14:44–49.

103. Ferenczy A, Choukroun D, Falcone T, et al. The effect of cervical loop electrosurgical excision on subsequent pregnancy outcome: North American experience. Am J Obstet Gynecol 1995;172:1246–1250.

104. Linares AC, Storment J, Rhodes-Morris H, et al. A comparison of three cone biopsy techniques for evaluation and treatment of squamous intraepithelial lesions. J Gynecol Tech 1997;3:151–156.

105. Denehy TR, Gregori CA, Breen JL. Endocervical curettage, cone margins, and residual adenocarcinoma in situ of the cervix. Obstet Gynecol 1997;90:1–6.

106. Wolf JK, Levenback C, Malpica A, et al. Adenocarcinoma in situ of the cervix: significance of cone biopsy margins. Obstet Gynecol 1996;88:82–86.

107. Poynor EA, Barakat RR, Hoskins WJ. Management and follow-up of patients with adenocarcinoma in situ of the uterine cervix. Gynecol Oncol 1995;57:158–164.

108. Sherman ME, Kelly D. High-grade squamous intraepithelial lesions and invasive carcinoma following the report of three negative Papanicolaou smears: screening failures or rapid progression? Mod Pathol 1992;5:337.

109. Brown JV, Peters WA, Corwin DJ. Invasive carcinoma after cone biopsy for cervical intraepithelial neoplasia. Gynecol Oncol 1991;40:25–28.

110. Ostor AG. Natural history of cervical intraepithelial neoplasia: a critical review. Int J Gynecol Pathol 1993;12:186–192.

111. Webb MJ. Invasive cancer following conservative therapy for previous cervical intraepithelial neoplasia. Colposc Gynecol Laser Surg 1985;1:245.

112. Rellihan MA, Dooley DP, Burke TW, et al. Rapidly progressing cervical cancer in a patient with human immunodeficiency virus infection. Gynecol Oncol 1990;36:435–438.

113. Schwartz LB, Carcangiu ML, Bradham L, et al. Case report. Rapidly progressive squamous cell carcinoma of the cervix coexisting with human immunodeficiency virus infection: clinical opinion. Gynecol Oncol 1991;41:255–258.

114. Wright TC, Moscarelli RD, Dole P, et al. Significance of mild cytologic atypia in women infected with human immunodeficiency virus. Obstet Gynecol 1996;87:515–519.

115. Fink MF, Fruchter RG, Maiman M, et al. The adequacy of cytology and colposcopy in diagnosing cervical neoplasia in HIV-seropositive women. Gynecol Oncol 1994;55:133–137.

116. Maiman M, Fruchter RG, Guy L, et al. Human immunodeficiency virus infection and invasive cervical carcinoma. Cancer 1993;71:402–406.

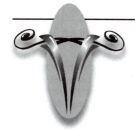

Dysfunctional Uterine Bleeding

JOHN C. PETROZZA
KAREN POLEY

Abnormal uterine bleeding is a common complaint in women of all ages. It can be a confusing picture for the physician because there are multiple reasons for its etiology, each with its own treatment modality.

PATHOPHYSIOLOGY OF MENSES

Menstrual bleeding occurs after the withdrawal of estrogen and progesterone. In each cycle where there is no implantation of a fertilized egg, there is demise of the corpus luteum, and hormonal support of the endometrium is withdrawn. Prostaglandins PGE_2 and $PGF_{2\alpha}$ rise during menses and are believed to play a role in the vasoconstriction of the spiral arterioles. Spiral arterioles supply the superficial two thirds of the endometrium. Vasoconstriction of these vessels results in ischemic breakdown of the superficial endometrium. The superficial endometrium sloughs, leaving the lower one third of the endometrium, the basalis layer, behind. The basalis layer is important in the regeneration of endometrium, which occurs in response to estrogen stimulation early in the next cycle. During menses, hemostasis is achieved through vasoconstriction and clotting over the endometrial surface.

Normal menstrual flow occurs at regular intervals of 28 days. The range of cycle length is between 21 and 35 days. The number of cycles occurring between menarche and menopause is approximately 400 to 500. The average menses lasts 4 to 6 days. The normal amount of blood loss ranges from 20 to 60 mL. A loss of more than 80 mL is considered abnormal and is sufficient to cause anemia. Approximately 10% of women suffer from true menorrhagia. The amount of iron lost with each normal menses is 13 mg. Approximately 70% of all blood loss during menses occurs during the first 2 days (1). There is great variation in menstrual characteristics between women but very little between cycles in an individual. If a woman reports significant change in her menses, this should be investigated.

The following are definitions of commonly used terms describing abnormal uterine bleeding:

- *Oligomenorrhea*—cycle length greater than 35 days
- *Polymenorrhea*—cycle length less than 21 days
- *Amenorrhea*—absence of menses for at least 6 months, or three cycles
- *Menorrhagia*—increased flow or duration of flow occurring at regular intervals or loss of more than 80 mL
- *Metrorrhagia*—bleeding occurring at irregular intervals
- *Menometrorrhagia*—increased flow or duration of flow occurring at irregular intervals
- *Postmenopausal bleeding*—bleeding occurring more than 12 months after the last menstrual period

241

DETERMINATION OF BLOOD LOSS

The determination of the amount of menstrual flow is very difficult for both the patient and physician. Counting the number of pads or tampons is not really sufficient because each may have very different absorption characteristics. Hallberg et al. (1) found that 40% of women with flow greater than 80 mL considered their menstrual loss to be small or moderate, whereas in women with loss of less than 20 mL, 14% thought their flow was heavy. Hallberg and Nilsson (2) described a precise technique for the objective measurement of blood loss, the alkaline hematin method. This technique is frequently used in research but has never become popular for routine use.

In 1990, Higham et al. (3) developed the most objective test to date to determine the amount of menstrual blood flow. Patients would record the type of pad they were using and the amount of blood coverage on each pad with each change. These recordings would then be converted to a diary score. A score of 100 was validated as being equivalent to a menstrual egress of 80 mL, or menorrhagia. However, the menstrual effluent is not composed entirely of blood. Fraser et al. (4) determined the percentage contribution of blood to total menstrual discharge. The mean contribution from whole blood was 36%, but the range was between 1.6 and 81%, with the remainder of menstrual discharge consisting of endometrial fluid. The ratio of blood to fluid changes with the use of different contraceptive methods, decreasing with oral contraceptive pills and increasing with the use of an intrauterine device (IUD). This variation in composition of menstrual discharge is likely to contribute to the difficulty in estimation of amount of menstrual bleeding.

DIFFERENTIAL DIAGNOSIS OF ABNORMAL UTERINE BLEEDING

The differential diagnosis of abnormal uterine bleeding is extensive and varies with the age of the patient. Dysfunctional uterine bleeding can consist of oligomenorrhea or prolonged excessive bleeding. It is a diagnosis of exclusion, made only after all other causes have been eliminated. It occurs commonly at the extremes of the reproductive ages, specifically, during the postmenarche and perimenopausal time periods. Although usually associated with anovulation, it does sometimes occur with ovulation. Chronic anovulation can be associated with polycystic ovarian syndrome, adult-onset congenital adrenal hyperplasia, development of premature ovarian failure, or thyroid or prolactin disorders. In the reproductive-age woman, abnormal bleeding must be considered a complication of pregnancy until proven otherwise. Because history may not be reliable, a urine or serum pregnancy test should be obtained in all women of reproductive age. Bleeding may be secondary to an ectopic pregnancy, threatened abortion, subinvolution of a placental site, placental polyp, or trophoblastic disease.

Systemic diseases can be associated with abnormal uterine bleeding. Liver or renal failure can be complicated by uterine bleeding because of alterations in the metabolism and excretion of hormones. Liver disease causes increased free estrogen and hypothrombinemia and decreased production of fibrinogen and clotting factors. Endocrine disorders, such as thyroid disease, adrenal hyperplasia, or prolactinemia, can result in changes in menstrual pattern. Hypothyroidism is frequently associated with menorrhagia, whereas hyperthyroidism is often associated with amenorrhea.

An adolescent with a previously undiagnosed coagulopathy usually presents with significant bleeding at, or soon after, menarche. Claessens and Cowell (5) found that 19% of adolescents requiring hospitalization due to menorrhagia had a coagulopathy. A bleeding disorder, such as von Willebrand's disease, can cause menorrhagia and is often overlooked as a possible cause of abnormal bleeding. Disorders of platelet number or function can also present as abnormal uterine bleeding. Examples include idiopathic thrombocytopenic purpura, disseminated intravascular coagulation, sepsis, leukemia, aplastic anemia, hypersplenism, and thrombocytopenia or platelet dysfunction secondary to medications. Women with coagulopathies frequently have marked blood loss with menses. Fraser et al. (6) reported that the average blood loss in women with various coagulopathies is 400 mL per menses. Iatrogenic causes of abnormal uterine bleeding include contraceptives, hormones, and other medications. The copper IUD, Depo-Provera, and Norplant are all associated with an initial increase in the amount of bleeding. Long-term use of progestin-only contraceptives is also associated with breakthrough bleeding. Ginseng has some estrogenic activity and has been associated with abnormal bleeding (7). Other medications altering the menstrual pattern include digitalis, phenytoin, tranquilizers, antidepressants and other psychotropic drugs, and corticosteroids. Anticoagulants in the therapeutic range usually do not cause excessive bleeding; however, if the dosage is too high, the patient may experience an increase in menstrual flow.

Reproductive tract pathology of many types may cause abnormal bleeding. Trauma to the vulva, vagina, or cervix can result in bleeding. An infection, such as cervicitis or endometritis, can be the cause, usually in the form of intermenstrual bleeding, and should be treated with the appropriate antibiotic. A polyp in the cervix usually results in spotting or postcoital bleeding. An endometrial polyp, however, can result in significant bleeding, either intermenstrual or menorrhagia. Endometriosis or adenomyosis can also contribute to abnormal uterine bleeding. Endometriosis has been associated with premenstrual spotting; adenomyosis may cause menorrhagia.

Fibroids are benign tumors of the uterus, arising from smooth muscle, which occur in 30% of women. They can result in symptoms such as pain, infertility, and abnormal bleeding or may be entirely asymptomatic. One third of fibroids cause abnormal bleeding, usually in the fourth to fifth decade of life. The fibroids that are commonly related to significant menorrhagia are located in the submucous position. The reason the myoma in this position causes heavier bleeding is not entirely clear. One theory is that it results in an abnormal venous pattern, with stasis and a change in venous drainage. A submucous fibroid increases the surface area of the endometrium and disrupts the vascular supply to the endometrium in the area over the fibroid.

Endometrial hyperplasia is proliferation of glands of irregular size and shape, with crowding of the glands and an increase in the gland-to-stroma ratio, which occurs in response to unopposed estrogen stimulation. Endometrial hyperplasia can be divided into two groups: with and without atypia. Hyperplasia with atypia refers to the presence of atypical cells lining the glands, showing a loss of polarity, prominent nucleoli, and enlarged pleomorphic nuclei. Hyperplasia with atypia has a tendency to recur after treatment and has a higher chance of developing into endometrial adenocarcinoma (8). Less than 2% of women diagnosed with hyperplasia without atypia progress to adenocarcinoma, but 23% of women having hyperplasia with atypia develop adenocarcinoma (9).

Malignancy along the reproductive tract causes bleeding. Vulvar, vaginal, or fallopian tube malignancies rarely cause bleeding as a significant symptom, but cervical or uterine malignancies frequently cause bleeding. An estrogen-producing ovarian tumor could result in bleeding through estrogen stimulation of the endometrium.

There are 33,000 new cases of endometrial adenocarcinoma each year. The median age at diagnosis is 61. Postmenopausal bleeding must be considered as endometrial adenocarcinoma until proven otherwise. Risk factors for endometrial adenocarcinoma are obesity, nulliparity, late menopause, hypertension, and diabetes.

Women with prolonged exposure to unopposed estrogen are at increased risk of developing adenocarcinoma. This may occur through exogenous administration, such as hormone replacement of estrogen without a progestin, or through prolonged anovulation. Women who are anovulatory secondary to polycystic ovary syndrome have an increased risk of developing endometrial cancer. Endometrial malignancy usually occurs in the postmenopausal period, but 20 to 25% of cases occur in premenopausal women and 5% are diagnosed in women under the age of 40.

Bleeding may come from another site and may be confused with uterine bleeding. A careful history and physical should distinguish these cases. Bleeding from the urinary or gastrointestinal tracts should always be ruled out.

PATHOPHYSIOLOGY OF DYSFUNCTIONAL UTERINE BLEEDING

Alterations in the normal hormonal sequence of the menstrual cycle can result in dysfunctional bleeding. There are three types of hormonal changes resulting in bleeding: estrogen withdrawal, estrogen breakthrough, and progestin breakthrough.

An example of estrogen withdrawal is midcycle bleeding. The fall in estrogen just before ovulation may be enough to cause bleeding in some women. This type of bleeding is also seen after surgical removal of the ovaries. This type of bleeding resolves with addition of estrogen.

Estrogen breakthrough bleeding may be the mechanism in the patient with prolonged amenorrhea followed by profuse bleeding. When there is anovulation and failure of the corpus luteum to develop, there is no progesterone produced, and estrogen stimulation of the endometrium continues. Unopposed estrogen stimulation results in disorderly, vascular, and fragile tissue. The structure of the endometrium is unstable, necrosis eventually occurs, and bleeding follows. This does not occur uniformly. As hemostasis occurs in one area through vasoconstriction and platelet plugging, another area may start to bleed. Continued unopposed estrogen can eventually result in hyperplasia or endometrial cancer.

Progestin breakthrough bleeding can be found in women who have been on long-term progestin therapy, such as with Depo-Provera or Norplant. In these patients, the ratio of progestin to estrogen is too high, the endometrium becomes atrophic, and bleeding occurs at irregular intervals. This type of bleeding also responds well to estrogen therapy.

Prostaglandins play a role in the control of bleeding and hemostasis in the endometrium. Prostacyclin is associated with decreased platelet aggregation, whereas thromboxane is associated with increased platelet aggregation. The normal menstrual cycle has a concurrent rise in both PGE_2 and $PGF_{2\alpha}$. The ratio of the vasoconstrictor $PGF_{2\alpha}$ to PGE_2, a vasodilator, increases during menses. Women with ovulatory dysfunctional uterine bleeding have imbalances in prostaglandins. In these women, there is a disproportionate increase in the concentration of PGE_2, causing vasodilation to predominate. This may result in menorrhagia.

EVALUATION OF ABNORMAL UTERINE BLEEDING

A thorough history is the first step in evaluating a patient with abnormal uterine bleeding. Medical, gynecologic, family, and menstrual histories are obtained and a sexual history and details of current contraceptive use. Details regarding the character of bleeding should be elucidated, including the time of onset, duration of bleeding, frequency of bleeding, interval between bleeds, and the presence of intermenstrual bleeding. The pattern of bleeding, regular or irregular, should be noted. The patient should attempt to estimate the severity of the bleeding, although the patient's estimation of blood loss is usually poor. If the patient reports large clots or greater than 7 days of bleeding, it is safe to assume true menorrhagia. The patient should be asked about any associated symptoms, such as pain. It is helpful for the patient to keep a written menstrual diary. Consideration should be given to the occurrence of any trauma or sexual abuse. A patient who describes other sites of bleeding, such as gingival bleeding, epistaxis, or easy bruising, may have a bleeding disorder. The patient should be asked about their diet and any recent weight loss or gain. Clues that may point to an eating disorder include counting calories, excessive exercise, or distorted body image, such as the very thin patient who feels she is obese. Strenuous exercise can cause anovulation with resulting estrogen breakthrough bleeding. The history can help determine if the patient is ovulatory or anovulatory. If she describes regular intervals of bleeding, preceded by moliminal symptoms, she is likely to be ovulatory.

A focused physical examination should be performed, keeping in mind the information obtained during the history. Vital signs are important to rule out hypovolemia. The general examination should include palpation of the thyroid gland and breast examination. Hirsutism or acne would suggest hyperandrogenism. Galactorrhea would point to hyperprolactinemia. Bruises or petechiae may suggest a bleeding disorder, thrombocytopenia, or platelet dysfunction. Evidence of an eating disorder may suggest hypothalamic dysfunction. Clues to this diagnosis on physical examination include low weight, callouses on the back of the hand secondary to induced vomiting, and/or orange palms from a diet consisting of vegetables high in beta-carotene. The patient with anorexia nervosa may exhibit hypotension and bradycardia. Bulimics may also have cardiac arrhythmias and/or enlarged parotid glands. Patients with polycystic ovarian disease typically are obese and hirsute, although this is not true in all cases. Physical findings in the patient with Cushing's syndrome include truncal obesity, purple striae, moon facies, and a "buffalo hump." Proximal muscle weakness is also common and can be noted by observing difficulty when the patient rises from her chair.

The next step in the evaluation is a pelvic examination. The vulva, vagina, and cervix should be inspected carefully to rule out a traumatic lesion, foreign body, or tumor. Inspection of the cervix may reveal evidence of a cervicitis, cervical erosion, or a cervical polyp. A current Papanicolaou smear needs to be documented, and cultures of the cervix for gonorrhea and chlamydia can may be helpful. On bimanual examination, evidence of an enlarged or irregularly shaped uterus and any adnexal mass should be sought. An irregular shape might indicate fibroids, whereas a diffusely enlarged tender uterus is often associated with adenomyosis. Cervical motion tenderness would point to infection.

Laboratory studies should be individualized for each patient. Initial studies for all patients should include a hemoglobin/hematocrit; platelet count; and, in all reproductive-age women, a urine β human chorionic gonadotropin (β-hCG). Modern immunoassays are sensitive to the level of 20 to 50 IU/L. This level is sufficient to detect a pregnancy as early as the first missed menses. Serum iron or a serum ferritin level to assess iron stores may be helpful to confirm a suspected iron-deficiency anemia. A mean corpuscular volume less than 80 indicates a microcytic anemia. In a patient where a coagulopathy is suspected, platelets, prothrombin time, activated partial thromboplastin time, and a bleeding time are helpful. These studies will detect almost all blood dyscrasias. Thyroid-stimulating hormone (TSH) level should be checked in the patient with symptoms suggesting hypothyroidism. In an asymptomatic patient, an elevated ultrasensitive TSH level is suggestive of hypothyroidism, which has also been associated with abnormal uterine bleeding. It is unusual for a young healthy woman in her teens to mid-30s to have an ultrasensitive TSH level greater than 3.5 μIU/mL. A level higher than this is suggestive of subclinical hypothyroidism and should be further evaluated with more extensive thyroid testing. A patient with suspected anovulation should have TSH and prolactin levels drawn. A prolactin level should also be checked in a woman with galactorrhea. Liver function tests, blood urea nitrogen, and creatinine levels can be ordered to rule out liver or renal disease. The patient with evidence of hyperandrogenism, such as hirsutism, should have dehydroepiandrosterone sulfate, testosterone, and 17-hydroxyprogesterone levels checked. Polycystic ovarian disease is often, but not always, characterized by a luteinizing hormone:follicle-stimulating hormone ratio of 3:1. An elevated FSH level of at least 30 IU/L would indicate premature ovarian failure in a woman less than 40 years of age. In a patient with suspected Cushing's syndrome, the best test to detect this is a 24-hour urinary free cortisol, although a dexamethasone suppression test may be more reliable in a potentially noncompliant patient.

IMAGING STUDIES

Helpful imaging studies include transvaginal ultrasound, hysterosalpingogram, saline infusion sonogram, and office diagnostic hysteroscopy.

Ultrasound

Transvaginal ultrasound is a quick and well-tolerated examination. This can be used to assess the structure of the uterus and examine the adnexa and to measure the thickness of the endometrial stripe. Transvaginal ultrasound is performed using a 5.0-MHz transvaginal probe. The transabdominal ultrasound may provide more information about the body of the uterus when there is an enlarged uterus secondary to adenomyosis or fibroids. In a postmenopausal woman with bleeding, an endometrial stripe with a maximal thickness of greater than 5 mm is suspicious for endometrial hyperplasia (10, 11). A thinner stripe (less than 4 mm) is associated with endometrial atrophy, which is a primary cause of uterine bleeding in postmenopausal women (11, 12). Evaluation of the endometrial stripe thickness in a postmenopausal woman may be helpful in determining those who would benefit from endometrial sampling, especially in those women in whom office sampling was not possible. In a study of 205 women with postmenopausal bleeding, Granberg et al. (11) concluded that screening with transvaginal ultrasound and using a cutoff of 5 mm results in a positive predictive value of 87% in identification of endometrial abnormality. Use of 5 mm as a cutoff for curettage would have avoided invasive procedures in 70% of these women. Many other studies comparing the use of transvaginal ultrasound with hysteroscopy and endometrial sampling have confirmed its benefit as a screening tool, especially in postmenopausal women with bleeding. An abnormal or inconclusive ultrasound should be followed by further evaluation of the uterine cavity and endometrial sampling (13, 14).

Saline Infusion Sonography

Saline infusion sonography, or sonohysterography, is a variation of transvaginal ultrasound where saline is injected into the endometrial cavity to provide contrast to the endometrium and also to distend the uterine cavity. The examination is well tolerated by patients without the use of anesthesia, with most reporting little or no discomfort. After placement of a speculum, the cervix is washed, and a thin plastic catheter, such as a Soule's insemination catheter, is advanced through the cervical canal to the fundus using a long Kelly clamp or forceps. This catheter is only 5.3 Fr, and no cervical dilation is required for insertion. The speculum is removed, a transvaginal ultrasound probe is positioned, and a small amount of saline, approximately 30 to 60 mL, is then injected into the cavity while observing with real-time ultrasound. Patients with recent endometrial biopsies or a history of pelvic infection(s) may warrant prophylactic antibiotics, although this is not advocated in all cases. Occasionally, especially in grand multiparous patients, a hysterosalpingogram balloon catheter must be used to prevent leakage of the saline through the cervical os and to allow adequate distention of the uterine cavity. The inflation of the balloon causes a moderate degree of discomfort. Usually, if the use of this catheter is anticipated, premedication with a nonsteroidal drug is beneficial. Indications for saline infusion sonography include further evaluation of abnormal or inconclusive results on transvaginal ultrasound or hysterosalpingogram and evaluation of menorrhagia not responsive to medical therapy.

Goldstein (15) reported a series of 21 perimenopausal women undergoing saline infusion sonography in 1994. They were able to reliably distinguish between women with minimal endometrial tissue whose bleeding could be treated with hormonal therapy and women with significant tissue who required further evaluation with biopsy. They could also reliably distinguish between endometrial polyps and submucous myomas, something transvaginal ultrasound alone had not been able to do well (Fig. 10.1). They concluded saline infusion sonography could eliminate the need for diagnostic hysteroscopy. Saline infusion sonography can be used to triage these patients to either operative or medical treatment. Cullinan et al. (16) described saline infusion sonography as the most accurate technique for detecting submucous myomas and for the evaluation of their size, location, and intrauterine extension. This is very useful information to have before attempting surgical excision of the myoma and also for determining the procedure of choice.

Widrich et al. (17) compared the results of saline infusion sonography with of-

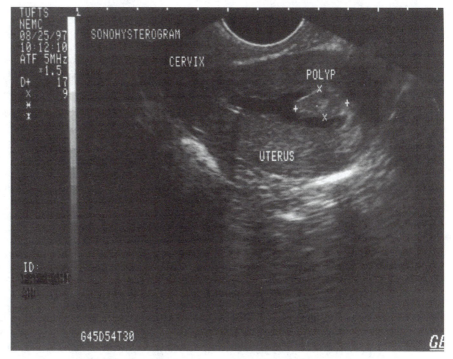

FIGURE 10.1. Sonohysterogram depicting a submucosal polyp.

fice hysteroscopy in a group of 130 women. They found the sensitivity of saline infusion sonography to be 96% and the specificity to be 88%. The findings and diagnoses were not significantly different between the two methods. The saline infusion sonogram was an accurate and well-tolerated method for evaluation of dysfunctional uterine bleeding. Saline infusion sonography caused less discomfort for patients than office hysteroscopy. This study indicates that saline infusion sonography is an especially helpful study for physicians who do not have office hysteroscopy available to them. In this regard, the use of saline infusion sonography could decrease the need for an invasive operating room procedure.

Hysterosalpingogram

Hysterosalpingogram is a study using contrast dye to fill the uterine cavity and fallopian tube lumens while observing with fluoroscopy. The primary indication for hysterosalpingogram is assessment of tubal patency in the infertile patient, although information about the uterine cavity is also provided. Hysterosalpingogram is an excellent way to diagnose uterine malformations. Other defects of the uterine cavity, such as myomas, polyps, or synechiae, can also be diagnosed, although these defects may have similar appearances.

After placement of a speculum, the cervix is cleansed and then numbed with a 2% lidocaine jelly or an analgesic spray (Hurricane spray). The anterior lip of the cervix is grasped with a single-tooth tenaculum. A Jarcho cannula is then advanced through the cervix and held firmly in place. Alternatively, a special hysterography cannula or pediatric Foley may be advanced through the cervix to inject the dye. These devices have small balloons that may obscure part of the cavity and should be avoided, if possible. An oil- or water-based dye may be used. The dye should be injected slowly. Approximately 3 to 6 mL of dye will fill the uterus and tubes. The injection of dye may cause the patient some cramping. This can be diminished by taking a prostaglandin synthetase inhibitor 30 minutes before the procedure. Straightening the uterus by pulling down on the cervix or pushing the cervix into the abdominal cavity may be helpful to see the entire uterine cavity. It is imperative that a trained gynecologist perform the procedure for rapid assessment of this nonstatic test and for patient comfort. Visualizing the uterine cavity during the initial instillation of dye offers the most information. As more dye fills the uterine cavity, small polyps, fibroids, or synechiae may be obscured. In a series of 139 patients, preoperative hysterosalpingogram and hysteroscopy were compared with pathologic findings at the time of surgery. Only 50% of the hysterosalpingogram findings were correct, whereas 86% of the hysteroscopic findings were correct (18). Frequently, abnormal hysterosalpingograms must be followed by hysteroscopy or sonohysterography for definitive diagnosis. Hysteroscopy and sonohysterography are superior to hysterosalpingography in the diagnosis of uterine pathology causing abnormal bleeding (19).

Hysteroscopy

Diagnostic office hysteroscopy has become an important tool for the physician evaluating abnormal uterine bleeding. It allows direct visualization of the uterine cavity, with accurate detection of endometrial polyps and submucous fibroids. Hysteroscopy is useful to rule out an anatomic cause for abnormal bleeding in a woman who has failed medical treatment of dysfunctional bleeding. It is contraindicated only in women who have a history of recent or current pelvic infection or are pregnant. Unfortunately, office hysteroscopy may not be available to all physicians.

Operative hysteroscopy is usually performed in an operating room under regional or general anesthesia. Instruments available include scissors, biopsy forceps, or graspers. Electrosurgical instruments include the rollerball or bar, which provides a uniform coagulating current, and the loop electrode, which can be used to shave the endometrium or fibroid(s). Additionally, the fiberoptic laser can be used through the hysteroscope. Further discussion of operative hysteroscopy as treatment can be found later in this chapter.

The rigid hysteroscope is the most commonly used hysteroscope and is the preferred type for operative procedures. The rigid diagnostic hysteroscope is 3 to 5.5 mm in diameter and approximately 25 cm long. A small amount of cervical dilatation may be required for the 5- to 5.5 mm scopes. The operative hysteroscope is 5.5 to 8 mm in diameter and requires dilation of the cervix. The lens on the hysteroscope may have a 0°, 12°, 20°, or 30° angle. The 30° lens allows an expanded field of view with rotation of the hysteroscope. The 12° scope is preferred by many physicians because of its panoramic view of the uterine cavity, often helpful when doing extensive ablation procedures, teaching residents, or learning hysteroscopy for the first time. The flexible hysteroscope is smaller in diameter (approximately 3 mm) and may be more comfortable for the patient. This may have an operative channel to allow directed biopsies; however, more extensive procedures are limited. The view with a flexible hysteroscope is less panoramic, yet most newer scopes have a flexible distal tip that allows the operator to visualize difficult areas in the cornua. A third type of hysteroscope is the contact hysteroscope. This is a rigid scope, consisting of a single glass column, which requires direct contact with the tissue. No distention medium or fiberoptic light source is required. The panoramic view is not possible with this hysteroscope.

Hysteroscopy can be safely performed in an office setting. If possible, hysteroscopy should be performed in the early to mid proliferative phase because the endometrium is thinner at this time. Bimanual examination reveals the position of the uterus, which helps to avoid perforation of the uterus with the hysteroscope. Office hysteroscopy can often be performed without any anesthesia; however, some patients may require local anesthesia or light sedation with diazepam. After a speculum is placed in the vagina, the cervix is washed with Betadine or a bacteriocidal soap. Cervical anesthesia can then be administered by paracervical block or topical application of 2% xylocaine jelly or Hurricane spray. The paracervical block is performed using approximately 10 mL of 1% lidocaine. With a small needle, 1% lidocaine with epinephrine is infiltrated submucosally at the junction of the vagina and cervix at 5, 7, 10, and 2 o'clock. Before injection, the needle is pulled back to avoid intravascular injection. Once the anesthetic has been injected, it takes several minutes for it to take its full effect.

The tip of the hysteroscope should be inserted just into the cervical canal. The distention medium should be allowed to distend the canal and uterine cavity as the scope is slowly advanced under direct visualization. In our experience, most uterine perforations occur when the hysteroscope is inserted blindly, and we have thus adopted the direct visualization technique. The mucosa of the canal should be inspected because a cervical polyp may be a cause of bleeding. Once the cavity is reached, careful survey of the entire cavity is performed. Both tubal ostia should be visualized.

Carbon dioxide is the traditional distention medium of choice in the office setting, although fluid distention may be used. If using carbon dioxide, a Hysteroflator is required to measure the flow rate of the gas and the intrauterine pressure. The flow rate required is between 40 and 60 mL/min. The normal intrauterine pressure required is 40 to 60 mm Hg, although if the tubes are blocked bilaterally, the intrauterine pressure may rise to 200 mm Hg. The advantages of carbon dioxide include its rapid absorption and relative safety. One disadvantage is the loss of the view with bleeding or bubbles. There is also a very rare risk of embolism and circulatory collapse if there are exposed blood vessels. The risk of embolism is reduced through the use of the Hysteroflator, which limits flow to less than 100 mL/min and keeps intrauterine pressure below 200 mm Hg (20). If the gas is leaking through the cervix, the tenaculum can be replaced to narrow the cervical os. Currently, many diagnostic hysteroscopes allow for fluid distention either with a intravenous tubing set up to a fluid bag and then to the inflow port or via instillation directly with a fluid-filled syringe into the inflow port. Usually, only a minimal amount of fluid is used, and the threat for fluid overload is minimal.

Fluid distention media are more often used for operative hysteroscopy, including electrolyte solutions, such as normal saline or lactated Ringer's, and nonelectrolyte solutions, such as 1.5% glycine or high-molecular-weight dextran (Hyskon). The electrolyte solutions are used for diagnostic procedures, but when bleeding occurs, the solution and blood mix, making visualization difficult. Extensive continuous flushing is required to avoid this problem. Also, operative procedures using electrocautery cannot be performed because electrolyte solutions conduct electricity. The nonelectrolyte solutions can be used for diagnostic and operative procedures and do not conduct electrical current. Bleeding is less likely to cause visualization problems because the solution and blood do not mix. Usually only small amounts of dextran solution are required. Excess absorption of dextran can lead to pulmonary edema and disseminated intravascular coagulation.

Observation of fluid intake and output is always important. A fluid deficit of 1000 mL or more with any hypotonic solution is associated with a significant risk of fluid overload and hyponatremia. This is usually associated with long operative procedures or those involving resection of large amounts of tissue. In continuous flow systems, the outflow port should be attached directly to the suction canisters. Attaching the suction tubing only to the drape "catch bag" often leads to erroneous results because a lot of fluid may end up on the floor or on sheets/drapes. Many companies offer fluid management systems that monitor the amount of fluid deficit and display the number directly onto the operative screen. These instruments are worth the investment. Electrolytes should be checked in the recovery room in any patient where fluid overload is suspected. Hyponatremia can lead to cerebral edema, seizures, and/or death. Treatment with furosemide may be necessary in severe cases, but in an otherwise healthy woman, diuresis occurs in a matter of hours with normalization of electrolytes. Measurement of preoperative electrolytes is not needed because it is the absolute sodium level that is critical rather than sodium change.

Complications of hysteroscopy are uncommon. In addition to the complications related to the distention media that have already been mentioned, possible complications include perforation of the uterus or infection. Perforation can be avoided by never advancing the hysteroscope without good visualization at the tip. If bleeding has occurred, advancement should be avoided until the view has cleared with the flow of the distention media. A midline perforation of the uterus rarely causes any further problems, but a lateral perforation can result in damage to major vessels and significant bleeding, requiring further surgery. If perforation occurs while using an operative instrument, damage to the bowel or bladder may occur. If hysteroscopy is not performed in a woman with suspected pelvic infection, infection after the procedure is rare. Any woman who is at risk for bacterial endocarditis should receive prophylactic antibiotics. In a study of 276 patients, Gimpelson and Rappold (21) reported that hysteroscopy with directed biopsy revealed more accurate results than dilation and curettage (D&C) of the uterine cavity. Hysteroscopy and curettage agreed in 223 cases, and hysteroscopy provided more information in an additional 44 cases. Of these cases, 236 hysteroscopies were performed in the office setting. Office hysteroscopy is a safe, well-tolerated, and rapid examination that can be used as a first-line diagnostic modality. In a series of 149 patients, Towbin et al. (22) found a higher sensitivity and specificity compared with transvaginal ultrasound in the diagnosis of pathology (79% versus 54% and 93% versus 90%). These numbers were determined by comparing the results of ultrasound and hysteroscopy with pathology specimens obtained at subsequent procedures. Fedele et al. (23) found that mapping of myomas is more precise with ultrasound than hysteroscopy but that ultrasound was poor in distinguishing a myoma from a polyp. The combination of examinations can then help the physician determine whether a fibroid can be removed by hysteroscopy or whether it requires abdominal myomectomy or hysterectomy.

ENDOMETRIAL SAMPLING

Endometrial sampling is indicated in any patient where there is concern regarding the possibility of endometrial hyperplasia or endometrial adenocarcinoma. The risk factors for endometrial adenocarcinoma include obesity, advancing age, nulliparity, hypertension, and diabetes mellitus. A patient of any age who has had prolonged exposure to unopposed estrogen is at risk for endometrial hyperplasia and should undergo endometrial sampling. This includes a patient with prolonged anovulation due to polycystic ovarian syndrome or other causes or a patient who has received estrogen replacement without progestin. The patient with polycystic ovarian syndrome has a threefold increased risk of developing endometrial adenocarcinoma over her lifetime. An obese woman may have excessive peripheral production of estrogen. Another source of excessive estrogen could be an estrogen-secreting tumor of the ovary or adrenal. Also, any woman over 35 with abnormal uterine bleeding deserves an endometrial biopsy because 20 to 25% of cases of endometrial carcinoma occur in patients before menopause. In postmenopausal women with bleeding, one study found 7% had endometrial adenocarcinoma and 15% had endometrial hyperplasia upon sampling (24).

In the past, D&C was the main method of sampling the endometrium. Development of office sampling techniques, using small, flexible, disposable devices, has largely replaced this procedure as a method of histologic evaluation. D&C can miss lesions, such as polyps or submucous fibroids, 10% of the time (25). Gimpelson and Rappold (21) found that 47 lesions were missed in 512 hysterectomies done after D&C, for a false-negative rate of 10%. Stock and Kanbour (26) examined 50 hysterectomy specimens done after curettage and found inadequate sampling in most specimens. Less than one half of the endometrial surface was sampled in 60% of hysterectomy specimens.

Various disposable biopsy devices using suction are available. The Pipelle and Z-sampler are the most convenient and create suction by removal of an internal piston (27). The Vabra aspirator requires an electric suction unit. Other devices generate suction through a syringe attachment. The Vabra aspirator, one of the earliest office techniques, was compared with the D&C and was found to obtain adequate tissue for diagnosis and to cost less, to be more convenient, and to be associated with fewer complications, such as hemorrhage, perforation, or infection (28). Grimes (28) compared 13,598 diagnostic D&Cs with 5951 Vabra suction biopsies and found the suction device to be less expensive; more convenient, safe, and accurate; and with fewer complications. One study comparing the Vabra aspirator with the Pipelle found each device obtained sufficient tissue for correct diagnosis in 89% of women, but the Pipelle was less painful and obtained more tissue (29). D&C is associated with higher complication rates, such as hemorrhage, infection, and perforation. McElin et al. (30) reported uterine perforation in 0.63% of patients undergoing D&C. The perforation rate with endometrial biopsy is only 0.1 to 0.2% (31). Prophylaxis for bacterial endocarditis is not required for endometrial biopsy (32).

The endometrial biopsy is performed in the office setting and, if done correctly, should be of minimal discomfort for a short period of time to the patient. Office sampling is more convenient for the patient and physician than D&C in the operating room. Sampling devices currently available cause minimal discomfort. The office endometrial biopsy may not be possible in some women who have developed cervical stenosis or who cannot tolerate the examination. In these cases, women should then undergo sampling by hysteroscopy and D&C. A negative pregnancy test is required before endometrial sampling in a woman of reproductive age. After placement of the speculum, the cervix is prepped in a sterile manner. A topical anesthetic, such as xylocaine jelly or Hurricane spray, is then applied to both the exocervix and endocervix. A tenaculum is placed on the anterior lip. The biopsy instrument, such as the Pipelle, is then advanced through the cervical canal to the fundus. The Pipelle is only 3.1 mm in diameter and therefore does not require any cervical dilation. The insertion and activation may cause some cramping, which can be decreased by taking an antiprostaglandin before the procedure. The piston is then removed, pulling tissue into the cannula. The Pipelle is then rotated as it is removed from the uterine cavity. Once the Pipelle is inserted into the cavity, it should not take longer than 10 seconds to complete the procedure. Always make sure that enough tissue is obtained for an adequate pathologic analysis; it is always easier to take more time to get more tissue than to bring the patient back for a repeat procedure. The tissue is then placed in formalin. Multiple areas of endometrium should have a biopsy taken when trying to diagnose hyperplasia or adenocarcinoma.

TREATMENT OF ABNORMAL UTERINE BLEEDING

Treatment should be individualized to the diagnoses made after history, physical, laboratory, and imaging studies. The goals of management include stopping the bleeding, correcting any resultant anemia, and preventing recurrence. Whenever anemia is diagnosed, oral supplementation of iron should be started. Management of abnormal uterine bleeding depends on the suspected etiology and the age of the patient. If a specific cause for abnormal bleeding can be identified, then treatment should center around that cause. The management of selected causes of abnormal bleeding are discussed.

Ectopic pregnancies can cause life-threatening intraabdominal hemorrhage and often require surgical management. When ectopic pregnancies are identified early, they can be managed with methotrexate. Other complications of pregnancy such as abortion may require D&C or may be managed expectantly. Trophoblastic disease requires D&C and may require chemotherapy for complete treatment. Systemic diseases are managed depending on the underlying cause. Long-term problems with abnormal bleeding related to chronic disease can be controlled well with a progestin-releasing IUD. In the case of a blood dyscrasia, the patient should be referred to a hematologist. The treatment of the most common form of von Willebrand's disease is desmopressin, a synthetic analog of arginine vasopressin. It is supplied in an intranasal or intravenous form. The intranasal form can be self-administered by the patient. No blood products are necessary, avoiding the transmission of blood-borne infections. Idiopathic thrombocytopenic purpura may be managed with corticosteroids, intravenous immunoglobulin, or splenectomy, depending on the severity of the disease.

Abnormal bleeding caused by the use of a specific medication should resolve once the offending drug is discontinued. Progestin-only contraceptive use is sometimes complicated by breakthrough bleeding. Adding estrogen controls the bleeding. For example, conjugated estrogens, 1.25 mg/day, or estradiol, 2 mg/day, for 7 days controls breakthrough bleeding in a patient receiving Depo-Provera or Norplant.

Endometrial hyperplasia without atypia can be treated with progestins. The patient should be cycled with 10 mg of medroxyprogesterone acetate (Provera), or a similar progestin, for 12 days/mo, or 5 mg of Provera for 14 days/mo. This should be done for 3 months and then another biopsy of the endometrium should be taken. A patient who has endometrial hyperplasia with atypia should undergo a hysteroscopy with curettage to rule out coexisting adenocarcinoma. In patients with atypical hyperplasia, the risk of coexisting adenocarcinoma is approximately 35% (9). If possible, the patient should be managed surgically because this will more likely progress to endometrial cancer. If the patient refuses hysterectomy or desires future fertility, she should be managed aggressively with high-dose progestins and undergo endometrial biopsy every 3 months. Commonly used progestin regimens for this situation include medroxyprogesterone acetate (Provera), 30 mg/day, or megestrol (Megace), 20 mg/day.

Structural causes of bleeding, such as a polyps or myoma, can be removed surgically. Removal of endometrial polyps and submucous fibroids can be accomplished through hysteroscopic resection. Fibroid removal can be achieved through hysteroscopic myomectomy, transabdominal myomectomy, or by hysterectomy. In the case of myomectomy, pretreatment with a gonadotropin-releasing hormone (GnRH) agonist allows any current anemia to resolve, shrink the fibroid, induce endometrial atrophy, and decrease the risk of bleeding during the procedure in those cases with multiple large fibroids. The decreased blood loss may not be of clinical significance (e.g., need for blood transfusion), but preoperative use of GnRH agonists does seem to be of benefit if the pretreatment uterine volume is greater than 600 cm^3 (33). Some surgeons do not recommend using a GnRH agonist preoperatively, claiming that it alters the fibroid's pseudocapsule, thus making it harder to dissect out during a myomectomy.

Treatment of dysfunctional uterine bleeding can be divided into surgical and nonsurgical methods. Once other causes of bleeding have been ruled out, dysfunctional uterine bleeding can almost always be managed medically.

Medical Treatment of Abnormal Uterine Bleeding

Hormonal Treatment

Heavy uterine bleeding in the patient who is not hemodynamically unstable may be treated with high-dose estrogens. Treatment with high-dose estrogen allows rapid regrowth of endometrium. High-dose estrogen acts to increase fibrinogen and factors V and IX; it also promotes aggregation of platelets and clotting at the capillary level. DeVore et al. (34) published a randomized prospective trial comparing intravenous Premarin with placebo in the treatment of abnormal bleeding. In patients with suspected dysfunctional uterine bleeding, bleeding stopped more rapidly in the women treated with intravenous Premarin. They found significantly more patients' bleeding resolved after the second dose of Premarin, with doses given 3 hours apart, than with placebo.

Intravenous administration of high-dose conjugated estrogen (Premarin) is as efficacious as oral intake of high-dose estrogen. Intravenously, the dose is 25 mg every 4 hours until the bleeding stops. The oral regimen may be given as 1.25 mg conjugated estrogen (Premarin) or 2 mg estradiol (Estrace) every 4 hours for 24 hours; it is then given as a single daily dose for 7 to 10 days. If bleeding continues past 12 to 24 hours, a D&C is indicated. A progestin needs to be started at the same time as the high-dose estrogen. The progestin should be continued for 5 to 10 days, after which the patient should expect a withdrawal bleed. After the withdrawal bleed, the patient should be cycled on oral contraceptive pills or medroxyprogesterone acetate (Provera), 10 mg/day orally, for 10 days a month. Complications of high-dose estrogen treatment include the increased risk of thrombosis. The risks and benefits of high-dose estrogen for heavy bleeding in patients with a history of thrombosis must be weighed carefully by the patient and her physician. High-dose estrogen may cause nausea and vomiting in some patients, which can be avoided with concurrent use of antiemetics.

Chronic dysfunctional uterine bleeding can be treated with progestins. The typical scenario for a chronically anovulatory woman is oligomenorrhea with occasional episodes of heavy bleeding. Progestins can be used to stop a heavy episode of bleeding, and continued monthly use helps to regulate cycles and to prevent recurrence of heavy bleeding. Progestins act as antiestrogens. They stop the growth of the endometrium and promote the support and organization of estrogen-primed endometrium. When the progestin is later withdrawn, sloughing of the tissue to the basalis layer occurs. This may be a heavy bleed, but there should be rapid cessation of bleeding. Progestins stimulate the conversion of estradiol to estrone, which is less potent and rapidly excreted from the cell. Progestins also inhibit estrogen receptor augmentation, limiting the effects of estrogen on the endometrial tissue.

Patients should be cycled monthly with medroxyprogesterone acetate using 10 mg/day orally for 10 days a month. This results in an organized shedding of the endometrium, the "medical curettage." If patients are placed on long-term continuous progestins, the side effects may include fatigue, weight gain, mood changes, and changes in lipid profile. Cyclic progestins can be used to regulate menses in women with oligomenorrhea and with menorrhagia.

Women can also be cycled on oral contraceptive pills, which is especially useful if contraception is desired. During the initial episode of bleeding, the cessation of bleeding can be induced by dosing of the oral contraceptive, one pill two to four times daily for 5 to 7 days, with the flow usually stopping on days 2 to 4 of treatment. This should be followed by a withdrawal bleed, and then standard cycling of the oral contraceptive can be started, one pill daily for at least three cycles. Variations of the dosing tapers have been described. We tend to judge the severity of the bleeding, starting with one pill four times daily for heavy bleeding and two pills daily for mild bleeding and continuing this regimen until the bleeding lessens, usually in 48 hours. Once the bleeding has decreased, the medication is tapered down over the ensuing 7 days, until patients are on one pill a day. Nausea is also a problem on this regimen, and an antiemetic is often invaluable for compliance. When oral contraceptives are continued for the long term, the amount of flow is decreased by 60% (35).

In a patient who has had prolonged bleeding, there may be a raw basalis layer. When endometrial sampling is attempted in these patients, minimal tissue is obtained. Patients who have been on long-term treatment with progestins, with either medroxyprogesterone acetate (Provera) or contraceptives such as Norplant or Depo-Provera, may experience bleeding secondary to an atrophic endometrium. The initial treatment is with estrogen to build up the endometrium. Dosing is 1.25 mg of conjugated estrogen or 2 mg oral estradiol for 7 days. When the patient with chronic anovulatory dysfunctional uterine bleeding desires pregnancy, treatment with clomiphene citrate is started. This medication induces ovulation and regulates cycles.

Intrauterine Device

Dysfunctional uterine bleeding can be treated with an IUD containing a progestin, either progesterone or levonorgestrel. The levonorgestrel IUD is not currently available in the United States, although it is used in some European countries. The progestational agent is released directly against the endometrium. With long-term use, there is a significant decrease in the amount of menstrual flow. After 12 months of use of the levonorgestrel-releasing IUD, there is a 96% decrease in flow (36). There is a 65% decrease in blood loss after 12 months use of the progesterone-releasing IUD, Progestasert (37). The progestin-releasing IUD is a good option for use in dysfunctional uterine bleeding related to chronic illness. Milsom et al. (36) compared the use of the levonorgestrel-releasing IUD, flurbiprofen (an antiprostaglandin), and tranexamic acid (an antifibrinolytic). The IUD reduced blood loss to well below 80 mL. The average monthly blood loss before treatment was 203 mL, and after 12 months of use, the average blood loss was 9 mL. Neither of the other two medications decreased the blood loss to below 80 mL.

Antiprostaglandins

Antiprostaglandins, or nonsteroidal anti-inflammatory drugs, are prostaglandin synthetase inhibitors that work by inhibiting the synthesis of cyclic endoperoxidases and by blocking the action of prostaglandins directly at their receptor sites. Several different prostaglandin inhibitors have been shown to be effective in the treatment of menorrhagia. These medications are especially useful in women with ovulatory dysfunctional uterine bleeding, where there has been a reported 20 to 50% decrease in blood loss (38, 39). How these medications work in reducing blood loss is not completely understood. These medications have the added benefit of reducing dysmenorrhea.

Compared with women who have normal menses, women with menorrhagia have higher levels of the prostaglandins PGE_2 and $PGF_{2\alpha}$ in their endometrium, with a relatively larger increase in PGE than $PGF_{2\alpha}$ (40). As mentioned previously, PGE_2 mediates vasodilation, whereas $PGF_{2\alpha}$ causes vasoconstriction. Antiprostaglandins affect the balance between PGE and $PGF_{2\alpha}$ and between thromboxane (a vasoconstrictor) and prostacyclin (a vasodilator). Treatment duration should consist of the first 3 days of menses or throughout menses. There are minimal gastrointestinal side effects with intermittent use, although their use would be contraindicated in women with existing peptic ulcer disease. Their use is also contraindicated in women with bronchospastic disease or an allergy to aspirin. Suggested regimens include mefenamic acid (Ponstel) 500 mg three times a day, ibuprofen (Motrin, Advil, Nuprin, Rufen) 400 mg three times a day, meclofenamate sodium (Meclomen) 100 mg three times a day, or naproxen sodium (Anaprox) 275 mg every 6 hours after a loading dose of 550 mg.

Vargyas et al. (38) conducted a double-blind, placebo-controlled, crossover study looking at the use of antiprostaglandins in the treatment of women with menorrhagia. The antiprostaglandin used in this study was meclofenamate sodium, which was given 100 mg orally three times a day. Mean blood loss decreased from 141 to 69 mL during treatment cycles. A reduction in blood loss was documented in 26 of 29 patients (38).

Other Medications

GnRH agonists induce a "medical menopause." They are good for short-term use, but long-term use results in hypoestrogenism, causing hot flushes and eventually osteoporosis. If use is continued after 6 months, add-back therapy with estrogen is required to prevent bone loss. Once add-back therapy is started, however, the control of the abnormal bleeding may not be as good. GnRH agonists are available in injectable, intranasal, or subcutaneous implant forms. The depot injectable forms are effective for 1 to 3 months. The subcutaneous implant is good for 1 month and will resorb into the tissue, eliminating the need for removal. The intranasal form is the most cost-effective method and, because of its short duration of action, allows the patient to discontinue its use with no lingering side effects. However, it may not be the best choice for a noncompliant patient.

Danazol (Danocrine) is an androgenic steroid that results in marked reduction of blood loss but is expensive and has significant side effects. The most common side effects limiting the use of danazol include weight gain and acne. Irreversible deepening of the voice has also been reported. It has adverse effects on the lipid profile, causing a decrease in high-density lipoprotein and an elevation in low-density lipoprotein. The usual dosage is 200 to 400 mg/day for 12 weeks (41). One advantage of danazol, compared with GnRH agonists, is its bone-sparing properties.

Ergot derivatives are used effectively in postpartum hemorrhage but have no effect in the nonpregnant uterus. Nilsson and Rybo (35) demonstrated the lack of improvement in blood loss with the use of methylergobaseimmaleate, a compound similar to methylergonovine maleate (Methergine), in dysfunctional uterine bleeding.

Antifibrinolytics are strong inhibitors of fibrinolysis. Examples include ϵ-aminocaproic acid (Amicar), tranexamic acid, and para-aminomethylbenzoic acid. In the same study by Nilsson and Rybo (35), women treated with antifibrinolytic agents showed an approximately 50% decrease in blood loss. The use of these medications is limited by side effects, including nausea, dizziness, diarrhea, headache, abdominal pain, and allergic reaction. Antifibrinolytics have an associated increased risk of thrombosis and are contraindicated in women with a history of thrombotic events.

These medical therapies are frequently used in combination with hormonal methods for the best control of blood loss. For example, combining the use of oral contraceptives with antiprostaglandins results in further reduction of blood loss than either method alone.

Surgical Therapy

In a patient who is hemodynamically unstable, D&C, with or without blood transfusion, is indicated. Curettage results in quick cessation of bleeding. This procedure will not correct the underlying problem, and menorrhagia may resume as soon as the next cycle. Follow-up with subsequent medical therapy is indicated.

Surgical therapy should be considered in women who have completed childbearing when medical therapy has failed. A D&C can also be considered in the older patient where a sampling of endometrium is desired. However, blind curettage results in missing a large portion of the endometrium in most patients and may possibly miss a pathologic lesion.

Hysteroscopy

Hysteroscopy is used for diagnosis and treatment. As previously described, office hysteroscopy is used mainly for diagnostic purposes; however, more modern office hysteroscopes have added the ability to provide continuous flow of the distention media, allowing an improved operative field and the opportunity to do minor operative procedures such as polypectomies, lysis of thin adhesions, directed biopsies, and separation of septums. Operative hysteroscopy is an outpatient procedure, usually performed in the operating room under general or regional anesthesia. With the introduction of smaller diameter operative hysteroscopes (5.5 to 7 mm), many of these procedures can be done under conscious sedation. This procedure is superior to a D&C because it allows the direct visualization of the uterine cavity with identification and resection of lesions, such as myomas or polyps. Small polyps or fibroids can be removed with the use of grasping forceps and scissors, whereas the removal of larger myomas requires the use of laser or electrocautery. In resection of lesions, the excision is carried down to the level of the surrounding epithelium. If deeper resection is attempted, there is a risk of developing perforation or hemorrhage. If a deeper resection is anticipated, a laparoscopy is used to visualize the procedure. Various distention mediums have been described for use with operative hysteroscopy, including dextran 70, normal saline, Ringer's lactate, and 1.5% glycine. Electrocautery cannot be used in an electrolyte solution such as saline. The amount of solution used must be measured carefully because the absorption of a large amount can result in complications such as fluid overload or hyponatremia. A volume deficit of greater than 1000 mL has been associated with electrolyte imbalances. There are several current fluid-monitoring systems on the market that allow the operator a continuous reading of their fluid parameters during a hysteroscopic procedure, reducing substantially the risk of fluid overload. Townsend et al. (42) looked specifically at women who had postmenopausal bleeding for at least 6 months. The combination of diagnostic and operative hysteroscopy was successful in controlling postmenopausal bleeding in 90% of women who had submucous myomas and polyps.

Endometrial Ablation

Another alternative in the woman with dysfunctional uterine bleeding is endometrial ablation. The goal of endometrial ablation is to destroy the endometrium. The result is a significant reduction in the amount of bleeding or, in many women, amenorrhea. This procedure is indicated if the patient refuses hysterectomy or if there are contraindications to major surgery. Patients must also not desire any further pregnancies. However, the use of ablation in any patient who has completed childbearing is increasing. Advantages of ablation include efficacy, low morbidity, rapid recovery, and safety in high-risk patients. The cost of hysteroscopic treatment, including endometrial ablation and hysteroscopic myomectomy, is significantly less than that of hysterectomy, both abdominal and vaginal (43).

Endometrial ablation is traditionally an outpatient procedure performed in the operating room using hysteroscopic guidance. Endometrial sampling before the procedure is important to rule out malignancy. Pretreatment with drugs causing endometrial atrophy improves results. Options for pretreatment include GnRH agonists, danazol, or progestins. GnRH agonists have been reported to cause adequate endometrial atrophy with minimal edema. Pretreatment for only 1 month is usually sufficient (44). Also, a suction curettage just before ablation has been shown to be equally effective for medical pretreatment (45). In our experience, however, pretreatment with a GnRH agonist allows a more efficient surgical procedure with less residual endometrial tissue buildup on the rollerball or loop (46). Complications of the procedure are rare but include perforation, hemorrhage, and electrolyte disturbances related to excessive absorption of the distention medium. Systematic ablation of the endometrium can be accomplished under direct visualization by laser (neodymium:yttrium-aluminum-garnet laser) or thermal destruction with electrocautery, although this is cumbersome and more time consuming. Recently, a uterine balloon therapy system (Thermachoice, Gynecare, Inc., Menlo, CA) was given U.S. Food and Drug Administration approval for marketing. The system consists of a controller with power cord, a single-use sterile catheter, and umbilical cable (Fig. 10.2). A latex balloon at the end of the catheter is inserted into the uterus and filled with 2 to 30 mL of sterile 5% dextrose in water and heated to 87°C for 8 minutes. The balloon pressure is maintained at a constant 160 to 180 mm Hg. The heated balloon causes thermal ablation of the uterine lining, resulting in scarring that eliminates or reduces bleeding (Fig. 10.3). Six-month data on 245 women in the United States suggested comparable success rates to the more traditional endometrial ablation, with less skill needed and less operative time (Myer, unpublished observations). More importantly, it has the potential to be an office procedure, since only minimal sedation is needed and there is no risk for fluid overload.

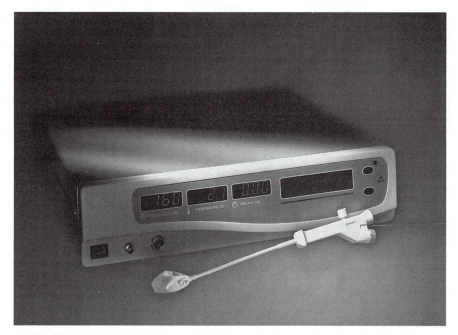

FIGURE 10.2. Thermachoice uterine balloon device (power source and catheter).

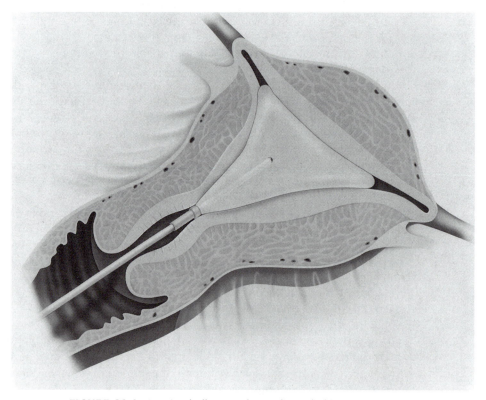

FIGURE 10.3. Uterine balloon catheter distended in uterine cavity.

Endometrial ablation done in the operative suite may be successfully accomplished using electrocautery with a wire loop resectoscope, rollerball resectoscope, or ball end electrode (47–50). The ball end electrode allows easier access to the cornual area of the uterus. Although laser ablation has been successfully used, ablation with rollerball or electrocautery is easier to learn and less time consuming to perform (47).

In recent years, several large series of patients have been published confirming safety and success with the use of endometrial ablation. Excellent results are reported in 90 to 95% of patients with the use of all techniques. A large series of patients who underwent ablation using laser was described by Garry et al. (51), who found a 92% rate of reduced or absent flow. In 1996, Baggish and Sze (52) reported the procedure as safe and reliable in a series of 568 patients (401 using laser, 167 using electrocautery). Amenorrhea was achieved in 65% of patients, and bleeding was reduced in another 30%. There was a 5% failure rate. Also in 1996, Rankin and Steinberg (53) described a series of 400 patients who underwent endometrial resection. There was no preprocedure suppression of endometrium, and the procedure was performed with electrocautery, using either a wire cutting loop or a rollerball. There was an 82% patient satisfaction rate after the procedure, with a total of 92% of patients satisfied after a second procedure. Amenorrhea was achieved in 50% of patients, and 90% reported improvement.

The long-term effects of endometrial resection are not known. There is a risk of concealing a nest of endometrium behind scar tissue, with subsequent development of a malignancy in that tissue; however, this has not been confirmed in follow-up studies (54). Careful preprocedure evaluation should minimize this risk.

Hysterectomy

A hysterectomy is a reasonable alternative in women where other pathology is associated, such as pelvic organ prolapse, fibroids, or other mass. Hysterectomy is obviously a definitive method of treatment for abnormal bleeding, but there are significant risks of morbidity and mortality (55).

TREATMENTS FOR SPECIFIC AGE GROUPS

Adolescents

Anovulatory cycles are very common in the postmenarchal period. The hypothalamic-pituitary-ovarian axis is not mature until positive feedback of estrogen on the hypothalamus develops. Until this time, cycles are anovulatory. The adolescent requiring treatment for anovulatory bleeding should receive cycling with progestins, 10 mg medroxyprogesterone acetate for 10 days a month for 3 to 6 months. The patient should be reevaluated after treatment. When the hypothalamic-pituitary-ovarian axis matures and cycles become ovulatory, treatment may no longer be needed. In the adolescent where birth control is desired, oral contraceptive pills can be used to regulate cycles.

Claessens and Cowell (56) found that 19% of adolescents who required hospitalization for heavy vaginal bleeding had a coagulopathy. Menorrhagia is frequently the first evidence of the coagulopathy. The most common diagnosis was idiopathic thrombocytopenic purpura, followed by von Willebrand's disease. Bleeding disorders are important diagnoses to consider in the adolescent age group.

Another very important diagnosis to consider in the adolescent is that of pregnancy-related complications. A serum or urine pregnancy test should always be included in the workup of an adolescent.

Reproductive Age but Anovulatory

The patient with chronic anovulation, secondary to polycystic ovarian disease or other causes, can be regulated using monthly progestins or oral contraceptive pills. The combination of two or more medical therapies may be required for adequate control of bleeding. In the anovulatory patient who desires pregnancy, ovulation can be induced using clomiphene citrate.

Perimenopause and Postmenopause

The perimenopausal or postmenopausal patient with abnormal bleeding must be considered to have endometrial adenocarcinoma until proven otherwise. Endometrial sampling must be performed in this age group. If the office biopsy is inconclusive, hysteroscopic-directed biopsies must be done. Once malignancy has been ruled out, the perimenopausal patient can be started on hormonal therapy. Anovulation is often the cause of irregular bleeding as the woman approaches menopause. These patients can be successfully treated with sequential hormone replacement consisting of 0.625 mg of conjugated estrogen on days 1 to 25 of the month and medroxyprogesterone acetate 10 mg/day on days 15 to 25. An alternative to this treatment in the nonsmoking patient is to use low-dose oral contraceptive pills. This should only be prescribed in nonsmoking patients because of the increased risk of myocardial infarction in smokers. To determine when the woman on oral contraceptive pills has passed into menopause, an FSH level should be checked on day 6 or 7 of the pill-free week. When this level is elevated, the woman can be switched to hormone replacement. Another option is to continue cyclic withdrawal, using medroxyprogesterone acetate 10 mg/day for 10 days each month until there is no evidence of a withdrawal bleed. At this point, there is no longer estrogen stimulation of the endometrium, and the woman can safely be switched over to hormone replacement therapy.

The postmenopausal woman on hormone replacement therapy who presents with abnormal bleeding always requires investigation. Although endometrial atrophy is the most common cause of bleeding in these patients, endometrial adenocarcinoma must be ruled out.

CLINICAL NOTES

- Normal menses lasts 4 to 6 days and incurs a blood loss of 20 to 60 mL. About 70% of blood loss occurs in the first 2 days. A loss of more than 80 mL may cause anemia. Ten percent of women suffer true menorrhagia.
- The diagnosis of dysfunctional uterine bleeding is a diagnosis of exclusion, made only after all other causes have been eliminated.
- Causes of abnormal bleeding include reproductive tract pathologies or malignancies, systemic diseases, coagulopathies, and various medications.
- Approximately 20% of adolescents hospitalized for menorrhagia have an underlying coagulopathy. The average blood loss in women with various coagulopathies is 400 mL per menses.
- Three types of hormonal changes result in abnormal bleeding: estrogen withdrawal (often seen as midcycle bleeding), estrogen breakthrough (seen with anovulation or unopposed estrogen), and progestin breakthrough (seen with long-term progestin therapy).
- Evaluation of abnormal bleeding includes a thorough history and physical examination, including a pelvic examination, and laboratory tests. A hemoglobin/hematocrit, platelet count, and urine β-hCG in all women of reproductive age should be done along with any individualized tests.

- Ultrasound is a useful adjunct in the evaluation of abnormal uterine bleeding. In a post-menopausal woman with bleeding, an endometrial stripe less than 4 mm thick is associated with endometrial atrophy. A thicker endometrial stripe should be further evaluated.
- Sonohysterography is a transvaginal ultrasound with infusion of normal saline into the endometrial cavity to provide contrast to and distention of the cavity. It is a useful tool to distinguish between endometrial polyps and submucous myomas.
- Endometrial sampling is indicated in any patient where there is concern regarding the possibility of endometrial hyperplasia or adenocarcinoma. A patient of any age who has had prolonged exposure to unopposed estrogen is at risk for endometrial hyperplasia and should undergo endometrial sampling. Any woman over 35 with abnormal uterine bleeding deserves an endometrial biopsy because 20 to 25% of endometrial carcinoma cases occur in patients before menopause.
- Office sampling techniques are adequate for obtaining tissue for biopsy and have fewer complications than D&C. For women who have stenosis or who are unable to tolerate the office biopsy, sampling by hysteroscopy and D&C is indicated.
- Endometrial hyperplasia without atypia can be treated with progestins such as medroxy-progesterone acetate (Provera) 5 mg for 14 days each month. Patients with atypia should undergo hysteroscopy with D&C to rule out existing adenocarcinoma. If there is no adenocarcinoma and the patient refuses surgical therapy, she may be managed with high-dose progestins such as medroxyprogesterone acetate (Provera) 30 mg/day or megestrol (Megace) 20 mg/day.
- In patients with heavy uterine bleeding but no hemodynamic instability, high-dose oral estrogen may be used. Common doses are 1.25 mg conjugated estrogen (Premarin) or 2 mg estradiol (Estrace) every 4 hours for 24 hours. It is given as a single daily dose for 7 to 10 days thereafter. Intravenous estrogen may also be used, although it is not more efficacious than oral administration. It is given as conjugated estrogen (Premarin) 25 mg every 4 hours until the bleeding stops. If bleeding continues past 12 to 24 hours, a D&C is indicated. A progestin is started at the same time as the high-dose estrogen and continued for 5 to 10 days, after which a withdrawal bleed may occur. After the withdrawal bleed, the patient should be started on either oral contraceptive pills or a monthly progestin.
- Chronic abnormal bleeding due to anovulation may be treated with monthly progestins or oral contraceptives.
- Patients with long-term treatment with progestins (atrophic bleeding) or who have had prolonged bleeding (a raw basalis layer) should be treated with estrogen for 7 to 10 days to build up the endometrium.
- Antiprostaglandins have been shown to be efficacious in the treatment of menorrhagia. Treatment should be given for the first 3 days of menses or throughout menses. Combining their use with oral contraceptives results in further reduction of blood loss than either method alone.
- In a patient who is hemodynamically unstable because of uterine bleeding, a D&C, with or without transfusion, is indicated. Although this results in cessation of the bleeding, it will not correct the underlying problem, and menorrhagia may occur again as soon as the next cycle.
- Surgical therapy should be considered in women who have completed childbearing and in whom medical therapy for dysfunctional uterine bleeding has failed. Options include hysteroscopy, endometrial ablation, or hysterectomy.
- Anovulatory cycles are common in the adolescent. Cyclic progestins or oral contraceptives may be used for treatment.
- The perimenopausal or postmenopausal patient with abnormal bleeding must be considered to have endometrial adenocarcinoma until proven otherwise. Endometrial sampling must be performed in this age group. Once malignancy or premalignant conditions have been ruled out, hormonal therapy may be considered. Anovulation is a common cause of irregular bleeding as the woman approaches menopause. Sequential hormone replacement therapy may be used, although it does *not* provide contraception, or, in appropriately selected patients, oral contraceptives may be started.

References

1. Hallberg L, Hogdahl A, Nilsson L, et al. Menstrual blood loss—a population study. Acta Obstet Gynecol Scand 1966;45:320–351.
2. Hallberg L, Nilsson L. Determination of menstrual blood loss. Scand J Clin Lab Invest 1964;16:244–248.
3. Higham JM, O'Brien PM, Shaw RW. Assessment of menstrual blood loss using a pictorial chart. Br J Obstet Gynaecol 1990;97:734–739.
4. Fraser IS, McCarron G, Markham R, et al. Blood and total fluid content of menstrual discharge. Obstet Gynecol 1985;65:194.
5. Claessens EA, Cowell CL. Acute adolescent menorrhagia. Am J Obstet Gynecol 1981;139:377.
6. Fraser IS, McCarron G, Markham R, et al. Measured menstrual blood loss in women with menorrhagia associated with pelvic disease or coagulation disorder. Obstet Gynecol 1986;68:630.
7. Hopkins MP, Androff L, Benninghoff AS. Ginseng face cream and unexplained vaginal bleeding. Am J Obstet Gynecol 1988;159:1121.
8. Ferenczy A, Gelfand M. The biologic significance of cytologic atypia in progestogen-treated endometrial hyperplasia. Am J Obstet Gynecol 1990;160:126–131.
9. Kurman RJ, Kaminski PF, Norris HJ. The behavior of endometrial hyperplasia. A long-term study of "untreated" hyperplasia in 170 patients. Cancer 1985;56:403–412.
10. Goldstein SR, Nachtigal M, Snyder JR, et al. Endometrial assessment by vaginal ultrasonography before endometrial sampling in patients with postmenopausal bleeding. Am J Obstet Gynecol 1990;163:119–123.
11. Granberg S, Wikland M, Karlsson B, et al. Endometrial thickness as measured by endovaginal ultrasonography for identifying endometrial abnormality. Am J Obstet Gynecol 1991;164:47–52.
12. Grimes D. Diagnostic dilation and curettage: a reappraisal. Am J Obstet Gynecol 1982;142:1–6.
13. Emanuel MH, Verdel MJ, Wamsteker K, et al. A prospective comparison of transvaginal ultrasonography and diagnostic hysteroscopy in the evaluation of patients with abnormal uterine bleeding: clinical implications. Am J Obstet Gynecol 1995;172:547–552.
14. Dijkhuizen FP, Brolman H, Potters AE, et al. The accuracy of transvaginal ultrasonography in the diagnosis of endometrial abnormalities. Obstet Gynecol 1996;87:345–349.
15. Goldstein SR. Use of ultrasonohysterography for triage of perimenopausal patients with unexplained uterine bleeding. Am J Obstet Gynecol 1994;170:565–570.
16. Cullinan JA, Fleischer AC, Kepple DM, et al. Sonohysterography: a technique of endometrial evaluation. Radiographics 1995;15:501–514.
17. Widrich T, Bradley LD, Mitchinson AR, et al. Comparison of saline infusion sonography with office hysteroscopy for the evaluation of the endometrium. Am J Obstet Gynecol 1996;174:1327–1334.
18. Barbot J. L'Hysteroscopie de contact. Obstet Gynecol Clin North Am 1995;22:591–602.
19. Baggish MS, Barbot J, Valle RF, eds. Diagnostic and Operative Hysteroscopy, A Text and Atlas. Chicago, IL: Year Book Medical Publishers Inc., 1989:147–155.
20. Lindeman JH, Mohr J. CO_2 hysteroscopy: diagnosis and treatment. Am J Obstet Gynecol 1976;124:129.
21. Gimpelson RJ, Rappold HO. A comparative study between panoramic hysteroscopy with directed biopsies and dilation and curettage. Am J Obstet Gynecol 1988;158:489–492.
22. Towbin NA, Gviazda IM, March CM. Office hysteroscopy versus transvaginal ultrasonography in the evaluation of patients with excessive uterine bleeding. Am J Obstet Gynecol 1996;174:1678–1682.
23. Fedele L, Bianchi S, Dorta M, et al. Transvaginal ultrasonography versus hysteroscopy in the diagnosis of uterine submucous myomas. Obstet Gynecol 1991;77:745.

24. Lidor AB, Isamajovich B, Confino E, et al. Histopathological findings in 226 women with postmenopausal uterine bleeding. Acta Obstet Gynecol Scand 1986;65:41–43.

25. Word B, Gravlee LC, Wideman GL. The fallacy of simple uterine curettage. Obstet Gynecol 1958;12:642.

26. Stock RJ, Kanbour A. Pre-hysterectomy curettage: an evaluation. Obstet Gynecol 1975;45:537.

27. Chambers JT, Chambers SK. Endometrial sampling: When? Where? Why? With what? Clin Obstet Gynecol 1992;35:28–39.

28. Grimes DA. Diagnostic dilation and curettage: a reappraisal. Am J Obstet Gynecol 1982;142:1.

29. Kaunitz AM, Masciello A, Ostrowski M, et al. Comparison of endometrial biopsy with the endometrial Pipelle and Vabra aspirator. J Reprod Med 1988;33:427.

30. McElin TW, Bird CC, Reeves BD, et al. Diagnostic dilation and curettage. Obstet Gynecol 1974;17:205.

31. Kaunitz AM, Masciello A, Ostrowski M. Comparison of endometrial biopsy with the endometrial Pipelle and Vabra aspirator. J Reprod Med 1988;33:427.

32. Dajani AS, Taubert KA, Wilson W, et al. Prevention of bacterial endocarditis: recommendations by the American Heart Association. JAMA 1997;277:22.

33. Friedman AJ, Rein MS, Harrison Atlas D. A randomized, placebo-controlled, double-blind study evaluating the efficacy of leuprolide acetate depot in the treatment of uterine leiomyomata. Fertil Steril 1989;51:251.

34. DeVore GR, Owens O, Kase N. Use of intravenous Premarin in the treatment of dysfunctional uterine bleeding—a double-blind randomized control study. Obstet Gynecol 1982;59:285–291.

35. Nilsson L, Rybo G. Treatment of menorrhagia. Am J Obstet Gynecol 1971;110:713.

36. Milsom I, Andersson K, Andersch B, et al. A comparison of flurbiprofen, tranexamic acid, and a levonorgestrel-releasing intrauterine device in the treatment of idiopathic menorrhagia. Am J Obstet Gynecol 1991;164:879–883.

37. Bergqvist A, Rybo G. Treatment of menorrhagia with intrauterine release of progesterone. Br J Obstet Gynaecol 1983;90:255–258.

38. Vargyas JM, Campeau JD, Mishell DA. Treatment of menorrhagia with meclofenamate sodium. Am J Obstet Gynecol 1987;157:944.

39. Fraser IS, Pearse C, Shearman RP, et al. Efficacy of mefenamic acid in patients with a complaint of menorrhagia. Obstet Gynecol 1981;58:543.

40. Willman EA, Collins WP, Clayton SG. Studies in the involvement of prostaglandins in uterine symptomatology and pathology. Br J Obstet Gynaecol 1976;83:337.

41. Chimbira TH, Anderson ABM, Naish C, et al. Reduction of menstrual blood loss by danazol in unexplained menorrhagia: lack of effect of placebo. Br J Obstet Gynaecol 1980;87:1152–1158.

42. Townsend DE, Fields G, McCausland A, et al. Diagnostic and operative hysteroscopy in the management of persistent postmenopausal bleeding. Obstet Gynecol 1993;82:419–421.

43. Brumsted JR, Blackman JA, Badger GJ, et al. Hysteroscopy versus hysterectomy for the treatment of abnormal uterine bleeding: a comparison of cost. Fertil Steril 1996;65:310–316.

44. Serden SP, Brooks PG. Preoperative therapy in preparation for endometrial ablation. J Reprod Med 1992;37:679–681.

45. Gimpelson RJ, Kaigh J. Mechanical preparation of the endometrium prior to endometrial ablation. J Reprod Med 1992;37:691–694.

46. Petrozza JC, DeCherney AH. Electrosurgical endometrial ablation. In: Diamond MP, Osteen KG, eds. Endometrium and Endometriosis. Malden, MA: Blackwell Science, 1997:285–293.

47. Goldrath MH, Fuller TA, Segal S. Laser photovaporization of endometrium for the treatment of menorrhagia. Am J Obstet Gynecol 1981;140:14–19.

48. DeCherney AH, Diamond MP, Lavy G, et al. Endometrial ablation for intractable uterine bleeding: hysteroscopic resection. Obstet Gynecol 1987;70:668–670.

49. Vancaille TG. Electrocoagulation of the endometrium with the ball-end resectoscope. Obstet Gynecol 1989;74:425–427.

50. Townsend DE, Richart RM, Paskowitz RA, et al. "Rollerball" coagulation of the endometrium. Obstet Gynecol 1990;76:3310–3313.

51. Garry R, Erian J, Grochmal SA. A multicenter collaborative study into the treatment of menorrhagia by Nd-YAG laser ablation of the endometrium. Br J Obstet Gynaecol 1991;98:357–362.

52. Baggish MS, Sze EH. Endometrial ablation: a series of 568 patients treated over an 11-year period. Am J Obstet Gynecol 1996;174:908–913.

53. Rankin L, Steinberg LH. Transcervical resection of the endometrium: a review of 400 consecutive patients. Br J Obstet Gynaecol 1992;99:911–914.

54. Copperman AB, DeCherney AH, Olive DL. A case of endometrial cancer following endometrial ablation for dysfunctional uterine bleeding. Obstet Gynecol 1993;82:640–642.

55. Dicker RC, Greenspan JR, Strauss LT, et al. Complications of abdominal and vaginal hysterectomy among women of reproductive age in the United States. Am J Obstet Gynecol 1992;138:880–892.

56. Claessens EA, Cowell CL. Acute adolescent menorrhagia. Am J Obstet Gynecol 1986;68:630.

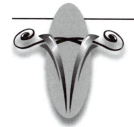

C H A P T E R   1 1

Hirsutism

STEVEN STRONG

Hirsutism describes the presence of male-pattern hair growth in a woman. Excess facial and body hair is caused by the action of androgens on androgen-sensitive hair follicles. This socially distressing complaint is commonly encountered by all practitioners who care for women. The presentation may vary in degree, distribution, and chronicity. A thorough history and physical examination, supplemented in select cases with hormonal evaluations, distinguishes between the more commonly benign and rarely sinister underlying causes. The use of oral contraceptives (OCs) has been the cornerstone of treatment in most cases, and several new medications have recently been evaluated.

PHYSIOLOGY

Androgen Production and Metabolism

The main circulating androgens in women are androstenedione, dehydroepiandrosterone (DHEA), dehydroepiandrosterone sulfate (DHEA-S), testosterone, and 5α-dihydrotestosterone (DHT). Among these, only testosterone and DHT have androgenic activity at the target cell.

Androstenedione is produced by both the zona reticularis of the adrenal gland and in the ovary, approximately 1 mg/day from each source. About 5% of androstenedione is converted in peripheral tissues to testosterone. DHEA is produced mainly in the adrenal, with smaller amounts from the ovary, and is peripherally converted in lesser quantities to testosterone. DHEA-S arises entirely from the adrenal gland.

The normal female produces about 0.3 mg/day of testosterone. One third to one half of testosterone is secreted *directly* from the ovary and the remainder is converted peripherally from androstenedione and DHEA so that approximately two thirds of the total daily testosterone production is accounted for by the ovaries. In most hirsute women, the ovary is the major source of excess testosterone, due to both increased direct secretion and increased production of androstenedione for peripheral conversion (1).

Only about 1% of circulating testosterone is free, with 80 to 85% tightly bound to sex hormone-binding globulin (SHBG) and the remainder weakly bound to albumin. The free and albumin-bound fractions are biologically active. Hepatic synthesis of SHBG increases in response to estrogens and decreases in response to androgens, obesity, corticosteroids, and acromegaly. Most hirsute women have significantly decreased levels of SHBG. Consequently, there is a substantial increase in bioavailable testosterone.

In hair follicles and other target tissues, testosterone is converted by 5α-reductase to DHT, a biologically more potent androgen. The production of DHT depends on the amount of circulating testosterone, the amount directly secreted and that peripherally converted from androstenedione and DHEA, and the 5α-reductase activity in the target tissue (2). DHT is metabolized to 3α-androstenediol, which is then conjugated to 3α-androstenediol glucuronide. Testosterone is metabolized to the 17-ketosteroids androsterone and etiocholanolone, which are excreted in the urine.

Hair Growth

The pilosebaceous unit consists of a hair canal, sebaceous glands, a dermal papilla, and an arrector pili muscle. Hair growth occurs during the anagen phase when there is a proliferation of epidermal cells in contact with the dermal papilla, causing elongation and keratinization of the hair column. This is followed by involution of the matrix cells, the catagen phase. A resting period, the telogen phase, follows, and the existing hair is shed at the initiation of the next anagen phase. Hair length is determined by the length of the anagen phase, and the occasional appearance of shedding corresponds to increased synchrony of the individual hair follicles.

There are three different types of hair. Lanugo is the lightly pigmented, short, thin, loosely attached hair that covers the fetus. Vellus hair is soft lightly pigmented hair that covers the body during the prepubertal years. Thick, coarse, and highly pigmented terminal hair occurs only on the scalp and eyebrows before puberty. At adrenarche, pubic and axillary hair transforms from vellus to terminal hair in response to adrenal androgens. Hirsutism, an increase in male-pattern hair growth, is caused by a transformation from vellus to terminal hair in the androgen-dependent follicles of the face, chest, lower abdomen, lower back, medial thighs, and pubic area. The amount of terminal hair growth, and thus the severity of the hirsutism, depends on the degree of androgen increase, the 5α-reductase activity in the pilosebaceous unit, and the density of hair follicles. Follicle density and 5α-reductase activity are genetically determined and vary significantly between ethnic groups.

ETIOLOGY

Hirsutism may result from an increase in circulating androgens of ovarian, adrenal, or exogenous origin or from an increase in target hair follicle sensitivity to normal levels of androgen due to excess 5α-reductase activity. In addition to hirsutism, excess androgen may result in acne, oily skin, increased libido, and alopecia. Virilization describes the effects of pronounced hyperandrogenism with extreme hirsutism, clitoromegaly, deepening of the voice, and increased muscle mass. Hyperandrogenic chronic anovulation and idiopathic hirsutism account for most cases, although care must be taken to exclude more sinister causes (Table 11.1).

TABLE 11.1. Etiologies of Hirsutism and Virilization

Ovarian	Hyperandrogenic chronic anovulation
	Androgen-producing tumors
	Stromal hyperthecosis
	Luteoma of pregnancy/hyperreactio luteinalis
Skin	Idiopathic
Adrenal	Late-onset 21-hydroxylase deficiency
	Cushing's syndrome
	Androgen-producing tumors
Exogenous	Drugs

Hyperandrogenic Chronic Anovulation

Chronic anovulation with hyperandrogenism affects 5 to 10% of women in developed countries and accounts for greater than one third of all cases of anovulation. Stein and Leventhal (3) first described a syndrome of obesity, oligomenorrhea, hirsutism, and enlarged polycystic ovaries in 1935. As the complex hormonal alterations that give rise to this syndrome have been elucidated, many authors proposed that the term hyperandrogenic chronic anovulation replace the traditional polycystic ovary syndrome (PCO). Indeed, several authors showed that only 70 to 80% of women with menstrual irregularity and elevated androgens and as many as 25% of normal women have sonographically confirmed polycystic ovaries (4, 5). In addition, although obesity in conjunction with PCO is common, it is not always present for anovulation and hirsutism to occur. The term hyperandrogenic chronic anovulation is also supported in the most recent American College of Obstetricians and Gynecologists (ACOG) technical bulletin (6).

Patients with hyperandrogenic chronic anovulation often present with a gradual onset of symptoms of androgen excess and menstrual irregularity that usually begin perimenarcheally, although sometimes they may follow a period of weight gain. If these women began OCs shortly after menarche, they may report the onset of symptoms upon discontinuation of the pill. Acne and mild to moderate hirsutism are common, but the occasional woman will exhibit severe hirsutism and alopecia. Anovulation usually presents as oligomenorrhea but varies from amenorrhea to metrorrhagia.

Although the precise initiating factor is not clear, several interrelated endocrinologic abnormalities have been described. A tonically elevated level of luteinizing hormone (LH) exists, resulting from either an increased pulsatility of gonadotropin-releasing hormone (GnRH) or heightened sensitivity of the anterior pituitary to normal GnRH levels (7). The tonic elevation of LH increases the production of testosterone and androstenedione in ovarian theca cells. Some of this testosterone and androstenedione is converted to estrone peripherally, resulting in an increase in estrogen levels. This elevation of circulating androgens inhibits production of SHBG in the liver, resulting in increased amounts of bioavailable non-SHBG-bound testosterone. The decreased SHBG also results in an increase in *bioavailable* estradiol. This inhibits follicle-stimulating hormone (FSH) release from the pituitary and may even increase the pulsatility of GnRH (contributing to tonically elevated LH levels). FSH depression results in decreased aromatase activity in the granulosa cells so that little of the excess androgen is converted to estradiol and most is released into the circulation. Persistently low FSH levels allow the recruitment of multiple early follicles, but a dominant follicle is not permitted to mature, thus giving rise to anovulation and polycystic ovaries.

Although patients with hyperandrogenic chronic anovulation suffer from symptoms of androgen excess, it is important to realize they are also exposed to tonically elevated levels of estrogen. As mentioned above, estrogen levels are increased in two ways in hyperandrogenic chronic anovulation: the decrease in SHBG results in increased amounts of bioavailable estrogen and conversion of testosterone and androstenedione peripherally results in increased levels of estrone. This chronic exposure to relatively unopposed levels of estrogen increases the risk of endometrial hyperplasia and/or endometrial carcinoma in these patients.

Insulin resistance is common in women with hyperandrogenic anovulation and has even been shown in anovulatory adolescents (8). Elevated serum insulin levels may manifest as acanthosis nigricans, a velvety gray-brown skin discoloration, usually at the neck, axilla, and groin. Several recent reports addressed the link between hyperandrogenism and insulin resistance (9). The action of insulin-like growth factor

1 (IGF-1) at its receptor augments LH-induced androgen production. Because of the homology between insulin and IGF-1, insulin also acts on the IGF-1 receptor to increase androgen synthesis. In addition, insulin decreases granulosa cell production of IGF-1-binding protein, resulting in increased free IGF-1, and directly inhibits hepatic SHBG production. Researchers demonstrated a decrease in circulating androgens when serum insulin levels were decreased with diazoxide (Hyperstat), metformin (Glucophage), or troglitazone (Rezulin) (10–12). Although one study found that suppressing androgen levels with a GnRH analog partially reversed insulin resistance in nonobese patients with PCO, others have been unable to confirm that hyperandrogenemia contributes to insulin resistance (13).

Obesity, affecting 50 to 80% of women with hyperandrogenic anovulation, contributes to the endocrinologic alterations in several ways (14). Increased android obesity worsens insulin resistance (15). Obesity is also associated with a decrease in SHBG and an increase in peripheral conversion of androgens to estrone (16).

In addition to hirsutism and menstrual irregularity, women with hyperandrogenic anovulation are subject to serious long-term health risks. Chronic unopposed estrogen can lead to endometrial hyperplasia and adenocarcinoma (17). A higher incidence of hypertension and diabetes has been noted in women treated for PCO (18). Recent studies addressed the association between increased cardiovascular risk and hyperandrogenism. Both elevated androgens and insulin resistance correlate with decreased high-density lipoprotein, increased triglycerides, and increased very-low-density lipoprotein. These alterations confer a higher risk of coronary artery disease (19–21). Current evidence suggests that insulin resistance is the more important modifier of cardiovascular risk and that hyperandrogenism plays a smaller role or may only be a marker for hyperinsulinemia (22).

Variation in the severity of hirsutism depends on the increase in bioavailable testosterone, on follicle density, and the level of 5α-reductase activity in the skin. A study of Japanese women diagnosed with PCO revealed levels of circulating androgens, SHBG, and serum insulin similar to those in Caucasian women with PCO, but hirsutism was uncommon in the Japanese women (23). Analysis of androgen levels in oligo-ovulatory women in the United States without hirsutism has shown that 19% have elevations in free testosterone and that the testosterone level correlated with the degree of menstrual irregularity (24). Whether these women are subject to similar long-term sequelae remains to be determined. For a graphic display of these interrelated endocrinologic processes, see Figure 11.1.

Idiopathic Hirsutism

More than one third of women with hirsutism ovulate regularly. Because serum androgen levels in these women are most often normal, this has been called idiopathic hirsutism. Seen in certain ethnic groups and within certain families, hirsutism is gradual in onset and menses are regular. Increased 5α-reductase activity causing a local increase in DHT has been demonstrated in the skin of these women (25). This entity should therefore be considered one of enhanced peripheral conversion of testosterone to DHT.

Because DHT is metabolized rapidly to androstenediol glucuronide, many authors attempted to measure 5α-reductase activity by measuring androstenediol glucuronide (26). Assessment of the clinical utility of this measurement is mixed (27). Androstenediol precursors arise primarily from the adrenal gland, and most glucuronidation occurs in the liver (28). Use of the 5α-reductase inhibitor finasteride (Proscar) has resulted in a decrease in serum androstenediol glucuronide along with a reduction in hirsutism (29–32).

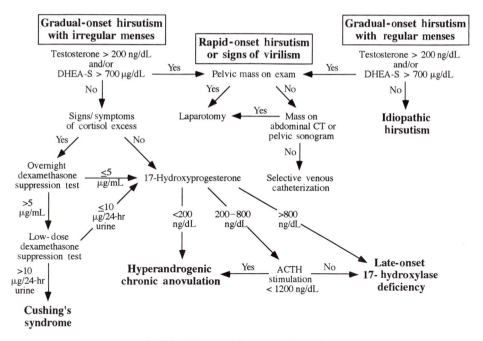

FIGURE 11.1. Evaluation of hirsutism.

Late-Onset 21-Hydroxylase Deficiency

Congenital adrenal hyperplasia is an inherited disorder of cortisol synthesis usually caused by a defect in the 21-hydroxylase enzyme and less commonly by defects in the 11β-hydroxylase or 3β-hydroxysteroid dehydrogenase enzymes. In the classic form, ambiguous genitalia and virilism occur in affected females. This is due to an accumulation of the 21-hydroxylase substrate 17-hydroxyprogesterone (17-OHP) that is converted to androstenedione and DHEA. A deficiency in aldosterone results in salt wasting in 75% of cases. The incidence of classic congenital adrenal hyperplasia is one in 1400 births.

A milder enzymatic defect results in a delay of symptoms until after puberty and so has been referred to as nonclassic congenital adrenal hyperplasia, late-onset congenital adrenal hyperplasia, or late-onset 21-hydroxylase deficiency (LOHD). The overall frequency is 0.1 to 1%, although it has been found in between 3 and 9% of hirsute women. Affected women present nearly identically to those with hyperandrogenic chronic anovulation with gradually worsening hirsutism and menstrual irregularity beginning in the perimenarcheal time period. Nearly all women with LOHD have oligomenorrhea or amenorrhea (33). Hirsutism varies from mild to severe, but virilization is rare. Although earlier reports stated that these patients are often tall in childhood and short in adulthood, as seen in those afflicted with the classic form of the disease, larger series showed that short stature is uncommon (34).

Mutations at the gene locus for 21-hydroxylase on chromosome 6 may result in an enzyme with minimal or no activity (the severe allele) or partial activity (the mild allele). Homozygotes for the severe allele suffer from classic congenital adrenal hyperplasia. Homozygotes for the mild allele or compound heterozygotes with one mild and one severe allele manifest LOHD. Women with cryptic adrenal hyperplasia, a carrier state with one mild or one severe allele, have no symptoms and are discovered only by DNA or biochemical analysis.

Patients may be screened for LOHD by measuring serum 17-OHP levels. The 17-OHP level must be drawn in the morning because of variation in response to the diurnal pattern of corticotropin (ACTH). If the level of 17-OHP is greater than 800 ng/dL, LOHD is present. If the level is less than 200 ng/dL, an enzyme defect does not account for the presence of hirsutism. If the level is less than 800 ng/dL but greater than 200 ng/dL, an ACTH stimulation test should be performed. For this test, basal serum levels of 17-OHP are drawn in the morning and 1 hour after an infusion of 25 μg of synthetic ACTH. A level of 17-OHP greater than 1200 ng/dL in response to ACTH establishes a diagnosis of LOHD.

There is disagreement regarding the need to screen for LOHD. Treatment of LOHD depends on the patients desires and concerns. For women most bothered by hirsutism, antiandrogens (such as spironolactone [Aldactone] or cyproterone) are superior to glucocorticoids for therapy. For women desirous of pregnancy, Clomid is superior to glucocorticoids in the induction of ovulation, although many women do have resumption of ovulatory cycles and arrest of hirsutism when treated with dexamethasone 0.5 mg nightly. Women with LOHD who become pregnant may choose to undergo genetic counseling and testing for paternal carrier status so that antenatal glucocorticoid therapy can be initiated for female fetuses at risk for classic 21-hydroxylase deficiency.

Cushing's Syndrome

Cushing's syndrome is a persistent increase in cortisol secretion. Cortisol excess may result from pituitary ACTH production (Cushing's disease), ectopic ACTH production by tumors, cortisol-secreting adrenal tumors, or, rarely, cortisol-secreting ovarian tumors. Women are affected five times as frequently as men, and the mean age at onset is 33 years. Findings include central obesity with moon facies, a dorsal cervical fat pad (buffalo hump), striae, ecchymoses, muscle weakness, hypertension, osteoporosis, and glucose intolerance. Of hirsute women, only those with other signs or symptoms suggestive of cortisol excess should be screened for Cushing's syndrome.

An overnight dexamethasone suppression test should be performed initially. A single dose of 1 mg dexamethasone is taken at bedtime, and plasma cortisol is measured at 8 AM. A value less than 5 μg/dL excludes Cushing's syndrome. Obese patients have false-positive rates as high as 13%. If the level is above 5 μg/dL, a low-dose suppression test is performed in which 0.5 mg of dexamethasone is given every 4 hours for 2 days. Failure to suppress the 24-hour urinary free cortisol below 10 μg on the second day establishes the diagnosis of Cushing's syndrome but does not determine the precise etiology.

Androgen-Producing Tumors

Androgen-secreting tumors as a cause of hirsutism or virilism are extremely rare. Suspicion should be aroused when signs of severe hirsutism or virilization rapidly progress over the course of several months.

Although Sertoli-Leydig and hilus cell tumors account for fewer than 1% of ovarian neoplasms, they are the only ovarian tumors that frequently produce excess testosterone. One third of Sertoli-Leydig and three fourths of hilus cell tumors produce very high levels of testosterone, resulting in virilization. The patient usually notes the onset of oligomenorrhea followed by amenorrhea, acne, and hirsutism within a few months. This rapidly progresses to temporal balding, deepening of the voice, clitoromegaly, and breast atrophy. Sertoli-Leydig cell tumors occur most often in women under 30 years of age. They are usually unilateral well-differentiated tumors, and 85% are palpable by the time symptoms are produced. Hilus cell tumors are almost always benign, usually occur after menopause, and are not palpable.

Adrenal cortical carcinoma has an incidence of about 1 in 1 million. Five percent of women with adrenal carcinoma have hirsutism. Benign adrenal adenomas may cause hirsutism, although this is rare. Functioning tumors may produce signs and symptoms relating to excess production of androgens, mineralocorticoids, and/or glucocorticoids. About half of women with adrenal tumors producing hirsutism also manifest Cushing's syndrome.

A testosterone level of 200 ng/dL has traditionally been used as a threshold for further evaluation of a possible ovarian or adrenal neoplasm. A DHEA-S level of greater than 700 μg/dL has been used as a marker for adrenal tumors. However, case series have been reported in which several patients with adrenal cortical carcinoma had levels of testosterone and DHEA-S that were elevated but fell below these cutoffs (35). Therefore, the presence of severe and rapidly progressing virilism, along with any increase in androgen levels, should dictate a search for ovarian or adrenal tumors, regardless of the absolute levels.

When an androgen-producing neoplasm is suspected, a pelvic examination, pelvic sonogram, and a computed tomography of the adrenals are the most important diagnostic procedures needed. Dexamethasone suppression has been used to establish adrenal versus ovarian origin and distinguish tumor from nontumor. However, this test is nether as sensitive nor as specific as radiologic imaging. Because selective catheterization of adrenal and ovarian veins is technically difficult, it should be reserved for those patients in which the presence of a tumor is strongly suspected but radiologic studies are negative.

Ovarian Stromal Hyperthecosis

Ovarian stromal hyperthecosis is an uncommon benign disorder in which the ovaries produce large amounts of testosterone. The ovaries are bilaterally enlarged and nests of luteinized theca cells are seen on microscopic examination.

Menstrual irregularity is observed first, followed by gradually increasing hirsutism. Signs of hirsutism progress gradually, as in hyperandrogenic chronic anovulation, but when left untreated may result in more severe masculinization with temporal balding, deepening of the voice, and clitoromegaly. Signs and symptoms may appear early in life or may not appear until after the menopause. Although the severe virilization and testosterone elevation (often above 200 ng/dL) can mimic an androgen-producing tumor, symptoms usually progress much more slowly than those from neoplastic causes.

The diagnosis should be suspected in the presence of severe hirsutism, elevated testosterone levels, and enlarged ovaries. It is confirmed by histopathologic examination. Treatment usually has been bilateral oophorectomy, but there has been recent success with GnRH agonists (36). It must be stressed that a response to GnRH agonists should not be used to exclude a diagnosis of tumor because testosterone production by some Sertoli-Leydig cell tumors are suppressed by these medications (37).

Pregnancy-Related Conditions

Two rare conditions specific to pregnancy can result in hirsutism or virilism. Luteoma of pregnancy, a solid ovarian enlargement that produces large amounts of testosterone, results from an exaggeration of the normal luteinization reaction of the ovary. Hyperreactio luteinalis is a benign cystic enlargement of the ovary associated with high levels of human chorionic gonadotropin. These lesions regress post-partum but may recur in subsequent pregnancies. Although virilization of a female fetus has been reported, androgen levels in the umbilical cord are usually normal because of the high capacity of the placenta to convert androgens to estrogen (38).

Drugs

Several medications are associated with androgenic side effects. Oral and parenteral testosterone, alone or in combination with estrogen, has been used in postmenopausal and oophorectomized women to increase libido (39). Danazol (Danocrine) is some-times used in the treatment of endometriosis and mastodynia. Systemic absorption of topical testosterone in the treatment of lichen sclerosus can cause elevated testos-terone levels, and a few case reports documented severe virilization as a result (40). Various anabolic steroids bring about masculinization in addition to other serious health risks. Although the progestin components of OC pills are 19-nortestosterone derivatives and retain some androgenic activity, the very low doses in current formula-tions are unlikely to cause hirsutism. Hypertrichosis, an increase in non-androgen-dependent hair, can be seen with cyclosporin (Sandimmune, Neoral), diazoxide (Hy-perstat), minoxidil (Loniten), and phenytoin (Dilantin).

EVALUATION

The etiology of hirsutism in most cases may be determined with a careful history and physical examination. A concerned sympathetic approach is important because hir-sutism can greatly affect a woman's sense of femininity, attractiveness, and social ac-ceptance. Because treatment must be undertaken for many months before results appear, a trusting relationship is necessary for the patient to persist in therapy.

The duration and extent of hirsutism are critical in distinguishing common be-nign causes, usually with early onset and gradual progression, from rare sinister causes, usually with rapid progression of severe hirsutism over several months. The presence of other symptoms of androgen excess, acne or alopecia, should be elicited. If cosmetic measures such as shaving, plucking, or use of depilatories are practiced, noting the frequency aids in assessing severity and measuring treatment effectiveness. A menstrual history establishes the likelihood of ovulation. A thorough medication history can exclude iatrogenic causes. A family history may reveal a fa-milial pattern of hirsutism or point to the possibility of hydroxylase deficiency. A re-view of symptoms is important to look for evidence of cortisol excess.

The location and degree of hair growth should be noted at the physical exami-nation and carefully recorded. Several scoring systems have been created to grade hirsutism. The system by Ferriman and Gallwey (41) assesses hair in each of nine an-drogen-sensitive body areas on a scale of 0 to 4 with total scores above 8 or 10 defin-ing clinically significant hirsutism (Fig. 11.2 and Table 11.2). An alternative is the Lorenzo method (42), in which hair growth is graded on the chin and anterior neck, upper lip, chest, abdomen, thighs, and forearms. Signs of virilization, including breast atrophy and clitoromegaly, often indicate an androgen-producing neoplasm. An adnexal or abdominal mass suggests an ovarian or adrenal tumor. Acanthosis ni-gricans should raise the suspicion of insulin resistance. Signs of cortisol excess war-rant testing for Cushing's syndrome.

After the initial history and physical examination, further evaluation is guided by dividing hirsute women into three categories: those with a gradual onset of hir-sutism and regular menses, those with a gradual onset of hirsutism and irregular menses, and those with a rapid onset of hirsutism or signs of virilism.

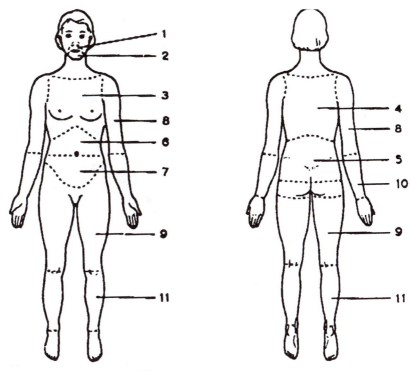

FIGURE 11.2. Demarcation of 11 sites used for numerically grading amount of hair growth—anterior and posterior views. (Reprinted with permission from Ferriman D, Gallwey J. Clinical assessment of body hair growth in women. J Clin Endocrinol Metab 1961;21:1440–1447. © The Endocrine Society.)

TABLE 11.2. Definition of Hair Gradings at 11 Sites[a]

Site	Grade	Definition
Upper lip	1	Few hairs at outer margin
	2	Small moustache at outer margin
	3	Moustache extending halfway from outer margin
	4	Moustache extending to midline
Chin	1	Few scattered hairs
	2	Scattered hairs with small concentration
	3 and 4	Complete cover, light and heavy
Chest	1	Circumareolar hairs
	2	With midline hair in addition
	3	Fusion of these areas, with three-quarters cover
	4	Complete cover
Upper back	1	Few scattered hairs
	2	Rather more, still scattered
	3 and 4	Complete cover, light and heavy
Lower back	1	Sacral tuft of hair
	2	With some lateral extension
	3	Three-quarters cover
	4	Complete cover

continued

TABLE 11.2. (continued) Definition of Hair Gradings at 11 Sites[a]

Site	Grade	Definition
Upper abdomen	1	Few midline hairs
	2	Rather more, still midline
	3 and 4	Half and full cover
Lower abdomen	1	Few midline hairs
	2	Midline streak of hair
	3	Midline band of hair
	4	Inverted V-shaped growth
Arm	1	Sparse growth affecting not more than one quarter of limb surface
	2	More than this; cover still incomplete
	3 and 4	Complete cover, light and heavy
Forearm	1, 2, 3, 4	Complete cover of dorsal surface: 2 grades of light and 2 of heavy growth
Thigh	1, 2, 3, 4	As for arm
Leg	1, 2, 3, 4	As for arm

Reprinted with permission from Ferriman D, Gallwey J. Clinical assessment of body hair growth in women. J Clin Endocrinol Metab 1961;21:1440–1447. © The Endocrine Society.
[a]Grade 0 at all sites indicates absence of terminal hair.

Gradual-Onset Hirsutism and Regular Menses

The gradual onset of mild to moderate hirsutism with regular menses supports a diagnosis of idiopathic hirsutism with increased peripheral conversion of testosterone to DHT. Although a neoplastic cause is extraordinarily unlikely, serum levels of testosterone and DHEA-S may be assessed for reassurance. For a summary of evaluative treatment plans for these categories, see Figure 11.3.

Gradual-Onset Hirsutism and Irregular Menses

A woman with long-standing hirsutism and irregular menses likely has hyperandrogenic chronic anovulation. Serum testosterone and DHEA-S are useful in ruling out ovarian or adrenal tumors. The serum testosterone level may be mildly elevated or even normal. However, the decrease in SHBG in hirsute women greatly increases the amount of bioavailable testosterone. Measurement of the free or non-SHBG-bound testosterone level is unnecessary because the presence of hirsutism alone is evidence that an excess in biologically active testosterone exists. Although the LH level is typically elevated, the normal range for LH is broad and the LH:FSH ratio is highly variable so that neither the LH level itself nor the LH:FSH ratio adds useful information (7). A morning 17-OHP level should be drawn to screen for LOHD because its presentation is often similar to that of hyperandrogenic chronic anovulation.

Anovulation is evaluated with a thyroid-stimulating hormone and prolactin level. If amenorrhea is present, a progestin challenge is added. With long-standing anovulation, an endometrial biopsy should be performed to rule out endometrial hyperplasia or carcinoma from unopposed estrogen stimulation. The association of hyperandrogenic chronic anovulation and lipid abnormalities warrants a lipid profile. Because insulin resistance plays a significant role in the pathogenesis of hyperandrogenism, glucose tolerance should be evaluated, especially if acanthosis nigricans is found.

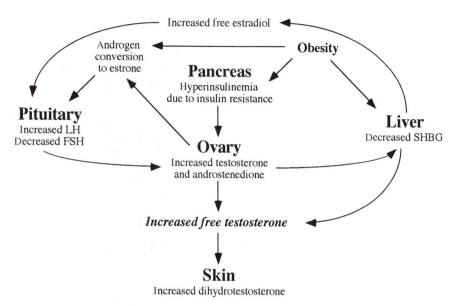

FIGURE 11.3. Hormonal and biochemical interactions in hyperandrogenic chronic anovulation.

Rapid-Onset Hirsutism or Virilism

The rapid progression of severe hirsutism or virilism over several months suggests an androgen-producing tumor. Androgen levels are usually very high but may be only slightly elevated. In about half of all cases of adrenal tumors, patients exhibit features of Cushing's syndrome. Most androgen-producing ovarian tumors are palpable on pelvic examination. If a tumor is suspected, a pelvic sonogram and an abdominal computed tomography should be obtained. Suppression and stimulation testing have little value in distinguishing an ovarian from an adrenal source (43). When there is a marked elevation in androgen level and the radiologic studies fail to localize a source, selective venous catheterization may be performed.

TREATMENT

The treatment of uncommon causes of hirsutism is usually straightforward. Androgenic medications should be discontinued. Hyperreactio luteinalis and luteoma resolve postpartum so expectant management and cosmetic measures are used. Ovarian tumors require surgical removal, most often a total abdominal hysterectomy and bilateral salpingo-oophorectomy, although a unilateral adnexectomy may be performed for a unilateral well-differentiated Sertoli-Leydig tumor in a woman who wishes to preserve fertility. Adrenal tumors are removed operatively. Bilateral salpingo-oophorectomy has traditionally been performed for ovarian stromal hyperthecosis. Although successful treatment of stromal hyperthecosis with a GnRH analog has recently been reported in four postmenopausal women, further follow-up is needed to assess long-term efficacy (36, 44). In most remaining cases of hirsutism, treatment involves suppressing ovarian or adrenal androgen production and blocking androgen action at the skin, either by competitively inhibiting androgen receptors or by inhibiting 5α-reductase.

TABLE 11.3. Treatment of Hyperandrogenism

WEIGHT LOSS	Flutamide
	Ketoconazole
MEDICATIONS	Glucocorticoids
Combined oral contraceptives	
Progesterone	**COSMESIS**
GnRH analogs	Shaving
Spironolactone	Plucking
Cyproterone acetate	Depilatories
Finasteride	Electrolysis

Hyperandrogenic Chronic Anovulation

A summary of the multiple modalities of treatment is discussed in Table 11.3.

Weight Loss

Weight loss is an essential, although often underemphasized, element in treating patients with hyperandrogenic chronic anovulation who are obese. Obesity decreases serum SHBG levels and enhances insulin resistance, thereby increasing both total androgen production and the free fraction of testosterone.

Several studies demonstrated a rise in SHBG, a decrease in total and free testosterone, an improvement in Ferriman-Gallwey score, and a decrease in serum insulin in response to weight reduction (45, 46). In addition, the resumption of ovulation has been observed with regular menses and successful pregnancies (47). Although many therapies are effective in treating hirsutism, only weight loss has been proven beneficial in modifying the associated insulin resistance, hypertension, and lipid abnormalities. Advice on regular exercise and a sensible diet should be given.

Combined Oral Contraceptives

In hirsute women not currently desiring pregnancy, combined estrogen-progestin OC pills are inexpensive, easy to administer, and effective in reducing excess hair growth.

OCs act through several mechanisms to decrease the amount of bioavailable androgens and ameliorate hirsutism and acne. OCs suppress ovarian androgen production by suppressing LH, although the LH suppression is highly variable and the LH:FSH ratio is not affected. OCs increase SHBG levels, which results in decreased amounts of circulating free testosterone. Some studies found a greater rise in SHBG with OCs containing desogestrel or norgestimate.

Because of the length of the hair growth cycle, an observable decrease in hair growth requires at least 6 months of treatment. The addition of an antiandrogen improves the response, but prolonged treatment is still necessary. Acne usually responds more rapidly. Low-dose OCs are as effective as higher dose preparations. Multiphasic OCs are as effective as monophasic. OCs with low-dose levonorgestrel, which is known to cause acne at high doses, are equally beneficial in treating hirsutism. Newer OCs with desogestrel and norgestimate are often recommended because of their lower androgenic activity and because they are associated with a greater increase in SHBG. However, no studies have yet documented a clinical advantage for these third-generation OCs in the treatment of hirsutism.

Additional benefits of OCs include regulation of menses and a decreased risk of both endometrial hyperplasia and cancer. In chronically anovulatory women in whom OCs are contraindicated or unacceptable, periodic withdrawal bleeding should be induced with progestin to decrease these risks.

Gonadotropin-Releasing Hormone Agonists

GnRH agonists suppress pituitary gonadotropin secretion, resulting in decreased ovarian androgen production, and hence are effective in decreasing hirsutism. Gonadotropin suppression also causes a hypoestrogenic state that results in menopausal symptoms and decreased bone density. Estrogen, usually in the form of OCs, is often added to avoid bone demineralization.

A recent randomized trial comparing the combination of an OC and a GnRH agonist with either agent alone found that the GnRH agonist alone resulted in a greater reduction in Ferriman-Gallwey score at 6 months but also resulted in an unacceptable decrease in bone density. The GnRH agonist-OC combination resulted in a greater score reduction than the OC alone at 3 months, but at 6 months the decrease in Ferriman-Gallwey score was equivalent, indicating a more rapid initial response with the combination but overall equal efficacy (48). Others confirmed similar efficacy between the OC-GnRH agonist combination and OCs alone (49).

Because GnRH agonists are very expensive and their use in conjunction with OCs appears to add little additional long-term benefit, most women should be treated with an OC alone. Bisphosphonates have been shown to preserve bone density when given with a GnRH agonist so the combination of alendronate (Fosamax) and a GnRH agonist might be used where a contraindication to estrogen exists (50).

Cyproterone

Cyproterone acetate is a steroidal progestogen derived from 17-OHP. It is not approved for use in the United States but is marketed in other countries as a component of the contraceptives "Diane" (2 mg cyproterone acetate and 50 μg ethinyl estradiol) and "Dianette" (2 mg cyproterone acetate and 35 μg ethinyl estradiol). It decreases androgen production by suppressing LH secretion and competitively inhibits testosterone and DHT at their intracellular receptors.

A higher dose of cyproterone is commonly used for the treatment of hirsutism. Because of its progestational activity and long half-life, it is administered with oral ethinyl estradiol in a reversed sequential regimen, 50 to 100 mg of cyproterone on days 5 to 14 with 35 μg ethinyl estradiol on days 5 to 25. Significant improvement in hirsutism has been noted within 3 months with this high-dose regimen. Although some studies found that a 2-mg dose yields results similar to higher doses at 12 months, a faster initial response with the higher doses has been documented (51, 52).

Side effects include weight gain, edema, diminished libido, headache, nausea, fatigue, and mood swings (52). Overall, however, it is well tolerated. Rare cases of hepatotoxicity have been reported in women taking cyproterone, but a causal relationship has not been established.

Spironolactone

Spironolactone (Aldactone) is a synthetic steroidal aldosterone antagonist used as a potassium-sparing diuretic in the treatment of hypertension. Its antiandrogenic action is threefold. It competitively binds the DHT receptor, decreases androgen production by inhibiting cytochrome P450, and inhibits 5α-reductase activity. Of these mechanisms, competitive inhibition at the DHT receptor appears most important. In addition, spironolactone has weak progestational activity.

Spironolactone is administered in doses of 25 to 100 mg twice daily. Clinical improvement usually requires 6 months of treatment. Results have been noted as early as 3 months with the higher dose (200 mg/day), but side effects are also increased (53). Side effects are mild and include diuresis and fatigue. Significant hyperkalemia in patients without renal disease does not occur. Because of its progestational activity, irregular menses are common, with a 25% frequency seen with 100 mg/day and a frequency greater than 50% seen at 200 mg/day (54). There is a theoretic risk of feminization of a male fetus so that contraception is necessary.

The use of an OC with spironolactone regulates menses, further suppresses androgen production, and provides contraception. Studies with the OC-spironolactone combination demonstrate greater reductions in the Ferriman-Gallwey score than those with spironolactone alone, but the two regimens have not been compared in a single study (32, 55, 56). Daily OC use with spironolactone, 50 mg twice daily, has similar efficacy to the use of cyproterone, 50 mg/day, with ethinyl estradiol (56, 57).

Impressive efficacy, low risk profile, and low cost make spironolactone, in conjunction with an OC, a good choice for women with hyperandrogenic chronic anovulation.

Ketoconazole

Ketoconazole (Nizoral) is an imidazole derivative active as an antifungal. It suppresses both adrenal and ovarian synthesis of androgens by inhibiting 17,20-desmolase, 17-hydroxylase, and 11β-hydroxylase. Improvement may be seen in patients who complete at least 6 months of 400-mg/day therapy (58). There is a very high rate of discontinuation, however, because of frequent side effects of headache, nausea, fatigue, and loss of scalp hair (59). Serious hepatotoxicity has also been reported. Because of poor tolerability and risk of hepatotoxicity, ketoconazole should not be used long term or as a first-line agent.

Flutamide

Flutamide (Eulexin) is a nonsteroidal antiandrogen used in the treatment of prostatic cancer. It acts primarily by competitive inhibition at the DHT receptor. Although the affinity of flutamide for the DHT receptor is much less than that of spironolactone, its lack of progestational or mineralocorticoid activity allows it to be given in much higher doses. It also suppresses adrenal androgen production by inhibiting 17,20-desmolase. At a dose of 125 mg two or three times a day, flutamide is equally as effective as spironolactone (60). Minor side effects include dry skin and increased appetite. Drug-induced hepatitis has occurred in 0.5% of men receiving flutamide and has been reported in one woman being treated for hirsutism (61, 62). Because of the risk of drug-induced hepatitis and its high cost, flutamide is not recommended for the initial treatment of hirsutism.

Cimetidine

Cimetidine (Tagamet) blocks the type 2 histamine receptor and is prescribed for peptic ulcer and gastroesophageal reflux. Because of its weak affinity for the androgen receptors, it has been investigated as a treatment for hirsutism. Results have been disappointing with no clinical effect at doses up to 1200 mg/day (63). It is not recommended for the treatment of hirsutism.

Finasteride

Finasteride (Proscar) has also been used in the treatment of prostatic cancer. A 5α-reductase inhibitor, it blocks peripheral conversion of testosterone to DHT. A dose of 5 mg/day results in a reduction in Ferriman-Gallwey score along with a lowering of serum DHT and androstenediol glucuronide (29–32). Clinical efficacy is similar to spironolactone (32). Doses of up to 400 mg/day have been given in men without significant side effect. Because of potential teratogenic effects, reliable contraception is necessary.

Finasteride may be the drug of choice for hirsutism in the future with its lack of side effects and good clinical response. However, the medication is costly, and further experience is needed to ensure safety.

Glucocorticoids

Prednisone, 5 to 7.5 mg/day, or dexamethasone, 0.5 mg/day, suppresses adrenal androgen production. Glucocorticoids are often used as the first-line therapy for LOHD. Its efficacy in treating hirsutism in patients with hyperandrogenic chronic anovulation is inferior to that of OCs or spironolactone. The fact that the ovary is the major source of excess androgen in these patients probably accounts for the poor response. Weight gain and depression are frequent side effects, and its use may exacerbate insulin resistance.

Cosmetic Measures

There are several widely used methods for the temporary removal of unwanted hair. Depilatory creams remove hair by dissolving disulfide bonds. These creams sometimes cause skin irritation and allergic dermatitis. Shaving does not stimulate hair growth but does result in stubble, which gives the appearance of thicker coarser hair. In addition, shaving may further threaten a woman's sense of femininity and gender identity. Waxing is effective but may be time consuming and expensive.

Electrolysis involves permanent hair removal by destruction of the dermal papilla with electric current. Attempts at permanent hair removal without addressing the underlying hyperandrogenism are often in vain because new terminal hairs continue to be formed. Electrolysis is most useful after several months of medical therapy when there is no new terminal hair growth.

Idiopathic Hirsutism

Although the underlying biologic mechanism in idiopathic hirsutism is different from that of hyperandrogenic chronic anovulation, the treatment is similar. The use of OCs decrease hirsutism by reducing circulating androgens to subnormal levels so that less testosterone is available for conversion to DHT. Antiandrogens have been proven effective in treating idiopathic hirsutism (55). Spironolactone is a prudent choice and may be combined with an OC to enhance efficacy, avoid irregular uterine bleeding, and provide contraception. Finasteride has been shown to be effective in idiopathic hirsutism and may prove especially useful because it specifically addresses the apparent etiology of this disorder by inhibiting 5α-reductase.

Late-Onset 21-Hydroxylase Deficiency

Women with LOHD may be treated with dexamethasone, 0.5 mg/day, or prednisone, 5 mg/day. Glucocorticoid therapy suppresses ACTH-induced adrenal androgen production and has resulted in a decrease in hirsutism and a resumption of ovulatory cycles in some women. However, peripheral androgen blockade with cyproterone or spironolactone has been shown to be more effective than adrenal suppression (64).

Evaluation of Treatment

Treatment efficacy is best evaluated clinically. Useful measures include a reduction in the Ferriman-Gallwey score or a reduction in the amount of time spent in temporary hair removal. Subjective improvement may be noted in serial photographs. The amount of reduction in serum androgen levels does not correlate well with the magnitude of clinical improvement assessed by Ferriman-Gallwey score (29, 65). Therefore, measurement of serum androgens is usually not helpful.

CLINICAL NOTES

- Hirsutism is male-pattern hair growth in a woman. It results from the stimulation of hair follicles by excess androgens and may occur on the face, chest, lower abdomen, lower back, medial thighs, and pubic area.
- Androgens are produced in the ovary and adrenal glands. Testosterone, produced in the ovary and through peripheral conversion of androstenedione and DHEA, is converted in the skin to DHT, which stimulates terminal hair growth. In addition to hirsutism, acne and alopecia are often signs of hyperandrogenism.
- Women with a gradual onset of hirsutism and regular menses likely have idiopathic hirsutism that results from an increase in the conversion of testosterone to DHT by 5α-reductase.
- Women with a gradual onset of hirsutism and irregular menses likely have hyperandrogenic chronic anovulation (also known as PCO) in which the ovary produces excess androgens in response to tonically elevated LH.
- About 5% of women with a gradual onset of hirsutism and irregular menses have LOHD (also known as late-onset congenital adrenal hyperplasia) in which excess androgens are produced in the adrenal because of a defect in the enzyme 21-hydroxylase.
- Androgen-producing ovarian or adrenal tumors are rare and usually present with the rapid onset of severe hirsutism or signs of masculinization. Other uncommon causes of hirsutism include Cushing's syndrome, androgenic medications, ovarian stromal hyperthecosis, and luteoma or hyperreactio luteinalis of pregnancy.
- Studies for evaluation include testosterone and DHEA-S to rule out ovarian or adrenal tumors. In women with irregular menses, anovulation should be evaluated with thyroid-stimulating hormone and prolactin levels. A morning 17-OHP should be drawn to rule out LOHD. Radiologic imaging, an abdominal computed tomography, and a pelvic sonogram should be performed when the serum androgen levels are very high or there is a rapid progression of severe hirsutism.
- A combination of an OC to suppress ovarian androgen production and the antiandrogen spironolactone results in clinical improvement in about 6 months in most women with hyperandrogenic chronic anovulation or idiopathic hirsutism.

References

1. Chang R. Ovarian steroid secretion in polycystic ovarian disease. Semin Reprod Endocrinol 1984;2:244–248.
2. Rittmaster RS. Clinical relevance of testosterone and dihydrotestosterone metabolism in women. Am J Med 1995;98(suppl):17S–21S.
3. Stein I, Leventhal M. Amenorrhea associated with bilateral polycystic ovaries. Am J Obstet Gynecol 1935;29:181–191.
4. Farquhar C, Birdsall M, Manning P, et al. The prevalence of polycystic ovaries on ultrasound scanning in a population of randomly selected women. Aust N Z J Obstet Gynaecol 1994;34:67–72.

5. Polson D, Wadsworth J, Adams J, et al. Polycystic ovaries: a common finding in normal women. Lancet 1988;1:870–872.

6. Hyperandrogenic chronic anovulation. ACOG Tech Bull 1995;202:1–7.

7. Taylor A, McCourt B, Martin K, et al. Determinants of abnormal gonadotropin secretion in clinically defined women with polycystic ovary syndrome. J Clin Endocrinol Metab 1997;82:2248–2256.

8. Apter D, Butzow T, Laughlin G, et al. Metabolic features of polycystic ovary syndrome are found in adolescent girls with hyperandrogenism. J Clin Endocrinol Metab 1995; 80:2966–2973.

9. Nestler J. Role of hyperinsulinemia in the pathogenesis of the polycystic ovary syndrome, and its clinical implications. Semin Reprod Endocrinol 1997;15:111–122.

10. Nestler J, Barlascini C, Matt D, et al. Suppression of serum insulin by diazoxide reduces serum testosterone levels in obese women with polycystic ovary syndrome. Metabolism 1989;68:1027–1032.

11. Velazquez E, Mendoza S, Hamer T, et al. Metformin therapy in polycystic ovary syndrome reduces hyperinsulinemia, insulin resistance, hyperandrogenemia, and systolic blood pressure, while facilitating normal menses and pregnancy. Metabolism 1994;43:647–654.

12. Ehrmann D, Schneider D, Sobel B, et al. Troglitazone improves defects in insulin action, insulin secretion, ovarian steroidogenesis, and fibrinolysis in women with polycystic ovary syndrome. J Clin Endocrinol Metab 1997;82:2108–2116.

13. Moghetti P, Tosi F, Castello R, et al. The insulin resistance in women with hyperandrogenism is partially reversed by antiandrogen treatment: evidence that androgens impair insulin action in women. J Clin Endocrinol Metab 1996;81:952–960.

14. Douchi T, Ijuin H, Nakamura S, et al. Body fat distribution in women with polycystic ovary syndrome. Obstet Gynecol 1995;86:516–519.

15. Ferranini E, Natali A, Bell P, et al. Insulin resistance and hypersecretion in obesity. J Clin Invest 1997;100:1166–1173.

16. Bernasconi D, del Monte P, Meozzi M, et al. The impact of obesity on hormonal parameters in hirsute and non-hirsute women. Metabolism 1996;45:72–75.

17. Coulam C, Annegers J, Kranz J. Chronic anovulation syndrome and associated neoplasms. Obstet Gynecol 1983;61:403–407.

18. Dahlgren E, Johansson S, Lindstedt G. Women with polycystic ovary syndrome wedge resected in 1956–1965: a long term follow-up focusing on natural history and circulating hormones. Fertil Steril 1992;57:505–513.

19. Castelo-Branco C, Casals E, de Osaba M, et al. Plasma lipids, lipoproteins and apolipoproteins in hirsute women. Acta Obstet Gynecol Scand 1996;75:261–265.

20. Wild R, Painter P, Coulson P, et al. Lipoprotein lipid concentrations and cardiovascular risk in women with polycystic ovary syndrome. J Clin Endocrinol Metab 1985;61:946–951.

21. Wild R. Obesity, lipids, cardiovascular risk, and androgen excess. Am J Med 1995; 98(suppl):27S–32S.

22. Wild R, Alaupovic P, Givens J. Lipoprotein abnormalities in hirsute women: the association with insulin resistance. Am J Obstet Gynecol 1992;166:1191–1197.

23. Carmina E, Koyama T, Chang L, et al. Does ethnicity influence the prevalence of adrenal hyperandrogenism and insulin resistance in polycystic ovary syndrome. Am J Obstet Gynecol 1992;167:1807–1812.

24. Allen S, Potter H, Azziz R. Prevalence of hyperandrogenemia among non-hirsute oligoovulatory women. Fertil Steril 1997;67:569–572.

25. Mauvais-Jarvis P. Regulation of androgen receptors and 5α-reductase in the skin of normal and hirsute women. Clin Endocrinol Metab 1986;15:307–317.

26. Kirschner M, Samojlik E, Szmal E. Clinical usefulness of plasma androstanediol glucuronide measurements in women with idiopathic hirsutism. J Clin Endocrinol Metab1987;65:597–601.

27. Khoury M, Baracat E, Pardini D, et al. Serum levels of androstenediol glucuronide, total testosterone, and free testosterone in hirsute women. Fertil Steril 1994;62:76–80.

28. Rittmaster R. Androgen conjugates: physiology and clinical significance. Endocrinol Rev 1993;14:121–132.

29. Fruzzetti F, de Lorenzo D, Parrini D, et al. Effects of finasteride, a 5α-reductase inhibitor, on circulating androgens and gonadotropin secretion in hirsute women. J Clin Endocrinol Metab 1994;79:831–835.

30. Moghetti P, Castello R, Magnani C, et al. Clinical and hormonal effects of the 5α-reductase inhibitor finasteride in idiopathic hirsutism. J Clin Endocrinol Metab 1994;79:1115–1121.

31. Tolino A, Petrone A, Sarnacchiaro F, et al. Finasteride in the treatment of hirsutism: new therapeutic perspectives. Fertil Steril 1996;66:61–65.

32. Wong I, Morris R, Chang L, et al. A prospective randomized trial comparing finasteride spironolactone in the treatment of hirsute women. J Clin Endocrinol Metab 1995;80:233–238.

33. Panitsa-Faflia C, Batrinos M. Late-onset congenital adrenal hyperplasia. Ann N Y Acad Sci 1997;816:230–234.

34. Baskin H. Screening for late-onset congenital adrenal hyperplasia in hirsutism or amenorrhea. Arch Intern Med 1987;147:847–848.

35. Derksen J, Nagasser S, Meinders A, et al. Identification of virilizing adrenal tumors in hirsute women. N Engl J Med 1994;331:968–973.

36. Barth JH, Jenkins M, Belchetz PE. Ovarian hyperthecosis, diabetes and hirsuties in postmenopausal women. Clin Endocrinol (Oxf) 1997;46:123–128.

37. Pascale M, Pugeat M, Roberts M, et al. Androgen suppressive effect of GnRH agonist in ovarian hyperthecosis and virilizing tumours. Clin Endocrinol 1994;41:571–576.

38. Cohen D, Daughaday W, Weldon V. Fetal and maternal virilization associated with pregnancy. Am J Dis Child 1982;136:353–356.

39. Urman B, Pride S, Yuen B. Elevated serum testosterone, hirsutism, and virilism associated with combined androgen-estrogen hormone replacement therapy. Obstet Gynecol 1991;77:595–985.

40. Joura E, Zeisler H, Bancher-Todesca D, et al. Short-term effects of topical testosterone in vulvar lichen sclerosus. Obstet Gynecol 1997;89:297–299.

41. Ferriman D, Gallwey J. Clinical assessment of body hair growth in women. J Clin Endocrinol Metab 1961;21:1440–1447.

42. Lorenzo E. Familial study of hirsutism. J Clin Endocrinol Metab 1970;31:556–564.

43. Moltz L, Schwartz U. Gonadal and adrenal androgen secretion in hirsute females. Clin Endocrinol Metab 1986;15:229–245.

44. Deleted in proof.

45. Pasquali R, Antenucci D, Casimirri F, et al. Clinical and hormonal characteristics of obese amenorrheic hyperandrogenic women before and after weight loss. J Clin Endocrinol Metab 1989;68:173–179.

46. Crave J, Fimbel S, Lejeune H, et al. Effects of diet and metformin administration on sex hormone-binding globulin, androgens and insulin in hirsute and obese women. J Clin Endocrinol Metab 1995;80:2057–2062.

47. Guzick D, Wing R, Smith D, et al. Endocrinologic consequences of weight loss in obese hyperandrogenic women. Fertil Steril 1994;61:598–604.

48. Carr B, Breslau N, Givens C, et al. Oral contraceptive pills, gonadotropin-releasing hormone agonists, or use in combination for the treatment of hirsutism: a clinical research center study. J Clin Endocrinol Metab 1995;80:1169–1178.

49. Vegelli W, Testa G, Maggioni P, et al. An open randomized comparative study of an oral contraceptive containing ethinyl estradiol and cyproterone acetate with and without the GnRH analogue goserelin in the long-term treatment of hirsutism. Gynecol Obstet Invest 1996;41:260–268.

50. Mukherjee T, Barad D, Turk R, et al. A randomized, placebo-controlled study on the effect of cyclic etidronate therapy on the bone mineral density changes associated with six months of gonadotropin-releasing hormone agonist treatment. Am J Obstet Gynecol 1996;175:105–109.

51. Barth J, Cherry C. Cyproterone acetate for severe hirsutism: results of a double-blind dose-ranging study. Clin Endocrinol 1991;35:5–10.
52. Belisle S, Love F. Clinical efficacy and safety of cyproterone acetate in severe hirsutism: results of a multi-centered Canadian study. Fertil Steril 1986;46:1015–1020.
53. Lobo R, Shoupe D, Serafini P, et al. The effects of two doses on spironolactone on serum androgens and anagen hair in hirsute women. Fertil Steril 1985;43:200–205.
54. Helfer E, Miller J, Rose L. Side-effects of spironolactone therapy in the hirsute woman. J Clin Endocrinol Metab1988;66:208–211.
55. Barth J, Cherry C, Wojnarowska F, et al. Spironolactone is an effective and well tolerated systemic antiandrogen therapy for hirsute women. J Clin Endocrinol Metab 1995; 80:2966–2973.
56. Erenus M, Yucelten D, Gurbuz O, et al. Comparison of spironolactone-oral contraceptive versus cyproterone acetate-estrogen regimens in the treatment of hirsutism. Fertil Steril 1996;66:216–219.
57. O'Brien P, Cooper M, Murray P, et al. Comparison of sequential cyproterone acetate/estrogen versus spironolactone oral contraceptive in the treatment of hirsutism. J Clin Endocrinol Metab 1991;72:1008–1013.
58. Martikainen H, Heikkinen J, Ruokonen A, et al. Hormonal and clinical effects of ketoconazole in hirsute women. J Clin Endocrinol Metab 1988;66:987–991.
59. Venturoli S, Fabbri R, Prato L, et al. Ketoconazole therapy for women with acne and/or hirsutism. J Clin Endocrinol Metab1990;71:335–339.
60. Erenus M, Gurbuz O, Durmusoglu F, et al. Comparison of the efficacy of spironolactone versus flutamide in the treatment of hirsutism. Fertil Steril 1994;61:613–616.
61. Wysowski D, Fourcroy J. Flutamide toxicity. J Urol 1996;155:209–212.
62. Wallace C, Lalor E, Chik C. Hepatotoxicity complicating flutamide treatment of hirsutism. Ann Intern Med 1993;119:1150.
63. Golditch I, Price V. Treatment of hirsutism with cimetidine. Obstet Gynecol 1990;75: 911–913.
64. Spritzer P, Billaud L, Thalabard J, et al. Cyproterone acetate versus hydrocortisone treatment in late-onset adrenal hyperplasia. J Clin Endocrinol Metab 1990;70:642–646.
65. Carmina E, Lobo R. Peripheral androgen blockade versus glandular androgen suppression in the treatment of hirsutism. Obstet Gynecol 1991;78:845–849.

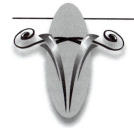

C H A P T E R   1 2

Premenstrual Syndromes

MEIR STEINER

Epidemiologic surveys estimated that as many as 75% of women of reproductive age experience some symptoms attributable to the premenstrual phase of the menstrual cycle (1). More than 100 physical and psychological symptoms have been reported (2). Most women are able to manage these symptoms through lifestyle changes and conservative therapies such as exercise and stress reduction. This phenomenon is often classified by the generic term of premenstrual syndrome and most often refers to any combination of symptoms appearing during the week before menstruation and resolving within a week of the onset of menses (3). Conversely, 3 to 8% of menstruating women report premenstrual symptoms of irritability, tension, dysphoria, and lability of mood that seriously interfere with their lifestyle and relationships (4–11). So disruptive are these symptoms that research diagnostic criteria have been developed for what is now labeled premenstrual dysphoric disorder. These criteria are published in the *Diagnostic and Statistical Manual of Mental Disorders,* 3rd revised and 4th editions (DSM-IV) (12, 13). Women who are found to meet the diagnostic criteria of premenstrual dysphoric disorder do not usually respond to conservative and conventional interventions and often seek out the expertise of a health professional.

ETIOLOGY

The etiology of premenstrual syndrome, and specifically of premenstrual dysphoric disorder, is still largely unknown. Attempts have been made to explain the phenomena in terms of biologic, psychological, or psychosocial factors, but most explanations failed confirmatory efforts by laboratory and treatment-based studies.

The role of female sex hormones in premenstrual dysphoric disorder has been considered of central importance. To date, however, studies attempting to attribute the disorder to an excess of estrogen, a deficiency of progesterone, a withdrawal of estrogen, or changes in estrogen:progesterone ratio have been unable to find specific differences between women with premenstrual dysphoric disorder and those without the disorder (14). Some investigators suggested that progesterone and progestogens may actually provoke rather than ameliorate the cyclical symptoms of premenstrual dysphoric disorder (15). The hypothesis that hormonal cyclicity is important in the etiology of premenstrual dysphoric disorder is, nevertheless, supported by several studies. Efforts to suppress ovulation with estradiol patches and cyclical oral norethisterone, use of gonadotropin-releasing hormone (GnRH) agonists, or surgical intervention via bilateral oophorectomy resulted in the disappearance of premenstrual mood disturbances and physical symptoms (16–25).

The current consensus seems to be that normal ovarian function (rather than hormone imbalance) is the cyclical trigger for premenstrual dysphoric disorder-related biochemical events within the central nervous system and other target tissues. A psychoneuroendocrine mechanism triggered by the normal endocrine events of the ovarian cycle seems to be the most plausible explanation (26). This viewpoint is attractive in that it encourages investigation of the neuroendocrine-modulated central neurotransmitters and the role of the hypothalamic-pituitary-gonadal axis in premenstrual dysphoric disorder. Of all the neurotransmitters studied to date, increasing evidence suggests serotonin may be important in the pathogenesis of premenstrual dysphoric disorder (27–31). Premenstrual dysphoric disorder also shares many features of other mood and anxiety disorders linked to serotonergic dysfunction (32–34). In addition, reduction in brain serotonin neurotransmission is thought to lead to poor impulse control, depressed mood, irritability, and increased carbohydrate craving—all mood and behavioral symptoms associated with premenstrual dysphoric disorder (35).

Reciprocity between fluctuations in ovarian steroids and serotonergic function has been established in animals, showing estrogen and progesterone influence central serotonergic neuronal activity. In the hypothalamus, estrogen induces a diurnal fluctuation in serotonin (36), whereas progesterone increases the turnover rate of serotonin (37).

More recently, several studies concluded that serotonin *function* may also be altered in women with premenstrual dysphoric disorder. Some studies used models of neuronal function (such as whole blood serotonin levels, platelet uptake of serotonin, and platelet tritiated imipramine [Tofranil] binding) and found altered serotonin function during all phases of the menstrual cycle (29, 38–41). Other studies that used challenge tests (with L-tryptophan, fenfluramine [Pondimin], and buspirone [BuSpar]) suggested abnormal serotonin function in symptomatic women but differed in their findings as to whether the response to serotonin is blunted or heightened (31, 42–45). These studies imply, at least in part, a possible change in 5-hydroxytryptamine (serotonin) (5-HT_{1A}) receptor sensitivity in women with premenstrual dysphoric disorder.

The current consensus is that women with premenstrual dysphoric disorder may be behaviorally or biochemically subsensitive or supersensitive to biologic challenges of the serotonergic system (46, 47). It is not yet clear whether these women present with a trait or state marker of premenstrual dysphoric disorder.

RISK FACTORS

Epidemiologic surveys from around the world continue to demonstrate convincingly that for adult women, the lifetime prevalence of mood disorders is substantially higher than it is among men. Most studies confirm the ratio of affected women to men is approximately 2:1, and this ratio is maintained across ethnic groups (48). The higher incidence of depression among women is primarily seen beginning at puberty and is less marked in the years after menopause (49). The relationship between premenstrual dysphoric disorder and other psychiatric disorders is complicated by the observation that a high proportion of women presenting with premenstrual dysphoric disorder have a history of previous episodes of mood disorders and that women with an ongoing mood disorder report premenstrual magnification of symptoms and an emergence of new symptoms (32, 50–55). Likewise, several family studies identified a concordance in rates of premenstrual tension between first-degree female family members (56–58).

PRESENTATION AND DIAGNOSIS

To aid in the study of menstrual cycle disorders, each menstrual cycle is characterized as containing two prominent phases: the follicular phase occurs after the onset of menses, and the luteal phase refers to the premenstrual interval. The temporal relationship between fluctuations in psychopathology and different phases of the menstrual cycle are well documented. It is therefore essential to ascertain whether the presenting premenstrual symptomatology is unique to the luteal phase or whether it is a worsening of an ongoing persisting physical or psychiatric disorder.

Unfortunately, investigators have yet to reach consensus on how to best define the follicular and luteal phases of the menstrual cycle. Some investigators use set days, others use cycle adjusted days, and other combinations also exist (Fig. 12.1). Although researchers are still defining the temporal boundaries of the follicular and luteal phase (59), a definition of the follicular phase as days 7 through 11 after onset of bleeding and the luteal phase as 6 days before bleeding through 2 days before bleeding seems most appropriate in clinical settings.

Another challenge in the delineation of premenstrual disorders is that most women report varying combinations of the most troubling symptoms. Some investigators attempted to divide the most prominent symptoms into physical and psychological domains; however, a complete separation is not possible. Measurement tools developed for depression and other mood disorders have not performed well in the diagnosis of premenstrual syndrome (60). A recent review identified at least 65 instruments developed specifically to measure various combinations of premenstrual symptoms. Generally, if an instrument has been tested for reliability and validity in this population, it is appropriate for both facilitating diagnosis and assessing treatment outcomes. There has yet to be consensus as to which instruments are most appropriate for diagnosis and measurement of treatment efficacy so most investigators use at least two or three of these instruments in their clinical trials (2).

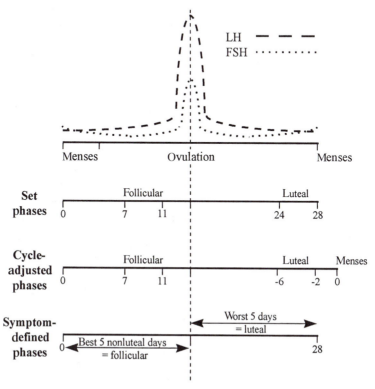

FIGURE 12.1. The follicular and luteal phases can be defined in various ways for research purposes. The cycle-adjusted phases illustrated in the middle graph seem most appropriate to clinical settings. *LH,* luteinizing hormone; *FSH,* follicle-stimulating hormone.

Women presenting with premenstrual complaints should be instructed to chart their symptoms daily over the course of several menstrual cycles to measure symptom changes within each cycle. The current emphasis is on prospective self-report instruments that are easy to administer and score without jeopardizing validity. The Daily Record of Severity of Problems (DRSP) assesses 20 symptoms associated with premenstrual dysphoric disorder and specifically measures functional impairment in work and social realms (61). The Premenstrual Record of Impact and Severity of Menstruation (PRISM) (62) and the Calendar of Premenstrual Experiences (COPE) (63) are detailed one-page calendars (Fig. 12.2) that have also been validated and used in clinical trials. These calendars allow respondents to rate a variety of physical and psychological symptoms, indicate negative and positive life events, and record concurrent medications and track menstrual bleeding and cycle length.

As a result of the lack of objective diagnostic tests for premenstrual syndrome or premenstrual dysphoric disorder, a complete history must be collected in these women. In addition to a retrospective history of the premenstrual symptomatology, this interview should also include a complete review of physical systems (including gynecologic and endocrinologic symptoms, allergies) and medical disorders and a psychiatric history and a detailed review of family history for mental illness. Because the symptoms of anemia and thyroid disease often mirror those of premenstrual syndrome or premenstrual dysphoric disorder, the patient should undergo laboratory studies if there is any hint of an underlying medical cause for the symptoms. In addition, women who are suspected to meet criteria for premenstrual dysphoric disorder should be assessed by their physician at least once during each cycle phase to ensure that the patient subjectively endorses phase-appropriate mood symptoms that support their daily charting (minimal or no symptoms during follicular phase and/or lifestyle-impairing symptoms during the luteal phase) (Table 12.1).

In using the DSM-IV (13) criteria for premenstrual dysphoric disorder (Table 12.2), criterion C is crucial in excluding any current psychiatric or medical illness or episode. The other essential features of the DSM-IV premenstrual dysphoric disorder criteria are the cyclicity of symptoms and the emphasis on core mood symptoms (criterion A), the requirement that the symptoms must interfere markedly with lifestyle (criterion B), and, most importantly, that the disorder must be confirmed prospectively by daily ratings for at least two menstrual cycles (criterion D). Prospective daily rating of symptoms is now the only acceptable means of confirming a provisional DSM-IV diagnosis of premenstrual dysphoric disorder.

The DRSP, PRISM, and COPE daily calendars contain the core symptoms and most additional symptoms considered for the DSM-IV diagnosis of premenstrual dysphoric disorder. In using one of the daily calendars, the clinician must identify a priori the patient's chief complaints and the symptoms to be followed throughout treatment. Daily symptoms are rated by the patient using scales ranging from none (for a score of 0) to severe (for a score of 7 on the PRISM or 3 on the COPE). Scores for the symptoms of interest are added for the 5 follicular days and the 5 luteal days and these total phase scores are then compared.

Investigators have typically followed a diagnostic severity criterion that is applied in addition to the criteria listed for premenstrual dysphoric disorder in the DSM-IV. Conventionally, an increase in symptom scores (worsening) of at least 30% from follicular to luteal phase scores within a single cycle is required to meet premenstrual dysphoric disorder diagnostic criteria (64). More recently it has been suggested that within-cycle worsening of at least 50% is necessary to confirm diagnosis and merit psychopharmacologic intervention (65). The within-cycle percent change is calcu-

Instructions for Completing the PRISM Calendar

1. Prepare the calendar on the first day of menstruation. Considering the first day of bleeding as day 1 of your menstrual cycle, enter the corresponding calendar date for each day in the space provided.

   e.g., Day of menstrual cycle.

   Month: _____   Date: | 1 | 2 | 3 | 4 |

2. Each evening, at about the same time, complete the calendar column for that day as described below:

Bleeding:	Indicate if you have had bleeding by shading the box above that day's date ▉; for spotting use an (x).
Symptoms:	If you do not experience any symptoms, leave the corresponding square blank. If present, indicate the severity by entering a number from 1 (mild) to 7 (severe).
Lifestyle impact:	If the listed phrase applies to you that day, enter an (x).
Life events:	If you experienced one of these events that day, enter an (x).
	Experiences: For positive (happy) or negative (sad/disappointing) experiences unrelated to your symptoms, specify the nature of the events on the back of this form.
	Social activities: This implies such events as a special dinner, show or party, etc. involving family or friends.
	Vigorous exercise: This implies participation in a sporting event or exercise program lasting more than 30 minutes.
Medication:	In the bottom five rows, list medication used, if any, and indicate days when they were taken by entering an (x).

(continued)

FIGURE 12.2. Premenstrual Record of Impact and Severity of Menstruation (PRISM). (Reprinted with permission from Reid RL. Premenstrual syndrome. Curr Probl Obstet Gynecol Fertil 1985;8:1–57.) *(continued)*

Study Number						Baseline weight on Day 1 _____ lbs. or kg. (circle one)

	Bleeding																																			
Day of Menstrual Cycle Month: Date:		1	2	3	4	5	6	7	8	9	10	11	12	13	14	15	16	17	18	19	20	21	22	23	24	25	26	27	28	29	30	31	32	33	34	35
SYMPTOMS																																				
Irritable																																				
Fatigue																																				
Inward anger																																				
Labile mood (crying)																																				
Depressed																																				
Restless																																				
Anxious																																				
Insomnia																																				
Lack of control																																				
Edema or rings tight																																				
Breast tenderness																																				
Abdominal bloating																																				
Bowels: const. (c) loose (l)																																				
Appetite: up ^ down v																																				
Sex drive: up ^ down v																																				
Chills (C) / sweats (S)																																				
Headaches																																				
Crave: sweets, salt																																				
Feel unattractive																																				
Guilty																																				
Unreasonable behavior																																				
Low self-image																																				
Nausea																																				
Menstrual cramps																																				
LIFESTYLE IMPACT																																				
Aggressive towards others	Physically																																			
	Verbally																																			
Wish to be alone																																				
Neglect housework																																				
Time off work																																				
Disorganized, distractible																																				
Accident prone/clumsy																																				
Uneasy about driving																																				
Suicidal thoughts																																				
Stayed at home																																				
Increased use of alcohol																																				
LIFE EVENTS																																				
Negative experience																																				
Positive experience																																				
Social activities																																				
Vigorous exercise																																				
MEDICATIONS																																				

FIGURE 12.2.—*continued*

TABLE 12.1. Workup of the Woman with Premenstrual Symptoms

HISTORY, PAYING SPECIAL ATTENTION TO
History of present illness
Review of systems (especially gynecologic and endocrine)
Past medical history
Past psychiatric history
Family history (especially psychiatric disorders)

PHYSICAL EXAMINATION

SCREENING LABORATORY TESTS, IF INDICATED BY HISTORY OR PHYSICAL
Hemoglobin
Thyroid-stimulating hormone

SELF-REPORT CALENDAR, FILLED OUT BY PATIENT FOR AT LEAST TWO CYCLES
Daily Record of Severity of Problems (DRSP), or
Premenstrual Record of Impact and Severity of Menstruation (PRISM), or
Calendar of Premenstrual Experiences (COPE)

MOOD SYMPTOMS, ASSESSED SUBJECTIVELY BY THE PHYSICIAN
During follicular phase (at least once)
During luteal phase (at least once)

TABLE 12.2. Summary of Premenstrual Dysphoric Disorder Criteria

A. Symptoms must occur during the week before menses and remit a few days after onset of menses.
   Five of the following symptoms must be present and include at least one from numbers 1, 2, 3, or 4.
   1. Depressed mood or dysphoria
   2. Anxiety or tension
   3. Affective lability
   4. Irritability
   5. Decreased interest in usual activities
   6. Concentration difficulties
   7. Marked lack of energy
   8. Marked change in appetite, overeating, or food cravings
   9. Hypersomnia or insomnia
   10. Feeling overwhelmed
   11. Other physical symptoms, i.e., breast tenderness, bloating
B. Symptoms must interfere with work, school, usual activities, or relationships
C. Symptoms must not merely be an exacerbation of another disorder (major mental disorder, personality disorder, or general medical condition)
D. Criteria A, B, and C must be confirmed by prospective daily ratings for at least two cycles

Adapted from American Psychiatric Association. Diagnostic and Statistical Manual of Mental Disorder, 4th ed. Washington, DC: American Psychiatric Association, 1994:717–718.

lated by subtracting the follicular score from the luteal score, dividing by the luteal score and multiplying by 100:

$$[(\text{luteal score} - \text{follicular score}) \div (\text{luteal score})] \times 100\% \quad (\text{Eq. 1})$$

Thus, a patient presenting with a mean follicular score of 20 and luteal score of 50 would demonstrate a within-cycle symptom increase of 60%. A change of this proportion demonstrates the cyclicity of symptomatology and is typical of women who meet criteria for premenstrual dysphoric disorder.

Upon completion of the two-cycle prospective diagnostic assessment phase, women may qualify for one of the following diagnostic categories.

Premenstrual Dysphoric Disorder

Women who receive this diagnosis meet criteria for premenstrual dysphoric disorder only, they have no other concurrent psychiatric disorder(s) or unstable medical condition(s), but may have a history of a past psychiatric disorder. When they chart symptoms daily for two cycles, their chief complaints include one of four core symptoms and at least 5 of 11 total symptoms (Table 12.2). Their symptoms have occurred with most menstrual cycles during the past year and have interfered with social or occupational roles. Their symptoms demonstrate clear worsening premenstrually and remit within a few days after the onset of the follicular phase. In addition, worsening between the follicular and luteal phases must be at least 30%.

Premenstrual Syndrome

Women who receive this diagnosis do not meet all DSM-IV criteria for premenstrual dysphoric disorder but do demonstrate symptom exacerbation premenstrually. Symptoms may include mild psychological discomfort and feelings of bloating and weight gain, breast tenderness, swelling of hands and feet, various aches and pains, poor concentration, sleep disturbance, and change in appetite. Only one symptom is required for this diagnosis, although the symptoms must be restricted to the luteal phase of the menstrual cycle, reach a peak shortly before menstruation, and cease with the menstrual flow or soon after (3).

Premenstrual Magnification

Women who receive this diagnosis may meet most of the criteria for premenstrual syndrome or premenstrual dysphoric disorder but are in the process of being assessed for or have been identified with a current major psychiatric disorder or an unstable medical condition (66). Medical disorders that are commonly exacerbated during the luteal phase include migraine headaches, allergies, asthma, seizures, and genital herpes. Psychiatric conditions that can be magnified include depression, anxiety, panic, bulimia, substance abuse, mania, and psychosis (67).

Other Psychiatric Diagnosis Only

These women do not demonstrate premenstrual symptoms that meet criteria for premenstrual dysphoric disorder but do meet DSM-IV criteria for another psychiatric disorder. Women meeting criteria for intermittent depressive disorder or cyclothymia may also fall into this category, where the cyclical nature of their symptoms does not necessarily match the phases of their menstrual cycle.

No Diagnosis

In these women, the diagnosis of premenstrual syndrome or premenstrual dysphoric disorder cannot be made and medical, gynecologic, and psychiatric screening is negative. These women experience disruptive symptoms that tend to occur throughout the cycle. It is often difficult to delineate the exact problem. Careful examination of the entire diary, especially the follicular phase, and discussion with the patient may show low-grade psychiatric or medical problems such as situational, vocational, or marital stress; irritable bowel syndrome; chronic fatigue syndrome; headache; fibromyalgia or other pain syndromes; and sleep disorders.

Applying these criteria to women who seek help for premenstrual complaints will facilitate the clinician in planning management interventions.

TREATMENT

Women who present with premenstrual magnification of a major psychiatric disorder, personality disorder, or general medical disorder should be treated for the primary disorder at the discretion of the supervising clinician. Referral to an appropriate specialist is often indicated for newly diagnosed disorders.

A wide range of therapeutic interventions has been tested in the treatment of premenstrual symptoms, from lifestyle changes to advanced hormonal treatment.

Conservative Therapies

It is prudent to start all women with premenstrual symptoms on a program of lifestyle changes (Table 12.3). For women who do not meet criteria for premenstrual syndrome, premenstrual dysphoric disorder, or other physical and psychological disorders, these conservative treatments are appropriate, and management without pharmacologic interventions should be encouraged. Unfortunately, there have been few randomized controlled trials to determine the efficacy of these conservative interventions. There is some evidence, however, to support that these patients may best respond to individual or group psychotherapy in combination with lifestyle changes (68, 69). Recommended dietary changes (especially during the luteal phase) should include the reduction or limitation of tobacco, chocolate, caffeine, and alcohol. Some women report improvement with small, frequent, complex carbohydrate meals with vitamin and mineral supplements (such as a daily multivitamin). Patients should be encouraged to decrease excess sodium in the diet when edema or fluid retention occurs and, if possible, to reduce or maintain weight to within 20% of their ideal weight. Regular exercise is important and particularly effective when combined with

TABLE 12.3. Conservative Treatment for Premenstrual Symptoms

CHARTING OF SYMPTOMS DAILY

DIET
Reduce or eliminate (especially in the luteal phase) salt, chocolate, caffeine, and alcohol
Small frequent complex carbohydrate meals
Vitamins and minerals in moderation

MODERATE, REGULAR AEROBIC EXERCISE

STRESS REDUCTION
Stress management course and/or counseling if necessary
Relaxation course or audio tape
Assertiveness course and/or marital counseling if necessary

SELF-HELP BOOKS, GROUPS IF AVAILABLE

the regular practice of stress management techniques. Patients should also be taught to review their own monthly diaries and identify triggers to symptom exacerbation.

Low-Risk Evidence-Based Therapies

Women who meet criteria for premenstrual syndrome should be encouraged to practice the lifestyle changes described above, but they may also respond to some of the tested conservative therapies (Table 12.4).

Vitamin B_6 has demonstrated mixed efficacy in clinical trials, with most trials demonstrating ambiguous or negative results using a wide range of dosing strategies from 50 to 500 mg daily (70). Studies reporting positive results used daily dosing of 100, 300, and 500 mg daily for two to four cycles (71, 72). Improvements in depression and irritability were reported by two studies (73). Because of reports of sensory neuropathy, dosing in clinical practice should not exceed 100 mg daily to be given during the last 2 weeks of each cycle.

Calcium (1000 mg daily) demonstrated significant improvement in negative affect, water retention, and pain compared with placebo in one clinical trial (74). No untoward side effects were reported with this dose.

Magnesium (360 mg daily) from the 15th day of the menstrual cycle to the onset of menstrual flow significantly improved premenstrual pain and negative affect in one randomized controlled trial (75).

Optivite (Otimox Corp., Torrance, CA) is a vitamin/mineral supplement. In one randomized controlled trial, subjects were randomized to 6 or 12 tablets of the supplement or placebo daily for three menstrual cycles and demonstrated significant treatment effects in physical symptoms and depression (76). No unusual side effects were reported. Clinically, up to six Optivite tablets daily during the luteal phase of the menstrual cycle may relieve symptoms.

Vitamin E (α-tocopherol) was administered in a randomized controlled trial to women with benign breast disease who scored the severity of their premenstrual symptoms before and after 2 months of vitamin E therapy (150, 300, or 600 IU/day versus placebo) (77). Significant improvements in physical symptoms and depression were demonstrated by all three treatment groups compared with placebo. Vitamin E therapy can safely begin at 400 IU daily.

Primrose evening oil (γ-linolenic acid) has not demonstrated efficacy superior to placebo in randomized trials and should not be recommended as treatment for premenstrual syndrome or premenstrual dysphoric disorder (78).

Naproxen sodium (Anaprox) improved premenstrual behavioral changes in one randomized trial when taken 7 days premenstrually (79) and menstrual migraine specifically in another randomized trial when it was taken on a daily basis (80).

Mefenamic acid (Ponstel) was superior to placebo for improving physical and

TABLE 12.4. Low-Risk Evidence-Based Treatment for Premenstrual Symptoms

	Dosage
Vitamin B_6	100 mg/day
Calcium	1000 mg/day
Magnesium	360 mg/day (14 days before menses)
Optivite	Up to 6 tablets day
Multivitamin	Per label directions
Vitamin E	400 IU/day

mood symptoms in one randomized trial; however, the use of this medication should be limited (7 to 10 days) because of gastric side effects (81).

Spironolactone (100 mg daily from day 12 of the menstrual cycle until the first day of the next menstrual cycle) significantly reduced bloating compared with placebo in one randomized controlled trial (82). The potential for diuretic abuse and the serious contraindication of potassium supplementation necessitates the use of this drug for severe symptoms only.

Bromocriptine (at least 5 mg daily) has demonstrated significant improvement in premenstrual mastodynia (83) but has not demonstrated efficacy with the mood symptoms associated with the premenstruum. Randomized controlled trial evidence suggests that a dosing range of 1.25 to 7.5 mg daily during the luteal phase of the menstrual cycle is appropriate for clinical use (83).

Women who continue to experience severe premenstrual symptoms after the commencement of lifestyle changes and the above conservative therapies may be considered for the pharmacologic treatment regimens indicated for premenstrual dysphoric disorder.

Pharmacotherapies

Therapeutic interventions for women who meet criteria for premenstrual dysphoric disorder and fail conservative therapies are available. These range from treatment of the most troublesome symptoms with psychotropic medications (Table 12.5) to hormonal therapy to eliminate ovulation (Table 12.6).

Listed below is a summary of the randomized controlled trial evidence for the most common therapies used to treat premenstrual dysphoric disorder. It is important to note that only studies that used prospective diagnostic criteria that could meet premenstrual dysphoric disorder classification have been cited (13).

Psychotropic Medications. Serotonin reuptake inhibitors have proven to be very successful in the treatment of premenstrual dysphoric disorder symptoms. Of the *selective* serotonin reuptake inhibitors, fluoxetine (Prozac), 20 mg/day, has been proven superior to placebo in several randomized trials (65, 84–87). One demonstrated the efficacy of fluoxetine (Prozac), 60 mg/day, although the improvement demonstrated by this group was not different than that demonstrated by women receiving 20 mg/day and the side-effect profile was significantly higher at the 60-mg dose (65). Sertraline

TABLE 12.5. Psychotropic Medications for Premenstrual Dysphoric Disorder and Premenstrual Syndrome Refractory to Conservative Treatment

	Dosage
Fluoxetine (Prozac)	20 mg/day
Sertraline (Zoloft)	50–150 mg/day
Paroxetine (Paxil)	10–30 mg/day
Clomipramine (Anafranil)	25–75 mg/day (14 days before menses)
Alprazolam (Xanax)	0.25–0.5 mg/day (6–14 days before menses)
Busiprone (BuSpar)	5 mg tid to 7.5 BID, with maximum of 20 TID or 30 BID daily (12 days before menses)

TABLE 12.6. Hormonal Therapies for Premenstrual Dysphoric Disorder Refractory to Other Treatment

	Dosage
GnRH AGONISTS	
Buserelin acetate	400–900 μg/day, intranasally
Nafarelin acetate (Synarel)	2 mg/mL daily, intranasally
Leuprolide (Lupron)	3.75–7.5 mg/mo, intramuscularly
plus	
ADD-BACK ESTROGEN AND PROGESTERONE	
Conjugated estrogen (Premarin)	0.625 mg/day (Monday to Saturday)
+	
Medroxyprogesterone (Provera)	Daily for 12 days every fourth menstrual cycle
or	
Transdermal estradiol	
Estraderm, Vivelle	0.05–0.1-mg patches (2 per week)
Climara	0.05–0.1-mg patches (1 per week)
+	
Progestogen (Provera) each cycle	10 mg days 1–12 each cycle or 5 mg days 1–14
ANDROGENIC AGENTS	
Danazol (Danocrine)	200–400 mg/day
ALTERNATIVE THERAPIES	
Progesterone, oral contraceptives	Demonstrated lack of efficacy

(Zoloft), 50 to 150 mg/day (88), and paroxetine (Paxil), 10 to 30 mg/day (89), also demonstrated efficacy in single randomized trials. Pilot studies demonstrated the efficacy of intermittent serotonin reuptake inhibitor dosing during the last 2 weeks of the menstrual cycle (90, 91). These findings, however, have yet to be confirmed by a large, randomized, controlled trial. The primarily serotonin tricyclic antidepressant reuptake inhibitor clomipramine (Anafranil) has also been proven superior to placebo in two randomized controlled trials. One study used 25 to 75 mg/day (92) and the other 25 to 75 mg/day for the luteal phase of each menstrual cycle (93). Thus, the serotonin reuptake inhibitors to date demonstrated their effectiveness in significantly improving the psychological and physical symptoms of premenstrual dysphoric disorder compared with placebo with only mild, mostly tolerable, side effects. The side-effect profile is similar among agents in the class, the most troublesome including headache, nausea/gastrointestinal upset, sleep disturbance/insomnia, tremulousness, sweating, dry mouth, and anorgasmia. These side effects can usually be managed through dosing changes, the use of intermittent versus daily dosing schedules, or by switching to other serotonin reuptake inhibitor compounds.

Anxiolytics have been tested for the treatment of premenstrual dysphoric disorder because of its mood disorder component. Alprazolam (Xanax) successfully alleviated the symptoms of premenstrual dysphoric disorder in several (94–97) but not all (98) randomized controlled trials. The risk of dependence and concerns regarding withdrawal prompted investigators to test the efficacy of alprazolam (Xanax) versus placebo when administered in the luteal phase only. Patient-modified dosing was allowed, and efficacious dosing ranged from 0.25 to 5.0 mg/day from 6 to 14 days before menstruation. One study also allowed women who demonstrated mild follicular symptoms to take this medication as needed during the follicular phase of the cycle (96). Sedation and drowsiness were the two most frequently identified side effects of this treatment. Significant improvements in mood and physical symptoms were reported for the positive studies. The $5-HT_{1A}$ receptor partial antagonist buspirone (BuSpar) has also demonstrated efficacy in one randomized controlled trial when administered at a mean daily dose of 25 mg for the 12 days before menstruation (99).

Hormonal Therapies. GnRH agonists can reversibly suppress the menstrual cycle, and this is often called "medical ovariectomy" or "medical menopause." GnRH agonists have proven to be very successful in improving mood in most, although not all, clinical trials. Unfortunately, the long-term use of GnRH agonists has been inhibited by the occurrence of side effects that mimic menopause and the potential for hypoestrogenism and osteoporosis. Preliminary evidence suggests that "add-back" therapy with low-dose estrogen and progesterone replacement therapy may prevent some side effects (22).

Intramuscular depot leuprolide (Lupron; 3.75 mg/mo) was significantly superior to saline placebo in one randomized controlled trial (16), whereas at a dose of 7.5 mg/mo it was not (100). GnRH agonist therapy significantly improved both mood and physical symptoms in many randomized controlled trials (16, 19–20, 22, 23, 100). In addition, monthly subcutaneous injections of the GnRH agonist goserelin (Zoladex; 3.6 mg) demonstrated a significant effect on physical symptoms but not mood symptoms when compared with placebo (101). Intramuscular leuprolide (Lupron), 3.75 to 7.5 mg/mo, or intranasal buserelin, 400 to 900 µg/day, are the most appropriate GnRH agonist treatments for clinical use.

The current indication for GnRH agonists requires that they not be used for longer than 6 months (cumulative) because of concerns about increased risk of osteoporosis and cardiovascular disease. It is not yet known how long one can prolong the treatment with GnRH agonists if hormone replacement therapy is concomitantly used. The most common add-back regimen consists of conjugated estrogen (Premarin), 0.625 mg/day (Monday to Saturday), and 5 mg medroxyprogesterone (Provera) daily for 14 days during every fourth menstrual cycle. Other add-back regimens have also been used.

Estradiol treatment can suppress ovulation and thus has been proven effective in reducing the symptoms of premenstrual dysphoric disorder, although adjunct progestogen therapy is necessary to prevent endometrial hyperplasia. Luteal phase-only administration of conjugated estrogen (Premarin) was ineffective in one randomized controlled trial (102); however, transdermal estradiol (Climara, Estraderm, Vivelle) or estradiol implants combined with luteal-phase norethisterone, medroxyprogesterone (Provera), or dydrogesterone improved physical and mood symptoms in three randomized controlled trials (25, 103, 104). Transdermal estradiol (Climara, Estraderm, or Vivelle) with low-dose progestogen daily from days 17 to 26 of each cycle is appropriate for clinical use.

Danazol (Danocrine) is a synthetic androgen, capable of suppressing the hypothalamic-pituitary-gonadal axis. Whereas the follicle-stimulating hormone and luteinizing hormone basal concentration levels remain normal in premenopausal women, danazol eliminates the midcycle surge of these hormones. Although danazol has proven superior to placebo in several randomized controlled trials (105–108), the adverse effect profile of this treatment is considerable and is the result of both its androgenic activity and antiestrogen properties. Tested doses include 100 to 400 mg/day, and both mood and physical symptoms improved significantly when compared with placebo. The most prominent side effect was altered menstrual cycle length, but at higher doses women can get acne, bloating, depression, and permanent lowering of the voice. One study of women with premenstrual syndrome found that danazol, 200 mg/day, from the onset of symptoms to the onset of menses significantly improved mood symptoms and bloating compared with placebo (109). Clinical dosing at 200 to 400 mg/day during symptoms is appropriate.

Progesterone has been shown to be no more effective than placebo in treating premenstrual syndrome or premenstrual dysphoric disorder symptoms in most trials and should not be used as a primary treatment for these disorders (97, 110–118).

Oral contraceptives suppress ovulation while maintaining menstruation with periodic steroid withdrawal. Oral contraceptives have side effects that are often similar to the symptoms of premenstrual syndrome or premenstrual dysphoric disorder. The one randomized controlled trial that tested oral contraceptives in this population was a negative study (119) that supported the conclusions of other less-rigorous studies. Until additional studies are done, oral contraceptives should not be used to treat premenstrual syndrome or premenstrual dysphoric disorder.

To date, no one intervention has proven to be effective for all women with premenstrual dysphoric disorder. Selective serotonin reuptake inhibitors and clomipramine (Anafranil) continue to prove efficacious in women with premenstrual dysphoric disorder who have failed conservative treatment and are currently the first treatment of choice. Alprazolam (Xanax) and buspirone (BuSpar) demonstrated efficacy in the reduction of psychological symptoms in randomized controlled trials, but side effects and the possibility of dependence inhibit maximum efficacy. The last line of treatment for women with premenstrual dysphoric disorder are the hormonal treatments, including the GnRH agonists with low-dose estrogen and progesterone add-back. Estradiol and danazol may also be effective, and gynecologic interventions such as oophorectomy may need to be considered (17, 18).

ASSESSMENT OF EFFICACY

Patients should be assessed every 2 weeks (i.e., during both the follicular and luteal phases) within the first month of commencing any therapy, and they should be instructed to continue to chart symptoms daily for at least two to three additional cycles. Dosing strategies vary, but most recent investigations demonstrated the efficacy of most therapeutic drugs at low doses. If efficacy has not been attained after several dose increases, alternative treatment options should be considered. There is increasing evidence that treatment effect is seen relatively quickly in this population. Therefore, if there is no change in symptomatology, an alternate therapy should be considered within two to three menstrual cycles. Continued symptom charting using a daily calendar helps to track efficacy, symptom response to dosing changes, symptoms upon termination of therapy, and side effects. For example, women who report headaches or nausea as side effects are often surprised to see that they rated these symptoms just as severe before commencing therapy.

Investigators have yet to reach a consensus on how to define efficacy. Clinically, the easiest way to define efficacy is by the reduction of luteal symptoms so that the luteal symptoms remit significantly or the within-cycle percent change (see Eq. 1) is less than 30%. In addition, instruments like the Clinical Global Impression-Efficacy Index are gaining popularity because the clinician can rate therapeutic effectiveness against side effects for an adjusted efficacy rating (120) (Fig. 12.3).

What has become obvious is that intervention alone cannot predict efficacy, and more consideration is now being given to past psychiatric history and to family psychiatric history, especially of mood disorders in the families of women with premenstrual dysphoric disorder.

CLINICAL GLOBAL IMPRESSIONS

INSTRUCTIONS: *Mark these items on General Scoring Sheet coded 01.*

Complete item 1 – SEVERITY OF ILLNESS at the initial and subsequent assessments. Items 2 and 3 may be omitted at the initial assessment by marking 0 – "Not Assessed."

Mark on the left half of the scoring sheet on rows 38–41.

ROW NO.	CLINICAL GLOBAL IMPRESSIONS
38	1. SEVERITY OF ILLNESS Considering your total clinical experience with this particular population, how mentally ill is the patient at this time? 0 = Not assessed 4 = Moderately ill 1 = Normal, not at all ill 5 = Markedly ill 2 = Borderline mentally ill 6 = Severely ill 3 = Mildly ill 7 = Among the most extremely ill patients

THE NEXT TWO ITEMS MAY BE OMITTED AT THE INITIAL ASSESSMENT BY MARKING "NOT ASSESSED" FOR BOTH ITEMS

39	2. GLOBAL IMPROVEMENT – Rate total improvement whether or not, in your judgment, it is due entirely to drug treatment. Compared to his condition at admission to the project, how much has he changed? 0 = Not assessed 4 = No change 1 = Very much improved 5 = Minimally worse 2 = Much improved 6 = Much worse 3 = Minimally improved 7 = Very much worse
40 & 41	3. EFFICACY INDEX – Rate this item on the basis of DRUG EFFECT ONLY. Select the terms that best describe the degrees of therapeutic effect and side effects and record the number in the box where the two items intersect. EXAMPLE: Therapeutic effect is rated as "Moderate" and side effects are judged "Do not significantly interfere with patient's functioning." Record 06 in rows 40 and 41.

THERAPEUTIC EFFECT	SIDE EFFECTS			
	None	Do not significantly interfere with patient's functioning	Significantly interfere with patient's functioning	Outweigh therapeutic effect
MARKED — Vast improvement. Complete or nearly complete remission of all symptoms	01	02	03	04
MODERATE — Decided improvement. Partial remission of symptoms	05	06	07	08
MINIMAL — Slight improvement which doesn't alter status of care of patient	09	10	11	12
UNCHANGED OR WORSE	13	14	15	16
Not Assessed = 00				

(continued)

FIGURE 12.3. Clinical Global Impression-Efficacy Index used to rate therapeutic effectiveness against side effects for an adjusted efficacy rating. *ECDEU,* early clinical drug evaluation unit.

Clinical Global Impressions (CGI), developed during the PRB collaborative schizo-phrenic studies, consists of three global scales (items) formatted for use with the General Scoring Sheet. Since the items are "universal," the CGI is included in both the Pediatric and Adult packets. Two of the items, Severity of Illness and Global Improvement, are rated on a 7-point scale, while the third, Efficacy Index, requires a rating of the interaction of therapeutic effectiveness and adverse reactions.

APPLICABILITY	For all research populations
UTILIZATION	For Severity of Illness: Once at pretreatment and at least one posttreatment assessment. Additional ratings are at the discretion of the investigator.
	For Global Improvement and Efficacy Index: No pretreatment (baseline) assessment is required. At least one posttreatment assessment should be made. Additional posttreatment ratings are at the discretion of the investigator.
TIME SPAN RATED	For Severity of Illness: Now or within the last week.
	For Global Improvement: Since admission to the study.
	For Efficacy Index: Now or within the last week.

CARD FORMAT—ITEMS CARD 01 = (19×, 2I1, I2)

Item	Column
Severity of Illness	20
Global Improvement	21
Efficacy Index	22–23

SPECIAL INSTRUCTIONS

The contexts under which the three CGI items are to be rated have been modified to increase the reliability and precision of the items. Veteran ECDEU raters should be alert to these new contexts.

Item 1—Severity of Illness—For this item, the modification for rating context is:

OLD	Considering your total clinical experience, how mentally ill is the patient at this time?
NEW	Considering your total clinical experience with this particular population, how mentally ill is the patient at this time?

The old version asked the rater to judge the severity of illness of a given subject in the context of that rater's total experience with all types of patients; i.e., regardless of diagnosis, chronicity, age, etc. The present version restricts the judgment within the range of the specific population under study. Thus, an anxious neurotic subject is judged in the context of the rater's experience with anxious neurotics, not, as was the case in the past, against a clinical background that may have included schizophrenics, brain-damaged, and depressive subjects as well as anxious ones.

FIGURE 12.3.—*continued*

Item 2—Global Improvement—The modification here involves the relationship between this item and Efficacy Index (Item 3). In the past, no distinction between TOTAL clinical improvement and that portion of the TOTAL that, in the opinion of the rater, is the direct result of the drug administered. The present contexts are:

Global Improvement
GLOBAL IMPROVEMENT—Rate total improvement whether or not, in your judgment, it is
due entirely to drug treatment.

Efficacy Index
EFFICACY INDEX—Rate this item on the basis of DRUG EFFECT ONLY.

In many studies, of course, TOTAL improvement and improvement due to drug will be one and the same; nevertheless, the new contexts allow a distinction to be made when it is present.

Raters are cautioned to observe the unique time span rated for Global Improvement. For most other ECDEU items, the time span to be rated is either a specified number of days or since the last rating. The time span for Global Improvement—at each and every rating—is "since admission to the project (study)," NOT from the last rating period.

Item 3—Efficacy Index—In addition to the contextual modification mentioned above, the matrix of therapeutic vs. side effects has been changed as follows:

THERAPEUTIC EFFECT	SIDE EFFECTS			
	None	Do not significantly interfere with patient's functioning	Significantly interfere with patient's functioning	Outweigh therapeutic effect
MARKED—Vast improvement. Complete or nearly complete remission of all symptoms	01	02	03	04
MODERATE—Decided improvement. Partial remission of symptoms	05	06	07	08
MINIMAL—Slight improvement that doesn't alter status of care of patient	09	10	11	12
UNCHANGED OR WORSE	13	14	15	16
Not Assessed = 00				

FIGURE 12.3.—*continued*

The new matrix has been made symmetrical (4 × 4) by combining two therapeutic cate-gories, "Unchanged" and "Worse" into one category. Category 4 of Side Effects has also been reworded.

Efficacy Index is an attempt to relate therapeutic effects and side effects. Therapeutic effect is regarded as gross profit; side effects, as cost. The Index, then, is analogous to net profit. The Index is derived by dividing therapeutic effect score by side effect score as follows:

	Side Effects			
Therapeutic Effect	None 1	No Significant Interference 2	Significant Interference 3	Out-weigh 4
4 Marked	4.00*	2.00	1.33	1.00
3 Moderate	3.00	1.50	1.00	0.75
2 Minimal	2.00	1.00	0.67	0.50
1 Unchanged or Worse	1.00	0.50	0.33	0.25

$$*\text{Example:} \quad \frac{\text{Therapeutic Score (4)}}{\text{Side Effect Score (1)}} = \text{Efficacy Index (4.00)}$$

The transformation procedure for Efficacy Index (EI) is:
Number Encoded = Transformed Score = EI

Number Encoded	Transformed Score	EI
01	41	4.00
02	42	2.00
03	43	1.33
04	44	1.00
05	31	3.00
06	32	1.50
07	33	1.00
08	34	0.75
09	21	2.00
10	22	1.00
11	23	0.67
12	24	0.50
13	11	1.00
14	12	0.50
15	13	0.33
16	14	0.25
00	00	0.00

Employing the cross-tabulation scheme to interpret EI, indices falling on the diagonal CB would indicate that the therapeutic and toxic effects of a treatment are equivalent. Those in the upper left quadrant would indicate some degree of "profit"—the profit increasing as

FIGURE 12.3.—*continued*

pole A is approached. The converse is true of indices falling in the lower right quadrant and, in fact, in all of the last column. The treatment with the greatest efficacy fills the cell at Pole A; the worst, at Pole D. The cell at Pole C contains the "insert" treatment. Pole B represents a paradoxical and "theoretical" cell—not one likely to be encountered in the real world.

DOCUMENTATION
  a. Raw score printout
  b. Means and standard deviations
  c. Frequencies and cross-tabulations
  d. Variance analyses

FIGURE 12.3.—*continued*

SUMMARY

The recent inclusion of research criteria for premenstrual dysphoric disorder in the DSM-IV validates the findings that some women in their reproductive years have extremely distressing emotional and behavioral symptoms premenstrually and should help clinicians recognize these women. The diagnosis of premenstrual syndrome is primarily reserved for milder physical symptoms and minor mood changes occurring before menses. Premenstrual magnification occurs when physical and/or psychological symptoms of a concurrent psychiatric and/or medical disorder are magnified during the premenstruum.

To apply the DSM-IV criteria for premenstrual dysphoric disorder, women must chart symptoms daily for two cycles and their chief complaints must include one of four core symptoms (irritability, tension, dysphoria, and lability of mood) and at least 5 of 11 total symptoms. The symptoms should have occurred with most menstrual cycles during the past year and have interfered with social or occupational roles. In addition, the charting of troublesome symptoms should demonstrate clear worsening premenstrually and remit within a few days after the onset of menstruation. Changes in symptoms from the follicular to luteal phase should be at least 30% to make a diagnosis of premenstrual dysphoric disorder and worsening between the follicular and luteal phases should increase by at least 50% to warrant pharmacologic treatment.

It is important to exclude the possibility that the presentation is of a different major psychiatric or medical problem with premenstrual onset. The relationship between premenstrual dysphoric disorder and other psychiatric disorders is further complicated by the observation that a high proportion of women presenting with premenstrual dysphoric disorder have a history of previous episodes of mood disorders and that women with a continuing mood disorder report premenstrual magnification of symptoms and an emergence of new symptoms.

Treatment options range from conservative measures, such as diet, exercise, or stress management, to treatment with psychotropic medications. For the more extreme cases, hormonal or surgical interventions to eliminate ovulation may be necessary therapies. Taken together, these data indicate that treatment may be accomplished by either eliminating the hormonal trigger or by reversing the sensitivity of the serotonergic system.

CLINICAL NOTES

Etiology

- Normal ovarian function is the cyclical trigger for premenopausal symptoms. Evidence suggests that serotonin may be the neurotransmitter involved.

Risk Factors

- Prior or ongoing mood disorder and affected first-degree family members may predispose a woman to premenstrual dysphoric disorder.

Presentation and Diagnosis

- DSM-IV lists criteria for premenstrual dysphoric disorder (Table 12.2). Women who do not meet these criteria may be categorized with premenstrual syndrome, premenstrual magnification (of a psychiatric or medical condition), other psychiatric diagnosis only, or no diagnosis.

Treatment

- Conservative treatment is used for all patients, including those with premenstrual complaints but no diagnosis.
- Low-risk/evidence-based modalities, including vitamins and nonsteroidal anti-inflammatories, are used for women with premenstrual syndrome or premenstrual dysphoric disorder.
- Psychotropics such as serotonin reuptake inhibiting antidepressants or anxiolytics may be useful for women with premenstrual dysphoric disorder or for other conditions refractory to conservative treatment.
- Hormonal therapies should be reserved for refractory premenstrual dysphoric disorder patients because of the adverse effects associated with "medical menopause." Oral contraceptives are not effective for premenstrual dysphoric disorder.

Assessment of Efficacy

- Patients should continue charting their symptoms. If on pharmacologic therapy, the physician should evaluate them during both the follicular and luteal phases of at least one cycle.

References

1. Johnson SR. The epidemiology and social impact of premenstrual symptoms. Clin Obstet Gynecol 1987;30:367–376.
2. Budeiri DJ, Li Wan Po A, Dornan JC. Clinical trials of treatment of premenstrual syndrome: entry criteria and scales for measuring treatment outcomes. Br J Obstet Gynaecol 1994;101:689–695.
3. World Health Organization. Mental, Behavioral and Developmental Disorders. Tenth Revision of the International Classification of Diseases (ICD-10). Geneva: World Health Organization, 1992.
4. Haskett RF, DeLongis A, Kessler RC. Premenstrual dysphoria: a community survey. Proceedings of the American Psychiatric Association Annual Meeting, Chicago, 1987.
5. Johnson SR, McChesney C, Bean JA. Epidemiology of premenstrual symptoms in a nonclinical sample. I. Prevalence, natural history and help-seeking behavior. J Reprod Med 1988;33:340–346.
6. Rivera-Tovar AD, Frank E. Late luteal phase dysphoric disorder in young women. Am J Psychiatry 1990;147:1634–1636.
7. Andersch B, Wendestam C, Hahn L, et al. Premenstrual complaints. Prevalence of premenstrual symptoms in a Swedish urban population. J Psychosom Obstet Gynaecol 1986;5:39–49.

8. Merikangas KR, Foeldenyi M, Angst J. The Zurich Study. XIX. Patterns of menstrual disturbances in the community: results of the Zurich Cohort Study. Eur Arch Psychiatry Clin Neurosci 1993;243:23–32.

9. Ramcharan S, Love EJ, Fick GH, et al. The epidemiology of premenstrual symptoms in a population based sample of 2650 urban women. J Clin Epidemiol 1992;45:377–378.

10. Freeman EW, Sondheimer K, Weinbaum PJ, et al. Evaluating premenstrual symptoms in medical practice. Obstet Gynecol 1985;65:500–505.

11. O'Brien PMS, Abukhalil IEH, Henshaw C. Premenstrual syndrome. Curr Obstet Gynecol 1995;5:30–37.

12. American Psychiatric Association. Diagnostic and Statistical Manual of Mental Disorders. 3rd ed. Washington, DC: American Psychiatric Association, 1987:367–369.

13. American Psychiatric Association. Diagnostic and Statistical Manual of Mental Disorders. 4th ed. Washington, DC: American Psychiatric Association, 1994:717–718.

14. Roca CA, Schmidt PJ, Bloch M, et a. Implications of endocrine studies of premenstrual syndrome. Psychiatr Ann 1996;26:576–580.

15. Hammarback S, Backstrom T, Holst J, et al. Cyclical mood changes as in the premenstrual tension syndrome during sequential estrogen-progestogen postmenopausal replacement therapy. Acta Obstet Gynecol Scand 1985;64:393–397.

16. Brown CS, Ling FW, Andersen RN, et al. Efficacy of depot leuprolide in premenstrual syndrome: effect of symptom severity and type in a controlled trial. Obstet Gynecol 1994;84:779–786.

17. Casper RF, Hearn MT. The effect of hysterectomy and bilateral oophorectomy in women with severe premenstrual syndrome. Am J Obstet Gynecol 1990;162:105–109.

18. Casson P, Hahn PM, Van Vugt DA, et al. Lasting response to ovariectomy in severe intractable premenstrual syndrome. Am J Obstet Gynecol 1990;162:99–105.

19. Hammarback S, Backstrom T. Induced anovulation as treatment of premenstrual tension syndrome: A double-blind cross-over study with GnRH-agonist versus placebo. Acta Obstet Gynaecol Scand 1988;67:159–166.

20. Hussain SY, Massil JH, Matta WH, et al. Buserelin in premenstrual syndrome. Gynecol Endocrinol 1992;6:57–64.

21. Mezrow G, Shoupe D, Spicer D, et al. Depot leuprolide acetate with estrogen and progestin add-back for long-term treatment of premenstrual syndrome. Fertil Steril 1994; 62:932–937.

22. Mortola JF, Girton L, Fischer U. Successful treatment of severe premenstrual syndrome by combined use of gonadotropin-releasing hormone agonist and estrogen/progestin. J Clin Endocrinol Metab 1991;72:252A–252F.

23. Muse KN, Cetel NS, Futterman LA, et al. The premenstrual syndrome: effects of a "medical ovariectomy." N Engl J Med 1984;311:1345–1349.

24. Smith RN, Studd JW. Estrogens and depression in women. In: Lobo RA, ed. Treatment of the Postmenopausal Woman: Basic and Clinical Aspects. New York: Raven, 1993:129–135.

25. Watson NR, Studd JW, Savvas M, et al. Treatment of severe premenstrual syndrome with estradiol patches and cyclical oral norethisterone. Lancet 1989;2:730–732.

26. Rubinow DR, Schmidt PJ. The treatment of premenstrual syndrome: forward into the past. N Engl J Med 1995;332:1574–1575.

27. Steiner M, Lepage P, Dunn E. Serotonin and gender specific psychiatric disorders. Int J Psychiatry Clin Pract 1997;1:3–13.

28. Rapkin A. The role of serotonin in premenstrual syndrome. Clin Obstet Gynecol 1992;35:629–636.

29. Rojansky N, Halbreich U, Zander K, et al. Imipramine receptor binding and serotonin uptake in platelets of women with premenstrual changes. Gynecol Obstet Invest 1991; 31:146–152.

30. Steiner M. Female-specific mood disorders. Clin Obstet Gynecol 1992;35:599–611.

31. Yatham LN. Is 5-HT$_{1A}$ receptor subsensitivity a trait marker for late luteal phase dysphoric disorder? A pilot study. Can J Psychiatry 1993;38:662–664.

32. Endicott J. The menstrual cycle and mood disorders. J Affect Disord 1993;29:193–200.

33. Pearlstein TB, Frank E, Rivera-Tovar A, et al. Prevalence of axis I and axis II disor-

ders in women with late luteal phase dysphoric disorder. J Affect Disord 1990; 20:129–134.

34. Wurtman JJ. Depression and weight gain: the serotonin connection. J Affect Disord 1993;29:183–192.

35. Meltzer HY. Serotonergic dysfunction in depression. Br J Psychiatry 1989;155:25–31.

36. Cohen IR, Wise PM. Effects of estradiol on the diurnal rhythm of serotonin activity in microdissected brain areas of ovariectomized rats. Endocrinology 1988;122:2619–2625.

37. Ladisich W. Influence of progesterone on serotonin metabolism: a possible causal factor for mood changes. Psychoneuroendocrinology 1977;2:257–266.

38. Ashby CR Jr, Carr LA, Cook CL, et al. Alteration of platelet serotonergic mechanisms and monoamine oxidase activity on premenstrual syndrome. Biol Psychiatry 1988;24:225–233.

39. Rapkin AJ, Edelmuth E, Chang LC, et al. Whole blood serotonin in premenstrual syndrome. Obstet Gynecol 1987;70:533–537.

40. Steege JF, Stout AL, Knight DL, et al. Reduced platelet tritium-labeled imipramine binding sites in women with premenstrual syndrome. Am J Obstet Gynecol 1992;167:168–172.

41. Taylor DL, Mathew RH, Ho BT, et al. Serotonin levels and platelet uptake during premenstrual tension. Neuropsychobiology 1984;12:16–18.

42. Bancroft J, Cook A, Davidson D, et al. Blunting of neuroendocrine responses to infusion of L-tryptophan in women with perimenstrual mood change. Psychol Med 1991;21:305–312.

43. Bancroft J, Cook A. The neuroendocrine response to d-fenfluramine in women with premenstrual depression. J Affect Disord 1995;36:57–64.

44. Fitzgerald M, Malone K, Li A, et al. Blunted serotonin response to fenfluramine challenge in premenstrual dysphoric disorder. Am J Psychiatry 1997;154:556–558.

45. Steiner M, Yatham L, Coote M, et al. Serotonergic dysfunction in premenstrual dysphoric disorder. Psychiatry Res 1998 (in press).

46. Halbreich U, Tworek H. Altered serotonergic activity in women with dysphoric premenstrual syndromes. Int J Psychiatry Med 1993;23:1–27.

47. Leibenluft E, Fiero PL, Rubinow DR. Effects of the menstrual cycle on dependent variables in mood disorders research. Arch Gen Psychiatry 1994;51:761–781.

48. Weissman MM, Olfson M. Depression in women: implications for health care research. Science 1995;269:799–801.

49. Weissman MM, Bruce ML, Leaf PJ, et al. Affective disorders. In: Robins LN, Regiers DA, eds. Psychiatric Disorders in America. New York: Free Press, 1991:53–80.

50. Harrison WM, Endicott J, Nee J, et al. Characteristics of women seeking treatment for premenstrual syndrome. Psychosomatics 1989;30:405–411.

51. Fava M, Pedrazzi F, Guaraldi GP, et al. Comorbid anxiety and depression among patients with late luteal phase dysphoric disorder. J Anxiety Disord 1992;6:325–335.

52. McLeod DR, Hoehn-Saric R, Foster GV, et al. The influence of premenstrual syndrome on ratings of anxiety in women with generalized anxiety disorder. Acta Psychiatr Scand 1993;88:248–251.

53. Bancroft J, Rennie D, Warner P. Vulnerability to perimenstrual mood change: the relevance of a past history of depressive disorder. Psychosom Med 1994;56:225–234.

54. Kaspi SP, Otto MW, Pollack MH, et al. Premenstrual exacerbation of symptoms in women with panic disorder. J Anxiety Disord 1994;8:131–138.

55. Graze KK, Nee J, Endicott J. Premenstrual depression predicts future major depressive disorder. Acta Psychiatr Scand 1990;81:201–206.

56. Condon JT. The premenstrual syndrome: a twin study. Br J Psychiatry 1993;162:481–86.

57. Kendler KS, Silberg JL, Neale MC, et al. Genetic and environmental factors in the aetiology of menstrual, premenstrual and neurotic symptoms: a population based twin study. Psychol Med 1992;22:1–16.

58. Freeman EW, Sondheimer SJ, Rickels K. Effects of medical history factors on symptoms severity in women meeting criteria for premenstrual syndrome. Obstet Gynecol 1988; 72:236–239.

59. Schnurr PP, Hurt SW, Stout AL. Consequences of methodological decisions in the di-

agnosis of late luteal phase dysphoric disorder. In: Gold JH, Severino SK, eds. Premenstrual Dysphorias: Myths and Realities. Washington, DC: American Psychiatric Press, 1994:715–718.

60. Haskett RF, Steiner M, Osmun JN, et al. Severe premenstrual tension: delineation of the syndrome. Biol Psychiatry 1980;15:121–139.

61. Endicott J, Harrison W. The daily record of severity of problems. Available from Dr. Endicott, New York State Psychiatric Institute, Biometrics Unit, 722 West 168th Street, New York, NY 10032.

62. Reid RL. Premenstrual syndrome. Curr Probl Obstet Gynecol Fertil 1985;8:1–57.

63. Mortola JF, Girton L, Beck L, et al. Diagnosis of premenstrual syndrome by a simple, prospective, and reliable instrument: the calendar of premenstrual experiences. Obstet Gynecol 1990;76:302–307.

64. National Institute of Mental Health. NIMH Premenstrual Syndrome Workshop Guidelines. Rockville, MD: National Institute of Mental Health, 1983.

65. Steiner M, Steinberg S, Stewart D, et al. Fluoxetine in the treatment of premenstrual dysphoria. N Engl J Med 1995;332:1529–1534.

66. Steiner M, Wilkins A. Diagnosis and assessment of premenstrual dysphoria. Psychiatr Ann 1996;26:571–575.

67. Pearlstein TB. Hormones and depression: what are the facts about premenstrual syndrome, menopause and hormone replacement therapy. Am J Obstet Gynecol 1995; 173:646–653.

68. Morse C, Dennerstein L, Farrell E, et al. A comparison of hormone therapy, coping skills training and relaxation for the relief of premenstrual syndrome. J Behav Med 1991;14:469–489.

69. Christensen AP, Oei TP. The efficacy of cognitive behaviour therapy in treating premenstrual dysphoric changes. J Affect Disord 1995;33:57–63.

70. Kleijnen J, Ter Riet G, Knipschild P. Vitamin B6 in the treatment of premenstrual syndrome—a review. Br J Obstet Gynaecol 1990;97:847–852.

71. Abraham GE, Hargrove JT. Effect of vitamin B6 on premenstrual tension syndromes: a double blind crossover study. Infertility 1980;3:155–165.

72. Barr W. Pyridoxine supplements in the premenstrual syndrome. Practitioner 1984; 228:425–427.

73. Doll H, Brown S, Thurston A, et al. Pyridoxine (vitamin B6) and the premenstrual syndrome: a randomized crossover trial. J R Coll Gen Pract 1989;39:364–368.

74. Thys-Jacobs S, Ceccarelli S, Bierman A, et al. Calcium supplementation in premenstrual syndrome: a randomized crossover trial. J Gen Intern Med 1989;4:183–189.

75. Facchinetti F, Borrella P, Sances G, et al. Oral magnesium successfully relieves premenstrual mood changes. Obstet Gynecol 1991;78:177–181.

76. London RS, Bradley L, Chiamori NY. Effect of a nutritional supplement on premenstrual symptomatology in women with premenstrual syndrome: a double-blind longitudinal study. J Am Coll Nutr 1991;10:494–499.

77. London RS, Murphy L, Kitlowski KE, et al. Efficacy of alpha-tocopherol in the treatment of premenstrual syndrome. J Reprod Med 1987;32:400–404.

78. Budeiri DJ, Li Wan Po A, Dornan JC. Is evening primrose oil of value in the treatment of premenstrual syndrome? Control Clin Trials 1996;17:60–68.

79. Facchinetti F, Fioroni L, Sances G, et al. Naproxen sodium in the treatment of premenstrual syndromes: a placebo controlled study. Gynecol Obstet Invest 1989; 28: 205–208.

80. Sances G, Martignoni E, Fioroni L, et al. Naproxen sodium in menstrual migraine prophylaxis: a double-blind placebo controlled study. Headache 1990;30:705–709.

81. Mira M, McNeil D, Fraser IS, et al. Mefenamic acid in the treatment of premenstrual syndrome. Obstet Gynecol 1986;68:395–398.

82. Vellacott ID, Shroff NE, Pearce MY, et al. A double blind, placebo controlled evaluation of spironolactone in the premenstrual syndrome. Curr Med Res Opin 1987;10:450–456.

83. Andersch B. Bromocriptine and premenstrual symptoms: a survey of double blind trials. Obstet Gynecol Surv 1983;38:643–646.

84. Stone AB, Pearlstein TB, Brown WA. Fluoxetine in the treatment of late luteal phase dysphoric disorder. J Clin Psychiatry 1991;52:290–293.

85. Menkes DB, Taghavi E, Mason PA, et al. Fluoxetine's spectrum of action in premenstrual syndrome. Int Clin Psychopharmacol 1993;8:95–102.

86. Wood SH, Mortola JF, Chan YF, et al. Treatment of premenstrual syndrome with fluoxetine: a double-blind, placebo-controlled crossover study. Obstet Gynecol 1992;80: 339–344.

87. Su TP, Schmidt PJ, Danaceau, et al. Fluoxetine in the treatment of premenstrual dysphoria. Neuropsychopharmacology 1997;16:346–356.

88. Yonkers KA, Halbreich U, Freeman E, et al. Symptomatic improvement of premenstrual dysphoric disorder with sertraline treatment: a randomized controlled trial. JAMA 1997;278:983–988.

89. Eriksson E, Hedberg MA, Andersch B, et al. The serotonin reuptake inhibitor paroxetine is superior to the noradrenaline reuptake inhibitor maprotiline in the treatment of premenstrual syndrome. Neuropsychopharmacology 1995;12:167–176.

90. Smoller JW, Halbreich U. Intermittent luteal phase sertraline treatment of dysphoric premenstrual syndrome. Biol Psychiatry 1997;41:120S.

91. Steiner M, Korzekwa M, Lamont J, et al. Intermittent fluoxetine dosing in the treatment of women with premenstrual dysphoria. Psychopharmacol Bull 1997;33:771–774.

92. Sundblad C, Modigh K, Andersch B, et al. Clomipramine effectively reduces premenstrual irritability and dysphoria: a placebo controlled trial. Acta Psychiatr Scand 1992;85:39–47.

93. Sundblad C, Hedberg MA, Eriksson E. Clomipramine administered during the luteal phase reduces the symptoms of premenstrual syndrome. Neuropsychopharmacology 1993;9:133–145.

94. Smith S, Rinehart JS, Ruddock VE, et al. Treatment of premenstrual syndrome with alprazolam: results of a double-blind, placebo-controlled, randomized crossover clinical trial. Obstet Gynecol 1987;70:37–43.

95. Harrison W, Endicott J, Nee J. Treatment of premenstrual dysphoria with alprazolam. Arch Gen Psychiatry 1990;47:270–275.

96. Berger CP, Presser B. Alprazolam in the treatment of two subsamples of patients with late luteal phase dysphoric disorder: A double-blind, placebo-controlled crossover study. Obstet Gynecol 1994;84:379–385.

97. Freeman EW, Rickels K, Sondheimer SJ, et al. A double-blind trial of oral progesterone, alprazolam, and placebo in the treatment of severe premenstrual syndrome. JAMA 1995;274:51–57.

98. Schmidt PJ, Grover GN, Rubinow DR. Alprazolam in the treatment of premenstrual syndrome: A double-blind, placebo-controlled trial. Arch Gen Psychiatry 1993;50:467–473.

99. Rickels K, Freeman E, Sondheimer S. Buspirone in the treatment of premenstrual syndrome (letter). Lancet 1989;1:777.

100. Helvacioglu A, Yeoman R, Hazelton JM, et al. Premenstrual syndrome and related hormonal changes. J Reprod Med 1993;38:864–870.

101. West CP, Hillier H. Ovarian suppression with the gonadotrophin-releasing hormone agonist goserelin (Zoladex) in management of the premenstrual tension syndrome. Hum Reprod 1994;9:1058–1063.

102. Dhar V, Murphy BE. Double-blind randomized crossover trial of luteal phase estrogens (Premarin) in the premenstrual syndrome (PMS). Psychoneuroendocrinology 1990; 15:489–493.

103. Magos AL, Brincat M, Studd JWW. Treatment of the premenstrual syndrome by subcutaneous oestradiol implants and cyclical oral norethisterone: placebo controlled study. BMJ 1986;292:1629–1633.

104. Smith RN, Studd JW, Zamblera D, et al. A randomized comparison over 8 months of 100 micrograms and 200 micrograms twice weekly doses of transdermal oestradiol in the treatment of severe premenstrual syndrome. Br J Obstet Gynaecol 1995;102:475–484.

105. Hahn PM, VanVugt DA, Reid RL. A randomized, placebo-controlled crossover trial of danazol for the treatment of premenstrual syndrome. Psychoneuroendocrinology 1995;20:193–209.

106. Gilmore DH, Hawthorn RJ, Hart DM. Danol for premenstrual syndrome: a preliminary report of a placebo-controlled double-blind study. J Int Med Res 1985;13:129–130.

107. Deeny M, Hawthorn R, McKay-Hart D. Low dose danazol in the treatment of premenstrual syndrome. Postgrad Med J 1991;67:450–454.

108. Watts JF, Butt WR, Edwards RL. A clinical trial using danazol for the treatment of premenstrual tension. Br J Obstet Gynaecol 1987;94:30–34.

109. Sarno AP, Miller EJ, Lundblad EG. Premenstrual syndrome: beneficial effects of periodic, low-dose danazol. Obstet Gynecol 1987;70:33–36.

110. Freeman E, Rickels K, Sondheimer SJ, et al. Ineffectiveness of progesterone suppository treatment for premenstrual syndrome. JAMA 1990;264:349–353.

111. Rapkin A, Chang LH, Reading AE. Premenstrual syndrome: a double blind placebo controlled study of treatment with progesterone vaginal suppositories. J Obstet Gynecol 1987;7:217–220.

112. Sampson GA. Premenstrual syndrome: a double-blind placebo controlled trial of progesterone and placebo. Br J Psychiatry 1979;135:209–215.

113. Maddocks S, Hahn P, Moller F, et al. A double-blind placebo-controlled trial of progesterone vaginal suppositories in the treatment of premenstrual syndrome. Am J Obstet Gynecol 1986;154:573–581.

114. Kirkham C, Hahn PM, VanVugt DA, et al. A randomized double-blind, placebo-controlled, cross-over trial to assess the side effects of medroxyprogesterone acetate in hormone replacement therapy. Obstet Gynecol 1991;78:93–97.

115. West CP. Inhibition of ovulation with oral progestins: effectiveness in premenstrual syndrome. Eur J Obstet Gynaecol Reprod Biol 1990;34:119–128.

116. Dennerstein L, Morse C, Gotts G, et al. Treatment of premenstrual syndrome: a double-blind trial of dydrogesterone. J Affect Disord 1986;11:199–205.

117. Dennerstein L, Spencer-Gardner C, Gotts G, et al. Progesterone and the premenstrual syndrome: a double-blind, cross-over trial. BMJ 1985;290:1617–1621.

118. Chan A, Mortola JF, Wood SH, et al. Persistence of premenstrual syndrome during low-dose administration of the progesterone agonist RU486. Obstet Gynecol 1994;84:1001–1005.

119. Graham CA, Sherwin BB. A prospective treatment study of premenstrual symptoms using a triphasic oral contraceptive. J Psychosom Res 1992;36:257–266.

120. Guy W. ECDEU Assessment of Manual for Psychopharmacology. Publication no. (Adm.) 76–338 (revised). Rockville, MD: NIMH Public Department of Health, Education and Human Welfare, 1976:217–222.

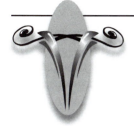

C H A P T E R   1 3

Chronic Pelvic Pain

JOHN F. STEEGE

Chronic pelvic pain is generally defined as pain present in the pelvis more often than not for 6 months or longer. It may be cyclic or continuous in nature. Pain that is present at least 5 days/month occurs in 12% of women of reproductive age and is the reason for hysterectomy in approximately 12% of such procedures (1, 2). Approximately half of all operative laparoscopies are performed to investigate problems with pain, many of those chronic in nature (3, 4).

As a multifactorial disease, chronic pelvic pain often challenges the best of clinicians. When organic pathology is detected, its precise relationship to the production of symptoms is often uncertain. The longer the pain has gone on, the more likely treatment is prolonged and perhaps incompletely successful. For the surgically oriented gynecologist, this problem can be especially frustrating. Surgical solutions are not always apparent, and pain may persist despite a satisfactory anatomic result.

This chapter focuses on new information about pain pathways that may help to explain some of these phenomena. It reviews basic elements of history and physical examination pertinent to the various diagnoses and sources of chronic pelvic pain. A review of criteria for consultation with other specialties and referral for tertiary care are also presented.

PATHWAYS OF PAIN PERCEPTION

Nociceptive signals emerging from pelvic visceral structures travel cephalad through one or more of several routes (5). ("Nociceptive signals" are peripheral nerve impulses that are destined to produce negatively perceived sensations; "pain" is a brain interpretation of sensations indicative of real or potential tissue damage.) Sympathetic afferent signals arising from the uterus, cervix, and immediately adjacent portions of the uterosacral, broad, and round ligaments travel via the inferior and superior hypogastric plexuses to the sympathetic chain. From there they go to the T10-T12 levels of the spinal cord. Additional sensation may be provided through the nervi erigentes, or pelvic nerves, which cross the pelvic floor and ultimately join the S2-S4 segments of the spinal cord. Fibers from both the sympathetic and parasympathetic systems traverse Frankenhäuser's plexus and the uterovesical ganglion.

Neuroanatomic work performed in the last century elucidated these pathways, and clinical neurophysiologic work has validated the significance of most of these. What is not always fully appreciated is the degree of biologic variability that exists among women. A better understanding of this variability may provide useful clinical information in the future as we attempt to understand unusual pain patterns.

The gate control theory, developed by Melzack and Wall in the 1950s and early 1960s, provides a model to help explain some of the variability in clinical pain patterns (6). It is a useful model of integration of physical and psychological processes into a single scheme. The major contribution of this theory was to suggest that higher centers in the brain have the capacity to *physiologically* down- or upregulate the spinal cord. This regulation may determine the degree to which peripheral nociceptive signals travel cephalad to reach conscious perception.

Building on this theory, further neurophysiologic research has focused on these spinal cord mechanisms (7). It is now known that there are several categories of narcotic receptor sites both in the brain and in the spinal cord. In addition, the spinal cord appears to have receptors for local anesthetics and numerous other neurotransmitter-like substances.

Two clinically important concepts emerge from this evidence: centralization of pain and spinal cord "wind-up" (8). Centralization of pain is said to occur when after extended periods of peripheral nociceptive signal production, changes seem to occur at the spinal cord level that result in ongoing signals sent to the brain despite the dramatic decrease or even absence of peripheral nociception. That is, the brain and spinal cord take over even when the best therapeutic efforts have been made to reduce signals from damaged tissue peripherally. Medical management of the central neurotransmitter processes would seem to be the most appropriate therapeutic intervention for pain that has become centralized.

Spinal cord wind-up occurs when repeated, low-level, nociceptive stimuli from the periphery elicit progressively more dramatic responses from second-order neurons at the spinal cord level even though the intensity of the stimuli may remain constant or even be diminished. This phenomenon has been well demonstrated in acute pain models at the animal level (9). There is considerable speculation regarding the impact of this process on chronic pain systems.

Although acute and chronic pain are quite different physiologic processes, some lessons learned from acute pain management apply well to the management of chronic pain. For example, studies regarding the impact of preemptive analgesia on acute postoperative pain suggest that the ideal interim postoperative pain regimen is multifaceted. The ideal regimen interrupts the nociceptive signals at the peripheral tissue level, blocks receptor sites within the spinal cord, and alters the central perception of pain (10). In many chronic pain situations, this is also the ideal regimen. Treatments need to be applied at the peripheral tissue level and include pharmacologic measures directed toward spinal cord and central mechanisms as well.

EVALUATION OF CHRONIC PAIN SYNDROMES

History

The diagnosis of chronic pelvic pain is made on the basis of a careful and detailed clinical history. Physical examination supplies additional detail(s) and confirmation of diagnoses, but in most cases, if uncertainty remains, more historical questions need to be asked. A very detailed history enables the physician and patient to formulate a well-designed intervention, especially one that involves surgical treatment.

The history of the present illness should include the character, intensity, radiation, and daily chronologic pattern of the pain. Some useful generalizations about pain patterns associated with particular kinds of pelvic pathology are listed in Table 13.1.

When pain is prolonged and chronic, it may remain confined to its original site and intensity. All too often, however, the anatomic site of the pain becomes less distinct and symptoms originating in surrounding organ systems may join the original complaint. For example, a woman who starts with a problem limited to endometriosis may develop functional bowel symptoms and discomforts related to excessive contraction of the pelvic floor musculature. When taking a history of a chronic pain prob-

TABLE 13.1. Typical Pain Patterns and Descriptors

Pain Type	History	Physical Examination
Endometriosis	Gradual progression from dysmenorrhea to continuous pain Deep dyspareunia	Tenderness in implant areas
Pelvic congestion	Luteal phase increase Afternoon, evening increase Deep dyspareunia Relieved by lying down "Heavy," "aching"	BLQ and central pelvic pain Tender at ovarian points, broad ligaments
Levator spasm	"Falling out" pressure sensation Afternoon, evening increase Midvaginal dyspareunia Radiates to low back Minimal cyclicity Relieved by lying down	Tender to palpation increased by contraction
Piriformis spasm	Pain on arising, climbing stairs, driving car	Pain on external thigh rotation; palpated externally or transvaginally
Adhesions	Starts 3–6 mo after surgery Localized to adhesions pulling, tugging	Vague thickening Pain on visceral motion

Reprinted with permission from Steege JF. Office assessment of chronic pelvic pain. Clin Obstet Gynecol 1997;40:554–563.
BLQ, bilateral lower quadrant.

lem, it is useful to pay attention to the precise chronology of the addition of each component of the pain. Asking this type of detailed question allows the clinician to deduce if the pain intensity is increasing despite relatively stable pathology.

In many instances, taking this type of complete history requires more than one visit. Once the clinician decides that they are dealing with a significant chronic pain problem, the patient should be prepared to attend several visits before the evaluation is complete.

The clinician needs to understand the impact the pain has had on the patient as an individual, on her relationships, and on her work capacities. The emotional components may be evaluated by the clinician's own history and possibly by psychometric evaluation or by psychological consultation. The purpose of psychometric instruments is to draw attention to particular problems, such as depression, that might not easily emerge from an interview. Their purpose is not to make psychiatric diagnoses; that responsibility remains with the clinician. Personality profiles can serve to define an individual's strengths and weaknesses but do not yield specific diagnoses. Taken as a whole, these instruments convey to the patient your interest in knowing as much about her as possible before beginning treatment.

The clinician must also ask about past or present experiences with physical and/or sexual abuse. Many studies suggest that histories of abuse are more common in women referred to tertiary care specialty clinics for pelvic pain (11). In the primary care setting, this association is also present but is substantially weaker (12). In some cases, a history of abuse serves as a trigger for referral, whereas in other cases, referral is done only if the history is accompanied by complicated psychosocial problems. Women with histories of particularly traumatic or prolonged abuse may develop somatization disorder and/or posttraumatic stress disorder. These women may exhibit dissociative reactions during examination, appearing to have "drifted off" and becoming withdrawn and noncommunicative (13).

Having obtained a history of sexual or physical abuse, the clinician is confronted with a dilemma: Is the abuse etiologically related to the person's pain? Or, is it an unfortunate, but unrelated, aspect of her life? The full impact of physical and/or sexual abuse in an individual's history requires careful assessment. Great care must be taken so that appropriate medical and surgical attention to organic disease is not undermined by overemphasis of a relationship between the patient's pain and her past history.

Physical Examination

The data provided by the history and observations made during the history-taking process provide focus for the physical examination. Before and during the history, the clinician may have the opportunity to observe posture, stance, gait, and sitting behavior. For example, a person with levator spasm will often sit forward on the chair and rest more of her weight on one buttock or the other. Sitting perfectly straight often aggravates the pain from this disorder.

The abdominal examination in a woman with chronic pelvic pain may be more informative if done in the following manner. Ask the patient to point to the area of pain with one finger and outline and circle the area involved. Ask her then to press as hard as she feels it is necessary to elicit the pain she experiences. Done in this manner, the impact of her anxiety about being examined may be diminished and a more accurate assessment of tissue sensitivity obtained.

The abdominal wall should then be systematically palpated by the examiner's index finger in an effort to identify local spots of tenderness, or "trigger points." If these areas are found, the patient is asked to contract the abdominal wall by either raising her head or one leg off the table without assistance. If focal pain is exacerbated by this maneuver, there is a reasonable probability that a trigger point or other myofascial abdominal wall component is present. If the pain is reduced, a visceral source is more likely; if the pain is unchanged, then the maneuver is not diagnostic. A diagrammatic record of the examination findings is valuable.

Specific elements of the musculoskeletal examination should be performed to look for piriformis spasm and/or psoas muscle pain. The piriformis forms a muscular bed for the sacral plexus of nerves in the pelvis. With her hip and knee partially flexed, ask the patient to externally rotate each thigh against resistance. Pain with this maneuver suggests piriformis spasm. In the lateral decubitus position, the hip is actively and passively extended and flexed. Pain with these maneuvers suggests a psoas muscle origin. Further elements of the musculoskeletal screening examination are discussed elsewhere (14) (Table 13.2)

The pelvic examination in the patient with chronic pelvic pain is more informative when performed in a careful stepwise fashion. Meticulous attention is paid to each potential contributing organ system. First, place one index finger in the vaginal introitus and ask for voluntary contraction and relaxation. Inability to exert conscious control of the bulbocavernosus muscles suggests vaginismus. This diagnosis should, of course, be corroborated by additional history. The presence of good vol-

TABLE 13.2. Musculoskeletal Screening Examination for Chronic Pelvic Pain

Observation/Maneuver	Typical Abnormal Findings
Gait, stance	Scoliosis
Lateral standing view	One extremity externally rotated
Sitting	Exaggerated kyphosis-lordosis
With supine flexion of one hip, observe other hip (Thomas test)	Raised up on one buttock (levator spasm)
External rotation of the thigh against resistance (sitting, supine, or during pelvic examination)	Contralateral hip flexes, indicating hip flexor contracture
Psoas flexion and extension	Pain on external rotation indicates piriformis syndrome
Digital vaginal examination	Limited extension and/or pain with flexion indicates psoas shortening and/or spasm
	Pain indicates levator spasm

untary control during pelvic examination does not exclude the diagnosis of vaginismus that may occur during sexual situations (15).

Extending the index finger beyond the bulbocavernosus muscle, one can usually palpate the levator muscles on the right and left sides at approximately the 4:30 and 7:30 o'clock positions. In the asymptomatic person, a sense of pressure is experienced. When levator spasm is present, gentle palpation on these muscles may reproduce the patient's sense of pelvic pressure (a "falling out" sensation) and/or the pain of dyspareunia. Further verification is obtained when the symptom is exacerbated by voluntary contraction of the levators.

The next step is to press directly on the coccyx, reaching it by going around the rectum on either side. External palpation of the coccyx combined with this maneuver normally allows it to rotate over an approximate 30° angle. This is normally not a painful maneuver. If pain is present, it may be related to coccydynia or adjacent levator spasm.

The piriformis muscle can be tested by the maneuvers described earlier. When these maneuvers suggest piriformis spasm, this can be further confirmed on pelvic examination. The belly of the piriformis can be easily felt transvaginally when the thigh is externally rotated against resistance. When palpation of the piriformis muscle belly reproduces pain, then spasm is likely to be present. A false-positive interpretation of this maneuver can occur if intrinsic cul-de-sac disease is present, because the vaginal examination finger must traverse this area to reach the piriformis muscle (Fig. 13.1).

The anterior vaginal wall, urethra, and bladder trigone should be examined either before or after the muscular examinations just described, depending on the clinical situation. In general, it is best to examine the (likely) nontender areas first. This technique helps minimize the tendency to experience pressure as pain once pain has been elicited. In many cases, the clinician can make the presumptive diagnosis of chronic urethritis, trigonitis, or interstitial cystitis on the basis of careful history combined with focused digital examination. If complex therapeutic interventions are being contemplated, then cystoscopic confirmation of these presumptive diagnoses should first be obtained. In asymptomatic patients, pressure on the bladder base creates only urinary urgency without replicating the clinical pain.

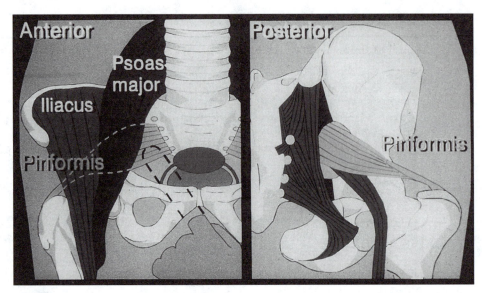

FIGURE 13.1. Palpation of the piriformis muscle during vaginal examination. (Reprinted with permission from Barton PM. Piriformis syndrome: a rational approach to management. Pain 1991:47:345–352.)

Unimanual single-digit transvaginal examination should continue by testing the intrinsic sensitivity of the cervix to palpation and traction. The adnexal areas are then examined in a similar manner, first unimanually and then by adding the abdominal hand. Separating the bimanual examination into three discrete steps (unimanual vaginal examination alone, unimanual external examination of lower abdomen alone, and then examining the pelvis bimanually) helps distinguish internal visceral pain from pain originating from the abdominal wall.

Rather than following a rigid sequence, speculum examination should be done at a time when it makes the most sense, depending on the type of pain under consideration. For example, in the patient with a history suggesting posthysterectomy vaginal apex pain, it is probably wisest to complete the muscular examination and the adnexal palpation *before* insertion of the speculum. In this manner, the areas more likely to be nontender are examined before the speculum directly touches the potentially sensitive vaginal apex.

In contrast, if the history suggests an adnexal source of pain, then the pelvic examination should begin with the speculum examination (as is traditionally done). The speculum examination is then followed by a pelvic musculoskeletal examination, leaving the adnexal examination for last. The adnexal areas are examined in the traditional bimanual fashion, proceeding from the midline out to the pelvic sidewall in small incremental steps to localize the area of tenderness as accurately as possible. Throughout this portion of the examination, the clinician should ask whether any tenderness elicited reproduces the pain of her chief complaint.

Rectovaginal examination remains an essential component of the complete pelvic examination. Insertion of the rectal finger causes the least discomfort if the middle finger is placed gently at the anus and exerts slow gentle pressure. Some clinicians are taught that having the woman bear down will facilitate insertion of the finger. When most patients bear down, however, they do a Valsalva maneuver and simultaneously contract the voluntary portion of the anal sphincter. This causes an increase in discomfort and makes digital insertion more difficult. The rectal finger should advance as far as possible, ideally reaching the hollow of the sacrum. In this manner, the entire floor of the posterior cul-de-sac can be thoroughly evaluated for the presence of irregularities or nodularity that might imply the presence of deep infiltrating endometriosis. To fully evaluate the uterosacral ligaments, a rectovaginal examination is done. The uterosacral ligaments can be more accurately assessed by putting the cervix on traction in an anterior direction with the tip of the vaginal finger while palpating the stretched uterosacral ligaments with the rectal finger.

After palpation of the uterosacral ligaments, the bimanual portion of the examination is repeated with sequential palpation with the rectovaginal hand, the abdominal hand, and both hands together. When examining areas that are tender, it is useful to pause and inform the patient that examination of the tender area will only last for a count of "one, two, three, . . . " and will only begin when she feels ready. By time limiting this portion of the examination and allowing the woman to determine when it will commence, the examination is made more tolerable for the patient. When tenderness is elicited, the clinician should ask whether this reproduces the clinical pain the patient is experiencing.

Office Diagnostic Procedures

Trigger-point injections have been well established as a diagnostic and therapeutic technique (16, 17). Multiple types of local anesthetics (e.g., 1% lidocaine or 0.25% bupivacaine) have been used with none demonstrably superior to any other. The pain of injection can be substantially reduced by adding sodium bicarbonate (1 mL/10 mL of 1% lidocaine; 0.2 mL/30 mL of 0.25% bupivacaine). A 27-gauge tuberculin needle or a 25-gauge 1.5-inch needle is preferable for injection. If the abdominal wall trigger points can be blocked successfully, then the pelvic examination might be repeated to better understand the contributions of intrapelvic pathology to the patient's pain.

Similarly, local injection can be used to anesthetize the vaginal apex tissue in an effort to determine whether this tissue is intrinsically sensitive or whether pain elicited from vaginal cuff palpation on bimanual examination emanates from intrapelvic pathology.

Transvaginal ultrasound examination provides very useful information in evaluating acute pelvic pain. Unfortunately, it is less contributory for the evaluation of chronic pelvic pain complaints. The occasional exceptions to this generalization are noted as individual pelvic pain syndromes and are discussed below.

SPECIFIC PELVIC PAIN SYNDROMES

Endometriosis

Certain historical stigmata signal the possibility that endometriosis may be present. Severe dysmenorrhea during adolescence with worsening in early adult life should suggest this etiology. With endometriosis, the duration of severe dysmenorrhea may also change. In cases of primary dysmenorrhea not due to endometriosis, the typical pattern is for the first day of menses to be the most painful. This is followed by a roughly 50% reduction in pain on the second menstrual day. If endometriosis develops, the duration of the more severe menstrual cramps may lengthen and the severe dysmenorrhea may last into the second or third menstrual days. The next change may be the appearance of premenstrual pain, ultimately followed by pain present for almost all of the menstrual month but with continuing premenstrual and menstrual exacerbations. Deep dyspareunia may join the picture at any point along the way, usually appearing perimenstrually at first.

Early in the disease of endometriosis, physical examination may not detect any abnormalities, but when endometriosis is at a stage where deep dyspareunia and severe dysmenorrhea are present, the examination may reveal focal cul-de-sac tenderness and nodularity of the uterosacral ligaments. Increased attention has been paid recently to deep infiltrating endometriosis in the cul-de-sac of Douglas that may not be readily visualized during laparoscopy (18, 19). The chances of detecting palpable nodularity may be increased by examining the patient during menstruation. At this point, the nodularity may be more palpable and more tender.

Recent investigations suggested more than one subtype of endometriosis (19). There are two common varieties of endometriosis: one with multiple peritoneal implants, predominantly in the cul-de-sac or on the ovaries, and a second variety appearing primarily as intraovarian disease, or endometriomas. The intraovarian variety is not frequently associated with dysmenorrhea and pelvic pain and is often diagnosed by an incidental finding of ovarian enlargement. Pain may appear if the endometrioma(s) becomes quite large.

A third variety, quite distinct from the other two, consists primarily of deep cul-de-sac disease. Laparoscopy in such cases may reveal only the mildest signs of peritoneal abnormality, with the bulk of the disease hidden in the retroperitoneal space next to the rectum and at the vaginal apex. This last variety has been called vaginal adenomyosis by some authors (20). It has been described as potentially due to a müllerian anomaly rather than resulting from retrograde menstruation (Sampson's theory). Diagnosis of deep infiltrating cul-de-sac endometriosis can be quite difficult. Although history and pelvic examination may be suggestive, the use of special magnetic resonance imaging (MRI) techniques may be necessary to accurately detect this disorder. Treatment is thought to be primarily surgical, because sex steroid receptor patterns are different in this type of disease when compared with more typical peritoneal disease (21).

Other physical findings of endometriosis may include a fixed retroverted uterus and generalized pelvic tenderness. Differentiating this diagnosis from chronic pelvic inflammatory disease or other forms of pelvic masses may be difficult.

With the possible exception of new approaches using MRI techniques, imaging studies in general are not very useful in the diagnosis of endometriosis. Transvaginal ultrasound may detect cystic enlargement of the ovaries, but endometriomas may have a variety of different ultrasonic appearances, none of which are unique to this disorder.

Medical management of this disorder most reasonably starts with cyclic oral contraceptives. Continuous oral contraceptives may be used as well, thus avoiding the discomforts of regular menstruation. To go beyond this first order of therapy is to ask the patient to incur significantly greater expense, side effects, and disruption of her normal endocrinologic milieu. For these reasons, most authorities advocate laparoscopic confirmation of the diagnosis before embarking on more intrusive medical therapies such as danazol (Danocrine), continuous high-dose progestins, or gonadotropin-releasing hormone (GnRH) agonists (Table 13.3).

Until recently, surgical treatment of minimal and mild endometriosis by laparoscopic methods was thought to be equivalent to medical management in improving fertility. However, a recent randomized trial demonstrated a more rapid accomplishment of the desired pregnancy after laparoscopic treatment of the disorder when compared with expectant therapy (22). Similar comparisons of medical and surgical treatments of endometriosis for the purpose of pain relief have not been performed.

Various opinions exist about the appropriate technique for laparoscopic treatment of endometriosis. Electrocoagulation or laser treatment of superficial implants

TABLE 13.3. Medications Used in Conjunction with GnRH Agonists

Norethindrone	Estrogen + progestin (continuous)
Etidronate	Estrogen + progestin (cyclic)
Norethindrone + etidronate	Calcitonin
Estrogen (oral and transdermal)	Calcium
	Medroxyprogesterone acetate

Reprinted with permission from Metzger DA. An integrated approach to the management of endometriosis. In: Steege JF, Metzger DA, Levy BS, eds. Chronic Pelvic Pain: An Integrated Approach. Philadelphia: WB Saunders, 1997.

is regarded as sufficient for very small foci of disease. When confluent collections of implants are noted or when active red or purple lesions are found, some surgeons prefer laser vaporization for definitive therapy. Others believe that excision of the entire area of involved peritoneum is the only way to adequately remove the disease to its depths (19). When extensive areas of peritoneum are removed, however, severe peritoneal adhesions may be the sequelae. This may result in trading endometriosis as the pain etiology for adhesive disease.

Women dealing with endometriosis may also develop some chronic pain syndromes described below, such as pelvic congestion, musculoskeletal problems, and/or irritable bowel syndrome (IBS). Careful attention to the nature and chronology of symptoms usually allows separate consideration and treatment of these disorders.

Pelvic Adhesions

Intra-abdominal adhesions are found in approximately 30% of autopsied women older than 60 years of age (23). In asymptomatic women undergoing laparoscopic tubal sterilization, adhesions are found in approximately 12% of the women (24). Among women undergoing laparoscopy for chronic pelvic pain, adhesions are found between 45 and 90% of the time (25).

Studies of the impact of adhesiolysis on chronic pelvic pain have been relatively limited. Uncontrolled series suggest that 65 to 85% of treated women obtained significant relief 8 to 12 months after surgery (26, 27). One randomized trial showed adhesiolysis by laparotomy to be superior to diagnostic laparoscopy only in the small percentage of women with dense bowel adhesions (28). This latter study did not evaluate the impact of the laparoscopic approach to adhesiolysis.

These results suggest that certain types of adhesions may play an etiologic role in chronic pelvic pain but by no means are they always responsible for pain generation. The clinician is left with the challenge of providing a balanced interpretation of the role of adhesions in pain causation and the role of adhesiolysis in the overall pain management plan. Future studies using microlaparoscopic pain mapping under conscious sedation may provide additional information regarding the particular types of adhesions that are most important in pain generation.

The clinical diagnosis of adhesions is quite difficult. It is possible to assess the relative mobility of the pelvic viscera during examination, but adhesions can only be strongly suspected when they are quite extensive. Transvaginal ultrasound is another way to evaluate the mobility of the pelvic organs, but it has low sensitivity and specificity in predicting the presence of adhesions. Sophisticated imaging studies, such as computed tomography and MRI, are ineffective in diagnosing adhesions; the gold standard for diagnosing adhesive disease remains diagnostic laparoscopy.

After laparoscopic adhesiolysis, adhesions start to reform within 1 to 2 weeks after surgery. Pain may not recur for another several months. The mechanism of this delay is uncertain, but strong possibilities include the time necessary for adhesive tissue to become well collagenized and contract and the time required for neural ingrowth. The overall prevalence of nerve tissue in adhesions is uncertain, as is its role in pain generation.

In summary, treatment of adhesions in some cases may play an important role in the management of chronic pelvic pain. In many situations it is wisest to simultaneously direct treatment efforts to other visceral and somatic sources of the pain and to the affective components to bring about the best resolution.

Adenomyosis

Adenomyosis is a condition in which endometrial glands and stroma grow within the myometrium, usually without direct connection to the endometrium. For true pathologic diagnosis, these glands and stroma must be present three high-powered fields below the basal layer of the endometrium. Adenomyosis is an extremely common condition, generally thought to be present in parous women in their 30s and 40s. Its relationship to symptoms is uncertain, because it may be present in as many as 30% of women, most of whom are asymptomatic (29). Its role as a post-hoc justification for hysterectomy in a woman with an otherwise anatomically normal pelvis makes it the focus of significant controversy.

Traditionally, the diagnosis has only been possible by histologic examination of the uterine wall. Transvaginal ultrasound, MRI, and myometrial needle biopsy have all been used in an effort to make a preoperative diagnosis. Although these efforts are encouraging, they lack sufficient resolution and standardized criteria and technique to explain or quantify the pathophysiologic process or relationship between histologic changes and clinical symptoms.

On a clinical basis, it may be useful to use serial pelvic examinations, possibly in combination with transvaginal ultrasound, in evaluating the potential role for adenomyosis as the etiologic source of the woman's pelvic pain. A woman who has a truly substantial amount of this disease often demonstrates substantial cyclic changes in the size, consistency, and tenderness of the uterine fundus. In the follicular phase, the uterus is smaller and firmer, whereas immediately premenstrually it is enlarged as much as over 1.5-fold over its baseline and is extremely tender and much softer in consistency.

Pharmacologic therapy has been attempted with continuous oral contraceptives, luteal-phase progestins, danazol (Danocrine), or GnRH agonists. Although success has not been confirmed by clinical trials, there are patients who report that luteal-phase medroxyprogesterone acetate (Provera) provides sufficient reduction of pain and diminution of menometrorrhagia. When these therapies are successful, the clinician must decide whether their long-term use makes practical and clinical sense.

Whether hysterectomy is appropriate for this condition is a matter of considerable debate, especially in the current era of managed care. The condition is not life threatening, and when medical therapy works, the discussion of further surgery centers primarily around quality of life issues. In this case, as in many others, the discussion of medical necessity leaves off, and the discussion of personal preferences and cultural expectations begins.

Pelvic Congestion

Over the past 50 years, this syndrome, and its many different names, has been widely described in the literature. Discomfort has been associated with distention of abnormal pelvic veins. In the early literature, a variety of other pathologic findings were attributed to the process (30, 31). More recent studies indicate the venous distention itself is primarily responsible for the production of symptoms (32, 33).

As much or more than any other gynecologic disorders related to pain, it is in this instance that mind-body interactions have been most intensely debated. Early publications by Taylor described a population of women with enlarged pelvic veins who had otherwise normal pelvic anatomy but whose psychosocial histories divulged a high prevalence of early deprivation and abuse. He described increases in vascular pelvic congestion (measured by increases in vaginal blood flow detected photometrically) that occurred only during interviews dealing with stressful topics (30, 31). Using similar methodology, however, a later investigator described the same phenomenon in pain-free control subjects (34).

Documentation of pelvic varices has been primarily demonstrated by transuterine venography (35). In this procedure, radiopaque aqueous contrast material is injected into the uterine fundus transvaginally and radiographs are taken at closely spaced intervals to document the passage of this contrast through the pelvic veins. Scoring criteria have been developed (36).

The symptom pattern associated with this disorder includes a sensation of pressure low in the pelvis that worsens during the course of the day, and a subset of women experience deep dyspareunia and menorrhagia. Bladder irritability and altered bowel habits are also found in some series, thus confusing the diagnostic picture (30, 31). Its prevalence is uncertain, because reports from experts on pelvic congestion may reflect a higher incidence than what is true for the general population (30, 31). Given the complexity of this disorder, prescription and assessment of therapeutic measures must be done carefully.

Concrete physical examination findings in this disorder are limited. Beard et al. places emphasis on the detection of pain at the "ovarian point" (32, 33). This is located two thirds of the way from the anterior, superior, iliac spine to the umbilicus. Tenderness in this area may be present in women without other evidence of this disorder, and therefore this sign may not be consistently diagnostic. Bimanual examination reveals a "doughy" consistency to the parametrial areas, and the patient reports these areas as the most sensitive areas in the pelvis. Examination in the premenstrual period may demonstrate substantial change in consistency of this area when compared with a follicular phase examination.

Diagnostic laparoscopy often misses this diagnosis. Laparoscopy is usually performed early in the day with the patient in Trendelenburg position. Attempts have been made to examine the pelvis laparoscopically with the patient in reverse Trendelenburg position using a volume of irrigating fluid to float the bowels out of the way. This approach has not been systematically studied or validated. Diagnostic ultrasound is being evaluated for this disorder, but the technique has been difficult to standardize (37).

Pelvic congestion has been treated by suppressing the menstrual cycle. One study using GnRH agonists with estrogen and progestin add-back therapy did not demonstrate relief (38). Oral contraceptives have been similarly ineffective (39). In contrast, continuous high-dose medroxyprogesterone acetate (Provera; 30 mg/day) in combination with a six-session course of psychotherapy has produced a minimum 50% improvement in three fourths of the women in one study (40). The psychotherapy focused on stress management and establishment of a better understanding of mind-body interactions. Medroxyprogesterone acetate (Provera) alone showed similar benefits when compared with placebo, but the duration of the effect was much greater when medical therapy was combined with counseling.

Surgical therapy traditionally involved hysterectomy (41). In the most severe cases, bilateral salpingo-oophorectomy is also recommended. Less radical approaches have included ligation of individual varices, although this has proven relatively unsuccessful. Other techniques are individual ovarian vein ligation or ligation of the entire infundibular pelvic ligament, with the literature describing a modest effect from this latter approach (42).

Although surgical therapy or intense medical therapy remains the mainstays of treatment, pharmacologic therapy with progestins and behavioral methods of stress reduction are central to an effective treatment plan.

Irritable Bowel Syndrome

The symptoms of IBS are frequently misinterpreted as being of gynecologic origin. The International Consensus Criteria (43) require that abdominal pain be relieved by defecation or associated with a change in the frequency or consistency of stools; in addition, two or more of the following symptoms must be present:

- Altered stool frequency
- Altered stool form
- Dyschezia or urgency
- Passage of mucus
- Bloating

Alternative etiologies can be ruled out with flexible sigmoidoscopy, stool Guaiac testing, and hematologic tests that screen for immunologic problems or thyroid dysfunction.

The differential diagnosis includes lactose intolerance, bacterial overgrowth of the small intestine, chronic intestinal pseudoobstruction, inflammatory bowel disease, diverticular disease, levator ani syndrome (proctalgia fugax), and/or endometriosis affecting the bowel (Table 13.4).

There appears to be a fairly strong association of IBS with dysmenorrhea (44). IBS is more common in women who have undergone hysterectomy in the absence of identifiable gynecologic pathology than in women who underwent hysterectomy for pathology (45).

In rectal manometric studies, approximately 40 to 60% of IBS patients report pain at levels of distention below the range of normal values (46). Although controversial, this observation may serve as a marker for IBS when combined with other clinical indicators. This lowered pain threshold may reflect a difference in the sensitivity of peripheral stretch receptors or pain afferent pathways. Attempts have been made to correlate these physiologic observations with measures of psychological stress or affective change, with mixed results (46, 47). In addition to the "visceral hyperalgesia" phenomenon suggested by these studies, IBS patients may have increased colonic motility and abnormal small bowel motility as well (48, 49). None of these physiologic markers is specific enough to be used as a single diagnostic sign of IBS. Fifty to 85% of patients with IBS report that psychological stress exacerbates their bowel symptoms (47). One study found that 53% of women with IBS referred to tertiary care centers had a history of previous sexual abuse compared with 37% of those referred with other organic diagnoses. This same pattern is not seen at a primary care level (50).

The medical management choices for IBS are dictated by the predominant symptom(s) (Table 13.5). If diarrhea is the major symptom, a variety of antispasmodic medications such as diphenoxylate (Lomotil), hyoscyamine (Levsin, Donnatal), and dicyclomine (Bentyl) are used. Desipramine (Norpramin) or other tricyclic antidepressants are also effective and have the added benefit of treating the chronic pain syndrome component of the problem.

TABLE 13.4. Differential Diagnosis of Painful Gastrointestinal Disorders That May Present as Pelvic Pain

Disorder	Symptoms	Diagnostic Test
Lactose intolerance test	Cramping pain, flatulence after milk products	Lactose tolerance
Small bowel bacterial overgrowth and diarrhea	Postprandial bloating	Hydrogen breath test
Chronic intestinal pseudoobstruction	Migratory abdominal pain	Small bowel motility study
Inflammatory bowel disease	Copious diarrhea, sometimes bloody	Endoscopy, x-ray contrast studies
Diverticulosis	Pain, diarrhea	Endoscopy, contrast studies
Bowel endometriosis	Pain with bowel movements, and/or alteration of bowel function	Endoscopy, laparoscopy

TABLE 13.5. Pharmacologic Treatment of Irritable Bowel Syndrome

Symptom	Drug	Daily Dose	Major Side Effects
Diarrhea	Loperamide (Imodium)	Titrate: 4 mg average	Constipation
	Diphenoxylate HCl	20 mg	Euphoria, sedation, dry mouth, constipation
	Hyoscyamine sulfate (Levsin, Donnatal)	<1.5 mg	Dry mouth, blurred vision, dizziness
	Dicyclomine HCl (Bentyl)	80–160 mg	Dry mouth, blurred vision, dizziness
	Desipramine HCl (Norpramin)	150 mg	Dry mouth, sedation, confusional states, hypertension, hypotension, constipation
	Trimipramine maleate (Surmontil)	50 mg	Dry mouth, sedation, confusional states, hypertension, hypotension, constipation
Constipation	Fiber from any source	≥30 g	Bloating, abdominal pain
	Lactulose (Chronulac, Duphalac)	10–30 g	Bloating
	Sorbitol	10–30 g	Bloating
	Cisapride (Propulsid)	40–80 mg	Dizziness, headaches

Constipation is best treated by increased fiber and water intake. Lactose and sorbitol are effective but increase abdominal bloating. A very effective, but more expensive, treatment is cisapride (Propulsid), although it may manifest side effects of dizziness and headaches.

For general pain treatment, the serotonin reuptake inhibitors have not been widely explored, although one study suggests that serotonin [5-hydroxytryptamine (5-HT$_3$)] receptor antagonists (such as granisetron HCl [Kytril]) lower the increased pain sensitivity seen in IBS patients (51).

Psychological treatments for IBS have included relaxation training, cognitive behavioral therapy, hypnosis, and individual psychotherapy. Each modality has research studies that support efficacy, and some studies have used them in one or more combinations (52, 53).

As a matter of practicality, the first-line approach for severe IBS includes dietary change, increased fiber and water intake, an anticholinergic for diarrhea-predominant patients, and tricyclic antidepressants when pain is the major complaint. If these interventions fail, mental health referral should be considered.

Musculoskeletal Problems

Three basic categories of musculoskeletal pain may contribute to or create pelvic pain:

1. Dysfunction of the levator ani and/or piriformis muscle(s)
2. Musculoskeletal dysfunction that is secondary to a primary gynecologic source of pain
3. Musculoskeletal dysfunction that is the primary source of pelvic pain but mimics a gynecologic problem

Levator Ani Spasm

Spasm of the levator ani muscle(s) is perhaps one of the most frequently overlooked findings in the patient with pelvic pain. Historically, the person describes a sensation of her pelvis "falling out," which is worse later in the day. The pain commonly radiates to the lower back or sacral area and may increase premenstrually. This premenstrual increase is less dramatic than that seen with endometriosis or pelvic congestion. The spasm may be relieved by lying down and is aggravated by defecation. Pelvic examination reveals tenderness specific to the levator muscles. This is most readily elicited by vaginal palpation of the pelvic floor in the 4:30 and 7:30 o'clock directions with the index finger. To amplify the finding, ask for voluntary contraction of the pelvic floor, such as what might occur during attempts to hold back defecation. The patient should then be asked how closely any discomfort mimics her chief complaint.

In this setting, it may be helpful to teach pelvic floor muscle relaxation exercises. The patient is asked to tighten the pelvic floor for a count of "one" or "two" and relax for a count of "seven" or "eight." In essence, these are "reverse" Kegel exercises. The patient is counseled that when she is standing and notes this sense of pelvic pressure, if she simply lets it "fall out," this will relax the pelvic floor.

Piriformis Muscle Spasm

The piriformis muscle originates in the lateral margin of the sacrum and passes through the greater sciatic notch to attach to the greater trochanter of the femur. Its function is to assist in external rotation of the thigh. When this muscle is in spasm, the patient may notice pain upon first arising and starting to walk, with climbing stairs, or with driving a car. The pain is present regardless of time of day and phase of the menstrual cycle.

Upon physical examination, the pain is elicited by externally rotating the entire leg in the supine position or externally rotating the thigh against resistance while transvaginally palpating the piriformis muscle during this maneuver. When cul-de-sac pathology is present, the transvaginal palpation of the piriformis may yield a false-positive result. In addition to being associated with initial gynecologic problems, piriformis syndrome may develop as a result of athletic injury or other inflammatory conditions such as trochanteric bursitis. As a normal anatomic variant, the sciatic nerve may traverse the belly of the piriformis in up to 20 to 30% of people. With this anatomic variant, when the piriformis goes into spasm, pseudosciatic symptoms may appear.

Treatment for the piriformis syndrome involves range of motion exercises, heat, local massage, deep ultrasound, and other physical therapy techniques. Continuous nonsteroidal anti-inflammatory drugs are useful as well and should perhaps be a first-line agent.

The second category of disorders, musculoskeletal dysfunctions that develop as a response to initial gynecologic problems, may include shortening and spasm of the psoas, shortening of the abdominal muscles, and/or a general abnormal posture including increased lumbar lordosis and an anterior tilt of the pelvis. The original gynecologic problem may promote splinting or cessation of exercise, leading to a muscle(s) of abnormal lengths (i.e., longer or shorter). This may induce tissue damage that results in the development of trigger points. Injection therapy for trigger points may not yield long-term results unless they are supplemented by physical therapy techniques aimed at reestablishing normal posture, muscle length, and muscular relaxation.

The musculoskeletal disorders listed above and others may develop primarily and not in response to other pain etiologies. When these problems are detected coincidentally with known gynecologic pathology, clinical judgment as to which component is the more likely originator of the pain disorder is difficult.

Urinary Tract Disorders

Problems of the bladder and urethra may be roughly grouped as anatomic, inflammatory, or functional. Whereas anatomic or structural urologic causes of chronic pelvic pain occur, most are either inflammatory or functional in nature.

Problems resulting from pelvic relaxation are the most common structural disorders of the urinary tract. A pronounced cystocele may result in urinary retention and chronic recurrent urinary tract infection. Ordinarily, the history and physical examination readily detects this anatomic problem. Postcoital antibiosis and voiding and, at times, daily antibiotic prophylaxis treat most cases of chronic infection. When possible, surgical repair of the cystocele is most appropriate.

A urethral diverticulum is a relatively infrequent cause of pelvic pain. A bulging mass underneath the urethra may be appreciated, although in many cases urethroscopy and/or a urethrogram with a double-balloon Davis catheter is needed. By history, the patient may report dribbling after she stands up after voiding. On examination, even if a bulge cannot be appreciated, an area of focal tenderness along the course of the urethra may be palpable.

Perhaps the largest overall category of bladder problems contributing to chronic pelvic pain are the inflammatory disorders. Chronic recurrent urinary tract infection is perhaps the most common, followed by chronic bacterial urethritis. In the latter disorder, clean-catch urine cultures may yield colony counts significantly less than 100,000 CFU/mL and are erroneously reported as "negative." Diagnosis can be made by historical reports of urethral pain and generalized tenderness to palpation along the entire urethra. A short course of antibiotics may help symptoms subside, but prolonged courses of 3 months or more are often needed to produce long-term relief. Urethral dilation is an outmoded treatment for chronic urinary tract infection but may have occasional application in refractory cases of chronic urethritis.

Much attention has been focused on the very difficult problem of interstitial cystitis. This disorder typically presents as frequency, nocturia, urgency, and suprapubic pain, often relieved by voiding. Dyspareunia is present in as many as 60% of female patients. The disorder may present in a mild intermittent form initially but may gradually progress to a more chronic and disabling pattern over several years.

The diagnosis of interstitial cystitis is made by cystoscopy and hydrodistention under general or regional anesthesia (54). The bladder is distended to 80 to 100 cm H_2O with gravity filling over a period of 1 to 2 minutes. After distention, the cystoscope typically reveals glomerulations that look like small petechiae or submucosal hemorrhages, fissures, and/or ulcers. Quantitatively, the diagnosis is made when these lesions appear in at least three quadrants of the bladder with at least 10 glomerulations per quadrant. Typically, total bladder capacity during anesthesia is reduced from a normal value of 1000 mL to between 550 and 650 mL. Bladder biopsy is done to rule out other diseases such as eosinophilia, cystitis, endometriosis, chronic cystitis, and carcinoma in situ. The hydrodistention process itself may reduce symptoms in 30 to 60% of patients.

Medical therapy for interstitial cystitis includes a host of oral and intravesical agents and general pain management techniques (Table 13.6). Overall response rates vary between 50 and 90% with about a third of responders relapsing over time.

Dietary therapy may contribute to management. This involves adequate food intake; avoidance of soft drinks, caffeine, and citrus juices; and a variety of other less well-substantiated recommendations (52).

Under the heading of functional disorders, chronic intermittent bladder spasm is an uncommon, but not rare, contributor to chronic pelvic pain. Ordinarily, the association with voiding and the suprapubic location of the pain makes the diagnosis. During pelvic examination, the bladder area may be somewhat tender, especially if the patient has just voided before the examination. Anticholinergic and antispasmodic agents (such as hyoscyamine sulfate [Levsin] or Donnatal) are good initial therapies, although the sedative side effects of these drugs complicate their use.

Bladder training or the bladder "drill" is often helpful in reducing the inherent irritability of the bladder in both interstitial cystitis and bladder spasm. In this exercise, the patient records the time of each urination over several days and then calculates the average interval. While maintaining a steady fluid intake throughout the day, the patient then voids on a schedule. She gradually increases the voiding interval over weeks or months. This accomplishes a gradual nontraumatic stretching of the bladder wall and, often, a reduction in symptoms.

Miscellaneous Causes

In addition to the above disorders, a whole host of uncommon and rare conditions may produce pelvic pain. The uncommon categories would include posthysterectomy entrapment of the ovary, ovarian remnant syndrome, and vaginal apex pain. The rarer disorders would include true peripheral neuropathies of the pelvis, traumatic neuromas, levator muscle tendinitis, and a variety of other focal pain syndromes of mixed etiology.

After hysterectomy, reapproximation of the pelvic peritoneum may result in en-

TABLE 13.6. Treatment Modalities in Interstitial Cystitis

NONSURGICAL	SURGICAL
Pharmacologic	*Endoscopic procedures*
Antihistamines	Hydrodistention
Anti-inflammatories	Transurethral resection and fulguration
Sodium pentosan polysulfate (Elmiron)	Neodymium:yttrium-aluminum
Anticholinergics	garnet laser
Intravesical	*Open surgical procedures*
Dimethyl sulfoxide (DMSO)	Denervation procedures
$DMSO_2$ (investigational)	Bladder augmentation procedures
DSMO cocktails	Urinary diversion
Silver nitrate	
Sodium oxychlorosene (Chlorpactin)	
Cystostat (investigational)	
Cromolyn (a mast cell inhibitor)	
(investigational)	
OTHER	
Electric stimulation	
Biofeedback	
Transcutaneous electric nerve stimulation	
Epidural block	
Bladder pillar block	

Reprinted with permission from Peters-Gee JM. Bladder and urethral symptoms. In: Steege JF, Metzger DA, Levy BS, eds. Chronic Pelvic Pain: An Integrated Approach. Philadelphia: WB Saunders, 1997.

casement of one or both ovaries in adhesion, sometimes at close proximity to the vaginal apex. During intercourse, percussion of the encased ovary can be quite painful. Incorporating the utero-ovarian ligament in the vaginal apex at the time of vaginal hysterectomy leads to a high frequency of postvaginal hysterectomy deep dyspareunia. For this reason, this surgical technique is no longer recommended. Although suppression of ovarian function may reduce the discomfort, surgical removal is often necessary.

The ovarian remnant syndrome is uncommon but not as rare as previously thought. Clinical series published in the past 10 years have prompted more frequent testing for, and hence diagnosis of, this condition (55–57). In a patient with ostensible bilateral salpingo-oophorectomy, the presence of functioning ovarian tissue is detected by withdrawing replacement hormones for 3 to 4 weeks and then determining the serum follicle-stimulating hormone (FSH) and estradiol levels. If the FSH level is well over 100 and estradiol levels are minimal, then it is highly unlikely that ovarian tissue is present. If premenopausal levels of these hormones are present, then hormonally functional ovarian tissue is present. Complete suppression of the remnant with a GnRH agonist helps to determine the degree to which the ovarian remnant contributes to the patient's pain. If the patient is sufficiently close to menopausal age, then suppression with a GnRH agonist may be continued until menopause is reached. If not, surgical intervention should be contemplated. With the best of surgical techniques, there is a 10 to 15% chance of recurrence of the ovarian remnant after careful excision.

After hysterectomy, the vaginal apex may be intrinsically sensitive in the occasional patient. Although granulation tissue can cause this problem in the early postoperative months, localized sensitivity sometimes remains for years thereafter, even after all postoperative inflammation has disappeared. This condition is detected by gently "walking" a cotton-tipped applicator over the vaginal apex during speculum examination. Often, one part of the vaginal apex is sensitive, whereas other parts are quite comfortable. A local block with 1% xylocaine mixed with sodium bicarbonate (0.3 mL of 0.9% sodium bicarbonate per 10 mL of 1% xylocaine) can accomplish transient and sometimes long-term relief. Blocking the area successfully confirms the diagnosis. Some patients can adequately cope with this disorder by using 2% xylocaine jelly and a vaginal applicator. Dose titration is important to accomplish comfortable intercourse without producing genital anesthesia for both partners. If these conservative modalities fail, then surgical revision of the vaginal apex may be helpful.

PSYCHIATRIC CONDITIONS INVOLVED WITH CHRONIC PELVIC PAIN

Once pain has become chronic, it has a very powerful emotional meaning to the patient and to her family and friends. When concise diagnosis proves elusive, anxiety and fear of the unknown pathologic process can aggravate both the intensity of the pain and the suffering that is its consequence.

When painful events happen to a person who has substantial emotional needs that are unmet, the combination of these circumstances may support the development of one of the following styles of interaction between family members and the patient (58):

1. The pain serves as a proxy for dysfunction in the family that is easier to tolerate than the dysfunctional relationships in the family.
2. The family acts as a reinforcer of the pain by nurturing and caring for the patient.
3. The patient uses the pain to control the family (with this pattern unwittingly reinforced by the family); and/or
4. The stress of the family life produces psychological effects that predispose the patient to stress and pain.

Even when these patterns are present or when obvious depression is present, this does not necessarily preclude the existence of organic pathology that requires medical and/or surgical therapy.

Much has been said and written about the association of depression with chronic pain of virtually any sort (59, 60). Depression, when associated with pain, may lower the pain threshold, thereby increasing sensitivity to pain, and may be associated with irritability and social withdrawal symptomatology rather than the more dramatic symptoms of overt sadness, sleeplessness, and suicidal ideation. In most instances, the depression can be seen as coevolving with the pain disorder, not as an etiologically important precursor.

Similarly, anxiety disorders may contribute substantially to the intensity of symptoms of pelvic pain but are rarely the sole etiologic agent of the pain. Comanagement with a mental health professional is usually desirable, although the interested and experienced primary care clinician can certainly manage medication approaches for these problems.

Finally, personality disorders, somatization, and hypochondriasis can accompany any of the pelvic pain disorders. A more complete discussion of these psychological aspects of chronic pain is presented elsewhere (61).

GENERAL PRINCIPLES OF PAIN MANAGEMENT

When confronted with chronic pelvic pain, the practitioner is challenged to present all possible modes of therapy in a balanced fashion. In addition, the health care provider must resist the tendency to attribute the entire symptom complex to a single disorder. It is useful to conduct a thorough educational session that creates a list of potentially contributing factors and outlines reasonable therapies. This list can be constructed only at the completion of a thorough history and physical examination and, possibly, after some preliminary diagnostic studies.

Even when surgery seems imperative, the clinician should resist the tendency to pursue maximal surgical treatment without consideration of treatment of other components. Pursuit of only one therapeutic modality reinforces the notion that chronic pelvic pain problems can be understood in an either/or fashion (i.e., they are *either* physically caused *or* psychologically based). In most situations, both realms are important to explore and treat, and overemphasis of one at the expense of the other is unproductive. For most, if not all, situations, this approach is applicable even when obvious organic pathology exists.

In addition to the specific therapies described for the conditions listed above, some general principles of medication management deserve review. An individual patient's problem list may require a pharmacologic approach to two or three conditions simultaneously. For example, the IBS may require dietary management with fiber and water additions, whereas the pain may require analgesia of either a narcotic or nonnarcotic variety, and a chronic pain syndrome may require antidepressant therapy. It is often useful to begin some or all of these medications in close proximity to each other, allowing only enough time between their initiations to evaluate the side effects accurately. Although this may result in polypharmacy initially, it is more likely to produce a greater degree of clinical improvement, thereby accomplishing a better, and perhaps quicker, return to normal function (62).

Narcotic medications can sometimes be used on a long-term basis in the carefully selected and monitored patient. Table 13.7 describes their general dose levels and common side effects. It is useful to have the patient sign a narcotics "contract," which is basically her promise to obtain controlled substances from only one physician and one pharmacy and to stick to a rigidly prescribed schedule.

Antidepressant medications have been a mainstay of chronic pain management of all types for many years. The best studied is amitriptyline (Elavil, Endep), commonly used in doses of 50 to 75 mg each night. If constipation is a major factor in the patient's pain, a selective serotonin uptake inhibitor such as sertraline (Zoloft) or paroxetine (Paxil) rather than amitriptyline is probably a better initial treatment because selective serotonin uptake inhibitors have fewer anticholinergic side effects.

The clinician dealing with chronic pain syndromes soon recognizes that complete success is often elusive. For the surgically oriented gynecologist who is used to a very high level of positive therapeutic outcome, this realization may prove frustrating. To survive, the successful clinician lowers his or her reward threshold when dealing with chronic pain patients but makes the commitment to continue the positive therapeutic relationship with the patient despite the frustrations involved. Early consultation with a specialist in chronic pain can often be fruitful and should provide the basis for an ongoing collaborative and therapeutic team approach.

TABLE 13.7. Narcotics Commonly Used in Chronic Pain Management

Drug Name	Usual Dose Range	Side Effects
Hydrocodone bitartrate with acetaminophen Lortab 2.5/500, 5/500, or 7.5/500 Vicodin 5/750 Lorcet 10/650 Lorcet Plus 7.5/650 (all are scored tablets)	5–10 mg hydrocodone either q6hr or q8hr Can use additional acetaminophen between doses to potentiate effect	Lightheadedness, dizziness, sedation, nausea and vomiting, and constipation. (These are common side effects of all narcotics.)
Oxycodone hydrochloride Percocet 5 mg with 325 mg acetaminophen Percodan 4.5 mg with 325 mg aspirin (also contains 0.38 mg oxycodone terephthalate)	1 tablet q6hr or q8hr Additional acetaminophen between doses may serve to potentiate effect.	Common effects.
Oxycodone controlled release OxyContin	10–40 mg q12hr	Common effects.
Methadone hydrochloride Dolophine 5- or 10-mg scored tablets	2.5 mg q8hr to 10 mg q6hr Commonly 15–20 mg qd	Common effects. Lower extremity edema or joint swelling may occur and require discontinuation. Concurrent use of desipramine may increase methadone blood level. Cautious use in patients on monoamine oxidase inhibitors.
Acetaminophen with codeine Tylenol No. 3, 300 mg acetaminophen with 30 mg codeine	1–2 tablets q6–8hr	Common effects. Constipation very likely. Nausea and vomiting more common than with other narcotics. More common allergy—rash.
Morphine sulfate MS Contin or Oramorph	15–60 mg q12hr; controlled-release tablets	Common effects. Higher doses increase risk of respiratory depression.
Fentanyl transdermal system Duragesic	25-μg patch, 1 q72hr Also available in 50 or 75 μg Always start with lowest dose	Common effects. Patch must be kept from heat sources, or dose may be increased. Extreme caution in patients on other central nervous system medications. Respiratory depression can result.

Reproduced with permission from Steege JF. General principles of pain management. In: Steege JF, Metzger DA, Levy BS, eds. Chronic Pelvic Pain: An Integrated Approach. Philadelphia: WB Saunders, 1997.

CLINICAL NOTES

- Chronic pelvic pain is pain present in the pelvis more often than not for 6 months or longer.
- Centralization of pain occurs when changes occur in the spinal cord that result in ongoing signals being sent to the brain despite the dramatic decrease or even absence of peripheral nociception.
- Spinal cord "wind-up" occurs when repeated low-level nociceptive stimuli from the periphery elicit progressively more dramatic responses from second-order neurons at the spinal cord level even though the intensity of the stimuli may remain constant or even be diminished.
- When pain is prolonged and chronic, the anatomic site of the pain may become less distinct and symptoms originating in surrounding organ systems may join the original complaint.
- Studies suggest an association between a history of abuse and chronic pelvic pain. Care must be taken not to automatically ascribe responsibility to this history for pain that is present.
- Examination of the patient with chronic pelvic pain should include a thorough abdominal examination.
- The sequence of the pelvic examination is determined by the nature, suggested source, and type of pain.
- Trigger points may be treated by injection of local anesthetics; this may also facilitate the pelvic examination.
- Possible pelvic sources for chronic pelvic pain include endometriosis, adhesions, adenomyosis, and pelvic congestion.
- Physical examination may not detect any abnormalities early in the disease of endometriosis, although detection of uterosacral nodularity may be enhanced by conduction of the pelvic examination during menstruation.
- Among women undergoing laparoscopy for chronic pelvic pain, adhesions are found between 45 and 90% of the time. Studies on the impact of adhesiolysis suggest laparotomy to be superior to laparoscopy only in cases of dense bowel adhesions.
- The diagnosis of adenomyosis requires histologic examination of the uterine wall. A woman with severe disease may demonstrate substantial cyclic changes in the size, consistency, and tenderness of the uterine fundus.
- The prevalence of pelvic congestion is uncertain and concrete physical findings are limited. Bimanual examination may reveal a "doughy" consistency to the parametrial areas.
- IBS may cause symptoms attributed to a gynecologic origin.
- There appears to be a fairly strong association of IBS and dysmenorrhea.
- The medical management of choice for IBS is determined by the predominant symptoms.
- Levator ani muscle spasm is a frequently overlooked finding in the patient with pelvic pain. If present, it may be helpful to teach pelvic floor relaxation exercises.
- Piriformis muscle spasm causes pain upon first arising and starting to walk, climbing stairs, and/or while driving. The pain is not related to time of day or phase of cycle. It may develop as a result of athletic injury or may be associated with other inflammatory conditions.
- Musculoskeletal dysfunctions may develop as a response to initial gynecologic problems.
- Urinary tract disorders may also cause pelvic pain; examples would include pelvic relaxation, urethral diverticulum, chronic urinary tract infections, and interstitial cystitis.
- Posthysterectomy pain may occur if the ovaries become encased in adhesions; dyspareunia may be present if the ovaries and/or ovarian adhesions are close to the vaginal apex.
- Other sources of posthysterectomy pain include ovarian remnant syndrome or hypersensitivity of the vaginal apex.
- Depression may be associated with chronic pelvic pain. Similarly, anxiety disorders, personality disorders, somatization, or hypochondriasis may also accompany a pelvic pain disorder.

- Treatment of a patient's pain may require a pharmacologic approach to two or three conditions simultaneously.
- Antidepressants, such as amitriptyline, have been a mainstay of chronic pain management of all types for many years. If the patient suffers constipation, a selective serotonin uptake inhibitor may be better initial therapy.

References

1. Jamieson DJ, Steege JF. The prevalence of dysmenorrhea, dyspareunia, pelvic pain, and irritable bowel syndrome in primary care practices. Obstet Gynecol 1996;87:55.
2. Graves EJ. National hospital discharge survey. Vital Health Stat 13 1992:112:1–62.
3. Hulka JF, Peterson HB, Phillips JM, et al. Operative laparoscopy: American Association of Gynecologic Laparoscopists 1991 Membership Survey. J Reprod Med 1993;38:569.
4. Steege JF, Metzger D, Levy B, eds. Chronic Pelvic Pain: An Integrated Approach. Philadelphia: WB Saunders, 1996.
5. Rogers RM Jr. Basic Pelvic neuroanatomy. In: Steege JF, Metzger D, Levy B, eds. Chronic Pelvic Pain: An Integrated Approach. Philadelphia: WB Saunders, 1996.
6. Melzack R. Neurophysiologic foundations of pain. In: Sternback RA, ed. The Psychology of Pain. New York: Raven Press, 1986:1.
7. Melzack R. Gate control theory: on the evolution of pain concepts. Pain Forum 1996; 5:128.
8. Cervero F. Visceral pain: mechanisms of peripheral and central sensitization. Ann Med 1995;27:235.
9. Melzack R. Gate control theory: on the evolution of pain concepts. Pain Forum 1996; 5:128.
10. Katz J. Pre-emptive analgesia: evidence, current status and future directions. Eur J Anaesthesiol Suppl 1995;10:8–13.
11. Walker EA, Katon W, Harrop-Griffiths J, et al. Relationship of chronic pelvic pain to psychiatric diagnosis and childhood sexual abuse. Am J Psychiatry 1988;145:75.
12. Jamieson D, Steege J. The association of sexual and physical abuse with pelvic pain complaints in a primary care population. Am J Obstet Gynecol 1997;177:1408.
13. Beitchman JH, Zuker KJ, Hood JE, et al. A review of the long-term effects of child sexual abuse. Child Abuse Negl 1992;16:101.
14. Baker PK. Musculoskeletal problems. In: Steege JF, Metzger D, Levy B, eds. Chronic Pelvic Pain: An Integrated Approach. Philadelphia: WB Saunders, 1997.
15. Lamont JA. Vaginismus. Am J Obstet Gynecol 1978;131:632.
16. Travell JG, Simmons DG. Myofascial Pain and Dysfunction: The Trigger Point Manual. 2nd ed. Baltimore: Williams & Wilkins, 1992.
17. Slocumb JC. Neurological factors in chronic pelvic pain: trigger points and the abdominal pelvic pain syndrome. Am J Obstet Gynecol 1984;149:536.
18. Koninckx PR, Martin D. Treatment of deeply infiltrating endometriosis. Curr Opin Obstet Gynecol 1994;6:231.
19. Koninckx PR, Meuleman C, Demeyere S, et al. Suggestive evidence that pelvic endometriosis is a progressive disease, whereas deeply infiltrating endometriosis is associated with pelvic pain. Fertil Steril 1991;55:759.
20. Donnez J, Nisolle M, Casanas-Roux F, et al. Rectovaginal septum endometriosis or adenomyosis: laparoscopic management in a series of 231 patients. Hum Reprod 1995; 10:630–635.
21. Donnez J, Nisolle M, Gillerot S, et al. Rectovaginal septum adenomyotic nodules: a series of 500 cases. Br J Obstet Gynaecol 1997;104:1014–1018.
22. Marcoux S, Maheux R, Berube S, et al. Laparoscopic surgery in infertile women with minimal or mild endometriosis. N Engl J Med 1997;337:217.
23. Weibel MA, Majno G. Peritoneal adhesions and their relation to abdominal surgery. Am J Surg 1973;126:345.
24. Kresch AJ, Seifer DB, Sachs LB, et al. Laparoscopy in the evaluation of pelvic pain. Obstet Gynecol 1973;64:672.

25. Steege JF: Adhesions and pelvic pain. In: Steege JF, Metzger D, Levy B, eds. Chronic Pelvic Pain: An Integrated Approach. Philadelphia: WB Saunders, 1997.

26. Steege JF, Stout AL. Resolution of chronic pelvic pain after laparoscopic lysis of adhesions. Am J Obstet Gynecol 1991;165:278.

27. Sutton C, MacDonald R. Laser laparoscopic adhesiolysis. J Gynecol Surg 1990;6:155.

28. Peters AA, Trimbos-Kemper GC, Admiraal C, et al. A randomized clinical trial on the benefit of adhesiolysis in patients with intraperitoneal adhesions and chronic pelvic pain. Br J Obstet Gynaecol 1992;99:59–62.

29. Vercellini P, Parazzini F, Oldani S, et al. Adenomyosis at hysterectomy: a study on frequency distribution and patient characteristics. Hum Reprod 1995;10:1160.

30. Taylor HC. Vascular congestion and hyperemia, their effect on structure and function in the female reproductive organs. Part II. The clinical aspects of the congestion-fibrosis syndrome. Am J Obstet Gynecol 1949;57:654.

31. Taylor HC. Vascular congestion and hyperemia, their effect on structure in the female reproductive organs. Part III. Etiology and therapy. Am J Obstet Gynecol 1949;57:654.

32. Beard RW, Highman JH, Pearce S, et al. Diagnosis of pelvic varicosities in women with chronic pelvic pain. Lancet 1984;2:946.

33. Beard RW, Reginald PW, Pearce S. Pelvic pain in women. BMJ 1986;293:1160.

34. Osofsky HJ, Fisher S. Pelvic congestion: some further considerations. Obstet Gynecol 1968;31:406.

35. Hughes RR, Curtis DD. Uterine phlebography: correlation of clinical diagnoses with dye retention. Am J Obstet Gynecol 1962;83:156.

36. Kaupilla A. Uterine phlebography with venous compression. A clinical and roentgenological study. Acta Obstet Gynaecol Scand 1970;49:33.

37. Giacchetto C, Cotroneo GB, Marincolo F, et al. Ovarian varicocele: ultrasonic and phlebographic evaluation. J Clin Ultrasound 1990;18:551.

38. Gangar KF, Stones RW, Saunder C, et al. An alternative to hysterectomy? GnRH analogue combined with hormone replacement therapy. Br J Obstet Gynaecol 1993;100:360.

39. Allen WM. Chronic pelvic congestion and pelvic pain. Am J Obstet Gynecol 1971;109:198.

40. Farquhar CM, Rogers V, Franks S, et al. A randomized controlled trial of medroxyprogesterone acetate and psychotherapy for the treatment of pelvic congestion. Br J Obstet Gynaecol 1989;96:1153–1162.

41. Beard RW, Kennedy RG, Gangar KF, et al. Bilateral oophorectomy and hysterectomy in the treatment of intractable pelvic pain associated with pelvic congestion. Br J Obstet Gynaecol 1991;98:988.

42. Rundqvist E, Sondholm LE, Larsson G. Treatment of pelvic varicosities causing lower abdominal pain with extraperitoneal resection of the left ovarian vein. Lancet 1984;1:339.

43. Thompson WG, Creed F, Drossman DA, et al. Functional bowel disease and functional abdominal pain. Gastroenterol Int 1992;5:75.

44. Crowell MD, Dubin NH, Robinson JC, et al. Functional bowel disorders in women with dysmenorrhea. Am J Gastroenterol 1994;89:1973.

45. Longstreth GF, Preskill DB, Youkeles L. Irritable bowel syndrome in women having diagnostic laparoscopy or hysterectomy. Relation to gynecologic features and outcome. Dig Dis Sci 1990;35:1285.

46. Lembo T, Munakata J, Mertz H, et al. Evidence for the hypersensitivity of lumbar splanchnic afferents in irritable bowel syndrome. Gastroenterology 1994;107:1686.

47. Drossman DA, Sandler RS, McKee DC, et al. Bowel patterns among subjects not seeking health care. Gastroenterology 1982;83:529.

48. Kellow JE, Gill RC, Wingate DL. Prolonged ambulant recordings of bowel motility demonstrate abnormalities in the irritable bowel syndrome. Gastroenterology 1990;98:1208.

49. Kellow JE, Phillips SF. Altered small bowel motility in irritable bowel syndrome is correlated with symptoms. Gastroenterology 1987;92:1885.

50. Drossman DA, Leserman J, Nachman G, et al. Sexual and physical abuse in women with functional or organic gastrointestinal disorders. Ann Intern Med 1990;113:828.

51. Talley NJ. 5-Hydroxytryptamine agonists and antagonists in the modulation of gastrointestinal motility and sensation: clinical implications. Aliment Pharmacol Ther 1992;6:273.

52. Drossman DA, Thompson WG. The irritable bowel syndrome: review and a graduated multi-component treatment approach. Ann Intern Med 1992;116:1009.

53. Guthrie E, Creed F, Dawson D, et al. A controlled trial of psychological treatment for the irritable bowel syndrome. Gastroenterology 1991;100:450–457.

54. Peters-Gee JM. Bladder and urethral syndromes. In: Steege JF, Metzger D, Levy B, eds. Chronic Pelvic Pain: An Integrated Approach. Philadelphia: WB Saunders, 1996.

55. Steege JF. Ovarian remnant syndrome. Obstet Gynecol 1987;70:64.

56. Pettit PD, Lee RA. Ovarian remnant syndrome: diagnostic dilemma and surgical challenge. Obstet Gynecol 1988;71:580.

57. Price FV, Edwards R, Buchsbaum HJ. Ovarian remnant syndrome: difficulties in diagnosis and treatment. Obstet Gynecol Surv 1990;45:151.

58. Payne B, Norfleet M. Chronic pain and the family: a review. Pain 1986;26:1.

59. Aronoff GM. Evaluation and Treatment of Chronic Pain. 2nd ed. Baltimore: Williams & Wilkins, 1992:57.

60. Talbott JA, Hales RE, Yudofsky SC. Textbook of Psychiatry. Washington, DC: American Psychiatric Press, 1988:409.

61. Bashford RA. Psychiatric illness. In: Steege JF, Metzger D, Levy B, eds. Chronic Pelvic Pain: An Integrated Approach. Philadelphia: WB Saunders, 1996.

62. Steege JF. General principles of pain management. In: Steege JF, Metzger D, Levy B, eds. Chronic Pelvic Pain: An Integrated Approach. Philadelphia: WB Saunders, 1996.

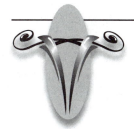

CHAPTER 14

Endometriosis

JOHN M. STORMENT
JOHN R. BRUMSTED

ENDOMETRIOSIS IN GENERAL

Since its original description in 1860, endometriosis has been considered a common disorder. It is one of the leading diseases encountered in clinical gynecology and a common cause for hysterectomy. Endometriosis is a condition characterized by ectopic endometrial glands and stroma. Endometriosis commonly presents as a progressive disease whose causes and rational treatment remains enigmatic. The literature on endometriosis is extensive but often contradictory or inadequate. This chapter reviews the current knowledge on the epidemiology, diagnosis, and treatment of endometriosis. In addition, endometriosis-associated infertility, recurrence, and appropriate hormone replacement after "definitive" surgery is covered.

Epidemiology

Standardized objective criteria for an accurate diagnosis of endometriosis are difficult to establish because the disease has a variable and nonspecific clinical presentation and natural history. Confirmation of the diagnosis requires laparoscopy or laparotomy. This makes data regarding the prevalence of endometriosis difficult to interpret. The variation in published incidence figures reflects diversity in the groups of women entered into the different studies (Table 14.1). Best estimates are that endometriosis is present in 5 to 10% of reproductive-age women and 25 to 35% of patients with infertility (1). Melis et al. (2) evaluated 305 premenopausal women undergoing surgery for infertility or benign gynecologic disease. Endometriosis was diagnosed in 24.9% of the total study population but was significantly higher in women with infertility, chronic pelvic pain, or benign ovarian cysts. Because endometriosis lesions are not always symptomatic, the mere *presence* of endometriosis is not a synonym for disease.

One group assessed the epidemiologic factors linked to endometriosis in infertile women (3). They compared 174 infertile women with 174 fertile women with laparoscopically proven endometriosis. Age at menarche; duration of menstrual flow; age at study; reproductive history, including previous abortion rate and infertility history; family history; and social class were similar in both groups. This report and others discredit prior studies indicating that endometriosis is seen more frequently in higher socioeconomic groups. There are little data of sufficient quality to show socioeconomic or ethnic differences in disease risk, thus refuting two common misperceptions: endometriosis is a disease afflicting only women over 30 who are career driven and it does not occur in women of African-American descent. There is a genetic basis of risk for endometriosis (4).

Pathogenesis

There are numerous theories proposed for the origin of endometriosis. No single theory can account for the location of the ectopic endometrium in all cases of en-

TABLE 14.1. Incidence of Endometriosis Depends on the Group of Women Entered into the Studies

Surgery (Indication)	Total	No. with Endometriosis	% with Endometriosis
Tubal anastomosis	1860	19	1
Tubal sterilization	3060	61	2
Vaginal hysterectomy	858	69	8
Abdominal hysterectomy	5511	606	11
Diagnostic laparoscopy (infertility)	724	116	16
Operative laparoscopy	2065	619	31
Diagnostic laparoscopy (teenager's pelvic pain)	140	74	53

Adapted from Wheeler JM. Epidemiology and prevalence of endometriosis. Infertil Reprod Med Clin North Am 1992;3:545.

dometriosis. For an in-depth discussion of the different theories proposed for the pathogenesis of endometriosis, there are several very thorough reviews (5–7). Theories for the histogenesis of endometriosis can be classified into three basic categories: transplantation of endometrial tissue via retrograde menstruation (Sampson's theory), coelomic metaplasia, and lymphatic or vascular transport of endometrial fragments. Sampson's theory of retrograde menstruation fails to explain why endometriosis affects such a small percentage of women, given that 75 to 90% of patients with patent tubes display retrograde flow (8). A role for immunologic factors influencing a woman's susceptibility for developing endometriosis has been proposed. One theory proposes that in women with decreased cellular immunity function, the endometriotic cells are "allowed" to implant and grow in ectopic sites (9). This altered cellular immunity may also partially explain the impaired fertility in some patients. Conclusions of studies regarding the role of cellular immunity have been inconsistent (10, 11). Genetic predisposition does appear to influence the development of disease (12). A woman whose sibling has endometriosis has a 6-fold increased risk and the daughter of a woman with endometriosis has a 10-fold increased risk of endometriosis compared with the general population. In one report, approximately 6 to 7% of first-degree female relatives of women with endometriosis had the disease compared with 1% in a control group (4).

Most endometrial implants are located in the dependent portions of the female pelvis. Two thirds of patients with endometriosis have ovarian involvement (13). Other common sites include the pelvic peritoneum; the anterior and posterior cul-de-sacs; and the uterosacral, round, and broad ligaments. However, endometriosis has been reported in almost every organ in the body, including the brain and lungs. The phenomenon of catamenial pneumothorax has been reported, whereby endometrial implants on the pleura may lead to recurrent pneumothorax at the time of menstruation. In the case of central nervous system implants, catamenial seizures have been reported (14–16). Any symptom(s) with a catamenial pattern of change and/or worsening should raise suspicion of being causally related to endometriosis.

Diagnosis

Classic symptoms of endometriosis include dysmenorrhea, dyspareunia, dyschezia, and/or a history of infertility. Few women present with all symptoms. Frequently, endometriosis presents as a diagnostic challenge to both the patient and physician. The diagnosis should be suspected in women who have pelvic pain or are infertile. The pain is thought to arise from enlargement of the implants stretching on the areas of fibrosis often found around the implants. (The implants not only enlarge in response to hormonal stimulation, they bleed into themselves, causing inflammation and fibrosis in the surrounding tissues.) Pain can be very diffuse or localized and of varying quality. A history of years of pain-free menses with a gradual onset and progressive worsening of dysmenorrhea is suggestive of endometriosis. Severe dysmenorrhea is often the only complaint. Symptoms can vary throughout the menstrual cycle or remain constant. Urinary tract complaints may indicate ureteral or bladder involvement and should be investigated as well. Low back pain and rectal pain may be due to endometriosis. The degree of pelvic pain is often unrelated to the severity or distribution of endometriosis (14, 17). Some studies, however, describe a very good correlation in the number of endometrial implants and the intensity of dysmenorrhea (18) (Table 14.2).

A history of factors that relieve and/or exacerbate the pain must be taken. Many patients derive significant relief from oral contraceptives, indicating that pain could be attributed to pelvic pathology. Although this finding is not uniform, it often helps in the management of this disease. A trial of a gonadotropin-releasing hormone (GnRH) agonist can also help in the diagnosis. If pain is improved, the pain is likely of reproductive tract origin (19). This approach can therefore allow both diagnosis and treatment to be achieved in one step and possibly avoid surgery.

Physical findings are as variable as subjective complaints. Uterosacral ligament tenderness and nodularity is very specific to endometriosis (20, 21). The finding of tenderness and nodularity of the uterosacral ligaments and/or cul-de-sac is present in only about one third of patients. Obliteration of the cul-de-sac in conjunction with fixed uterine retroversion implies extensive disease. Ovarian involvement may be accompanied with adnexal tenderness and palpable enlargement if endometriomas are present. Endometriomas are cystic structures usually filled with a chocolate-colored fluid. The presence of any adnexal mass should prompt the usual workup, including a pelvic ultrasound. Endometriomas have unique radiologic features that increase the accuracy of diagnosis. The specificity of transvaginal ultrasonography in differentiating endometriomas from other ovarian masses is approximately 90% (22).

Currently, laparoscopy is the standard approach to confirm the presence of endometriosis. Because endometriosis is a specific disease entity, the diagnosis should not be given to a patient unless direct visualization of implants is made at either laparoscopy or laparotomy. It is imperative that the surgeon is skilled in diagnosing the various appearances of implants and in excising or ablating the disease. Al-

TABLE 14.2. Correlation Between Severity of Dysmenorrhea and Likelihood of Endometriosis Being Present

Menstrual Pain	Relative Risk of Endometriosis
None	1.0
Mild	1.7
Moderate	3.4
Severe	6.7

Reprinted with permission from Cramer DW, Wilson E, Stillman RJ, et al. The relation of endometriosis to menstrual characteristics, smoking and exercise. JAMA 1985;225:1904.

though endometriosis is classically described as having either a "powder-burn" appearance or that of red lesions, implants may be black, blue, white, or even nonpigmented. Implants are usually multiple and, if a biopsy specimen is taken, are out of phase with the normal endometrium. Accurate staging of the disease is extremely important to allow comparison of results of various treatments and consistent exchange of information among clinicians.

CA-125 Assay

CA-125 is a glycoprotein expressed on the cell surface of some derivatives of coelomic epithelium (including endometrium) and has been used for monitoring patients with epithelial ovarian cancer. Serum CA-125 levels are often elevated in patients with advanced endometriosis and correlate with patients' responses to treatment (23–25). It was thought that CA-125 levels could be used for a marker of recurrence of the disease, but levels that decrease with medical therapy often return to pretherapy levels upon cessation of treatment, so the clinical utility of the CA-125 marker is limited (26). It is not sensitive enough to use as a screening test because CA-125 levels can be elevated in other benign conditions such as early pregnancy, acute pelvic inflammatory disease, leiomyomata, and menstruation.

Classification

Numerous classifications have been proposed for endometriosis. The primary objective of a classification system is to describe certain characteristics of a disease that will respond to treatment in a consistent manner (25). Most recently, a revised classification system of the American Society of Reproductive Medicine (ASRM) has been proposed based on the surgical findings of 469 patients (Fig. 14.1) (27). Although trends were apparent, this method has not proven to be a sensitive predictor of pregnancy after treatment. There is no method of categorizing endometriosis shown to accurately correlate pain with location and severity of endometriosis. Thus, efforts must continue to develop a useful method of staging this disease (28).

Treatment

There is considerable debate regarding effective treatment of endometriosis. There is no medical therapy to prevent this disease or to selectively destroy the endometrial implants. Medical and conservative surgical therapy (i.e., retention of the uterus and ovaries) must be viewed as palliative and not curative. Much controversy involves the appropriate treatments of minimal and mild disease. Severe disease is usually treated surgically unless the patient desires fertility, in which case in vitro fertilization (IVF) is a common intervention. Numerous trials addressed the question of optimal therapy for endometriosis. Only recently have well-designed, prospective, randomized, controlled studies been introduced to this debate. The presence of a control group that includes patients who do not receive any therapy for endometriosis is essential to demonstrate conclusively that treatment of endometriosis is better than expectant management.

It is imperative that the goal of therapy, either pain relief or improvement of fertility, is outlined before any plan is initiated. Many times this delineation is not clear-cut because infertile women may also complain of pelvic pain. It is important to recognize that the diagnosis of endometriosis in an infertile woman does not preclude the presence of other infertility factors for the couple. This is particularly applicable to minimal or mild endometriosis where there is no distortion of pelvic anatomy. For these patients, one reasonable course would be to treat other infertility factors that are present and if no conception occurs, proceed to the use of clomiphene citrate

AMERICAN SOCIETY FOR REPRODUCTIVE MEDICINE
REVISED CLASSIFICATION OF ENDOMETRIOSIS

Patient's Name _____ Date_____

Stage I   (Minimal) · 1-5
Stage II (Mild)   · 6-15
Stage III (Moderate) · 16-40
Stage IV (Severe)   · >40
Total_____

Laparoscopy_____ Laparotomy_____ Photography_____
Recommended Treatment_____
_____
Prognosis_____

PERITONEUM	ENDOMETRIOSIS	<1cm	1-3cm	>3cm
	Superficial	1	2	4
	Deep	2	4	6
OVARY	R Superficial	1	2	4
	Deep	4	16	20
	L. Superficial	1	2	4
	Deep	4	16	20

	POSTERIOR CULDESAC OBLITERATION	Partial		Complete
		4		40

	ADHESIONS	<1/3 Enclosure	1/3-2/3 Enclosure	>2/3 Enclosure
OVARY	R Filmy	1	2	4
	Dense	4	8	16
	L Filmy	1	2	4
	Dense	4	8	16
TUBE	R Filmy	1	2	4
	Dense	4*	8*	16
	L Filmy	1	2	4
	Dense	4*	8*	16

*If the fimbriated end of the fallopian tube is completely enclosed, change the point assignment to 16.

Denote appearance of superficial implant types as red [(R), red, red-pink, flamelike, vesicular blobs, clear vesicles], white [(W), opacifications, peritoneal defects, yellow-brown], or black [(B) black, hemosiderin deposits, blue]. Denote percent of total described as R___%, W___% and B___%. Total should equal 100%.

Additional Endometriosis: _____
_____
_____
_____

Associated Pathology: _____
_____
_____

To Be Used with Normal
Tubes and Ovaries

L   R

To Be Used with Abnormal
Tubes and/or Ovaries

L   R

(continued)

FIGURE 14.1. American Society of Reproductive Medicine revised classification of endometriosis.

STAGE I (MINIMAL)

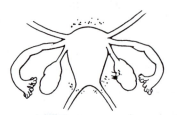

STAGE II (MILD)

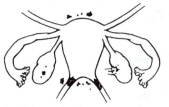

STAGE III (MODERATE)

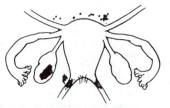

PERITONEUM
Superficial Endo – 1·3cm · 2
R. OVARY
Superficial Endo – <1cm · 1
Filmy Adhesions – <1/3 · 1
TOTAL POINTS 4

PERITONEUM
Deep Endo – >3cm · 6
R. OVARY
Superficial Endo – <1cm · 1
Filmy Adhesions – <1/3 · 1
L. OVARY
Superficial Endo – <1cm · 1
TOTAL POINTS 9

PERITONEUM
Deep Endo – >3cm · 6
CULDESAC
Partial Obliteration · 4
L. OVARY
Deep Endo – 1·3cm · 16
TOTAL POINTS 26

STAGE III (MODERATE)

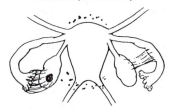

STAGE IV (SEVERE)

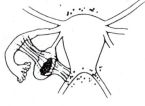

STAGE IV (SEVERE)

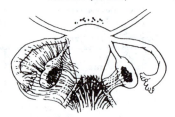

PERITONEUM
Superficial Endo – >3cm -4
R. TUBE
Filmy Adhesions – <1/3 · 1
R. OVARY
Filmy Adhesions – <1/3 · 1
L. TUBE
Dense Adhesions – <1/3 · 16*
L. OVARY
Deep Endo – <1 cm -4
Dense Adhesions – <1/3 -4
TOTAL POINTS 30

PERITONEUM
Superficial Endo – >3cm -4
L. OVARY
Deep Endo – 1·3cm - 32**
Dense Adhesions – <1/3 - 8**
L. TUBE
Dense Adhesions – <1/3 -8**
TOTAL POINTS 52

*Point assignment changed to 16
**Point assignment doubled

PERITONEUM
Deep Endo – >3cm · 6
CULDESAC
Complete Obliteration · 40
R. OVARY
Deep Endo – 1·3cm · 16
Dense Adhesions – <1/3 · 4
L. TUBE
Dense Adhesions – >2/3 · 16
L. OVARY
Deep Endo – 1·3cm · 16
Dense Adhesions – >2/3 · 16
TOTAL POINTS 114

Determination of the stage or degree of endometrial involvement is based on a weighted point system. Distribution of points has been arbitrarily determined and may require further revision or refinement as knowledge of the disease increases.

To ensure complete evaluation, inspection of the pelvis in a clockwise or counterclockwise fashion is encouraged. Number, size and location of endometrial implants, plaques, endometriomas and/or adhesions are noted. For example, five separate 0.5cm superficial implants on the peritoneum (2.5 cm total) would be assigned 2 points. (The surface of the uterus should be considered peritoneum.) The severity of the endometriosis or adhesions should be assigned the highest score only for peritoneum, ovary, tube or culdesac. For example, a 4cm superficial and a 2cm deep implant of the peritoneum should be given a score of 6 (not 8). A 4cm deep endometrioma of the ovary associated with more than 3cm of superficial disease should be scored 20 (not 24).

In those patients with only one adnexa, points applied to disease of the remaining tube and ovary should be multiplied by two. **Points assigned may be circled and totaled. Aggregation of points indicates stage of disease (minimal, mild, moderate, or severe).

The presence of endometriosis of the bowel, urinary tract, fallopian tube, vagina, cervix, skin etc., should be documented under "additional endometriosis." Other pathology such as tubal occlusion, leiomyomata, uterine anomaly, etc., should be documented under "associated pathology." All pathology should be depicted as specifically as possible on the sketch of pelvic organs, and means of observation (laparoscopy or laparotomy) should be noted.

Property of the American Society for Reproductive Medicine 1996

For additional supply write to: American Society for Reproductive Medicine,
1209 Montgomery Highway, Birmingham, Alabama 35216

FIGURE 14.1.—*continued*

and intrauterine insemination (IUI). (This assumes the patient had already been diagnosed with endometriosis and treated laparoscopically at the time. If no treatment was provided at the time of laparoscopy, repeat laparoscopy with the use of ablation or resection of implants should be considered.) The ideal treatment would provide pain relief *and* allow pregnancy to occur safely while on treatment. The section below reviews treatment options for endometriosis-associated infertility and pelvic pain. Treatment modalities for endometriosis can be classified into four major categories: expectant management, medical therapy, surgical therapy, and assisted reproductive technologies.

ENDOMETRIOSIS-ASSOCIATED INFERTILITY

Ten to 15% of infertile couples have endometriosis as the only identifiable cause, and 30 to 40% of women with the disease are infertile (29). Verkauf (30) prospectively described endometriosis in 38.5% of infertile patients compared with 5.2% of control subjects. Patients with even minimal endometriosis have decreased fecundity compared with normal control subjects (31, 32). Although these and other similar findings imply an association between endometriosis and infertility, doubts regarding a causal relationship remain. When adnexal adhesions alter tubo-ovarian anatomy, infertility is easily explainable, but in the presence of a few scattered peritoneal implants and no disruption of ovum pickup, an etiologic role is not as clear.

Proposed mechanisms for infertility associated with endometriosis include mechanical, peritoneal, immunologic, and ovulatory factors. Some authors suggested an association between endometriosis and spontaneous abortion; however, these data are purely observational and likely explained by other factors (33, 34). Alterations in tubal motility due to pelvic adhesions or elevated prostaglandins present in the peritoneal fluid are hypotheses to explain the decreased fecundity. Peritubal and periovarian adhesions can alter tubo-ovarian relationships essential for ovum pickup. Prostaglandins can cause dysmenorrhea, dyspareunia, and pelvic pain. They affect smooth muscle function and may interfere with tubal and uterine motility, resulting in altered transport of gametes or even implantation. Ectopic endometrial implants contain increased levels of prostaglandin F compared with normal endometrium, and some investigators reported a higher concentration of prostaglandins within the peritoneal fluid of patients with endometriosis (35, 36). Others found no difference in prostaglandin levels of peritoneal fluid in women with and without endometriosis (37). Because no study has definitively correlated impaired fertility with increased levels of prostaglandins, it remains speculative as an etiology.

Peritoneal fluid of patients with endometriosis contains increased number of activated macrophages (38). It had been thought that these macrophages might ingest sperm via phagocytosis, but further study failed to demonstrate a difference in the numbers of motile sperm in peritoneal fluid of patients with endometriosis versus those without (39, 40). Although no in vivo data support an adverse affect on fertility, these macrophages can serve as an additional source of prostaglandins and interleukin-1, possibly altering follicular rupture, tubal motility, and corpus luteum function.

Subtle defects in ovulation have also been attributed to endometriosis. Specifically, impaired folliculogenesis and luteinized unruptured follicle syndrome have been suggested as causes of decreased fertility (41, 42). Given that the diagnosis of follicle rupture is so difficult, even in normal ovulatory women, this correlation remains doubtful (43). McBean et al. (44) demonstrated an abnormal transition from follicular to luteal phase in endometriosis patients compared with control subjects.

The resulting abnormalities of oocyte release and progesterone production could be a contributing mechanism of infertility (44).

Fertilization and implantation rates have been compared between normal women and patients with endometriosis. Whereas some authors report a decreased fertilization rate in women with endometriosis, others show no correlation (45, 46). An increase in abnormal implantation rates has been reported in patients with endometriosis. This is theorized to be secondary to an embryotoxic environment created by endometriosis (47). Lessey et al. (48) described aberrant integrin expression in the endometrium of patients with endometriosis and proposed this as a possible cause of subfertility.

Treatment

Expectant Management

Lack of prospective controlled trials and agreement regarding the consistency of staging contributes to the uncertainty of whether endometriosis reduces fertility. The cumulative pregnancy rate after 5 years without treatment is 90% in women with minimal disease and is only slightly more in women without endometriosis (49). Based on these findings, many recommend a period of expectant management before any therapy (50). It is important to note that expectant treatment does not imply no treatment, and additional infertility factors such as ovulatory disorders should be diagnosed and treated. Compared with medical therapy, expectant management is less costly and avoids treatment-induced anovulation and medication-related side effects. The disadvantages of expectant management are that it does not specifically treat the endometriotic implants, and in most patients who fail to conceive with expectant management, progression of the disease may occur (51). Most studies that address treatment options first categorize patients according to the severity of disease. Classification of endometriosis based on the ASRM revised classification system requires laparoscopic evaluation, which is in itself an intervention. Marcoux et al. (52) presented the only prospective randomized trial comparing laparoscopic surgery with expectant management after minimal or mild disease had been diagnosed with laparoscopy. In contrast to other studies, they concluded that monthly fecundity of the laparoscopic surgery group was twice that of the expectant management group. However, the follow-up of these patients was only 36 weeks (52, 53). Most studies showing no difference between expectant management and surgery for minimal disease also demonstrate this initial increase in fecundity after surgery. With longer follow-up (2 years), however, it appears the difference in pregnancy rates is not significant. Thus, if time is a major factor (i.e., in patients older than 35 years old), it is reasonable to proceed with removal of endometriosis to obtain the most immediate improvement in pregnancy rate.

Medical Therapy

The most commonly used medical treatments for endometriosis-associated infertility include danazol (Danocrine), progestins, and GnRH agonists. Although use of ovulation-suppressive agents to treat patients with endometriosis may improve pelvic pain, they do not improve fecundity.

Danazol is a derivative of 17α-ethinyl testosterone. It produces a high-androgen low-estrogen environment that does not support the growth of endometriosis. Benefits of danazol include pain relief and prevention of disease progression (54). Discontinuation of the drug frequently leads to recurrence of symptoms. There is no apparent evidence supporting the use of danazol over expectant management in the treatment of infertility (55, 56).

Progestational agents have not been effective in the treatment of endometriosis-associated infertility (57, 58). Although some reports demonstrate higher pregnancy rates, these were not controlled studies (55). One randomized, double-blind, placebo-controlled study of luteal phase treatment with dydrogesterone (a synthetic progestogen) failed to show any improvement in pregnancy rates over a control group (59).

The GnRH agonist is the most recent type of medication introduced for the treatment of endometriosis. These medications are analogues of GnRH that have altered amino acid sequences to prolong their half-life and improve receptor binding (60). The use of a GnRH agonist in the treatment of endometriosis relies on its ability to downregulate the gonadotropins and create a hypoestrogenic environment that suppresses endometrial tissue growth. To date, no studies have shown an improved pregnancy rate using GnRH agonist versus danazol or expectant management in the treatment of endometriosis-associated infertility (61, 62).

Surgical Treatment

To appropriately assess the effect of surgical treatment of endometriosis on fertility, it is imperative to analyze the data with the proper methodology. Simple pregnancy rates are an inappropriate measure of success because of the variability in the length of patient follow-up. A reported 50% pregnancy rate has a vastly different meaning with 1 month of follow-up versus 1 year after therapy. A better approach is the use of life-table analyses to describe the resulting cumulative pregnancy rate (63). Life-table analysis is a statistical method that accounts for variable lengths of follow-up in a study population and for subjects lost to follow-up. It is frequently and appropriately applied to the study of infertility and fertility. A life-table analysis requires a well-defined starting point. In infertility studies this is most often the time when the couple registers with an infertility service. In addition, a distinct dichotomous end point must be defined. This is an end point that either occurs or does not and is usually defined as any pregnancy in studies of interest. Finally, the life-table must have a well-described and limited time interval.

Surgical treatment of severe disease has been shown by appropriate methodologic studies to improve pregnancy rates (64). Success of surgery is directly related to the severity of disease. Treatment of patients with moderate and severe endometriosis results in 60% and 35% pregnancy rates, respectively (63). Benefit from treatment of minimal and mild disease is less well established. Guzick and Rock (65) demonstrated a rapid rise in the cumulative pregnancy rate with endoscopic laser therapy, but a plateau is reached similar to that seen in other forms of treatment. Their study, however, did not compare surgery with expectant management. Marcoux et al. (52) described a significant improvement in surgery over expectant management in a randomized prospective trial. The duration of the study was only 36 weeks, and based on other trials, it is probable that this benefit is transient.

In summary, laparoscopic removal of minimal to mild endometriosis appears to have a benefit within the first 36 weeks after surgery. It is unknown if this improvement in pregnancy rate would be any different than expectant management over 1 to 2 years of follow-up. In addition, no study addressed whether the same immediate increase in pregnancy rates resulting from surgery could be obtained from more inexpensive medical management, such as ovulation induction with IUI. Treatment for severe endometriosis with either laparoscopic surgery or assisted reproductive technologies significantly improves pregnancy rates (66, 67).

Preoperative or postoperative medical therapy with hormonal suppression is not associated with any improvement in overall pregnancy rates when compared with surgical or medical treatment alone (68). Although one study demonstrated a small improvement in pregnancy rate with the use of postoperative danazol, the preponderance of evidence suggests no benefit (69–71).

For women not currently seeking pregnancy but diagnosed (incidentally) with mild endometriosis at the time of surgery, the need for treatment is controversial. For those incidentally diagnosed with more advanced disease (i.e., moderate or severe), the lesions should be treated at the time of surgery and consideration given to medical therapy with either a GnRH agonist, danazol (Danocrine), or medroxyprogesterone acetate (Provera) for 6 months, followed by continuous oral contraceptive use to avoid progression of the disease.

Advanced Reproductive Technologies

Because the benefit of conservative surgical treatment of patients with minimal disease still remains controversial, many physicians confronted with such cases have used advanced reproductive technology to bypass the unknown mechanism(s). For instance, if endometriosis is causing ovulatory dysfunction, treatment with ovulation induction should improve fecundity. If the infertility is secondary to tubal distortion from endometriosis, the use of IVF increases the chance of pregnancy.

Superovulation with clomiphene citrate or with human menopausal gonadotropin (hMG) has been used successfully to treat endometriosis-associated infertility (72–74). Results are not uniform, but it does appear that per cycle fecundity in women receiving superovulation and IUI is increased over expectant management. In women with documented mild endometriosis, clomiphene citrate/IUI provided improvement in pregnancy rates over expectant management but not as significant as that seen with hMG/IUI (74). In patients in whom clomiphene citrate/IUI is unsuccessful, hMG/IUI may be considered as the next step in treatment.

IVF should be reserved for patients failing to achieve pregnancy with the aforementioned less-invasive methods. As with other indications for IVF, such a decision must take into consideration the age of the couple, their wishes, and the duration of infertility. Most studies comparing the use of IVF with expectant management for all stages of endometriosis demonstrate a significant benefit for the treatment group (47, 75).

ENDOMETRIOSIS-ASSOCIATED PELVIC PAIN

Treatment

Optimal treatment of pelvic pain due to endometriosis is challenging. Expectant management, medical treatment with nonsteroidal anti-inflammatory drugs (NSAIDs) and/or hormonal therapies, and conservative or definitive surgery have all been used for treatment of pelvic pain secondary to endometriosis.

Before initiating any therapy, it is essential to complete a comprehensive history and physical examination. Other, perhaps additional, causes of pelvic pain, such as adhesions, leiomyomata, hernias, and gastrointestinal disease, should be sought. Routine laboratory tests and physical examination to exclude pelvic inflammatory disease or a sexually transmitted disease are important. Ovarian cancer, which rarely presents as chronic pelvic pain, and abnormalities of the ovary are generally detected by physical examination and/or ultrasonography.

Expectant Management

In a prospective, randomized, double-blind, controlled trial of laser laparoscopy in the treatment of stage I, II, or III disease, Sutton et al. (76) evaluated pelvic pain relief after laparoscopy. This study randomized 63 patients with pelvic pain and endometriosis at the time of laparoscopy to laser ablation of endometriotic implants and laparoscopic uterine nerve ablation or expectant management. The patients were unaware of the treatment allocated as was the nurse evaluating them at 3 and 6 months after surgery. Patients with stage II or III disease treated surgically demonstrated significant improvement in pain (74% of laser group versus 20% of expectant management group). There did not appear to be a significant difference between treatment and expectant management in patients with stage I disease. Because of the lack of proof of efficacy for treatment and the known surgical risks of complications or possible adhesion formation, how to address minimal disease encountered in a laparoscopy is a dilemma. Although expectant management of minimal disease is as effective as any other therapy, treating it may also slow or stop progression to a more severe stage.

Medical Treatment

Medical management of pelvic pain secondary to endometriosis includes symptomatic and hormonal therapy. Chronic, cyclic, pelvic pain symptoms of dysmenorrhea, dyschezia, and dyspareunia are characteristic of, although not unique to, endometriosis. Each patient needs to be carefully evaluated to identify the etiology of pelvic pain. The cyclicity of symptoms is not enough to exclude other causes of pain. To help delineate the nature of the pain, a trial of ovarian suppression with a GnRH agonist or danazol may be used. If pain is related to the reproductive tract, patients usually report symptomatic improvement after the first month of amenorrhea. If the frequency and intensity are unchanged, further evaluation of other organ systems is warranted (19).

Symptomatic management of endometriosis requires close interaction between the patient and her physician. Patients who are well informed and who understand their condition and the goals of treatment have a better response to symptomatic management. Various types of prostaglandin synthetase inhibitors can effectively control dysmenorrhea and endometriosis-associated pelvic pain (77). The severity of dysmenorrhea that women with endometriosis suffer does correlate with the amount of prostaglandins produced by the implants (78). To achieve optimal response, the use of the fenamate class of NSAIDs (meclofenamate [Meclomen], mefenamic acid [Ponstel]) is recommended. In one study, up to 80% of dysmenorrheic women reported improvement in symptoms using either a fenamate NSAID or indomethacin (Indocin) (79). Symptomatic therapy should begin 1 to 2 days before the onset of menses and continue for the duration of the menstrual process.

Hormonal treatment of endometriosis includes the use of oral contraceptives, danazol, progestins, gestrinone, mifepristone (RU-486), and GnRH agonists. Despite the histologic differences between endometrial implants and the endometrium, estrogen does stimulate the implants to grow; hence, hormonal therapy is used to interrupt the cycle of stimulation and bleeding. Oral contraceptives have been prescribed in a continuous fashion to promote decidualization of endometriotic implants with resulting pain relief in 75% of patients (19). There have been no comparative studies of monophasic versus triphasic oral contraceptives in the treatment of endometriosis, although some recommend the use of a more progestogenic pill for its androgen effects. Danazol has been used successfully in the treatment of endometriosis-associated pelvic pain. Danazol eliminates the midcycle surge of luteinizing hormone (LH) and follicle-stimulating hormone (FSH), lowers basal levels of FSH and LH, and suppresses ovarian steroidogenesis. As a result, estrogen and progesterone concentrations are decreased, thereby removing hormonal stimulation of endometriotic implants. Unfortunately, it also displaces testosterone from sex hormone-binding globulin, resulting in increased free serum testosterone, and this causes androgenic side effects to occur. Ultimately, danazol creates a high-androgen low-estrogen environment that does not allow growth or cyclical changes in the endometrial implants. Up to 90% of patients with minimal to moderate disease experience improvement in pain symptoms (80). Initial studies recommended a dose of 400 mg twice a day, but 400 mg/day appears to be just as effective (81, 82).

The induction of amenorrhea appears to correlate with an improved outcome of treatment. The patient must be told that the chances of spontaneous ovulation increase in doses of less than 600 mg. Treatment is initiated after menses, and patients should be advised to use barrier contraception for the first few months of therapy. We recommend an initial dose of 800 mg/day, and if side effects are intolerable, the dose can be decreased to 600 mg. Therapy is generally continued for 6 months. Women with small endometriomas may require slightly longer courses of therapy. If large endometriomas are present, these usually shrink after 6 to 9 months of therapy but will not disappear completely. Up to 80% of women experience side effects, including weight gain, fluid retention, acne, decreased breast size, hot flushes, muscle cramps, and emotional lability. In addition, danazol is associated with decreased high-density-lipoprotein levels. A baseline lipid profile is warranted to ensure that the patient does not have hyperlipidemia. Although symptomatic improvement is common, recurrence rates of up to 30% are reported in the first year after discontinuation of treatment (83). As danazol is hepatically metabolized, its use is contraindicated in women with liver disease. There is no contraindication to repeated courses of danazol. If the side effects are intolerable or if optimal effectiveness was not achieved, another treatment modality should be considered.

Progestins are also used to suppress ovarian function and are similar to danazol in their effectiveness in treating endometriosis (84, 85). Like danazol, progestins induce decidualization and subsequent atrophy in the implants. The progestin most commonly used to treat endometriosis is medroxyprogesterone acetate (Provera). The usual dosage is 10 to 30 mg/day orally of Provera or 40 mg/day of Megace. Monthly Depo-Provera (150 mg intramuscularly) is also effective and provides reliable contraception to the patient not interested in pregnancy. With oral progestin therapy, ovarian suppression is inconsistent, resulting in variable estrogen levels. Breakthrough bleeding is common and may be treated with ethinyl estradiol (20 µg/day) or conjugated estrogens (1.25 mg/day) for 1 to 2 weeks. Adverse lipid effects may be seen during therapy. Other side effects include depression, nausea, fluid retention, and breast tenderness. In light of the decreased cost, comparable efficacy, and more tolerable side effects of progestins in comparison with danazol, many clinicians prescribe this as first-line therapy for endometriosis-associated pelvic pain. A summary of the literature regarding progestin therapy for symptomatic endometriosis suggests that the efficacy for temporary relief is good and is comparable with other treatments with more side effects (86).

Antiprogestational agents, gestrinone and mifepristone, have been recently proposed as alternative agents for treatment of endometriosis (87). Currently, gestrinone is not available in the United States and mifepristone is available in research settings only. Only gestrinone has been evaluated in a randomized, double-blind, clinical trial (88). Gestrinone was as effective as the GnRH agonist in reducing pelvic pain in patients with documented endometriosis. Its side effects are similar to those seen with danazol. Recurrence at the 6-month follow-up interval was less with the gestrinone group. In addition, the bone mineral content was decreased by 3% in the GnRH agonist group compared with a 2% *increase* in the gestrinone group. High-density-lipoprotein levels have been reported to decrease with gestrinone therapy. The recommended dosage is 2.5 mg twice a week beginning on the first day of menses.

GnRH agonists have been demonstrated to be effective in treating chronic pelvic pain due to endometriosis (89, 90). These agents are effective against endometriosis because of their profound suppression of ovarian function and induced hypoestrogenic state. GnRH agonists decrease the secretion of FSH and LH. This diminishes production of ovarian steroids to the postmenopausal range within 6 weeks. Trials comparing the efficacy of GnRH agonists with danazol demonstrate equal efficacy in successfully alleviating pelvic pain. Hypoestrogenic side effects occur more frequently with GnRH agonists and androgenic side effects are more common with danazol. GnRH agonists should not be used in women with osteoporosis or other medical conditions causing accelerated demineralization of the bone.

The long-term consequence of the hypoestrogenic state caused by a GnRH agonist is a reduction in trabecular bone density (91). Trabecular bone is found in the distal radius and spine. The addition of progestin alone or in combination with low-dose estrogen (0.625 mg conjugated estrogens) has been proposed as an effective means of preventing hypoestrogenic symptoms, including loss of bone mineral density. Studies evaluated the impact of this "add-back" therapy on the efficacy of pain treatment (92). Those patients with osteoporosis risk factors (strong family history, Caucasian or Oriental race, thin, high alcohol intake, or low calcium intake) that cannot be modified should perhaps consider an alternative medicine with a bone-sparing effect.

During the first 1 to 2 weeks after initial administration of the GnRH agonists, there is a release of gonadotropins that causes an ovarian "flare-up" and resultant increased estradiol production. This flare response, which may exacerbate pain symptoms, can be minimized by initiating therapy on cycle day 1 or just before day 1 of expected menses (93). A pregnancy test should be performed before initiating therapy in the luteal phase. There are no data indicating that extremely low estrogen concentrations have a more pronounced effect on endometriosis than moderately depressed ones. Barbieri (94) proposed a so-called "therapeutic window" for the end-organ response to estrogen concentration. He determined that an estradiol concentration of 30 to 50 pg/mL is sufficient for reduction in endometriosis without causing deleterious bone loss. This provides a basis for estrogen add-back therapy. If no improvement from GnRH agonist is obtained, two possibilities exists. Either severe disease is present or, if treatment was begun empirically, no disease is present.

Surgical Treatment

The most common form of treatment for endometriosis is surgery (95). The goals of conservative surgery are to remove and/or destroy the endometriosis, lyse (any) adhesions, and to restore, as much as possible, normal pelvic anatomy. Most forms of endometriosis can be eliminated with laparoscopic intervention (76). Treatment of minimal or mild disease usually involves laser vaporization or electrocauterization of peritoneal implants. Complete excision of the peritoneum has also been described. Moderate forms of the disease, which include unilateral endometriomas and bilateral small ovarian cysts with limited adhesions, can also be treated successfully at endoscopy. Standard treatment for severe endometriosis, that is, bilateral large ovarian endometriomas attached by extensive dense adhesions, an obliterated cul-de-sac, and parametrial infiltration, depends on the laparoscopic expertise of the surgeon (96).

Success of laparoscopy is not necessarily related to stage of disease. In fact, one trial comparing expectant management versus laparoscopy demonstrated increased pain relief only in patients receiving laparoscopic treatment of stages II and III (76). This reiterates the need for a full diagnostic evaluation of patents suffering from

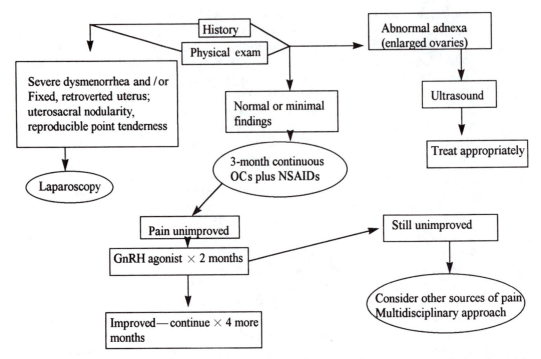

FIGURE 14.2. Clinical algorithm for the evaluation and management of chronic pelvic pain. *OC,* oral contraceptives.

chronic pelvic pain before surgery. Once laparoscopy is chosen as the treatment modality, the patient and surgeon must be prepared for all possible outcomes. Because of the expense and the imperfections in visualizing all endometriotic lesions, an initial empirical trial of GnRH agonist is frequently recommended (Fig. 14.2). If laparoscopy is chosen, it is important to inquire about the patient's expectations from surgery and her desire for future fertility and to establish a preoperative plan of treatment if severe disease is encountered (i.e., if conservative therapy versus hysterectomy and/or oophorectomy is to be done).

RECURRENCE OF ENDOMETRIOSIS

Endometriosis may recur after medical therapy, conservative surgical therapy, and even after castration (97). Recurrence rates in women treated with GnRH agonists were 37% for minimal disease and 74% for severe disease (98). These rates are similar for patients treated with danazol as well (99). The recurrence rate 5 years after conservative surgery is close to 40%. Compared with women treated with oophorectomy for endometriosis, patients undergoing hysterectomy with ovarian conservation have a 6.1 times greater risk of developing recurrent pain and an 8.1 times greater risk of reoperation (100, 101).

Hormone Replacement Therapy After "Definitive" Surgery

The potential for estrogen replacement therapy to reactivate residual endometriotic implants remains unclear. Some studies indicate that hormone replacement therapy does not stimulate recurrence of symptoms related to endometriosis, but others advocate delaying the initiation of hormone replacement therapy for up to 1 year (102, 103). In patients with moderate or severe disease immediately after hysterectomy and bilateral salpingo-oophorectomy, we prescribe combined estrogen/progestin therapy during the first 3 to 6 months postoperatively, and if no symptoms have occurred, we prescribe the initiation of estrogen alone. In rare cases of recurrent pain, progestins can be added to help diminish the pain. The addition of a progestational agent is sometimes recommended even after a hysterectomy because of reported cases of adenocarcinoma arising from endometriotic implants in women treated with unopposed estrogen (104, 105).

CLINICAL NOTES

Endometriosis in General

- Based on estimates, endometriosis affects 5 to 10% of reproductive-age women and 25 to 35% of women with infertility.
- Endometriosis does *not* primarily afflict women over 30 who are career driven and it *does* occur in women of African-American descent.
- Two thirds of women with endometriosis have ovarian involvement.
- Classic symptoms of endometriosis include dysmenorrhea, dyspareunia, dyschezia, and/or a history of infertility, but few women present with all symptoms.
- The degree of pelvic pain is not related to the severity or distribution of endometriosis, although there may be a correlation in the number of endometrial implants and the intensity of dysmenorrhea.
- Although uterosacral ligament tenderness and nodularity is specific to endometriosis, this finding is present in only about one third of patients and is usually present late in the course of the disease.
- The diagnosis of endometriosis requires direct visualization of lesions by laparoscopy or laparotomy.
- CA-125 is not a marker that can be reliably used for screening for endometriosis or for following response to therapy.
- The classification system most commonly used is that developed by the ASRM; neither it nor any other method of classification/staging has been proven to accurately correlate pain with location and severity of endometriosis.

Endometriosis-Associated Infertility

- Ten to 15% of infertile couples have endometriosis as the only identifiable cause and 30 to 40% of women with the disease are infertile.
- The cumulative pregnancy rate after 5 years of expectant management in women with minimal disease is 90%.
- Limited data show an increase in fecundity of women with minimal or mild endometriosis after laparoscopic surgical therapy compared with women undergoing expectant management, but this difference is not seen after 2 years of follow-up.
- To date, no studies have shown any difference in improved pregnancy rates in the medical therapy of endometriosis with danazol or GnRH agonists.
- Surgical treatment of moderate or severe disease has been shown to improve pregnancy rates by 60% and 35%, respectively.
- For women receiving superovulation and IUI, per cycle fecundity is increased over expectant management; IVF should be reserved for patients failing to achieve pregnancy after attempt(s) at superovulation and IUI.
- There are data to support the use of surgical therapy in patients with pelvic pain and moderate or severe endometriosis; the efficacy of surgical treatment of minimal endometriosis for pelvic pain is more controversial.

Endometriosis-Associated Pelvic Pain

- Of the NSAIDs used to treat endometriosis-related pelvic pain, the fenamate class (meclofenamate [Meclomen] or mefenamic acid [Ponstel]) or indomethacin (Indocin) is recommended.
- Oral contraceptives, prescribed in a continuous fashion, have resulted in pain relief in 75% of patients with endometriosis-related pain.
- If danazol (Danocrine) is used to treat endometriosis, an initial dose of 800 mg/day with a decrease to 600 mg/day is one recommended regimen. With doses of less than 600 mg/day, the chance of spontaneous ovulation is increased.
- Progestins such as medroxyprogesterone acetate (Provera), 10 to 30 mg/day; megestrol (Megace), 40 mg/day; or monthly Depo-Provera, 150 mg intramuscularly, may be used to treat endometriosis-related pain.
- Use of GnRH therapy with "add-back" estrogen and progesterone sufficient to maintain an estradiol concentration of 30 to 50 pg/mL may provide pain relief from endometriosis without incurring deleterious bone loss.

Recurrence of Endometriosis

- Rates of recurrence for women treated with GnRH agonists or danazol are approximately 35% for minimal disease and 75% for severe disease.
- The recurrence rate 5 years after treatment with conservative surgery is close to 40%.
- For patients with moderate or severe disease immediately after hysterectomy and bilateral oophorectomy, one regimen recommends combined estrogen/progestin therapy for 3 to 6 months. If no symptoms develop, estrogen alone is initiated thereafter.

References

1. Cramer DW. Epidemiology of endometriosis. In: Wilson EA, ed. Endometriosis. New York: Alan R Liss, 1987:5.
2. Melis GB, Ajossa S, Guerriero S, et al. Epidemiology and diagnosis of endometriosis. Ann N Y Acad Sci 1994;74:352–357.
3. Matorras R, Rodriguez F, Pijoan JI, et al. Epidemiology of endometriosis in infertile women. Fertil Steril 1995;63:34–38.
4. Simpson JL, Elias S, Malinack LR, et al. Heritable aspects of endometriosis I. Genetic studies. Am J Obstet Gynecol 1980;137:327.
5. Haney AF. Endometriosis: pathogenesis and pathophysiology. In: Wilson EA, ed. Endometriosis. New York: Alan R Liss, 1987:23–51.
6. Haney, AF. Etiology and histogenesis of endometriosis. In: Schenken RS, ed. Endometriosis: Contemporary Concepts in Clinical Management. Philadelphia: JB Lippincott, 1989:1–49.
7. Brosens I, Vasquez G, Deprest J, et al. Pathogenesis of endometriosis. In: Endometriosis. New York: Springer-Verlag, 1995:9–19.
8. Liu DT, Hitchcock A. Endometriosis: its association with retrograde menstruation, dysmenorrhea, and tubal pathology. Br J Obstet Gynaecol 1986;93:859–862.
9. Steele RW, Dmowski WP, Marmer DJ. Immunologic aspects of human endometriosis. Am J Reprod Immunol 1984;6:33.
10. Dmowski WP. Immunological aspects of endometriosis. Int J Gynaecol Obstet 1995;50(suppl 1):S3–S10.
11. Kennedy S, Mardon H, Barlow D. Familial endometriosis. J Assist Reprod Genet 1995;12:32–34.
12. Damewood MD. Pathophysiology and management of endometriosis. J Fam Pract 1993;37:68–75.
13. Franklin RR, Grunert GM. Extragenital endometriosis. In: Endometriosis. New York: Springer-Verlag, 1995:127–136.

14. Vercellini P, Trespidi L, Giorgi OD, et al. Endometriosis and pelvic pain: relation to disease stage and localization. Fertil Steril 1996;65:299–304.

15. Foster DC, Stern JL, Buscema J, et al. Pleural and parenchymal pulmonary endometriosis. Obstet Gynecol 1991;78:946.

16. Schorlemer GR, Battaglini JW. Pneumothorax in menstruating females. Contemp Surg 1982;20:53.

17. Fedele L, Parazzini F, Bianchi S, et al. Stage and localization of pelvic endometriosis and pain. Fertil Steril 1990;53:155.

18. Perper MM, Nezhat F, Goldstein H, et al. Dysmenorrhea is related to the number of implants in endometriosis patients. Fertil Steril 1995;63:500–503.

19. Dmowski WP. The role of medical management in the treatment of endometriosis. In: Endometriosis: Advanced Management and Surgical Techniques. New York: Springer-Verlag, 1995:229–240.

20. Matorras R, Rodriguez F, Pijoan JI, et al. Are there any clinical signs and symptoms that are related to endometriosis in infertile women? Am J Obstet Gynecol 1996;174:620–623.

21. Ripps B, Martin DC. Focal pelvic tenderness, pelvic pain and dysmenorrhea in endometriosis. J Reprod Med 1991;7:36.

22. Mais V, Guerriero S, Ajossa S, et al. The efficiency of transvaginal ultrasonography in the diagnosis of endometrioma. Fertil Steril 1993;60:776–780.

23. Ozaksit G, Caglar, T, Cicek N, et al. Serum CA125 levels before, during and after treatment for endometriosis. Int J Gynaecol Obstet 1995;50:269–273.

24. Barbieri RL, Niloff JM, Bast RC Jr, et al. Elevated serum concentrations of CA-125 in patients with advanced endometriosis. Fertil Steril 1986;45:630.

25. Schenken RS, Guzick DS. Revised endometriosis classification: 1996. Fertil Steril 1997;67:815–816.

26. Franssen AM, van der Heijden PF, Thomas CM, et al. On the origin and significance of serum CA-125 concentrations in 97 patients with endometriosis before, during, and after buserelin acetate, naferelin, or danazol. Fertil Steril 1992;57:974–979.

27. Guzick DS, Silliman NP, Adamson GD, et al. Prediction of pregnancy in infertile women based on the American Society of Reproductive Medicine's revised classification of endometriosis. Fertil Steril 1997;67:822–829.

28. Fedele L, Branchi S, Bocciolone L, et al. Pain symptoms associated with endometriosis. Obstet Gynecol 1992;79:767–769.

29. Burns WN, Schenken RS. Pathophysiology of endometriosis. In: Schenken RS, ed. Endometriosis: Contemporary Concepts in Clinical Management. Philadelphia: JB Lippincott, 1989:83–126.

30. Verkauf BS. The incidence, symptoms and signs of endometriosis in fertile and infertile women. J Fla Med Assoc 1987;74:671.

31. Toma SK, Stovall DW, Hammond MG. The effect of laparoscopic ablation on Danocrine on pregnancy rates in patients with stage I or II endometriosis undergoing donor insemination. Obstet Gynecol 1992;80:253.

32. Jansen RP. Minimal endometriosis and reduced fecundability: prospective evidence from an artificial insemination by donor program. Fertil Steril 1986;46:141–143.

33. Wheeler JM, Johnston BM, Malinak LR. The relationship of endometriosis to spontaneous abortion. Fertil Steril 1983;39:656–660.

34. Metzger DA, Olive DL, Stohs GF, et al. Association of endometriosis and spontaneous abortion: effect of control group selection. Fertil Steril 1986;45:18–22.

35. Moon YS, Leung PC, Yuen BH, et al. Prostaglandin F in human endometriotic tissue. Am J Obstet Gynecol 1981;141:344–345.

36. Badawy SZ, Cuenca V, Marshall L, et al. Cellular components in peritoneal fluid in infertile patients with and without endometriosis. Fertil Steril 1984;42:704–707.

37. Haney AF, Muscato JJ, Weiberg JB. Peritoneal fluid cell populations in infertility patients. Fertil Steril 1981;35:696.

38. Graf MJ, Dunaif A. Association of reproductive endocrine dysfunction with pelvic endometriosis. Semin Reprod Endocrinol 1985;3:319.

39. Muscato JJ, Hancy AF, Weinberg JB. Sperm phagocytosis by human peritoneal macrophages: a possible cause of infertility and endometriosis. Am J Obstet Gynecol 1982;144:503.

40. Stone SAC, Himsl K. Peritoneal recovery of motile and nonmotile sperm in the presence of endometriosis. Fertil Steril 1986;46:338.

41. Doody MC, Gibbons WE, Buttram VC Jr. Linear regression analysis of ultrasound follicular growth series: evidence for an abnormality of follicular growth in endometriosis patients. Fertil Steril 1988;49:47.

42. Brosens IA, Koninckx PR, Corvelyn PA. A study of plasma progesterone, estradiol, prolactin, and LH levels and the luteal phase appearance of the ovaries in patients with endometriosis and infertility. Br J Obstet Gynaecol 1978;85:246.

43. Portuondo JA, Pena L, Otaola C. Absence of ovulation stigma in the conception cycle. Int J Fertil 1983;28:52–54.

44. McBean JH, Blackman J, Brumsted JR. Abnormal ovulation in women with endometriosis (abstract P-168). Presented at the American Society of Reproductive Medicine, October 1997.

45. Mills MS, Eddowes HA, Cahill DJ, et al. A prospective controlled study on in-vitro fertilization, gamete intra-fallopian transfer and intrauterine insemination combined with superovulation. Hum Reprod 1992;7:490–494.

46. Jones HW Jr, Acosta AA, Andrews MC, et al. Three years of in vitro fertilization at Norfolk. Fertil Steril 1984;42:826–834.

47. Arici A, Oral E, Bukulmez O, et al. The effect of endometriosis on implantation: results from the Yale University in vitro fertilization and embryo transfer program. Fertil Steril 1996;65:603–607.

48. Lessey BA, Castelbaum AJ, Sawin SW, et al. Aberrant integrin expression in the endometrium of patients with endometriosis. J. Clin Endocrinol Metab 1994;79:643–649.

49. Badawy SZ, ElBakry MM, Samuel F, et al. Cumulative pregnancy rates in infertile women with endometriosis. J Reprod Med 1988;33:757–760.

50. Rodriguez-Escudero FJ, Neyro JL, Corcostegui B, et al. Does minimal endometriosis reduce fecundity? Fertil Steril 1988;50:3.

51. Thomas IJ, Cooke ID. Successful treatment of asymptomatic endometriosis: does it benefit infertile women? Br Med J 1987;294:1117–1119.

52. Marcoux S, Maheux R, Berube S. Canadian Collaborative Group on Endometriosis. Laparoscopic surgery in infertile women with minimal or mild endometriosis. N Engl J Med 1997;337:217–222.

53. Schenken RS, Malinak LR. Conservative surgery versus expectant management for the infertile patient with mild endometriosis. Fertil Steril 1982;37:183–186.

54. Dmowski WP, Cohen MR. Antigonadotropin (Danazol) in the treatment of endometriosis: evaluation of post-treatment fertility and three year follow–up data. Am J Obstet Gynecol 1978;130:41.

55. Hull ME, Moghissi KS, Magyar DF, et al. Comparison of different treatment modalities of endometriosis in infertile women. Fertil Steril 1987;47:40.

56. Seibel MM, Berger MJ, Weinstein FG, et al. The effectiveness of Danazol on subsequent fertility in minimal endometriosis. Fertil Steril 1982;38:534.

57. Tellima S. Danazol and medroxyprogesterone acetate inefficacious in the treatment of infertility in endometriosis. Fertil Steril 1988;50:872.

58. Moghissi KS, Boyce CR. Management of endometriosis with oral medroxyprogesterone acetate. Obstet Gynecol 1976;47:265–267.

59. Overton CE, Lindsay PC, Johal B, et al. A randomized, double-blind, placebo-controlled study of luteal phase dydrogesterone (Duphaston) in women with minimal to mild endometriosis. Fertil Steril 1994;62:701–707.

60. Henzl M. Gonadotropin-releasing hormone agonists in the management of endometriosis: a review. Clin Obstet Gynecol 1988;31:4.

61. Fedele L, Bianchi S, Arcaini L, et al. Buserelin versus danazol in the treatment of endometriosis associated infertility. Am J Obstet Gynecol 1989;161:871–876.

62. Marana R, Pailli FV, Muzii L, et al. GnRH analogs versus expectant management in minimal and mild endometriosis-associated infertility. Acta Eur Fertil 1994;25:37–41.

63. Olive DL, Lee KL. Analysis of sequential treatment protocols for endometriosis-associated infertility. Am J Obstet Gynecol 1986;154:613–619.

64. Olive DL, Martin DC. Treatment of endometriosis-associated infertility with CO_2 laser laparoscopy: the use of one- and two-parameter exponential models. Fertil Steril 1987; 48:18.

65. Guzick DS, Rock JA. A comparison of danazol and conservative surgery for the treatment of infertility due to mild or moderate endometriosis. Fertil Steril 1983;40:580.

66. Kodama H, Fukuda J, Karube H, et al. Benefit of in vitro fertilization for endometriosis associated infertility. Fertil Steril 1996;66:974–979.

67. Adamson GD, Pasta DJ. Surgical treatment of endometriosis-associated infertility: meta-analysis compared with survival analysis. Am J Obstet Gynecol 1994;171:1488–1505.

68. Donnez J, Nisolle M, Clerckx F, et al. Evaluation of preoperative use of danazol, gestrinone, lynestrenol, buserelin spray and buserelin implant, in the treatment of endometriosis associated infertility. Prog Clin Biol Res 1990;323:427–442.

69. Wheeler JM, Malinak LR. Postoperative danazol therapy in infertility patients with severe endometriosis. Fertil Steril 1990;53:407–410.

70. Telimaa S, Puolakka J, Ronnberg L, et al. Placebo-controlled comparison of danazol and high-dose medroxyprogesterone acetate in the treatment of endometriosis. Gynecol Endocrinol 1987;1:13–23.

71. Chong AP, Keene ME, Thornton NL. Comparison of three modes of treatment for infertility patients with minimal pelvic endometriosis. Fertil Steril 1990;53:407–410.

72. Fedele L, Bianchi S, Marchini M, et al. Superovulation with human menopausal gonadotropins in the treatment of infertility associated with minimal or mild endometriosis: a controlled randomized study. Fertil Steril 1992;58:28–31.

73. Simpson CW, Taylor PJ, Collins JA. A comparison of ovulation suppression and ovulation stimulation in the treatment of endometriosis-associated infertility. Int J Gynaecol Obstet 1992;57:597–600.

74. Kemmann E, Ghazi D, Corsan G, et al. Does ovulation stimulation improve fertility in women with minimal/mild endometriosis after laser laparoscopy? Int J Fertil Menopausal Stud 1993;38:16–21.

75. Soliman S, Davis S, Collins J, et al. A randomized trial of in vitro fertilization versus conventional treatment for infertility. Fertil Steril 1993;59:1239–1244.

76. Sutton CJ, Ewen SP, Whitelaw N, et al. Prospective, randomized, double-blind, controlled trial of laser laparoscopy in the treatment of pelvic pain associated with minimal, mild, and moderate endometriosis. Fertil Steril 1994;62:696–700.

77. Kauppila A, Ronnberg L. Naproxen sodium in dysmenorrhea secondary to endometriosis. Obstet Gynecol 1985;65:379–383.

78. Owens PR. Prostaglandin synthetase inhibitors in the treatment of primary dysmenorrhea: outcome trials reviewed. Am J Obstet Gynecol 1984;148:96.

79. Olive DL. Medical treatment: alternatives to danazol. In: Schenken RS, ed. Endometriosis: Contemporary Concepts in Clinical Management. Philadelphia: JB Lippincott, 1989: 189–211.

80. Koike H, Egawa H, Ohtsuka T, et al. Correlation between dysmenorrheic severity and prostaglandin production in women with endometriosis. Prostaglandins Leukot Essent Fatty Acids 1992;46:133.

81. Bayer SR, Siebel MM, Saffan DS, et al. Efficacy of danazol treatment for minimal endometriosis in infertile women: a prospective, randomized study. J Reprod Med 1988;33:179–183.

82. Dmowski WP, Kapetanakis E, Scommegna A. Variable effects of danazol on endometriosis at four low-dose levels. Obstet Gynecol 1982;59:408.

83. Bayer SR, Seibel MM. Medical treatment: danazol. In: Schenken RS, ed. Endometriosis: Contemporary Concepts in Clinical Management. Philadelphia: JB Lippincott, 1989:169–187.

84. Dmowski WP, Cohen MR. Antigonadotropin (danazol) in the treatment of endometriosis: evaluation of the post-treatment fertility and three year follow-up data. Am J Obstet Gynecol 1978;130:41.

85. Gunning JE, Moyer D. The effect of medroxyprogesterone acetate on endometriosis in the human female. Fertil Steril 1967;18:759–774.

86. Vercellini P, Cortesi I, Crosignani PG. Progestins for symptomatic endometriosis: a critical analysis of the evidence. Fertil Steril 1997;68:393–401.

87. Kettel LM, Murphy AA, Morales AJ, et al. Treatment of endometriosis with the antiprogesterone mifepristone. Fertil Steril 1996;65:23–28.

88. Gestrinone Italian Study Group. Gestrinone versus a gonadotropin-releasing hormone agonist for the treatment of pelvic pain associated with endometriosis: a multi-center, randomized, double-blind study. Fertil Steril 1996;66:911–919.

89. Adamson GD, Kwei L, Edgren RA. Pain of endometriosis: effects of nafarelin and danazol therapy. Int J Fertil Menopausal Stud 1994;39:215–217.

90. Rock JA, Truglia JA, Caplan RJ, et al. Zoladex (goserelin acetate implant) in the treatment of endometriosis: a randomized comparison with danazol. Obstet Gynecol 1993;82:198–205.

91. Dawood MY. Considerations in selecting appropriate medial therapy for endometriosis. Int J Gynaecol Obstet 1993;40(suppl):S29–S42.

92. Hurst BS, Schlaff WD. Treatment options for endometriosis: medical therapies. Infertil Reprod Clin North Am 1992;3:645–655.

93. Bergqvist IA. Hormonal regulation of endometriosis and the rationales and effects of gonadotrophin-releasing hormone agonist treatment: a review. Hum Reprod 1995;10:446–452.

94. Barbieri RL. Hormone treatment of endometriosis: the estrogen threshold hypothesis. Am J Obstet Gynecol 1992;166:740–745.

95. Olive DL, Schwartz LB. Endometriosis. N Engl J Med 1993;328:1759–1769.

96. Crosignani PG, Vercellini P, Biffignandi F, et al. Laparoscopy versus laparotomy in conservative surgical treatment for severe endometriosis. Fertil Steril 1996;66:706–711.

97. Koninckx PR, Lesaffre E, Meulaman C, et al. Suggestive evidence that endometriosis is a progressive disease, whereas deeply infiltrating endometriosis is associated with pelvic pain. Fertil Steril 1991;55:759–765.

98. Waller KG, Shaw RW. Gonadotropin-releasing hormone analogues for the treatment of endometriosis: long-term follow-up. Fertil Steril 1993;59:511.

99. The Nafarelin European Endometriosis Trial Group. Nafarelin for endometriosis: a large-scale danazol-controlled trial of efficacy and safety, with 1-year follow-up. Fertil Steril 1992;57:514.

100. Schmidt CL. Endometriosis: a reappraisal of pathogenesis and treatment. Fertil Steril 1985;44:157–173.

101. Wheeler JM, Malinak LR. Recurrent endometriosis: incidence, management, and prognosis. Am J Obstet Gynecol 1983;146:247–253.

102. Thom MH, Studd JW. Procedures in practice. Hormonal implantation. Br Med J 1980;280:848–850.

103. Malinak LR. Proceedings of the ICI Conference on Endometriosis, Cambridge, 1989. Carnforth, UK: Parthenon Press, 1990.

104. Reimnitz C, Brand E, Nieberg RK, et al. Malignancy arising in endometriosis associated with unopposed estrogen replacement. Obstet Gynecol 1988;71:444.

105. Heaps JM, Nieberg RK, Berek JS. Malignant neoplasms arising in endometriosis. Obstet Gynecol 1990;75:1023.

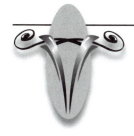

C H A P T E R   1 5

Infertility and Recurrent Pregnancy Loss

JOHN M. STORMENT
JOHN R. BRUMSTED

Infertility

Infertility is a condition affecting over five million couples annually with important medical, economic, and psychological implications (1). The care of the infertile couple must be based on an accurate assessment of factors affecting the fertility of both partners. The postponement of marriage and delay of pregnancy in marriage in the post-World War II generation are largely responsible for the increase in consultations for the evaluation of infertility (1). With the increased availability of services and improved diagnostic and therapeutic managements, more couples are now able to access infertility services.

EPIDEMIOLOGY

A couple is said to be infertile if they have been trying to achieve a pregnancy for more than 1 year without success. This definition is arbitrary, and many couples achieve pregnancy in over 12 months with no abnormalities and no outside intervention. Infertility is classified by the woman's history. Primary infertility implies no antecedent pregnancy, and secondary infertility is defined by a history of any pregnancy, including abortions and ectopic pregnancies.

Fecundity (f) is the most useful statistic pertaining to reproduction. It represents the probability of conception per month of effort and is calculated by dividing the number of conceptions (C) by the person-months of exposure (T):

$$f = C/T \qquad \text{(Eq. 15.1)}$$

It must be remembered that even in infertile populations, fecundity is almost never zero and for fertile couples is only approximately 0.20. Thus, it is useful to consider infertility as simply a reduction in fecundity to less than the general population. The evaluation of infertile couples should be designed to identify factors responsible for diminished fecundity, and treatment should be limited to therapy proven to restore fecundity toward normal. Counseling patients is made easier when tests and treatments are discussed using these terms.

Estimating the prevalence of infertility is not straightforward, in that inconsistencies in epidemiologic reports make it difficult to assess any trends in fecundity. Between 1965 and 1988, the prevalence appeared to remain stable at approximately 13% of U.S. women 15 to 44 years old (excluding surgically sterilized individuals). Approximately half of these couples will never succeed in having as many children as they wish (2). Although the prevalence of infertility has remained at approxi-

355

mately 13 to 15% of the U.S. population over the past 20 years, more couples are seeking medical and surgical services for impaired fecundity. The number of childless women 35 to 44 years old increased by over one million from 1982 to 1988 (3). Women were 2 to 3 years older in 1990 than in 1979 when they delivered their first child, and significantly more women never had a child (3).

The change in the distribution of primary and secondary infertility has had a direct impact on the use of fertility services because women with primary infertility are more likely to use medical services than are women with secondary infertility. Overall, about half of all infertile couples seek treatment, although only 25% obtain assistance from an infertility specialist (4). Approximately half of couples with infertility eventually conceive. Likelihood of conception is influenced by several factors, including the duration of fertility, the cause of infertility, and the age of the woman at the time of treatment.

Age and Infertility

A woman's fertility is known to decline after the age of 35. It is estimated that between 1980 and 2010, the number of U.S. women 35 to 45 years old will increase from 13 to 19 million. This alone will contribute to the increase in the number of women over age 35 seeking treatment for infertility. The gynecologist must be aware of age-related fecundity to properly counsel patients and must know when referral to a specialist should not be delayed.

The classic study of the Hutterites who live in Montana, the North and South Dakotas, and parts of Canada provides demographic information regarding natural fertility rates and aging (5). This sect is unique because contraception is denounced and, because of the arrangement of their community, there is no incentive to limit the size of families. Tietze (5) examined the demographics of this population to derive conclusions about natural fertility rates. The infertility rate was only 2.4%. A decline in fertility with age was demonstrated, with 11% of the women infertile by age 34, 33% infertile by age 40, and 87% infertile by age 45. The mean age at the last pregnancy was 41 years.

The decline in fertility as women age can be attributed to several factors (Fig.15.1). With aging there is an increase in the frequency of gynecologic and systemic disease, such as endometriosis, pelvic infection, leiomyomata, smoking, diabetes, and obesity. The potential for oocytes to be fertilized and develop normally is compromised with increasing age. Schwartz and Mayaux (6) reported on 2193 women with azoospermic husbands treated by donor insemination. The cumulative pregnancy rates were 73%, 74%, 62%, and 54% for age groups younger than 25 years ($n = 371$), 26 to 30 years ($n = 1079$), 31 to 35 years ($n = 599$), and older than 35 years ($n = 144$), respectively. The decline between age groups becomes significant at about age 35, and pregnancies are rarely reported after age 45.

Significant changes in ovarian and uterine physiology begin to occur at age 35. Before embarking on any infertility workup of women 35 years and older, proper counseling involving the risks of pregnancy loss with advancing maternal age is essential. The spontaneous abortion rate increases to approximately 30% at age 35. Among successful pregnancies, trisomies and other chromosomal disorders are significantly increased. The reasons include loss of oocyte integrity and decreased uterine receptivity after age 30 (7).

A prompt and full investigation of fertility status should be offered immediately to women in their late 30s complaining of difficulty conceiving so that any correctable conditions can be treated as soon as possible. Although it is difficult to se-

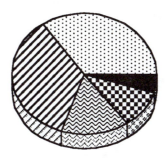

Tuboperitoneal 35%
Male 35%
Ovulatory 15%
Unexplained 10%
Other 5%

FIGURE 15.1. Causes of infertility among U.S. couples.

lect an arbitrary time at which no treatment should be offered, appropriate counseling should involve realistic expectations of conception based on the patient's age.

INVESTIGATION OF THE INFERTILE COUPLE

A standardized approach to the investigation of the infertile couple allows a complete evaluation of each potential cause of infertility. Consistent application of a standard algorithm (Fig. 15.2) provides useful information that can help eliminate unnecessary and costly diagnostic tests. Initially, obtaining a thorough history is essential to guide the remainder of the workup. There are many specific examples of when historical information is useful. Identification of an ovulatory patient can be made by eliciting a history of regular menstrual cycles and premenstrual molimina (8). Diethylstilbestrol (DES)-exposed women have a significantly higher incidence of primary infertility, even with a structurally normal reproductive tract. Smoking, marijuana, and cocaine can reduce fecundity in men and women (9). Some centers find it helpful to distribute a detailed questionnaire to patients before their first visit to obtain information that is sometimes difficult to express in an office interview.

The first office visit should include counseling regarding the couple's identifiable problems and provide a realistic estimate of likelihood for conception (Table 15.1). A discussion of the statistics associated with human reproduction is useful, pointing out that the probability of conception in an ovulatory cycle is only 25% under ideal circumstances (10). The time required for conception to occur in couples who attain pregnancy without medical intervention is shown in Figure 15.3.

After the initial discussion, a plan outlining appropriate laboratory testing should be reviewed. In addition, women with a negative rubella titer should be immunized, and human immunodeficiency virus testing should be offered to all couples. Folic acid can also be prescribed at this time to decrease the risk of fetal neural tube defects (11).

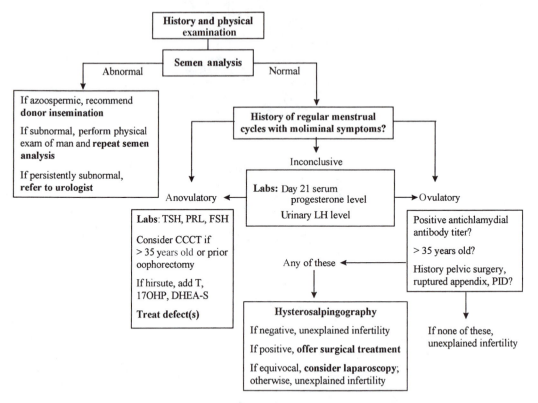

FIGURE 15.2. Infertility workup. *CCCT,* clomiphene citrate challenge test; *DHEA-S,* dehydroepiandrosterone sulfate; *FSH,* follicle-stimulating hormone; *17OHP,* 17-hydroxyprogesterone; *PID,* pelvic inflammatory disease; *PRL,* prolactin; *T,* testosterone; *TSH,* thyroid-stimulating hormone.

TABLE 15.1. Major Causes of Infertility and Treatment Outcomes

Cause of Infertility	Frequency (%)	Posttreatment Conception at 2 Years (%)
ANOVULATION	21	
Amenorrhea	7	96
Oligomenorrhea	14	78
ANATOMIC CAUSE		19
MALE FACTOR		
Oligospermia	15	11
Azoospermia	6	0
UNEXPLAINED CAUSES	28	72

Adapted from Hull MG, Glazener CM, Kelly NJ, et al. Population study of causes, treatment, and outcome of infertility. BMJ (Clin Res Ed) 1985;291:1693–1697.

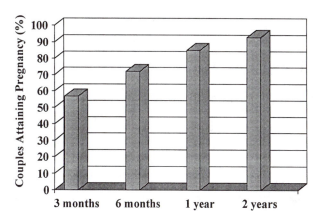

FIGURE 15.3. Natural history of conception. Within 2 years of unprotected intercourse, approximately 90% of average couples attain pregnancy. The remaining 10% are clinically defined as infertile. (Reprinted with permission from: Prevention of neural tube defects: results of the Medical Research Council Vitamin Study. MRC Vitamin Study Research Group. Lancet 1991;338:131–137.)

TABLE 15.2. Diagnostic Tests Commonly Used to Assess Impairment of Fecundability

ABNORMAL TEST RESULTS THAT HAVE A VALIDATED CORRELATION WITH IMPAIRED FECUNDABILITY[a]
Semen analysis
Assessment of tubal patency by hysterosalpingogram or laparoscopy
Laboratory assessment of ovulation

ABNORMAL TEST RESULTS THAT ARE NOT CONSISTENTLY CORRELATED WITH IMPAIRED FECUNDABILITY[b]
Postcoital test
Laparoscopic finding of minimal or mild endometriosis
Cervical mucus penetration test
Antisperm antibody assays
Zona-free hamster egg penetration test

ABNORMAL TEST RESULTS THAT DO NOT APPEAR TO BE CORRELATED WITH IMPAIRED FECUNDABILITY[c]
Endometrial biopsy for dating
Asymptomatic varicocele repair (infertility alone is not considered a symptom)
Falloposcopy

[a]In these diagnostic tests, when the test is unequivocally abnormal (azoospermia, bilateral tubal occlusion, or anovulation), fertility is definitely impaired without therapy.
[b]For these diagnostic tests, abnormal results are frequently associated with subsequent fertility without therapy.
[c]For these diagnostic tests, either there are data that confirm the lack of a correlation with pregnancy or such follow-up studies do not exist.

The evaluation should be individualized for each couple based on the initial history; a common approach may include laboratory assessment of ovulation, evaluation of reproductive tract anatomy, and semen analysis. Diagnosis of sterility is simple, but diagnosis of subfertility can be quite arduous. The difficulty is compounded by a lack of consensus regarding which diagnostic tests should be performed. The outcome of primary interest to the infertile couple is pregnancy, and the merit of diagnostic tests lies in their ability to predict this outcome (8). The European Society for Human Reproduction and Embryology provides recommendations for establishing a manner with which to evaluate infertility (12). In this practical way, we can divide the most commonly used diagnostic tests into three categories based on the correlation of an abnormal test result with impaired fecundability: valid correlation, inconsistent correlation, and not apparently correlated (Table 15.2). Treatment effectiveness can be assessed accurately only in randomized clinical trials because conception without therapy can occur in most subfertile couples over time.

FEMALE FACTOR INFERTILITY

Anovulatory Infertility

Ovulatory dysfunction and anovulation affect 15 to 25% of all infertile couples seeking therapy. Unfortunately, the only absolute proof of normal ovulation is a subsequent pregnancy. The process leading to ovulation is made up of several components, disruption of any of which can impede ovulation or the capacity of a mature oocyte to fertilize. Treatment of ovulation disorders remains one of the most successful of all infertility treatments (Table 15.1).

Evaluation

The woman who reports infrequent irregular menses and no moliminal symptoms (or who gives an unclear history of her menstrual cycles) should be evaluated for anovulation (Fig. 15.4). An understanding of normal hormonal events that regulate the ovulatory process is essential to determine which of the many tests devised for ovulation detection should be used. The trophic effects of both follicle-stimulating hormone (FSH) and luteinizing hormone (LH) result in maturation of ovarian follicles. Release of both FSH and LH from the anterior pituitary is controlled by gonadotropin-releasing hormone (GnRH), which is produced in the hypothalamus in a pulsatile fashion. The ovulatory process is characterized by a rapid midcycle rise in LH that culminates in the LH peak. A consensus from previous reports places the onset of the serum LH surge approximately 36 to 38 hours before ovulation (13). FSH also increases midcycle but to a lesser degree than does LH. The luteal phase is characterized by a rise in the concentration of progesterone with maximal concentration reached about 8 days after the LH peak. The menstrual cycle length is variable, with the variation residing in the follicular phase. The luteal phase is consistently 12 to 14 days.

When ovulation is uncertain from the history, tests should be done to determine if ovulation occurs. The amenorrheic or oligomenorrheic woman should have a workup and should be treated for the cause of her anovulation or infrequent ovulation, as discussed below. These same tests may be used to predict ovulation when necessary as part of assisted reproductive therapies.

Detection of greater than 2 ng/mL of plasma progesterone is documentation that ovulation has occurred. One report indicated that midluteal progesterone levels greater than 8.8 ng/mL were present in more than 95% of spontaneous conception cycles (14). The reliability of monoclonal antibody rapid assay tests for LH

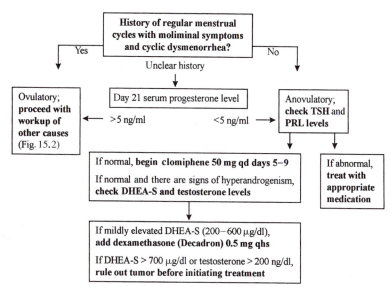

FIGURE 15.4. Workup for anovulatory infertility. *PRL,* prolactin; *TSH,* thyroid-stimulating hormone.

in the urine has been confirmed (15). There is a lag of approximately 4 to 6 hours between serum and urinary LH surges, and most surges begin between 5:00 am and 9:00 am. So more than 90% of ovulation episodes can be detected by a single urinary test performed that midafternoon or early evening (16). Basal body temperature charting has long been used because of its simplicity, but its variability and inconvenience restrict its efficacy as a diagnostic test. The World Health Organization (WHO) defines a shift in basal body temperature as three consecutive daily temperatures 0.4°F higher than the previous six daily temperatures. This is considered confirmation that ovulation has occurred (17). Physical release of the ovum probably occurs on the day before the first day of temperature elevation; hence, this test provides only retrospective evidence of ovulation.

Histologic evidence of secretory endometrium detected by endometrial biopsy is indicative of ovulation and corpus luteum formation. The endometrial biopsy is performed 2 to 3 days before the expected period. A good correlation has been noted between biopsy results, the time of the basal body temperature nadir, and midcycle LH surge, indicating this test is reliable for determining timing of ovulation (18). Disadvantages of endometrial sampling include expense and patient discomfort.

The use of transvaginal sonography is recognized as a reliable technique for monitoring follicular development. Ovulation is deemed to have occurred if the follicle reached a mean diameter of 18 to 25 mm and subsequently changed in sonographic density or demonstrated sonographic evidence of follicular collapse (19). However, its use as an initial diagnostic test for all infertile women does not appear to be cost effective.

Specific tests ordered to determine the cause of anovulation should depend partly on the physical examination of each patient (Fig. 15.4). Serum prolactin and thyroid-stimulating hormone are routine tests for all patients in whom the cause of anovulation is uncertain. In addition, determination of the serum FSH concentration identifies causes where amenorrhea is secondary to ovarian failure. It is reasonable to assess the gonadotropin levels on any patient in whom the cause of anovulation is not apparent but especially in women over age 30. In patients demonstrating significant signs of androgen excess, testosterone, dehydroepiandrosterone sulfate (DHEA-S), and 17-hydroxyprogesterone levels are necessary to rule out androgen-secreting tumors of either the ovary or adrenal or the possibility of late-onset congenital adrenal hyperplasia. In cases of amenorrhea, a progestin challenge test (medroxyprogesterone acetate [Provera] 10 mg daily for 10 days) can help to determine the etiology. When withdrawal bleeding occurs, the outflow tract is patent and sufficient estrogen production has stimulated endometrial growth. This is most indicative of polycystic ovary syndrome. When no withdrawal bleeding occurs and a normal outflow tract has been identified, the most likely etiology is hypothalamic dysfunction.

Classification and Treatment of Anovulatory Disorders

Classification of ovulatory disorders can be made based on the level of FSH and prolactin. The appropriate treatment is determined by the outcome of these tests.

Hypogonadotropic Anovulation. These patients demonstrate low FSH levels, normal prolactin concentrations, and no withdrawal bleeding after a progesterone challenge test. The most common type of hypogonadotropic hypogonadism is idiopathic. If causes such as anorexia, excessive exercise, or stress are elucidated, treatment with appropriate counseling should be initiated. If instead the cause is primary pituitary failure, ovulation induction with gonadotropins is indicated. Patients demonstrating panhypopituitarism also demonstrate other symptoms in addition to anovulation.

Patients with hypothalamic ovulatory failure can be treated with pulsatile GnRH and should be referred to a specialist. An alternative therapy involves the use of human menopausal gonadotropins (Pergonal), discussed in a separate section below. Pure FSH (Metrodin) is not indicated for patients with hypogonadotropic hypogonadism, as some LH is required for ovulation (20). Clomiphene citrate (Clomid, Serophene) is not an effective treatment for anovulation in these cases. Most treatments for hypothalamic ovulatory failure should be administered by specialists.

Normogonadotropic Anovulation. These patients have a normal FSH concentration (with either normal or high LH levels) and demonstrate withdrawal bleeding in response to the progesterone challenge test. Most patients have polycystic ovarian disease. In patients with body mass index greater than 30, where body mass index = weight (kg) ÷ height (m^2), weight loss is the initial recommended treatment. These patients show marked improvement in pregnancy rates with weight reduction alone and frequently need no further therapy (21). The initial pharmacologic treatment in this group is the antiestrogen clomiphene citrate (Clomid, Serophene). Clomiphene citrate is believed to interfere with the normal negative feedback of estradiol on the hypothalamic-pituitary axis (22). When this inhibitory effect is impeded, pituitary FSH and LH are increased. The increased FSH stimulates folliculogenesis by promoting proliferation of granulosa cells and increased intrafollicular estrogen production.

The recommended starting dose of clomiphene citrate is 50 mg/day beginning on cycle day 5 and continuing for a total of 5 days. In patients with irregular menses, medroxyprogesterone acetate (Provera) is commonly given at a dose of 10 mg daily and clomiphene citrate started on cycle day 5 after initiation of the withdrawal bleed. Documentation of ovulation is usually made with either urinary LH monitoring or a luteal progesterone level. If clomiphene citrate is taken on cycle days 5 through 9, ovulation usually occurs between days 15 and 18 (23). Therefore, the LH surge would begin about day 14. If there is no ovulation, the dose should be increased by 50-mg increments (to a maximum of 200 mg) until ovulation is achieved (Table 15.3). If

TABLE 15.3. Clomiphene Citrate (Clomid, Serophene) Use for Anovulatory Infertility

Clomiphene 50 mg PO QD, cycle days 5–9.

If ovulatory (detected by either urinary LH, serum luteal progesterone, or spontaneous menses), continue with same dose for 4–6 cycles.

If no ovulation, increase dose by 50 mg daily in next cycle, reassess as above, and increase dose by another 50 mg or continue dose as indicated in subsequent cycles.

If no ovulation on 150 mg, consider referral to reproductive endocrinologist for gonadotropin therapy. May also choose to increase to 200 mg daily, days 5–9, and assess ovulation.

ovulation occurs, that clomiphene citrate dose should be continued until pregnancy occurs or for four to six cycles. Ninety-five percent of conceptions with clomiphene citrate occurs within six ovulatory cycles (24).

Approximately 70% of women treated with clomiphene citrate for anovulatory infertility ovulate and 15 to 40% become pregnant (25). (The pregnancy rate depends on additional infertility factors.) The twin gestation rate is approximately 10% (26). There does not appear to be an increase in congenital malformations with clomiphene citrate use (27). Dickey et al. (28) observed a small increase in spontaneous abortions in patients using clomiphene citrate compared with spontaneous pregnancies (24 versus 20%). Dickey and Holtkamp (26) provided a more thorough review of clinical observations and pregnancy outcomes with clomiphene citrate use.

Failure to conceive on clomiphene citrate therapy prompts further investigation and therapy. In patients with a DHEA-S value greater than 2000 ng/mL, pregnancy rates may improve with the concurrent administration of dexamethasone (Decadron) 0.5 mg every morning. It is thought that suppression of the androgenic milieu may improve the response to clomiphene citrate therapy. In patients who ovulate in response to clomiphene citrate therapy but still do not conceive, there is a high incidence of other associated infertility factors (24). Before further therapy, it is essential that at least a semen analysis and a hysterosalpingogram are completed to rule out other causes of infertility. Failure to ovulate with 100 to 150 mg of clomiphene citrate may result from an abnormal LH surge, in which case the addition of 10,000 units of intramuscular human chorionic gonadotropin (hCG) timed with follicular ultrasounds may facilitate ovulation. Dominant follicles should approach a mean diameter of 18 to 20 mm before hCG administration during clomiphene citrate-induced cycles (29, 30).

The side effects of clomiphene citrate include hot flushes, abdominal bloating, breast discomfort, nausea and vomiting, visual changes, headache, and alopecia. These require discontinuation of treatment for only a small percentage of patients. If a patient does not ovulate or fails to conceive after 6 months of ovulatory cycles on clomiphene citrate treatment, the use of human gonadotropins, discussed in a separate section below, is usually the next step in therapy.

Hypergonadotropic Hypogonadism. This group includes all variants of ovarian failure and ovarian resistance. FSH concentrations are usually greater than 20 mIU/mL in repeated measurements (31). The patient usually displays hypoestrogenic signs and symptoms and does not respond to the progesterone challenge. If she is less than 40 years old, this indicates premature ovarian failure. In women less than 30 years old, a karyotype should be obtained to rule out the presence of a Y chromosome. If a Y chromosome is detected, extirpation of the gonads is warranted to prevent possible malignant transformation (32). Treatment of infertility in these patients requires assisted reproduction technologies.

Hyperprolactinemia.   The incidence of hyperprolactinemia in patients with secondary amenorrhea is 23% and in subjects with oligomenorrhea is 8%. The mechanism of anovulation is believed to be an impaired gonadotropin pulsatility and derangement of the estrogen-positive feedback effect on LH secretion in hyperprolactinemic patients (33). When prolactin levels exceed 20 to 25 ng/mL, the measurement should be repeated under basal conditions (i.e., early morning sampling). If it is still elevated, hypothyroidism should also be ruled out with a thyroid-stimulating hormone level. If prolactin is elevated in the absence of a thyroid disorder, imaging of the pituitary with a coned-down view of the sella turcica, computed tomography, or magnetic resonance imaging should be performed to diagnose empty sella, microadenoma, or macroadenoma. Computed tomography is most commonly used. Prolactin concentration can be increased by stress or normal breast or pelvic examination. These events may lead to false positives if the test is inappropriately timed.

The only approved medication for the treatment of hyperprolactinemia in the United States is bromocriptine (Parlodel). Bromocriptine is an ergot alkaloid derivative with dopamine receptor agonist activity that directly inhibits prolactin secretion. It is usually started at 1.25 mg orally at bedtime for 1 week and then increased to 2.5 mg twice daily. After 1 week on this dose (2.5 mg), ovulatory status should be evaluated. In the absence of ovulation, the dose can be increased in 1.25-mg increments (34). Once ovulation is established, the medication is maintained until the patient becomes pregnant. Bromocriptine is usually discontinued after a positive pregnancy test but can be used safely during pregnancy. Most patients who conceive do so within six ovulatory cycles, with the average being two cycles (35).

Bromocriptine has been advocated in the anovulatory patient with normoprolactinemic galactorrhea (36). In the absence of galactorrhea or an abnormal prolactin level, however, inadequate data remain to support the addition of bromocriptine to an ovulation-induction regimen.

Side effects of bromocriptine include nausea, headache, and faintness due to orthostatic hypotension. These effects are minimized by gradually increasing the dose. Taking it with food is recommended to avoid gastrointestinal side effects. Vaginal administration of bromocriptine has been associated with fewer side effects but with similar effectiveness (37).

Gonadotropin Therapy.   The human menopausal gonadotropin medications include Metrodin (75 IU FSH) and Pergonal (75 IU LH). Gonadotropin therapy can be used in hypogonadotropic hypogonadism (as discussed previously), although referral to a specialist for pulsatile GnRH therapy is the preferred treatment. Gonadotropin therapy may also be used for normogonadotropic anovulation after clomiphene citrate (Clomid, Serophene) failure. Gonadotropin therapy provides good per cycle and cumulative pregnancy rates in hypogonadotropic anovulation (25% and 91.2%, respectively) but carries a higher risk of multiple pregnancies and ovarian hyperstimulation. In normogonadotropic patients who failed to ovulate on clomiphene citrate, the per cycle and cumulative pregnancy rates are 8% and 21.4%, respectively (38, 39).

Intramuscular or subcutaneous injections of gonadotropin(s) are usually administered on cycle day 2. Follicular growth is monitored by ultrasound, and estradiol levels are followed daily until optimal stimulation has occurred, with subsequent injection of hCG to stimulate ovulation.

The incidence of multiple pregnancies with the use of human menopausal gonadotropins can be as low as 10% with careful monitoring, but rates as high as 40% are reported (39). Ovarian hyperstimulation syndrome is characterized by excessive weight gain, ascites, and intravascular depletion. Most patients with ovarian hyperstimulation syndrome have mild symptoms and can be managed as outpatients. There is no risk of teratogenic effects on the fetus.

Tuboperitoneal Infertility

Approximately 40% of all infertile women demonstrate an abnormality of the uterus, cervix, and/or fallopian tubes. To date, the best assessment of pelvic anatomic causes of infertility is with a thorough history and physical examination and a hysterosalpingogram (40). The hysterosalpingogram is the test of choice to assess uterine and fallopian tube contour and tubal patency and should be part of the standard evaluation of the infertile couple. Recently, the antichlamydial antibody titer has also been proposed as an integral part of the initial evaluation and workup (41). Once an anatomic abnormality is detected, the decision to proceed with reparative surgery or in vitro fertilization (IVF) should be based on the specific defect, the clinical and financial resources available, and the desires of the patient.

Evaluation

A history of pelvic inflammatory disease, ectopic pregnancy, septic abortion, ruptured appendix, and tubal and/or other pelvic surgery should prompt suspicion for a possible anatomic cause for infertility. Clearly, pelvic inflammatory disease has had the greatest impact on the increasing incidence of tubal infertility. The classic studies of Westrom (42) correlated the number of episodes of pelvic inflammatory disease with the subsequent infertility rate. An 11% incidence of involuntary infertility was associated with one episode of salpingitis, 23% after two episodes, and 54% after three or more episodes. Physical examination should be directed at detecting decreased mobility of adnexa and uterosacral nodularity to help predict the presence of extensive adhesive disease or endometriosis.

Antichlamydial Antibody Titer. Genital infection with *Chlamydia trachomatis* remains the single most important cause of tubal pathology. Damage to the ciliated epithelium from *Chlamydia* results in impaired tubal transport. Many cases go undetected and untreated because 50 to 80% of women with these infections are asymptomatic (43). Thus, even without a history of recognized salpingitis, subclinical disease is a common cause of decreased fertility. Because of this, serologic *C. trachomatis* antibody testing has been introduced as a means of detecting tuboperitoneal pathology.

Dabekausen et al. (41) prospectively compared hysterosalpingography with *C. trachomatis* antibody testing in predicting tubal factor infertility. A series of 211 patients were tested for *C. trachomatis* antibody and underwent a standard hysterosalpingogram. Results of each were compared with findings at laparoscopy. The antibody titer had a 74% sensitivity and 92% specificity in predicting tubal abnormalities at laparoscopy. Hysterosalpingography had only a 58% sensitivity and 77% specificity. The positive likelihood ratio for *C. trachomatis* IgG antibody testing was 9.1, indicating a patient with tubal factor infertility to be 9.1 times mores likely to have abnormal serology results than a patient without tubal factor infertility. This was superior to hysterosalpingography, which had a positive likelihood ratio of 2.6 in this study. In a meta-analysis evaluating all studies comparing *Chlamydia* antibody titers and laparoscopy for tubal disease, Mol et al. (44) confirmed that the discriminative capacity of antibody testing is at least as good if not better than the hysterosalpingogram.

Although tuboperitoneal pathology can result from other causes (previous surgery, endometriosis, or pelvic inflammatory disease from nonchlamydial microorganisms), *C. trachomatis* antibody testing is an important component of the standard infertility evaluation.

Hysterosalpingography. Hysterosalpingography is important in the diagnostic evaluation of the infertile female. It is the first-line radiologic examination and provides immediate information about the appearance of the endocervical canal, the uterine cavity, and the fallopian tube lumina. Ideally, the gynecologist should perform the examination, but often it is the radiologist who completes the hysterosalpingogram.

The procedure involves placing a single-tooth tenaculum on the anterior lip of the cervix followed by insertion of the infusion device attached to a syringe filled with 10 to 20 mL of contrast material. Usually only 5 to 10 mL of dye is needed to adequately evaluate the uterine cavity and tubal lumen. To allow full visualization of the uterine cavity, the speculum should always be removed before injection of radiocontrast. After attachment of the cannula, the contrast should slowly be injected under fluoroscopic observation. Traction should be applied to the cervix to bring the uterus parallel to the x-ray film. In the absence of proximal tubal obstruction, one should carefully observe filling of both fallopian tubes. Should one or both tubes fail to be visualized, prone positioning has been useful in allowing the contrast to fill the tubal lumens (45). Spill of contrast into the peritoneal cavity should be documented. Collection of dye around the distal tube that does not spill into the cavity with changing patient position may suggest peritubal adhesions. Rarely are more than three films needed. A preliminary scout film adds little to the interpretation of the study. A delayed film may be taken to demonstrate late spillage.

Various instruments have been designed for and other methods adapted to the performance of the hysterosalpingogram. A lidocaine paracervical block can sometimes decrease patient discomfort but is not routinely recommended. In parous women, a hysterosalpingogram balloon catheter (Ackrad Laboratories Inc., Cranford, NJ) may be required to prevent leakage of dye back through the cervix. Nonsteroidal anti-inflammatory drugs are frequently prescribed 30 minutes before the procedure to decrease uterine cramping during injection of the contrast. Prophylactic antibiotics (doxycycline [Vibramycin, Doryx] 100 mg twice a day for 3 days before the hysterosalpingogram) are warranted in women with a prior history of pelvic infection, specifically *Chlamydia* (46, 47).

The specific dye used has been the subject of many reports, most of which compared the therapeutic effects of water-based versus oil-soluble contrast media (48–51). Most, but not all, concluded that the ethiodized oil-soluble contrast media provides a slight advantage in improving the pregnancy rate for patients with unexplained infertility within the months after the procedure. Because of the rare possibility of granuloma formation with the oil-based dye, we generally use the Ethiodol therapeutically only after bilateral patency has been demonstrated with the water-soluble contrast.

Hysterosalpingography provides extremely useful information in the early evaluation of the infertile female, but its validity as a diagnostic tool has been questioned by several investigators. One meta-analysis of 20 studies comparing hysterosalpingography and laparoscopy for tubal patency and peritubal adhesions concluded its principal use should be to rule out tubal obstruction (52). If bilateral proximal occlusion is shown with a history of chlamydia, one could reasonably avoid laparoscopy and proceed with IVF. If it shows bilateral distal occlusion, with no hydrosalpinx, one might attempt tuboplasty. Hysterosalpingography can demonstrate congenital and acquired lesions of the uterus but is associated with high false-positive and false-negative rates, precluding its use as the sole method of diagnosing uterine anomalies (53). For assessment of the uterine cavity, many physicians are now using hysterosonography in lieu of hysterosalpingogram. When used in conjunction with a thorough history, physical examination, and antichlamydial antibody titers, hysterosalpingography is an important adjunct in the assessment of most anatomic causes of infertility.

Based on current evidence, we recommend that a hysterosalpingogram should be obtained in the workup for infertility in the following cases:

- Positive antichlamydial antibody titer
- History of pelvic inflammatory disease, pelvic surgery, or ruptured appendix
- Patient older than 35 years
- Greater than four cycles of treatment for anovulation without success

Postcoital Test. The postcoital test (also known as the Sims-Huhner test) provides information about the interaction between the sperm and cervical mucus. Despite its frequent use over the past century as a tool to evaluate cervical factor infertility, its validity as a predictor of future pregnancy has been debated. Some authors assert a strong association between the results of the postcoital test and pregnancy rates (54, 55), whereas others claim it merely confirms the occurrence of intercourse (56). A review of the current literature by Griffith and Grimes (56) concluded that this test suffers from lack of standard methodology, a lack of a uniform definition of normal, and unknown reproducibility.

Cervical factors as a cause of infertility may exist, but a valid test to correctly diagnose them has yet to be discovered. The postcoital test should never be a substitute for a semen analysis because morphology cannot be adequately evaluated in the postcoital test and the correlation between postcoital sperm motility and total motile sperm count (from semen analysis) departs from linearity in the lower range of sperm count values (57).

The postcoital test may be used if there is clinical suspicion of a hostile cervical factor (most likely immunologic in nature).

Office (Diagnostic) Hysteroscopy. Evaluating the uterine cavity for abnormalities responsible for infertility has traditionally been done with hysterosalpingography. However, because of the high false-positive rate of hysterosalpingogram findings (i.e., radiographic findings not confirmed at endoscopy), other modes for detecting intrauterine lesions have been proposed. Hysteroscopy performed in the operating room is the gold standard for identifying such lesions but carries the burden of added expense and need for anesthesia. Office hysteroscopy with carbon dioxide as the distention medium has been proposed as a method to detect endometrial abnormalities (58). This technique can complement the hysterosalpingogram in differentiating endometrial polyps from submucous myomas or validating the presence of intrauterine adhesions or congenital anomalies.

Sonohysterography. Fluid contrast ultrasound or sonohysterography has been proposed as a tool in the diagnosis of intrauterine lesions. In light of high false-positive rates with hysterosalpingography and office hysteroscopy, this technique has been proposed as an inexpensive alternative (59, 60). It involves the insertion of either a pediatric Foley or hysterosalpingogram catheter into the uterine cavity with subsequent introduction of sterile saline while visualizing with the transvaginal ultrasound. Findings at sonohysterography correlate well with confirmatory diagnosis at hysteroscopy (in the operating room) or after hysterectomy. Sonohysterography offers greater than 85% sensitivity and specificity in diagnosing intracavitary lesions

(61). Rubin et al. (60) reported a 64% incidence of intrauterine abnormalities in patients with primary infertility. Although it is still controversial whether these abnormalities are causal for the infertility, all patients should be screened for such lesions. Sonohysterography appears to be an effective modality to use for this screening.

Laparoscopy.   Laparoscopy was once included in the initial workup of the standard infertility evaluation. Because of expense and risk-to-benefit analyses, there appears little role for a diagnostic laparoscopy in the early evaluation of the infertile couple. Based on current evidence, only patients with a history and physical examination compatible with endometriosis, positive antichlamydial antibody titer, or abnormalities displayed on the hysterosalpingogram or other studies should undergo laparoscopy for infertility. Even then, the decision to proceed with either laparoscopy or IVF should be made on an individual basis. In older women, because of the rapid decline of fertility potential with advancing age, efforts should be directed toward the treatment method that provides the highest likelihood of success within the shortest time interval (62).

Treatment of Tubal Disease

When the clinician has completed the diagnostic evaluation of infertility, the next step is to estimate the baseline prognosis without therapy and then determine whether treatment can increase the likelihood of pregnancy. There is a wide range of tubal pathology in patients with documented sequelae of pelvic inflammatory disease. Proximal tubal disease, diagnosed most commonly by hysterosalpingogram, has historically been treated with laparotomy. Excision of the uterine cornua with reimplantation of the tube or reimplantation of the nondiseased proximal portion of the tube into the back of the uterus are two methods that have been described (63). More recently, hysteroscopic cannulation of the proximal tube has been reported and appears to be a promising technique. Early studies report a 30% pregnancy rate after cannulation (64). However, in the absence of a prospective trial, appropriate counseling should include informing the patient of the paucity of statistics for the success of this procedure.

The appropriate therapy for distal disease depends on a number of factors. Patient age, severity of distal disease, and availability of assisted reproductive technologies are all significant in determining prognosis of subsequent fertility. Several studies assessed pregnancy rates based on degree of tubal damage, seen at laparoscopy or indicated on the basis of hysterosalpingography (65, 66). The best prognostic factor was thickness of the tubal wall. Tubal diameters greater than 2.5 cm measured by hysterosalpingography is associated with a lower pregnancy rate (22%) than normal-diameter tubes (48%) (66). In women whose distal tubes have a diameter greater than 3 cm measured at laparoscopy, the prognosis for a term pregnancy after tubal reconstruction was extremely poor (16%) compared with patients with mild disease (80%) (65). If there was a hydrosalpinx greater than 2 cm diameter with a thick tubal wall, the prognosis for a term pregnancy after tubal reconstruction was extremely poor in these studies.

More recently, Dlugi et al. (67) reported on success of laparoscopic procedures for distal disease. Patients with repair of bilateral disease with neosalpingostomy had significantly lower 2-year pregnancy rates compared with patients with unilateral disease (9 versus 32.8%). They also concluded that with severe adhesive disease (American Fertility Society score greater than 23), pregnancy rates were significantly reduced. Eight of 113 patients underwent a second surgical procedure with an intrauterine pregnancy rate of 25%. Most reports agree that patients with severe tubal disease, as defined by the American Fertility Society (68) or Rock et al.'s criteria (69), have poor pregnancy rates after repair and that recommendations for IVF should be made. Although IVF and tuboplasty have not been compared in a formal prospective study, IVF appears to be superior to surgical intervention for women with severe tubal disease (70). IVF offers delivery rates of 15 to 20% per cycle and an overall delivery rate of greater than 70% of women with tubal factor infertility with four cycles of treatment. This is superior to surgery for severe disease (71).

Treatment of endometriosis-associated infertility has been the subject of many trials of therapy with ovulation suppression and laparoscopic ablation of endometriosis implants (72). The data suggest that surgical correction of moderate-to-severe disease is effective in improving pregnancy rates. One prospective randomized trial assessed whether laparoscopic treatment of minimal or mild endometriosis improved cumulative pregnancy rates over expectant management of similar disease and concluded that an improvement in pregnancy rate was evident 36 weeks after laparoscopy (73). However, longer follow-up of these patients may demonstrate that the difference is no longer seen and that the benefit of surgery is only transient. Long-term trials are still unavailable to make any conclusions about the benefit of treating minimal or mild endometriosis.

Treatment of Intrauterine Disease

Infertility due to leiomyomata is a diagnosis of exclusion primarily because their relationship to one another is so poorly understood. Before treating an asymptomatic fibroid in an infertile patient, all other causes of infertility should be addressed. The location of the myoma should be determined, as it appears that subserosal fibroids have no impact on fertility but can cause other gynecologic symptoms (74, 75). The size of the fibroid has been implicated as prognostic of conception rate (76). Most authors agree, however, that in the absence of an intrauterine filling defect and no history of pregnancy losses, fibroids less than 10 to 12 cm in the widest dimension should not be removed before documented reproductive failure. In patients with large fibroids (greater than 10 to 12 cm) and no losses, appropriate counseling is essential. The patient should be informed that the literature is deficient in appropriately conducted studies showing a definitive improvement in pregnancy rate with myomectomy. Myomectomy could be justifiable if all diagnostic tests reveal no other cause of infertility.

Asherman's syndrome (the presence of intrauterine adhesions usually resulting from a postpartum dilation and curettage) can result in infertility. Treatment with hysteroscopic resection has been reported to result in an 80% term pregnancy rate (77). For a more detailed discussion of Asherman's syndrome, refer to the section on recurrent pregnancy loss below.

Endometrial polyps, although frequently diagnosed by various imaging studies, have no clear association with infertility but should be removed if other gynecologic symptoms are present. If they are discovered incidentally at hysteroscopy, polypectomy is warranted for histologic analysis.

Special Topics in Female Infertility

Luteal Phase Deficiency

The luteal phase of the menstrual cycle is the period of time between ovulation and the onset of menses. The luteal phase is characterized by progesterone secretion by the corpus luteum. Most cases of luteal phase deficiency are attributed to inadequate secretion of progesterone; however, decreased endometrial response to progesterone can also result in a luteal phase deficiency (78).

Although a number of clinical tests have been proposed to diagnose luteal phase deficiency, they all suffer from lack of validation and standardization. Jordan et al. (79)

reviewed common clinical tests and compared them all with luteal integrated progesterone levels. Basal body temperature charting, luteal length, ultrasound measurement of follicular diameters, and timed endometrial biopsies all had lower sensitivities or specificities than luteal progesterone measurement. Because of the pulsatile nature of progesterone, three serum levels should be obtained from days 5 through 9 after ovulation. A sum of these values, the integrated progesterone, of less than 30 ng/mL would indicate a defect in the production of progesterone from the corpus luteum.

Despite improved diagnostic testing, it remains unproved that luteal phase support with progesterone or hCG supplementation offers any improvement in pregnancy rates (80). There still appears to be little evidence to justify testing for this disorder. Numerous trials comparing progesterone, clomiphene citrate (Clomid, Serophene), and gonadotropin therapy for luteal phase deficiency have been described. A disordered luteal phase is likely a reflection of abnormal follicular development and treatment should be directed at correction of folliculogenesis with either clomiphene citrate or gonadotropins.

Ovulation Induction and Ovarian Cancer Risk

Case reports of ovarian carcinoma in infertile women raised interest about a potential causative relationship between ovulation induction and cancer. Because ovarian cancer is a relatively rare disease and ovarian cancer associated with fertility drug use even more rare, examination of this connection is limited to case reports and retrospective case-control studies. Current available data fail to reveal a causal effect, although nulliparous women with refractory infertility may harbor a high risk of ovarian cancer irrespective of their use of fertility medication(s) (81). Close clinical surveillance of patients before, during, and after treatment of infertility is recommended. Some recommend a baseline ultrasound before any clomiphene citrate use, repeating an ultrasound with the onset of new and unexplained symptoms, and encouraging yearly examinations with the patient advising their physician(s) that they have taken clomiphene citrate in the past.

Treating Infertility in Women of Advanced Reproductive Age

Although age-related changes in fecundity have been documented in several populations, there is significant variability in the timing of onset of diminished reproductive potential for individual women. Since 1990 there has been a greater than 10-fold rise in the number of cases of IVF performed for women over 40 years (71). The use of both a day 3 (basal) FSH concentration and patient age can aid in determining prognosis for conception. Women ages 40 to 44 with a basal FSH below 25 IU/L had a clinical pregnancy rate of 5.2% and a livebirth rate of 1.9% (14/267) compared with a clinical pregnancy rate of 0% per cycle (0/135) in cases in which either basal FSH was 25 IU/L or higher or patients were 44 years of age or older (82). The clomiphene citrate challenge test is a very effective tool to detect diminished ovarian reserve and has been validated in assisted reproduction and the general infertility population (83). It involves measuring day 3 FSH and estradiol, administration of clomiphene citrate (Clomid, Serophene) from days 5 through 9, followed by repeat FSH on day 10. The test result is considered abnormal if either the basal or day 10 FSH level is above 25 IU/L. The rationale behind this test is that women with adequate ovarian reserve should develop a cohort of follicles producing adequate estradiol and inhibin to suppress the FSH. It is logical to first obtain a basal FSH in the infertile patient over age 30. If the result is less than 25 IU/L, a clomiphene citrate challenge test is warranted. If either the day 3 or day 10 level is elevated (greater than 25 IU/L), appropriate counseling of a poor prognosis for conception is warranted (less than 5% chance of conception).

MALE FACTOR INFERTILITY

At least 30 to 40% of all infertility is attributable to abnormalities of male reproductive function. For this reason, it is important to evaluate the male partner as an integral part of the infertility workup. The semen analysis should always be included as an initial screening test. A history of fathering a prior pregnancy is inadequate to rule out abnormalities of the semen. The quality limits designed to discriminate infertile from fertile men are constantly being reexamined and redefined. The WHO normal values are seen in Table 15.4 (84). These values help to identify patients who should not experience decreased fecundity. However, the predictive value of subnormal semen analysis parameters is limited except in the case of azoospermia. No diagnostic test of sperm function can unequivocally predict the potential for fertilization to occur.

Although many techniques have been proposed to further elucidate etiologies of male factor infertility, only the semen analysis has been proven to be a reproducible predictor of impaired fertility.

History and Physical Examination

During the initial history, the sexual habits of the couple should be ascertained. KY jelly or other lubricants can be spermatotoxic and result in impaired motility or count (85). Timing and frequency of intercourse should also be addressed. Some authors recommend intercourse every 48 hours during midcycle (86). A history of childhood illnesses, abnormal testicular development (specifically undescended testicles), or trauma to the genitourinary organs should also be obtained. Impaired testicular function may result from any generalized insult (viremia, fever). It takes approximately 72 days for the sperm to reach the caudal epididymis after the initiation of spermatogenesis, and the effects of any adverse events may not be demonstrated in the ejaculate for 1 to 3 months. A history of a delay in pubertal development and maturation can suggest an endocrinopathy such as hypogonadotropic hypogonadism or adrenal dysfunction. Other factors contributing to impaired spermatogenesis include a history of chemotherapy or radiation, tuberculosis, exposure to environmental toxins, or drugs (specifically sulfasalazine [Azulfidine], cimetidine [Tagamet], alcohol, marijuana, and/or exogenous androgenic steroids). Elevated temperatures also impair spermatogenesis and routine use of hot tubs should be discouraged.

A detailed clinical assessment should be performed with particular regard to the evaluation of the genitalia. The presence of hypospadias, abnormally small testes, or the presence of a varicocele should be noted. Testicular volumes in normal men are

TABLE 15.4. World Health Organization (84) Normal Values for Semen Analysis

Volume	≥2.0 mL
Sperm concentration	≥20 million/mL
Motility	≥50% with forward progression *or*
	≥20% with rapid progression within 60 min of ejaculation
Morphology	≥30% normal focus
White blood cells	<1 million/mL
Immunobead	<20% spermatozoa with adherent particles
Mixed agglutination reaction test	<10% spermatozoa with adherent particles

usually in excess of 15 mL and are frequently in excess of 30 mL. Assessment for varicocele should be performed with the patient in the supine and standing positions using the Valsalva maneuver. An enlarged prostate can suggest prostatitis, which could affect semen quality. Androgen deficiency may be evident by decreased body hair, gynecomastia, or eunuchoid proportions, and if any of these findings are present, an exploration of an endocrine abnormality is indicated.

Laboratory Evaluation

Semen Analysis

The most important laboratory investigation in male infertility is the semen analysis. Some authors recommend a period of abstinence for several days before collection to maximize the quality of the specimen (87). However, not abstaining from the normal frequency of ejaculation may be a more accurate reflection of semen quality during intercourse. We generally recommend a period of abstinence only if a repeat sample is needed because of oligospermia. Collection by masturbation into a sterile container is the most commonly recommended method, although coitus interruptus or a spermicidal-free condom can be used if the man cannot or will not masturbate. The specimen should be protected from temperature extremes and delivered to the laboratory within an hour of collection.

Interpretation of the results are important to the prognosis of future conception. These values (Table 15.4) help to identify patients who should not have decreased ability to induce pregnancy. However, unless there is azoospermia, the predictive value of subnormal semen parameters is limited (12). Morphology consistently seems to be a good predictor of fertilization. One report demonstrated marked decrease in fertilization when the normal morphology was below 40%, although the current WHO cutoff point is 30% (88). No single category in the semen analysis can be used as a sole predictor of fertility (89). Some reports combine the motility and count for a total motile count: (sperm/mL) $\times$ (% motile) $\times$ (volume in mL). This measurement is often used to evaluate a washed specimen for intrauterine insemination. Pregnancy rates are improved in specimens with a total motile sperm count that exceeds 5×10^6 (90).

Abnormalities of any parameter in the semen analysis warrants attention. However, treatment of such abnormalities remains unproved in enhancing the pregnancy rate of the involved couple. Therefore, before initiating any therapy, it is prudent to completely assess both partners involved.

Tests of Sperm Function

No functional test has yet been validated that can unequivocally predict the fertilization capacity of spermatozoa. (In other words, nothing is more predictive than a normal or abnormal semen analysis based on WHO criteria.) Despite this, many tests have been proposed and are used routinely in the assessment of male factor infertility.

Sperm Penetration Assay.   Mao and Grimes (91) reviewed the literature and analyzed this test's performance as a clinically useful examination. For predicting IVF failures, its sensitivity varies from 0.00 to 0.78 and specificity ranges from 0.51 to 1.00. Other studies claim it is of useful predictive value (92). Despite a trend in Mao and Grimes' data correlating the sperm penetration assay with long-term fertility potential, a result of 0% was associated with a pregnancy rate of 16%. Therefore, the validity, reproducibility, and utility of the sperm penetration assay are still yet undefined by available literature. Until further studies are completed that demonstrate accurate prognostic ability of this test, it should probably not be included in the assessment of the infertile couple.

Other Tests of Sperm Function. A variety of assays has been developed to evaluate the fertilizing capacity of the spermatozoa. These include the hemizona assay, in vitro tests of penetration into mucus, sperm mannose-ligand receptor levels, and measurement of the acrosome reaction, to name a few. Unfortunately, none have provided the clinician with a valid method to predict fecundity and therefore should be discouraged from clinical use.

Sperm Antibodies

Sperm are very immunogenic. Because sperm antibodies develop only after specific instances, testing should be limited to a distinct population. Men with a history of testicular trauma, vasectomy reversal, or who have evidence of clumping on the semen analysis are candidates for evaluation. An immunologic reaction directed against the sperm has been implicated as a cause of decreased motility (93). Diagnosis is usually made with the immunobead test to identify the presence of antibodies on the sperm. Various forms of treatment have been used, including antibiotics, immunosuppression, testosterone therapy, sperm washing and intrauterine insemination, IVF, and donor insemination. One effective method involves sperm washing and intrauterine insemination of washed sperm with or without concomitant ovulation induction. When compared with corticosteroid immunosuppression, intrauterine insemination is associated with a higher pregnancy rate with fewer side effects (94). If this is unsuccessful, IVF, with or without micromanipulation, should be considered.

Treatment Options for Male Factor Infertility

Approximately 6% of infertile men have conditions for which specific therapy of confirmed benefit is available (e.g., the treatment of hypogonadotropic hypogonadism) (95, 96). Therefore, carefully randomized studies are needed for the assessment of infertility treatment for most subfertile men whose fertility is impaired but does not completely preclude conception.

Varicocele Repair

Although varicoceles are associated with infertility, many men with varicoceles father children. The literature is replete with studies both supporting and opposing the view that the repair of varicoceles results in increased pregnancy rates. Because the repair is a surgical procedure, it is not possible to perform a double-blind controlled study. Evaluation of varicocelectomy and its effect on subsequent pregnancy rates is extremely difficult, and the current literature is flawed by inappropriate study designs and reporting. Most urologic studies fail to outline the evaluation of the female partners of the men in the studies.

Varicocelectomy does appear to have a beneficial effect on sperm density (97, 98). Some studies also report a favorable effect on fertility, although this is an inconsistent finding in the literature (99, 100). Based on available data, a definitive statement concerning the efficacy of varicocelectomy cannot be made. Some propose that surgical intervention should be recommended if the patient is symptomatic with pain or for couples with reduced sperm count and otherwise unexplained infertility (101, 102). Because a definitive statement regarding the effectiveness of varicocelectomy cannot be made, individualized approach is warranted with referral to a urologist when necessary.

TABLE 15.5. Preparation of Spermatozoa for Intrauterine Insemination (One Method)

The semen is collected by masturbation into a sterile container. After liquefaction, the ejaculate is placed into 10 mL of warmed Ham's 10 (GIBCO, Grand Island, NY) and centrifuged at 300 g for 10 min. If a pellet is not obtained, it is resuspended and spun for an additional 10 min. The supernatant is discarded, and the pellet is resuspended in roughly 0.3 mL of Ham's 10 solution. The sperm suspension is introduced into the uterine cavity with a pediatric feeding tube (C.R. Bard, Inc., Cranston, RI) after first confirming adequate count and motility.

Intrauterine Insemination

Treatment of male factor infertility with intrauterine insemination of prepared spermatozoa has been evaluated by a meta-analysis of eight reported trials in which pregnancy was an outcome measure (96). The odds ratio suggests no increase in fertility is obtained with the use of intrauterine insemination alone for therapy. However, when combined with gonadotropin-stimulated cycles, the addition of intrauterine insemination increased the pregnancy rates as much as 8% (103, 104).

Intrauterine insemination is performed after separation of motile from non-motile spermatozoa and other material in the seminal plasma that might have detrimental effects on fertilization. One procedure is described in Table 15.5. Although a variety of techniques have been used for sperm preparation for intrauterine insemination, the appropriate choice should be the one most familiar to and least time consuming for the physician. Despite the diversity of sperm preparations, no single method has proven superior in improving fecundity.

Other Therapies

Assisted reproductive technology provides additional therapies for couples with male factor infertility. Most recently, the advent of intracytoplasmic sperm injection provides a unique treatment opportunity for couples whose infertility is secondary to severe oligospermia. The clinical pregnancy rate per cycle is reported to be up to 30% in appropriately selected cases (105). Therapeutic donor insemination involves many emotional, ethical, and legal issues. The success rate varies between fresh and frozen samples, but in women under 30 years old, the 6-month cumulative pregnancy rates are approximately 40 to 50% for frozen specimens (106). The use of a fresh specimen for therapeutic donor insemination is discouraged because of the need for a quarantine period to ensure absence of any transmittable disease(s). Before insemination, the involved couple should be appropriately counseled regarding all pertinent legal and social issues involved with this procedure.

UNEXPLAINED INFERTILITY

Unexplained infertility is a diagnosis of exclusion. It is a term applied to an infertile couple for whom standard investigations (semen analysis, tubal patency assessment, and laboratory assessment of ovulation) yield normal results. It is estimated that 10 to 15% of infertile couples ultimately reach this clinical diagnosis.

Without treatment, up to 60% of couples with unexplained infertility will conceive within 3 years (107). After 3 years of infertility, the pregnancy rate without treatment decreases by 2% for every month (24% for each additional year) of infertility (108). Patient age is a critical factor in determining fecundity. Tietze (5) reported 11% of women at the age of 34 were infertile compared with 33% at age 40 and 87% by age 44. Thus, in women over 30 with greater than 3 years of unexplained infertility, spontaneous conception is unlikely. Up to 40% of patients with the diagnosis of unexplained infertility display abnormal clomiphene citrate challenge tests. This simple tool can therefore aid the clinician in determining which protocol, if any, to initiate and the length of treatment (109).

Treatment Options for Unexplained Infertility

In couples with unexplained infertility, no biologic abnormality is evident and thus only empirical treatments are relevant. The effectiveness of treatment can only be determined from properly performed randomized controlled trials. To date, there have been few such trials to examine the effect of treatment for these couples. Bromocriptine (Parlodel) and danazol (Danocrine) as empiric therapy have no effect on fecundity (8). Although psychological factors have been suggested as causative agents of unexplained infertility, there are no controlled trials showing counseling to be effective. Four trials, to date, have examined the use of clomiphene citrate (Clomid, Serophene) as empiric treatment, and the combined data suggest an improvement in fecundity (8). One of these trials revealed that the greatest relative increase resulted when clomiphene citrate was given to women who had been infertile for more than 3 years (110).

Intrauterine insemination when used in unstimulated natural cycles has been proposed as a means to increase fecundity in couples with unexplained infertility. Unfortunately, few studies demonstrate a clear benefit of intrauterine insemination alone. When used with clomiphene citrate, Deaton et al. (111) described significantly improved per-cycle fecundity (9.7%) compared with control subjects (3.3%). Clomiphene citrate, 50 mg, was administered during cycle days 5 through 9, and 10,000 units hCG intramuscularly was added when an estimated follicular diameter of greater than 18 mm on ultrasound was reached. An intrauterine insemination using washed sperm was performed 36 hours after the hCG injection. Although this regimen may augment fertility, treatment should be limited to three cycles. No pregnancies occurred during the fourth cycle in this study, and no other study demonstrated benefit of treatment beyond this interval.

Superovulation and intrauterine insemination have also been demonstrated to be of benefit in the treatment of unexplained infertility (112). Immunotherapy with corticosteroids has demonstrated additional benefit to couples treated with this combination therapy (113), but risks of serious complications, such as aseptic necrosis of the femoral neck, osteoporosis, and increased susceptibility to infection, preclude it from routine use. A detailed description of different gonadotropin regimens and various assisted reproductive technologies for the treatment of unexplained infertility is beyond the scope of this chapter. Based on available data, a rational treatment plan for affected couples includes up to three cycles of clomiphene citrate in combination with hCG and intrauterine insemination. If unsuccessful, the next steps would include superovulation with intrauterine insemination followed by IVF. A cumulative pregnancy rate of 40% can be achieved using this regimen (8).

Recurrent Pregnancy Loss

Traditionally, recurrent pregnancy loss has been defined as three consecutive spontaneous abortions. However, it is usually appropriate to initiate an evaluation of the couple after two such losses (114). Recognizing that the spontaneous cure rate is high and the probability of a subsequent successful pregnancy outcome is usually greater than 50%, the focus of the physician should be directed toward obtaining a thorough history and providing adequate counseling to the couple before initiating diagnostic tests or suggesting therapy.

EPIDEMIOLOGY

Of all recognized human pregnancies, 15 to 20% end in spontaneous abortion. The actual incidence of spontaneous pregnancy loss is greater when early unconfirmed pregnancies are included. One group tested daily urine specimens from 221 healthy women attempting to conceive with ultrasensitive hCG assays and determined that the total rate of pregnancy loss after implantation was 31% (115). These estimates do not include instances where fertilized oocytes fail to implant.

Statistics regarding pregnancy outcome are beneficial when counseling patients during early gestation. Regan et al. (116) studied the course of pregnancy in women with ultrasonographically confirmed intrauterine gestations. The overall incidence of spontaneous abortion was 12%, and half occurred before 8 weeks of gestation. The miscarriage rate was only 5% in primigravidas and 14% in multigravidas (117). Prior successful pregnancy was associated with a 5% loss, whereas women whose last pregnancy aborted had a subsequent loss 20% of the time. This increased to 24% in the women in whom all previous pregnancies ended in spontaneous abortions. Thus, the most relevant predictive factor for pregnancy outcome in a subsequent pregnancy is past reproductive history.

Poland et al. (118) also reported a 20% spontaneous abortion rate in women with one prior spontaneous abortion, but in women reporting three or more consecutive abortions, the chance of a subsequent loss increased to 50%. These figures are similar to those reported by James (119), who added that women with at least one live birth followed by three or more losses had only a 30% chance of subsequent pregnancy loss.

ETIOLOGY

The mere presence of an etiologic factor does not signify that it is the definitive cause of recurrent miscarriage. Determination and initiation of appropriate therapy should be based only on the expectation that eradication of identified risk factors will enhance the likelihood of a subsequent live birth.

Genetic Factors

Several large studies indicate that the incidence of a fetal chromosomal anomaly in first-trimester spontaneous abortions exceeds 50% (120, 121). In addition, 30% of second-trimester abortions and 3% of stillbirths demonstrate abnormal karyotypes. Most of these are due to errors in gametogenesis (chromosomal nondisjunction during meiosis), fertilization (triploidy), or the first division of the fertilized ovum (tetraploidy or mosaicism). Only about 5% are due to structural abnormalities such as translocation (117). Aneuploid conceptions are reported to occur more frequently in pregnancies subsequent to recurrent pregnancy loss compared with a control group (1.6 versus 0.3%) (122).

Autosomal trisomy (of chromosomes 13, 16, 18, 21, and 22) is the most common abnormal karyotype (50%) followed by monosomy X (20%), triploidy (15%), tetraploidy (10%), and structural abnormalities (5%). The most common monosomy is 45,XO (Turner's syndrome) (120).

Parental chromosomal abnormalities are an infrequent cause of recurrent pregnancy loss. The reported incidence of major chromosomal abnormalities in either parent varies from 3 to 5%. Half of these anomalies are due to balanced translocation and one fourth are due to Robertsonian translocation. Translocation and inversion are associated with a higher risk of pregnancy wastage and are indications for prenatal diagnosis in subsequent pregnancy (123). However, these couples should not be dissuaded from attempting further pregnancies.

Effect of Maternal Age

Advanced maternal age has been associated with an increased frequency of spontaneous abortion and with an increase in chromosomal defects (124). Studies in pregnancies derived from oocyte donation indicate that the age of the donor, and thus the age of the oocyte, is the most important factor in determining the risk of miscarriage (125). Decreased endometrial receptivity is relatively less important (126).

Müllerian Anomalies

Patients with recurrent miscarriage exhibit a higher than average incidence of uterine anomalies. The least frequent uterine anomaly, the unicornuate uterus, is associated with the greatest incidence of miscarriage (about 50%) (127). The most common uterine anomaly is the arcuate uterus, followed by the septate uterus, and then the bicornuate uterus. The septate or bicornuate uterus is associated with a 30% rate of pregnancy loss (128). It has been suggested that hysteroscopic resection of a septum thicker than 1 cm results in a subsequent successful delivery in more than 80% of ensuing pregnancies (129). However, there have been no prospective randomized trials to confirm this finding.

DES Exposure in Utero

Women exposed to DES during fetal life have impaired reproductive function compared with control subjects. The exact mechanism, although not fully understood, is thought to be a decreased surface area or altered shape of the endometrial cavity. No intervention, including prophylactic cervical cerclage, has been shown to decrease the overall rate of recurrent loss in these women.

Leiomyoma

Buttram and Reiter (130) established that a myomectomy performed for recurrent abortion decreased the loss rate from 40 to 20%. They recommended a myomectomy in women with recurrent pregnancy loss if no other causes could be found. They reiterated the notion that any fibroid greater than 2 cm is a potential cause of abortion. In the investigation of recurrent pregnancy loss, a transvaginal ultrasound is usually performed. If submucous or large intramural fibroids are present, a hysteroscopic resection or abdominal myomectomy is usually offered (131).

The nulliparous female with asymptomatic fibroids offers a clinical dilemma. It seems reasonable that if the fibroids involve a significant portion of the endometrium or compromise the tubal ostia, removal is warranted. Although not based on prospective data, Buttram and Reiter (130) advocated myomectomy for asymptomatic patients with uteri measuring greater than 12 weeks' size.

Incompetent Cervix

The classic description of the incompetent cervix is painless dilation of the internal os leading to pregnancy loss, usually in the second trimester. A history of excessive mechanical cervical dilation at the time of a prior dilation and curettage has been previously described as a cause of cervical incompetence, but it is now thought that, in most cases, it results from a congenital defect in the cervical tissue. The diagnosis is best made by a history of second trimester loss(es) accompanied by spontaneous rupture of membranes but without antecedent uterine contractions.

Asherman's Syndrome

Asherman's syndrome is usually suspected by history and/or characteristic filling defects on hysterosalpingography. The diagnosis is confirmed with hysteroscopy. Intrauterine adhesions are almost always related to a prior dilation and curettage after a pregnancy-related event. Symptoms include menstrual irregularities, infertility, and recurrent abortion. This syndrome is also associated with premature labor, abnormal placentation, and abnormal fetal lie. Many patients may be asymptomatic. The recommended treatment is lysis of the adhesions during hysteroscopy. The abortion rate has been reported to decrease as much as 80% after appropriate treatment (131). Some authors recommend placement of a pediatric Foley catheter in the uterine cavity with subsequent administration of conjugated estrogen (Premarin) 2.5 mg twice daily for 30 to 60 days after hysteroscopic resection. The Foley is removed 3 to 5 days after surgery. The use of prophylactic antibiotics for 1 week postoperatively, usually doxycycline (Vibramycin), is common. The last week of hormonal therapy, medroxyprogesterone acetate (Provera), 10 mg daily for 10 days, is added (132).

Endocrine Causes

Progesterone Deficiency

There is no established consensus on the pathophysiology of luteal phase defects, the method of diagnosis, or its proper treatment. Low hCG and progesterone levels after implantation appear to be the result, not the cause, of pregnancy loss in most cases. Although no randomized controlled trials have had sufficient statistical power to detect a benefit with the use of progesterone vaginal suppositories or intramuscular progesterone in preventing pregnancy loss, a meta-analysis of these studies indicates evidence to support progesterone therapy to decrease pregnancy loss (133). The discrepancy between various trials probably arises from the heterogeneity of causes of luteal inadequacy.

Treatment should be directed at restoring normal folliculogenesis and luteal support. Because of the emotional impact of pregnancy loss and despite a lack of supporting evidence, many clinicians offer empiric treatment with either clomiphene citrate (Clomid, Serophene; 50 mg/day orally on cycle days 5 to 9), progesterone suppositories (25 mg per vagina twice daily through 8 or 9 weeks gestation), or even placebo (117).

Abnormal Thyroid Hormone

Although the traditional workup of recurrent pregnancy loss includes evaluation of thyroid status, several large trials fail to demonstrate clear-cut data on the effects of hypothyroidism and spontaneous abortion. However, the high frequency of hypothyroidism justifies screening with a serum thyroid-stimulating hormone level (134).

Diabetes Mellitus

Diabetes mellitus is also traditionally mentioned in association with an increased abortion rate, but it has been determined in a controlled trial that diabetes with good glucose control (with diet or insulin) does not increase the risk of spontaneous abortion (135). Although oral agents are not prescribed in pregnancy, patients in good control with oral agents before conception will probably have improved outcomes as well. Diabetes with poor glycemic control is associated with an increased risk of early pregnancy loss, and there is a direct correlation between hemoglobin A_{1C} levels and the rate of abortion.

Immunologic Factors

Patients with antiphospholipid antibodies (lupus anticoagulants and anticardiolipin antibodies) are at increased risk for venous and arterial thrombosis resulting in an increased rate of spontaneous abortion and/or intrauterine fetal death. A study by Deleze et al. (136) found that of women with systemic lupus erythematosus and recurrent pregnancy loss, 80% had antiphospholipid antibodies, whereas only 15% of women with lupus but without recurrent pregnancy loss had similar antibodies. Overall, antiphospholipid antibodies are present in 10 to 15% of patients with recurrent pregnancy loss; anticardiolipin antibodies are more common than lupus anticoagulants. In patients with antiphospholipid antibodies, the fetal loss rate approaches 70%.

Several different treatment regimens have been studied, all with the goal to decrease the placental infarction, thrombosis, and fibrin deposition thought responsible for pregnancy loss. The most widely used regimen is prednisone (Deltasone, Orasone), 20 to 60 mg/day, with 80 mg aspirin, and this appears to improve pregnancy outcome significantly. Nevertheless, no prospective, randomized, double-blind, placebo-controlled trials have established that any of these regimens are effective in reducing loss.

The hypothesis that a shared major histocompatibility locus antigen (HLA) may cause failure of the maternal immune system to produce blocking antibodies has not been established as a cause of or an associated risk for pregnancy loss. Although one report demonstrated improved pregnancy outcome in patients immunized with paternal lymphocytes (77 versus 37%), the control group was not adequately matched. Furthermore, the success in the control group still did not approximate the success in most placebo trials (greater than 50%) (137). Therefore, it is not necessary to perform expensive HLA typing on couples with recurrent pregnancy loss, and immunotherapy should be performed only under experimental protocol with informed consent.

Infectious Factors

Various infectious agents have been postulated to be etiologic factors for abortion. However, they likely play only a coincidental role in spontaneous abortion because there have been no placebo-controlled trials proving benefit with antibiotic therapy.

Environmental Factors

Women who smoke more than 14 cigarettes per day have a 1.7 relative risk for spontaneous abortion (138). The influence of alcohol on abortion rate is very small, with only heavy users demonstrating a slightly increased risk. However, both smoking and alcohol have other adverse effects on organogenesis and should be avoided during pregnancy.

DIAGNOSIS, TREATMENT, AND COUNSELING

The expected probability of a woman having three consecutive miscarriages is 0.3 to 0.4%, but the actual incidence range is 0.4 to 0.7%, indicating a distinct cause of recurrent pregnancy loss in some patients. The abortuses of women with greater than three losses are more likely to be chromosomally normal. Regardless of the cause, women with greater than three losses and no liveborn children still have a greater than 50% chance of a successful pregnancy. These facts are essential in counseling couples suffering from recurrent pregnancy loss.

A diagnostic regimen (Table 15.6) should begin with a thorough history and physical examination with specific questions regarding exact gestational age at loss and any possible symptoms of cervical incompetence. Pertinent blood tests include thyroid-

TABLE 15.6. Workup for Recurrent Pregnancy Loss

HISTORY
Past reproductive history (including history of early pregnancy losses)
Previous uterine surgery (including dilation and curettage)
History of thyroid disease or uncontrolled diabetes
History of DES exposure
Exposure to cigarette smoke or environmental toxins
Alcohol intake

LABORATORY TESTS
Thyroid-stimulating hormone
Lupus anticoagulant or activated partial thromboplastin time and anticardiolipin
   antibody titers
Hemoglobin A_{1C} (if patient is diabetic)
Patient and partner karyotypes (optional)
Hysterosalpingogram or hysterosonogram

stimulating hormone, tests to detect lupus anticoagulant activity, and antiphospholipid antibodies. If the patient is a diabetic, a hemoglobin A_{1C} is useful to reflect the level of glucose control. A hysterosalpingogram or hysterosonogram should be performed to diagnose uterine anomalies. If these tests reveal no abnormalities, parental karyotypes can be performed. These tests are very expensive, however, and offer little on which to base a change in management, other than heightened genetic counseling and any appropriate studies during the subsequent pregnancy.

Sympathetic and frequent counseling has improved pregnancy outcome as much or more than any therapeutic intervention, especially in those patients in which an abnormality cannot be identified (139). Unexplained recurrent pregnancy loss is a very frustrating condition, both for the couple and for the practitioner. Many new, as of yet unproved, therapeutic modalities will arise as possible therapies. Therefore, it is imperative that an evidence-based approach as described here serves as a guideline for diagnosis and treatment.

CLINICAL NOTES • Infertility

Epidemiology

- Approximately 13% of U.S. women between the ages of 15 and 44, excluding sterilized women, are infertile. Approximately half of infertile couples eventually conceive.
- The probability of conception in an ovulatory cycle is about 25% under ideal circumstances.

Investigation of the Infertile Couple

- Of causes for infertility, in 40% of cases it is due to a male factor, in 40% of cases it is due to a female factor, and in 20% of cases there are both male and female contributing causes.
- Evaluation of an infertile couple should be individualized, and both the man and the woman need to be evaluated.

Female Factor Infertility

Anovulatory Infertility

- Ovulatory dysfunction and anovulation affect 15 to 20% of all infertile couples seeking therapy.

- Women with infrequent irregular menses should be evaluated for anovulation. If ovulation is uncertain from the history, tests are done to determine if ovulation occurs.
- Tests for ovulation include plasma progesterone levels, urinary LH tests, use of basal body temperature charts, endometrial biopsy, and/or transvaginal sonography.
- Laboratory tests ordered to determine the etiology of anovulation include thyroid-stimulating hormone and prolactin. When indicated, androgen levels and/or 17-hydroxy progesterone levels are obtained.
- In infertility due to hypogonadotropic anovulation, the FSH levels are low, the prolactin is normal, and there is no withdrawal bleed after a progesterone challenge test. Treatment may involve a GnRH pump or use of Pergonal.
- In infertility due to normogonadotropic anovulation, the FSH is normal and there is a withdrawal bleed in response to a progesterone challenge. Most patients have polycystic ovarian disease. Initial treatment is with Clomid, 50 mg/day, starting on cycle day 5 until and including day 9. About 70% of women treated ovulate, with 15 to 40% becoming pregnant. Failure to conceive may indicate the need for use of either dexamethasone, 0.5 mg each morning, or timed induced ovulation via hCG injections.
- In infertility due to hypergonadotropic hypogonadism, FSH levels are usually greater than 20 mIU/mL and there is no response to a progesterone challenge. In women under 40, this indicates premature ovarian failure. In a woman under 30, a karyotype must be done. Treatment involves assisted reproductive technologies.
- In infertility due to hyperprolactinemia, the basal morning prolactin levels exceed 20 to 25 ng/mL. If no concurrent thyroid disorder is present, imaging studies to rule out a prolactinoma must be done. Treatment is with bromocriptine (Parlodel), started at 1.25 mg orally at bedtime for 1 week and increasing thereafter to 2.5 mg orally twice daily. If ovulation still does not occur, the dose is increased in 1.25-mg increments.

Tuboperitoneal Infertility

- Forty percent of all infertile women demonstrate an abnormality of the uterus, cervix, and/or fallopian tubes. Assessment for these potential causes includes an extensive history and physical examination, hysterosalpingography, and some also advocate an antichlamydial antibody titer.
- Most studies show an improvement in pregnancy rates for patients with unexplained infertility with use of the oil-based dye in hysterosalpingography, although the possibility of granuloma formation exists. Some use the oil-based dye therapeutically but only after bilateral patency has been demonstrated with the water-soluble contrast.
- The postcoital test may be used if there is suspicion of a hostile cervical factor contributing to the infertility.
- The office hysteroscopy may be used to detect intrauterine lesions, although some prefer the hysterosonogram for this. Additionally, the hysterosonogram may be able to provide information regarding tubal patency, which the hysteroscopy does not.
- Laparoscopy should be reserved for patients with a history and physical compatible with endometriosis, a positive antichlamydial antibody titer, and abnormalities of the uterus and/or tubes noted on imaging studies.
- Proximal tubal disease was previously treated with laparotomy, although a new technique, hysteroscopic cannulation, shows great promise as an effective therapy.
- With distal tubal disease, the best prognostic factor for pregnancy is the thickness of the tubal wall. For diameters greater than 3 cm, the likelihood of term pregnancy after tubal reconstruction is very poor—only 16%. Most patients with severe tubal disease have poor pregnancy rates after repair, and recommendation for IVF should be made.
- The relationship between fibroids and infertility is poorly understood. Most agree that if the fibroid does not impinge on the uterine cavity (i.e., there is no filling defect on hysterosalpingography), there are no previous pregnancy losses, and they are less than 10 to 12 cm wide, no intervention is necessary. Myomectomy could be justifiable if all diagnostic tests show no other cause of the infertility.

- Treatment of Asherman's syndrome, intrauterine adhesions, results in an 80% term pregnancy rate. Therapy is done via hysteroscopic lysis of adhesions.

Special Topics in Female Infertility

- Controversy regarding the existence and/or clinical significance of luteal phase deficiency continues. It remains unproven if luteal phase support with progesterone or hCG supplementation improves pregnancy rates.
- Current data fail to reveal a cause and effect relationship between ovulation induction and ovarian cancer risk, but until the issue is more fully researched, close clinical surveillance of patients before, during, and after treatment of infertility with these agents is recommended. In the infertile patient over age 30, a basal FSH should be obtained. If it is less than 25 IU/L, a clomiphene citrate challenge test is done. If day 3 or 10 FSH levels are greater than 25 IU/L, the prognosis for conception is very poor.

Male Factor Infertility

- A semen analysis should always be included as an initial screening test for male factor infertility. A careful history and physical examination is done as well.
- The sperm penetration assay is done to attempt to assess sperm function. The validity, reproducibility, and utility of this test is still undefined by available literature, so it should probably not be included in the assessment of the infertile couple. No other tests of sperm function have provided clinicians with a valid method to predict fecundity and so should be discouraged from clinical use.
- For men with a history of testicular trauma, vasectomy reversal, or with clumping on the semen analysis, a test for sperm antibodies may be indicated. If antibodies are found, one effective method of therapy involves sperm washing and intrauterine insemination of the washed sperm either with or without ovulation induction. If this fails, IVF should be considered.
- Although varicoceles are associated with infertility, many men with varicoceles father children. Some propose that surgical intervention should be limited to men reporting pain with the varicocele or for couples with reduced sperm counts and otherwise unexplained infertility.
- The data indicate that treatment for male factor infertility via intrauterine insemination with washed sperm increases fertility only when combined with gonadotropin-stimulated cycles.
- For men with severe oligospermia, intracytoplasmic sperm injection may result in clinical pregnancy rates per cycle of up to 30%.

Unexplained Infertility

- Ten to 15% of infertile couples are ultimately diagnosed with unexplained infertility. Without treatment, up to 60% of couples with unexplained infertility will conceive within 3 years. A treatment regimen of clomiphene citrate for days 5 to 9, followed by hCG to induce ovulation, and performance of intrauterine insemination with washed sperm 36 hours later has shown to augment fertility. This regimen should not be used beyond three cycles because there is no benefit.
- Superovulation and intrauterine insemination have been demonstrated to be of benefit in the treatment of unexplained infertility. If this fails, IVF should follow.

CLINICAL NOTES • Recurrent Pregnancy Loss

- Defined as three pregnancy losses, all at no more than 20 weeks gestation. It is appropriate to initiate evaluation after two such losses.
- Abortions may be attributable to genetic factors, maternal age, müllerian anomalies,

uterine anomalies, endocrine causes, immunologic or environmental factors, or a cause may never be identified.

- Patients and physicians should be encouraged and patients should be counseled that women with three recurrent pregnancy losses still have a greater than 50% chance of successful pregnancy.

References

1. Mosher WD, Pratt EF. The demography of infertility in the United States. In: Asch RH, Studd JW, eds. Annual Progress in Reproductive Medicine. Pearl River, NY: Parthenon, 1993:37–43.
2. Mosher WD, Pratt WF. Fecundity and infertility in the U.S. 1965–82. National Center for Health Statistics Advance Data. Vital and Health Statistics. Washington, DC: Public Health Service, 1985:104.
3. Healy DL, Trounson AO, Andersen AN. Female infertility: causes and treatment. Lancet 1994;343:1539–1544.
4. Hirsch MB, Mosher WD. Characteristics of infertile women in the United States and their use of infertility services. Fertil Steril 1987;47:618–625.
5. Tietze C. Reproductive span and rate of reproduction among Hutterite women. Fertil Steril 1957;8:89–95.
6. Schwartz D, Mayaux MJ. Female fecundity as a function of age: results of artificial insemination in 2193 nulliparous women with azoospermic husbands. Federation CECOS. N Engl J Med 1982;306:404–406.
7. Collins JA, Crosignani PG. Unexplained infertility: a review of diagnosis, prognosis, treatment efficacy and management. Int J Gynaecol Obstet 1992;39:267–275.
8. Magyar DM, Boyers SP, Marshall JR, et al. Regular menstrual cycles and premenstrual molimina as indicators of ovulation. Obstet Gynecol 1979;53:411–414.
9. Hull MG, Glazener CM, Kelly NJ, et al. Population study of causes, treatment, and outcome of infertility. BMJ (Clin Res Ed) 1985;291:1693–1697.
10. Guttmacher AF. Factors affecting normal expectancy of conception. JAMA 1956;161: 855.
11. Prevention of neural tube defects: results of the Medical Research Council Vitamin Study. MRC Vitamin Study Research Group. Lancet 1991;338:131–137.
12. The European Society for Human Reproduction and Embryology (ESHRE) Workshops. Guidelines to the Prevalence, Diagnosis, Treatment and Management of Infertility, 1996. Hum Reprod 1996;11:1779–1802.
13. Fritz MA, McLachlan RI, Cohen NL, et al. Onset and characteristics of the midcycle surge in bioactive and immunoactive luteinizing periovulatory ovarian steroid hormone secretion. J Clin Endocrinol Metab 1992;75:489–493.
14. Hull MG, Savage PE, Bromham DR, et al. The value of a single serum progesterone measurement in the midluteal phase as a criterion of a potentially fertile cycle ("ovulation") derived from treated and untreated conception cycles. Fertil Steril 1982;37:355–360.
15. Miller PB, Soules MR. The usefulness of a urinary LH kit for ovulation prediction during menstrual cycles of normal women. Obstet Gynecol 1996; 87:13–17.
16. Batzer FR, Corson SL. Indications, techniques, success rates, and pregnancy outcome: new directions with donor insemination. Semin Reprod Endocrinol 1987;5:45–52.
17. World Health Organization. Temporal relationships between ovulation and defined changes in the concentration of plasma estradiol-17β luteinizing hormone, follicle stimulating hormone and progesterone. I. Probit analysis. Am J Obstet Gynecol 1980;138: 383–390.
18. Lundy LE, Lee SG, Levy W, et al. The ovulatory cycle: a histologic, thermal, steroid and gonadotropin correlation. Obstet Gynecol 1974;44:14–25.
19. Batzer FR. Ultrasonographic indices of ovulation. J Reprod Med 1986;31:764–769.
20. Balasch J, Miro F, Burzaco J. The role of luteinizing hormone in human follicle development and oocyte fertility: evidence from in-vitro fertilization in a woman with long-

standing hypogonadotropic hypogonadism and using recombinant human follicle stimulating hormone. Hum Reprod 1995;10:1678–1683.

21. Clark AM, Ledger W, Galletly C, et al. Weight loss results in significant improvement in pregnancy and ovulation rates in anovulatory obese women. Hum Reprod 1995;10: 2705–2712.

22. Kerin JF, Lieu JH, Phillipou G, et al. Evidence for a hypothalamic site of action of clomiphene citrate in women. J Clin Endocrinol Metab 1985;61:265–268.

23. March CM. Ovulation induction. J Reprod Med 1993;38:335–346.

24. Gysler M, March CM, Mishell DR, et al. A decade's experience with an individualized clomiphene treatment regimen including its effect on the postcoital test. Fertil Steril 1982;37:164–167.

25. Lobo RA, Granger LR, Davajan V, et al. An extended regimen of clomiphene citrate in women unresponsive to standard therapy. Fertil Steril 1982;37:762–766.

26. Dickey RP, Holtkamp DE. Development, pharmacology and clinical experience with clomiphene citrate. Hum Reprod Update 1996;2:483–506.

27. Shoham Z, Zosmer A, Insler V. Early miscarriage and fetal malformations after induction of ovulation (by clomiphene citrate and/or human menopausal gonadotropins), in vitro fertilization, and gamete intrafallopian tube transfer. Fertil Steril 1991;55:1–11.

28. Dickey RP, Taylor SN, Curole DN, et al. Incidence of spontaneous abortion in clomiphene pregnancies. Hum Reprod 1996;11:2623–2628.

29. Blacker CM. Ovulation stimulation and induction. Endocrinol Metab Clin North Am 1992;21:57–84.

30. Pepperell BJ. A rational approach to ovulation induction. In: Wallach EE, Kempers RD, eds. Modern Trends in Infertility and Conception Control. Vol. 3. Chicago: Year Book Medical Publishers, 1985:250–285.

31. Baird DT. Amenorrhoea, anovulation and dysfunctional uterine bleeding. In: Degroot LJ, ed. Endocrinology. Vol. 3. 3rd ed. London: WB Saunders, 1995:2059–2079.

32. Layman LC, Reindollar RH. The genetics of hypogonadism. Infertil Reprod Med Clin North Am 1994;1:53–68.

33. Matsuzaki T, Azuma K, Irahara M, et al. Mechanism of anovulation in hyperprolactinemic amenorrhea determined by pulsatile gonadotropin-releasing hormone injection combined with human chorionic gonadotropin. Fertil Steril 1994;62:1143–1149.

34. Collins JA, Hughes EG. Pharmacologic interventions for the induction of ovulation. Drugs 1995;50:480–494.

35. Al-Suleiman SA, Najashi S, Rahman J, et al. Outcome of treatment with bromocriptine in patients with hyperprolactinemia. Aust N Z J Obstet Gynaecol 1989;29:176–179.

36. Padilla SL, Person GK, McDonough PG, et al. The efficacy of bromocriptine in patients with ovulatory dysfunction and normoprolactinemic galactorrhea. Fertil Steril 1985;44:695–698.

37. Vermesh M, Fossum GT, Kletzky OA. Vaginal bromocriptine: pharmacology and effect on serum prolactin in normal women. Obstet Gynecol 1988;72:693–698.

38. Fluker MR, Urman B, Mackinnon M, et al. Exogenous gonadotropin therapy in World Health Organization groups I and II ovulatory disorders. Obstet Gynecol 1994;83:189–196.

39. March CM. Improved pregnancy rate with monitoring of gonadotropin therapy by three modalities. Am J Obstet Gynecol 1987;156:1473–1479.

40. Bahamondes L, Bueno JG, Hardy E, et al. Identification of main risk factors for tubal infertility. Fertil Steril 1994;61:478–482.

41. Dabekausen YA, Evers JL, Land JA, et al. *Chlamydia trachomatis* antibody testing is more accurate than hysterosalpingography in predicting tubal factor infertility. Fertil Steril 1994;61:833–837.

42. Westrom L. Incidence, prevalence, and trends of acute pelvic inflammatory disease and its consequences in industrialized countries. Am J Obstet Gynecol 1980;138:880–892.

43. Cetin MT, Vardar MA, Aridogan N, et al. Role of *Chlamydia trachomatis* infections in infertility due to tubal factor. Indian J Med Res 1992;95:139–143.

44. Mol BW, Dijkman B, Wertheim P, et al. The accuracy of serum chlamydial antibodies in the diagnosis of tubal pathology: a meta-analysis. Fertil Steril 1997;67:1031–1037.

45. Spring DB, Boll DA. Prone hysterosalpingography. Radiology 1980;136:235–236.

46. Stumpf PG, March CM. Febrile morbidity following hysterosalpingography: identification of risk factors and recommendations for prophylaxis. Fertil Steril 1980;33:487–492.

47. Pittaway DE, Winfield AC, Maxson W, et al. Prevention of acute pelvic inflammatory disease after hysterosalpingography: efficacy of doxycycline prophylaxis. Am J Obstet Gynecol 1983;147:623–626.

48. Rasmussen F, Lindequist S, Larsen C, et al. Therapeutic effect of hysterosalpingography: oil- versus water-soluble contrast media—a randomized prospective study. Radiology 1991;179:75–78.

49. Schwabe MG, Shapire SS, Haning RV Jr. Hysterosalpingography with oil contrast medium enhances fertility in patients with infertility of unknown etiology. Fertil Steril 1983;40:604–606.

50. Alper MM, Garner PR, Spence EH, et al. Pregnancy rates after hysterosalpingography with oil and water soluble contrast media. Obstet Gynecol 1986;68:6–9.

51. Mackey RA, Glass RH, Olson LE, et al. Pregnancy following hysterosalpingography with oil and water soluble dye. Fertil Steril 1971;22:504–507.

52. Swart P, Mol BW, van der Veen F, et al. The accuracy of hysterosalpingography in the diagnosis of tubal pathology: a meta analysis. Fertil Steril 1995;64:486–491.

53. Raziel A, Arieli S, Bukovsky I, et al. Investigation of the uterine cavity in recurrent aborters. Fertil Steril 1994;62:1080–1083.

54. Hull MG, Savage PE, Bromham DR. Prognostic value of the postcoital test: prospective study based on time-specific conception rates. Br J Obstet Gynaecol 1982;89:299–305.

55. Eimers JM, te Velde ER, Gerritse R, et al. The validity of the postcoital test for estimating the probability of conceiving. Am J Obstet Gynecol 1994;171: 65–70.

56. Griffith CS, Grimes DA. The validity of the postcoital test. Am J Obstet Gynecol 1990;62:615–620.

57. Collins JA, So Y, Wilson EH, et al. The postcoital test as a predictor of pregnancy among 355 infertile couples. Fertil Steril 1984;41:703–708.

58. Nagele F, O'Connor H, Daview A, et al. 2500 outpatient diagnostic hysteroscopies. Obstet Gynecol 1996,88:87–92.

59. Hutchins CJ. Laparoscopy and hysterosalpingography in the assessment of tubal patency. Obstet Gynecol 1977;49:325–327.

60. Rubin RD, Hurst BS, Schlaff WE. Predictive value of fluid contrast ultrasound (sonohysterography) in diagnosis of intrauterine lesions. Poster, P–121, American Society of Reproductive Medicine meeting, University of Colorado Health Sciences Center, Denver, 1996.

61. Ayida G, Chamberlain P, Barlow D, et al. Uterine cavity assessment prior to in vitro fertilization: comparison of transvaginal scanning, saline contrast, hysterosonography and hysteroscopy. Ultrasound Obstet Gynecol 1997;10:59–62.

62. Benadiva CA, Kligman I, David O, et al. In vitro fertilization versus tubal surgery: is pelvic reconstructive surgery obsolete? Fertil Steril 1995;64:1051–1061.

63. Musich JR, Behrman SJ. Surgical management of tubal obstruction of the uterotubal junction. Fertil Steril 1983;40:423–441.

64. Risquez F, Confino E. Transcervical tubal cannulation, past, present, and future. Fertil Steril 1993;60:211–226.

65. Schlaff WD, Hassiakos DK, Damewood MD, et al. Neosalpingostomy for distal tubal obstruction: prognostic factor and impact of surgical technique. Fertil Steril 1990;54:984–990.

66. Donnez J, Casanas-Roux F. Prognostic factors of fimbrial microsurgery. Fertil Steril 1986;46:1089–1092.

67. Dlugi AM, Reddy S, Saleh WA, et al. Pregnancy rates after operative endoscopic treatment of total (neosalpingostomy) or near total (salpingostomy) distal tubal occlusion. Fertil Steril 1994;62:913–920.

68. The American Fertility Society classification of adnexal adhesions, distal tubal occlusion, tubal occlusion secondary to tubal ligation, tubal pregnancies, müllerian anomalies and intrauterine adhesions. Fertil Steril 1988;49:944–955.

69. Rock JA, Katayama P, Martin EJ, et al. Factors influencing the success of salpingostomy techniques for distal fimbrial obstruction. Obstet Gynecol 1978;52:591–596.

70. Holst N, Maltau JM, Forsdahl F, et al. Handling of tubal infertility after introduction of in vitro fertilization: changes and consequences. Fertil Steril 1991;55:140–143.

71. Assisted reproductive technology in the United States and Canada: 1993 results generated from the American Society for Reproductive Medicine/Society for Assisted Reproductive Technology Registry. Fertil Steril 1995;64:13–21.

72. Hughes EG, Fedorkow DM, Collins JA. A quantitative overview of controlled trials in endometriosis-associated infertility. Fertil Steril 1993;59:963–970.

73. Marcoux S, Maheux R, Berube S. Laparoscopic surgery in infertile women with minimal or mild endometriosis. Canadian Collaborative Group on Endometriosis. N Engl J Med 1997;337:217–222.

74. Farrer-Brown G, Beilby JO, Tarbit MH. Venous changes in the endometrium of myomatous uteri. Obstet Gynecol 1971;38:743–751.

75. Deligdish L, Lowenthal M. Endometrial changes associated with myomata of the uterus. J Clin Pathol 1970;23:676–680.

76. Buttram VC Jr. Uterine leiomyomata—aetiology, symptomatology and management. Prog Clin Biol Res 1986;225:275–296.

77. Valle RF, Sciarra JJ. Intrauterine adhesions: hysteroscopic diagnosis, classification, treatment, and reproductive outcome. Am J Obstet Gynecol 1988;158:1459–1470.

78. Spirtos NJ, Yurewicz EC, Moghissi KS, et al. Pseudocorpus luteum insufficiency: a study of cytosol progesterone receptors in human endometrium. Obstet Gynecol 1985;65:535–540.

79. Jordan J, Craig K, Clifton DK, et al. Luteal phase defect: the sensitivity and specificity of diagnostic methods in common clinical use. Fertil Steril 1994;62:54–62.

80. Soliman S, Daya S, Collins J, et al. The role of luteal phase support in infertility treatment: a meta-analysis of randomized trials. Fertil Steril 1994;61:1068–1076.

81. Bristow RE, Karlan BY. Ovulation induction, infertility and ovarian cancer risk. Fertil Steril 1996;66:499–507.

82. Pearlstone AC, Fournet N, Gambone JG, et al. Ovulation induction in women age 40 and older: the importance of basal follicle stimulating hormone level and chronological age. Fertil Steril 1992;58:674–679.

83. Scott RT, Leonardi MR, Hofmann GE, et al. A prospective evaluation of clomiphene citrate challenge test screening of the general infertility population. Obstet Gynecol 1993;82:539–544.

84. World Health Organization. Laboratory Manual for the Examination of Human Semen and Sperm-Cervical Mucus Interaction. 3rd ed. Cambridge: Cambridge University Press, 1992:44–45.

85. Goldenberg RL, White R. The effect of vaginal lubricants on sperm motility in vitro. Fertil Steril 1975;26:872–872.

86. Fisch H, Lipshultz LI. Diagnosing male factors of infertility. Arch Pathol Lab Med 1992;116:398–405.

87. Matilsky M, Battino S, Ben-Ami M, et al. The effect of ejaculatory frequency on semen characteristics of normospermic and oligospermic men from an infertile population. Hum Reprod 1993;8:71–73.

88. Mahadevan MM, Trounson AO. The influence of seminal characteristics on the success rate of human in vitro fertilization. Fertil Steril 1984;42:400–405.

89. Bartoov B, Eltes F, Pansky M, et al. Estimating fertility potential via semen analysis data. Hum Reprod 1993;8:65–70.

90. Huang HY, Lee C, Lai Y, et al. The impact of the total motile sperm count on the success of intrauterine insemination with husband's spermatozoa. J Assist Reprod Genet 1996;13:56–63.

91. Mao C, Grimes DA. The sperm penetration assay: can it discriminate between fertile and infertile men? Am J Obstet Gynecol 1988;159:279–286.
92. Margalioth EJ, Feinmesser M, Navot D, et al. The long term predictive value of the zona-free hamster ova sperm penetration assay. Fertil Steril 1989;52:490–494.
93. Adeghe JH. Male subfertility due to sperm antibodies: a clinical overview. Obstet Gynecol Surv 1993;48:1–8.
94. Lahteenmaki A, Veilahti J, Hovatta O. Intrauterine insemination versus cyclic low dose prednisolone in couples with male antisperm antibodies. Hum Reprod 1995;10:142–147.
95. Nachtigall LB, Boepple PA, Pralong FP, et al. Adult-onset idiopathic hypogonadotropic hypogonadism—a treatable form of male infertility. N Engl J Med 1997;336:410–415.
96. O'Donovan PA, Vandekerckhove P, Lilford RJ, et al. Treatment of male infertility: is it effective? Review and meta-analysis of published randomized controlled trials. Hum Reprod 1993;8:1209–1222.
97. Gorelick JI, Goldstein M. Loss of fertility in men with varicocele. Fertil Steril 1993;59: 613–616.
98. Laven JS, Haans LC, Mali WP, et al. Effects of varicocele treatment in adolescents: a randomized study. Fertil Steril 1992;58:756–762.
99. Marks JL, McMahon R, Lipshultz LI. Predictive parameters of successful varicocele repair. J Urol 1986;136:609–612.
100. Madgar I, Weissenberg R, Lunenfeld B, et al. Controlled trial of high spermatic vein ligation for varicocele in infertile men. Fertil Steril 1995;63:120–124.
101. Schlesinger MH, Wilets IF, Nager HM. Treatment outcome after varicocelectomy: a critical analysis. Urol Clin North Am 1994;21:517–529.
102. Hargreave TB. Debate on the pros and cons of varicocele treatment: In favor of varicocele treatment. Hum Reprod 1995;10(suppl 1):151–157.
103. Gregoriou O, Vitoratos N, Papadias C, et al. Pregnancy rates in gonadotrophin stimulated cycles with timed intercourse or intrauterine insemination for the treatment of male subfertility. Eur J Obstet Gynaecol Reprod Biol 1996;64:213–216.
104. Melis GB, Pauletti AM, Ajossa S, et al. Ovulation induction with gonadotropins as sole treatment in infertile couples with open tubes: a randomized prospective comparison between intrauterine insemination and timed vaginal intercourse. Fertil Steril 1995;64:1088–1093.
105. Van Steirteghem A, Liu J, Nagy Z, et al. Use of assisted fertilization. Hum Reprod 1993; 8:1784–1785.
106. Shenfield F, Doyle P, Valentine A, et al. Effects of age, gravidity and male infertility status on cumulative conception rates following artificial insemination with cryopreserved donor sperm: analysis of 2998 cycles of treatment in one centre over 10 years. Hum Reprod 1993;8:60–64.
107. Lobo RA. Unexplained infertility. J Reprod Med 1993;38:241–249.
108. Crosignani PG, Collins J, Cooke ID, et al. Unexplained infertility. Hum Reprod 1993;8: 977–980.
109. Scott RT, Leonardi MR, Hofmann GE, et al. A prospective evaluation of clomiphene citrate challenge test screening of the general infertility population. Obstet Gynecol 1993;82:539–544.
110. Glazener CMA, Coulson C, Lambert PA, et al. Clomiphene treatment for women with unexplained infertility: placebo-controlled study of hormonal responses and conception rates. Gynecol Endocrinol 1990;4:75–83.
111. Deaton JL, Gibson M, Blackmer KM, et al. A randomized, controlled trial of clomiphene citrate and intrauterine insemination in couples with unexplained infertility or surgically corrected endometriosis. Fertil Steril 1990;54:1083–1088.
112. Dodson WC, Whitesides DB, Hughes CL Jr, et al. Superovulation with intrauterine insemination in the treatment of infertility: a possible alternative to gamete intrafallopian transfer and in vitro fertilization. Fertil Steril 1987;48:441–445.
113. Kim CH, Cho YK, Mok JE. The efficacy of immunotherapy in patients who underwent superovulation with intrauterine insemination. Fertil Steril 1996;65:133–138.

114. Berry CW, Brambati B, Eskes TK, et al. The Euro-Team Early Pregnancy (ETEP) protocol for recurrent miscarriage. Hum Reprod 1995;10:1516–1520.

115. Wilcox AJ, Weinberg CR, O'Connor JF, et al. Incidence of early loss of pregnancy. N Engl J Med 1988;319:189–194.

116. Regan L, Braude PR, Trembath PL. Influence of past reproductive performance on risk of spontaneous abortion. Br Med J 1989;299:541–545.

117. Mishell DR. Recurrent abortion. J Reprod Med 1993;38:250–259.

118. Poland BJ, Miller JR, Jones DC, et al. Reproductive counseling in patients who have had a spontaneous abortion. Am J Obstet Gynecol 1977;127:685–691.

119. James WH. On the possibility of segregation in the propensity to spontaneous abortion in the human female. Ann Hum Genet 1961;25:207–210.

120. McDonough PG. Repeated first-trimester loss: evaluation and management. Am J Obstet Gynecol 1985;153:1–6.

121. Boue J, Boue A, Lazar P. Retrospective and prospective epidemiological studies of 1500 karyotyped spontaneous human abortions. Teratology 1975;12:11–26.

122. Drugan A, Koppitch FC, Williams JC, et al. Prenatal genetic diagnosis following early pregnancy loss. Obstet Gynecol 1990;75:381–384.

123. De Braekeleer M, Dao TN. Cytogenetic studies in couples experiencing repeated pregnancy losses. Hum Reprod 1990;5:519–528.

124. Guerro R, Rojas OI. Spontaneous abortion and aging of human ova and spermatozoa. N Engl J Med 1975;293:573–575.

125. Levran D, Ben-Schlomo I, Dor J, et al. Aging of endometrium and oocytes: observations on conception and abortion in an egg donation model. Fertil Steril 1991;56:1092–1094.

126. Check JH, Askari HA, Fisher C, et al. The use of a shared donor oocyte program to evaluate the effect of uterine senescence. Fertil Steril 1994;61:252–256.

127. Heinonen PK, Saarikoski S, Pystynen P. Reproductive performance of women with uterine anomalies. Acta Obstet Gynaecol Scand 1982;61:157–162.

128. Buttram VC, Gibbons WE. Müllerian anomalies: a proposed classification (an analysis of 144 cases). Fertil Steril 1979;32:40–46.

129. Fedele L, Arcaini L, Parazzini F, et al. Reproductive prognosis after hysteroscopic metroplasty in 102 women: life table analysis. Fertil Steril 1993;59:768–772.

130. Buttram VC Jr, Reiter RC. Uterine leiomyomata: etiology, symptomatology, and management. Fertil Steril 1981;36:433–445.

131. Valle RF, Sciarra JJ. Intrauterine adhesions: hysteroscopic diagnosis, classification, treatment and reproductive outcome. Am J Obstet Gynecol 1988;158:1459–1470.

132. March CM, Israel R. Intrauterine adhesions secondary to elective abortion: hysteroscopic diagnosis and management. Obstet Gynecol 1976;48:422–424.

133. Goldstein P, Berrier J, Rosen S, et al. A meta-analysis of randomized control trials of progestational agents in pregnancy. Br J Obstet Gynaecol 1989;96:265–274.

134. Montoro M, Collea JV, Frasier SD, et al. Successful outcome of pregnancy in women with hypothyroidism. Ann Intern Med 1981;94:31–34.

135. Rosen B, Miodovnik M, Combs CA, et al. Preconception management of insulin-dependent diabetes: improvement of pregnancy outcome. Obstet Gynecol 1991;77:846–853.

136. Deleze M, Alarcon-Segovia D, Valdes-Macho E, et al. Relationship between antiphospholipid antibodies and recurrent fetal loss in patients with systemic lupus erythematosus and apparently healthy women. J Rheumatol 1989;16:768–772.

137. Mowbray JF, Gibbings C, Liddell H, et al. Controlled trial of treatment of recurrent spontaneous abortion by immunization with paternal cells. Lancet 1985;1:941–946.

138. Kline J, Stein ZA, Susser M, et al. Smoking: a risk factor for spontaneous abortion. N Engl J Med 1977;297:793–796.

139. Stray-Pedersen B, Stray-Pedersen S. Etiologic factors and subsequent reproductive performance in 195 couples with a prior history of habitual abortion. Am J Obstet Gynecol 1984;148:140–146.

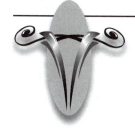

CHAPTER 16

Urogynecology

NICOLETTE S. HORBACH

Urogynecology encompasses the evaluation and treatment of conditions that adversely affect the lower genitourinary tract in women and produce an array of symptoms. Most commonly, these pelvic symptoms may be classified as due to urinary incontinence, pelvic organ prolapse, irritative bladder complaints, urinary retention, or a combination of these problems. These lower urinary tract disorders can produce profound psychosocial and financial impacts on affected women and their families. Women may experience embarrassment, depression, loss of self-esteem, loss of productivity, and, at times, social isolation because of their disease (1). Unfortunately, many women are reluctant to discuss their symptoms with a physician or find their physician ill-equipped to address these problems. It is incumbent on physicians to question their patients regarding symptoms of lower urinary tract dysfunction and to appropriately workup these symptoms.

URINARY INCONTINENCE

Urinary incontinence is defined by the International Continence Society as the "involuntary loss of urine which is objectively demonstrable and a social or hygienic problem" (2). Importantly, the leakage of urine must be clinically significant to the patient but not necessarily to the physician. Although studies vary, urinary incontinence has been reported to affect up to 26% of reproductive-age women and 30 to 42% of women in the postmenopausal years (3). A wide array of disorders can produce urinary incontinence, often with a myriad of overlapping and confusing symptoms. A thorough office evaluation can clarify the diagnosis in most patients and identify the remainder of women who require more sophisticated urodynamic or radiographic testing.

Differential Diagnosis

Urinary incontinence most commonly occurs when the pressure in the bladder exceeds the pressure in the urethra, excluding the act of micturition. Table 16.1 summarizes the factors associated with an increase in expulsive forces of the bladder, leading to incontinence. The most commonly encountered problem in this category is idiopathic detrusor instability due to uninhibited detrusor contractions, which primarily produce the symptom of urge incontinence. Bladder atony due to neurologic disease or bladder outlet obstruction (less common in women than men) result in urinary retention and may produce overflow urinary incontinence with elevated urinary postvoid residuals.

A decrease in retentive forces of the bladder leads to a decrease in urethral resistance to the flow of urine. A number of factors that may contribute to this problem are shown in Table 16.2. The primary symptom associated with a decrease in retentive forces of the bladder is stress incontinence. Office and laboratory investigations are necessary to confirm the presence of stress incontinence and to establish the diagnosis of genuine stress incontinence. Genuine stress incontinence is defined by the In-

TABLE 16.1. Etiologies of Active and Passive Increases of Expulsive Forces

Active	Passive
UNINHIBITED DETRUSOR CONTRACTIONS *Idiopathic*	**DECREASED BLADDER WALL COMPLIANCE** *Radiation fibrosis*
Neurologic Cerebrovascular disease Multiple sclerosis Parkinson's disease Senile dementia Meningomyelocele Tumors	*Intrinsic vesical disease* Recurrent infection Interstitial cystitis *Extrinsic pelvic disease*
Local Infection or irritation Foreign body (calculi, suture) Bladder tumors	**BLADDER ATONY** *Neurologic* Lower motor neuron lesion Automatic neuropathy
Pharmacologic Parasympathomimetics	*Endocrine* Hypothyroidism
Psychological	*Recurrent vesical overdistention*

TABLE 16.2. Etiologies of Decreased Retentive Forces

ANATOMIC Urethral hypermobility Decreased urethral closure pressure Decreased urethral length Postoperative urethral scarring (rigid urethra)	**PHARMACOLOGIC** α-Adrenergic blockers β-Adrenergic stimulators
PHYSIOLOGIC Pregnancy Menopause	**INFECTION** **NEUROLOGIC DISEASE**

ternational Continence Society as "the socially unacceptable, involuntary loss of urine that occurs when intravesical pressure exceeds maximum urethral pressure in the absence of detrusor activity" (2).

One of the most important causes of genuine stress incontinence is the anatomic relaxation of the supporting tissues of the urethra, bladder, and urethrovesical junction causing the proximal urethra to be displaced outside the intraabdominal cavity (4). This displacement may occur because of the effects of pregnancy and delivery or because of advancing age with its incumbent tissue changes (5, 6). In this situation, any increases in intraabdominal pressure with a stressful activity that normally should be transmitted equally to the urethra and bladder is transmitted appropriately to the bladder but suboptimally to the urethra. Thus, intravesical pressure exceeds intraurethral pressure with resultant leakage of urine.

Childbirth has also been reported to produce partial denervation of the nerves supplying the urethra because of stretching of the distal portion of the pudendal nerve during the pushing stage of labor for vaginal delivery (6, 7). Hypoestrogenic changes of the genitourinary system after menopause may contribute to stress incontinence by a number of mechanisms that prevent adequate closure of the urethra and lead to relaxation of the estrogen-dependent urethral and periurethral muscular tissue and connective tissue supports (8, 9).

Uncommon causes for urinary incontinence are the presence of a urinary fistula (ureterovaginal, vesicovaginal, or urethrovaginal), an ectopic ureter, or a urinary diverticulum. Fistulas or ectopic ureters traditionally cause continuous urinary leakage or constant wetness, which is relatively easily diagnosed. Urethral diverticulum may produce postmicturition dribbling as the urine that is trapped within the diverticular sac subsequently empties on standing. A diverticulum may also be diagnosed by the discovery of a painful suburethral mass or the development of recurrent urinary tract infections from chronic infections of the diverticulum.

Diagnosis

Considerable controversy exists in the literature regarding the optimal clinical investigation of patients with lower urinary tract symptoms, including urinary incontinence (10–20). At the very least, a detailed history and physical examination, residual urine measurement with urinalysis and culture, a stress test, assessment of urethrovesical junction mobility, and a cystometrogram should be done.

History

A detailed medical, gynecologic, and urologic history must be obtained in all women with lower urinary tract symptoms. A history of diabetes mellitus, thyroid disease, multiple sclerosis, prior cerebrovascular accidents, back pain, or back injuries suggests that the patient's symptoms may be due to an underlying neurologic abnormality. The patient's parity, mode of deliveries, and previous gynecologic procedures must be ascertained to determine any detrimental effects on lower urinary tract function. Commonly prescribed drugs that can affect the lower urinary tract are listed in Table 16.3. Alterations in the dosage or type of drug administered may be all that is required to alleviate the patient's symptoms.

Determination of the onset and duration of urinary symptoms is important in clarifying a patient's diagnosis. The abrupt onset of stress or urge incontinence may indicate an allergic or infectious process, whereas the gradual onset of symptoms, especially after oophorectomy or menopause, may imply estrogen deficiency. Involuntary loss of urine prompted by coughing, laughing, sneezing, vigorous physical activity, or a change in position is consistent with the diagnosis of stress incontinence but may also be seen on occasion in patients with detrusor instability. Based on history, stress incontinence is determined to be severe if the patient experiences urinary leakage in the supine position with a relatively empty bladder or requires continuous perineal pad protection. Except in severe cases, most women with genuine stress incontinence should be able to voluntarily interrupt their urinary stream during voiding.

Symptoms of urgency, frequency, nocturia, or urge incontinence may be reported in women with stress incontinence, detrusor instability, or a combination of both problems. Urgency is defined as a strong desire to void that is accompanied by the fear of impending urinary leakage or the fear of pain. The term "urinary fre-

TABLE 16.3. Common Medications Associated with Urinary Incontinence

MEDICATIONS THAT MAY CAUSE STRESS INCONTINENCE BY DECREASING URETHRAL SMOOTH OR SKELETAL MUSCLE TONE
α-Methyldopa (Aldomet)
Prazosin (Minipress)
Phenothiazines
Diazepam (Valium)
Sympathomimetics (decongestants)
Calcium channel blockers

MEDICATIONS THAT MAY CAUSE OVERFLOW INCONTINENCE WITH URINARY RETENTION BY RELAXATION OF THE DETRUSOR MUSCLE
Antihistamines
Anticholinergic therapies
Antidepressants
Antispasmodics

MEDICATIONS THAT MAY WORSEN URGE INCONTINENCE BY EXACERBATING DETRUSOR INSTABILITY
Alcohol
Caffeine

MEDICATIONS THAT MAY WORSEN URGE AND STRESS INCONTINENCE
Diuretics

quency" is used when the patient voids more than seven times in 24 hours, assuming a normal fluid intake. Nocturia is defined as being woken from sleep by the urge to void two or more times per night. The leakage of large volumes of urine or a history of nocturnal enuresis (bed wetting) suggests the presence of an unstable bladder. Table 16.4 contrasts the clinical history in patients with genuine stress incontinence and detrusor instability. Constant urinary leakage implies a functionless urethra, fistula, or ectopic ureter.

Although an accurate history is helpful in guiding the physician's diagnostic evaluation, therapeutic decisions should not be based on history alone. Lower urinary tract symptoms are notoriously nonspecific and overlapping (11–17). As previously discussed, patients with systemic or psychiatric disorders may present with urinary complaints without associated urologic disease. Numerous studies found that the diagnosis of genuine stress incontinence based on history alone is correct in only 50 to 88% of cases, underscoring the fact that history alone is unreliable for this diagnosis (18–20). Because the treatment of genuine stress incontinence traditionally involves surgery, it is essential that each incontinent patient undergo the appropriate office evaluation to establish a correct diagnosis and to detect any alternative nonsurgical explanations for her urinary leakage.

Urolog

A voiding diary or urolog is one of the most important aspects of a urogynecologic investigation (Fig. 16.1). Patients are sent home with a voiding chart and instructions and a measuring container that can fit on her toilet seat. She is asked to record the time and volume of her spontaneous voids over 24 to 72 hours. Additional informa-

TABLE 16.4. Comparison of Presenting Symptoms in Patients with Genuine Stress Incontinence and Detrusor Instability

Symptom	Genuine Stress Incontinence	Detrusor Instability
Precipitating factor	Cough, lift, exercise position change	Preceding urge, position change
Timing of leakage	Immediate	Delayed
Amount of leakage	Small→large	Large
Voluntary inhibition	Frequently	Possibly
Urgency, frequency	Occasionally	Yes
Nocturia	Rarely	Yes
Spontaneous remissions	No	Occasionally

VOIDING DIARY

Time	Amount Voided	Activity	Leak Volume	Urge Present	Amount/Type of Intake

FIGURE 16.1. Example of a voiding diary or urolog. Patients are instructed to complete the diary for 24 to 72 hours. (Reprinted with permission from Ostergard DR, Bent AK. Urogynecology and Urodynamics: Theory and Practice. 4th ed. Baltimore: Williams & Wilkins, 1996:682.)

tion regarding urgency before voids, frequency of incontinent episodes, activity precipitating incontinence, and the type and volume of fluid intake are also recorded. From this journal, vital information regarding the patient's normal voiding pattern, functional bladder capacity, and the severity of her incontinence episodes or irritative symptoms can be obtained. The findings from the urolog can be used to adjust fluid intake in older patients with nocturnal frequency or to begin a timed voiding schedule in a woman with detrusor instability. Occasionally, the voiding pattern may alert the clinician to the possibility of diabetes insipidus or anxiety-related diurnal frequency in a patient who sleeps through the night without problems. Thus, a urolog is an inexpensive noninvasive evaluation of lower urinary tract function that should be obtained early in the course of all urologic evaluations.

Physical Examination

Once a complete history is obtained, clinical evaluation of the lower urinary tract should begin with a screening neurologic examination to detect sensory or motor nerve dysfunction of the bladder or urethra. The T10 to S4 nerve roots are primarily responsible for control of micturition. An examination of the lower extremity functions dependent on these nerve roots provides indirect evidence regarding bladder function (Fig. 16.2). Motor function can be assessed by flexion and extension maneuvers against resistance at the ankle, knee, and hip. Pelvic floor muscle tone can be determined by voluntary contraction of the rectal sphincter and vagina. Normal sensation in the upper leg and perineal dermatomes confirms intact sensory innervation of the lower urinary tract. Finally, reflex contraction of the pelvic floor in response to light stroking of the anus or clitoris, seen as the "anal wink" reflex, and bulbocavernosus reflexes provide evidence of the integrity of the sacral reflex center. Findings suggestive of neurologic deficits should be referred for formal neurologic evaluation.

The pelvic examination should assess the patient's estrogen status and detect the presence of any concomitant pelvic relaxation. The urethra, trigone, and vagina are estrogen-dependent structures. Thus, hypoestrogenic changes of the vaginal mucosa indicate similar changes in the urethra and periurethral tissues. The resultant loss of urethral tone and connective tissue support may be corrected by vaginal estrogen replacement, preferably 1 g conjugated vaginal estrogen cream two to three times per week at bedtime. Vaginal estrogen may be required even in women on oral estrogen replacement.

Inspection of the anterior and posterior vaginal walls using the lower blade of a bivalve vaginal speculum facilitates the identification of any cystocele, rectocele, or enterocele. Although the extent of pelvic relaxation may influence the surgeon's choice of operative approach in patients with urinary leakage, a defect in the anterior vaginal wall support does not confirm the diagnosis of genuine stress incontinence. Fischer-Rasmussen et al. (14) reported no correlation between the presence of genital prolapse and the diagnosis of genuine stress incontinence (sensitivity 72%, specificity 46%). The possibility of a urethral diverticulum or urinary fistula must also be considered during the examination. Palpation of the urethra and bladder trigone may reveal tenderness consistent with acute or chronic inflammation of either structure. Bimanual examination should be performed to detect coexistent adnexal or uterine pathology.

A postvoid residual determination must be made to exclude the possibility of an atonic bladder and overflow incontinence. Bacteriuria also must be ruled out. The endotoxin produced by *Escherichia coli* may trigger abnormal detrusor activity, resulting in detrusor instability. It may also act as an α-adrenergic blocker, which would result in loss of urethral pressure and the subsequent development of stress incontinence (21). In one study, 4 of 12 women with stress incontinence and asymptomatic bacteriuria be-

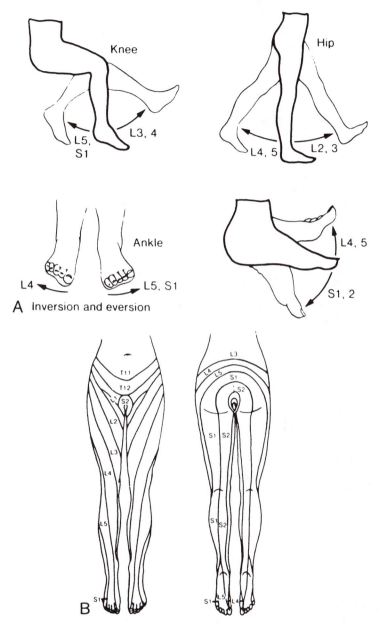

FIGURE 16.2. A. Patient maneuvers that assess the integrity of motor innervation of the lower extremities from T10 to S4. **B.** Sensory innervation of the lower extremities. (Reprinted with permission from Ostergard DR, Bent AK. Urogynecology and Urodynamics: Theory and Practice. 4th ed. Baltimore: Williams & Wilkins, 1996:101–102.)

come continent after antibiotic treatment, alleviating the need for surgical intervention (22).

Urethrovesical Junction Mobility

Because genuine stress incontinence is most often due to inadequate support of the urethrovesical junction with displacement of the proximal urethra and urethrovesical junction outside the abdominal cavity, an integral part of the workup for urinary incontinence is assessing the mobility of this tissue. A number of tests have been designed to ascertain the mobility of the proximal urethra and bladder base, including direct observation during pelvic examination, the Q-tip test, the beaded chain cystometrogram, a straining cystogram, and ultrasound evaluation (23–27). The Q-tip test appears to be the easiest objective method to determine this information. With the patient adequately prepped and in lithotomy position, a wooden Q-tip lubricated with 2% xylocaine jelly is inserted into the urethra through the urethrovesical junction. A resting angle is determined relative to the horizontal axis using an orthopedic goniometer. The patient is then asked to strain forcibly and to cough repetitively. A maximum straining angle of more than 30° from the horizontal axis is defined as a positive test and indicates significant mobility of the urethrovesical junction but does not necessarily confirm the diagnosis of stress incontinence.

Although the Q-tip test does not predict incompetence of the urethral sphincter, it does provide a noninvasive method for demonstrating excessive mobility of the urethrovesical junction in patients with suspected stress incontinence. Because the purpose of anti-incontinence procedures is to elevate the urethrovesical junction back to its normal intraabdominal position, it is essential that a defect in support of the junction is demonstrated before surgical intervention is contemplated. In patients with a negative Q-tip test, the diagnosis of genuine stress incontinence should be seriously questioned. More sophisticated radiographic or urodynamic studies are indicated before undertaking surgery in this group of patients.

Stress Test

Objective evidence of urinary leakage with stress is necessary to establish the diagnosis of genuine stress incontinence. The patient is asked to cough repetitively with a full bladder in the supine or standing position. Simultaneous loss of urine during coughing is highly suggestive of genuine stress incontinence. The stress test can easily be obtained at the beginning of the examination if the patient is asked to arrive at the office with a full bladder. Once the test is performed, the patient is asked to void. A stopwatch and measuring container are used to determine specific voiding parameters, and a postvoid residual volume is also measured. Alternatively, the stress test can be done at intervals during a cystometrogram to determine the volume at which leakage occurs.

Uroflowmetry

Uroflowmetry is a measurement of the urine volume voided and the time interval required for voiding. This test is used to detect gross voiding abnormalities preoperatively that may predispose a patient to prolonged voiding after anti-incontinence surgery (28). An average flow rate of less than 8 to 10 mL/sec indicates poor bladder contractility or urethral obstruction. Obstructive voiding patterns also may be seen in women with recurrent urinary tract infections, urethral spasms due to irritation to the urethra, or failure of the urethral muscles to relax during voiding (29, 30). Although uroflowmetry may be performed using an electronic uroflowmeter, the simplest method is to use a stopwatch and a measuring container that fits over the commode. The patient should void at least 200 mL for the test to be accurate. The average flow rate should be at least 10 mL/sec with postvoid residual of less than 50 mL to be considered normal.

Cystourethroscopy

Cystourethroscopy is an endoscopic evaluation of the urethral and vesical mucosa that can be performed in the office as a screening test. The procedure may also be undertaken in the operating room to facilitate a more extensive evaluation of the bladder, including bladder biopsies or bladder hydrodistention to treat interstitial cystitis. In the incontinent woman, the purpose of cystourethroscopy is to detect intrinsic bladder pathology such as fistulas or diverticula, tumors, foreign bodies, or nonfunctioning ureters. Not all incontinent women require cystourethroscopy. The procedure is indicated in the assessment of women who have failed prior incontinence surgery or in those with irritative bladder complaints to determine the site, and possible source, of inflammatory changes in the lower urinary tract.

Cystometry

Cystometry is a pressure-volume relationship recorded during bladder filling. The purpose of single-channel cystometry is to detect the presence of detrusor instability, which occurs in 8 to 63% of incontinent women (31). During cystometry, the first sensation of fluid in the bladder, maximum bladder capacity, and the presence of uninhibited detrusor contractions should be recorded. Detrusor instability is diagnosed when a true detrusor pressure rise of 15 cm H_2O or more occurs or when a true detrusor pressure rise of less than 15 cm H_2O occurs in the presence of urgency or urinary incontinence and reproduces the patient's presenting complaint (Fig. 16.3). Detrusor contractions of less than 15 cm H_2O may have clinical significance and may have been shown to cause urinary incontinence in 10% and urgency in 85% of patients (32). A gradual rise in intravesical pressure of at least 15 cm H_2O at normal bladder capacity indicates a hypertonic bladder. A hypotonic bladder is diagnosed when the maximum bladder capacity exceeds approximately 800 mL water.

Despite the widespread use of cystometry, the optimal technique for performing this test is unclear (33, 34). Questions remain regarding positioning of the patient; antegrade versus retrograde filling of the bladder; the use of water, saline, or carbon dioxide as the distention medium; the temperature of the medium; and rate of filling. Most studies are done using retrograde flow of saline (37°C) or carbon dioxide at a

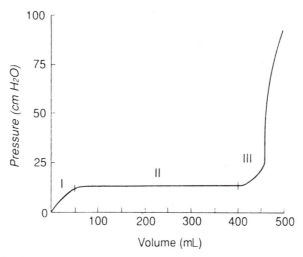

FIGURE 16.3. The three phases of a single-channel cystometrogram. *Phase I* is the small rise in intravesical pressure during the initial phase of filling. *Phase II* is the plateau phase characterized by an increase in bladder volume without a rise in bladder pressure. *Phase III* is the increase in intravesical pressure due to a detrusor contraction for voluntary voiding at the end of the study. (Reprinted with permission from Ostergard DR, Bent AK. Urogynecology and Urodynamics: Theory and Practice. 4th ed. Baltimore: Williams & Wilkins, 1996:116.)

flow rate of 50 to 100 mL/min. Although carbon dioxide cystometry may be easier and cleaner, it is less physiologic than water or saline as a distention medium. Carbon dioxide may irritate the bladder mucosa and mix with urine to form carbonic acid. As a gas, carbon dioxide is compressible, which may lead to less reproducible results.

If electronic equipment is unavailable to perform a single-channel cystometrogram, a number of more simplified techniques may be substituted. A Foley catheter can be inserted into the patient's bladder and attached to a catheter-tip syringe with the piston removed (Fig. 16.4). Fluid is gradually poured into the syringe (no more than 100 mL/min) such that the fluid level is constant. A rise in the fluid level associated with urgency or leakage is suggestive of detrusor instability. Alternatively, a spinal manometer may be used to determine intravesical pressure (Fig. 16.5). Supine, single-channel cystometry detects approximately 50 to 60% of patients with an unstable bladder (34–36). The accuracy of this test may be improved an additional 20 to 40% by performing the cystometrics

- To maximum bladder capacity
- In the standing position
- With the detrusor-provoking maneuvers of repetitive coughing and heel bounce

The reliability of single-channel cystometry compared with multichannel urodynamics has been debated extensively in the literature (31, 36). The reported advantage of multichannel cystometry is that artifactual increases in intravesical pressure due to a rise in intraabdominal pressure (e.g., Valsalva activity) can be recognized and subtracted out. This results in an accurate recording of true detrusor pressure. Thus, multichannel testing is thought to decrease the incidence of a false-positive diagnosis of detrusor instability (31, 35).

The use of multichannel urodynamics as the standard by which the accuracy of other tests is evaluated is controversial. It is well known that women with a history

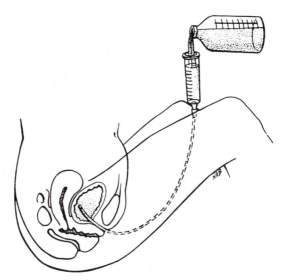

FIGURE 16.4. "Poor man's" cystometrogram for office evaluation of bladder filling function. With the patient in sitting or standing position with a catheter in the bladder, the bladder is filled by gravity by pouring sterile water into the syringe (no more than 100 mL/min). A rise in the fluid level associated with urgency or leakage is suggestive of detrusor instability. (Reprinted with permission from Walters MD, Karram MM. Clinical Urogynecology. St. Louis: CV Mosby, 1993:55.)

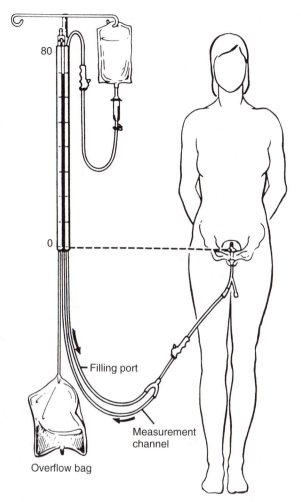

FIGURE 16.5. Spinal manometer used to determine intravesical pressure.

highly suggestive of detrusor instability may not demonstrate uninhibited contractions even during multichannel testing. Patients with detrusor instability may experience days without urinary leakage. Bhatia and Ostergard (37) suggested that ambulatory multichannel urodynamics is a more sensitive method of detecting detrusor abnormalities than standard urodynamic testing. In their study the diagnosis, based on multichannel urodynamics, was significantly revised in 60% of patients after continuous monitoring was performed. However, this testing is usually available only in special office settings.

Multichannel Urodynamics

Multichannel urodynamics are a group of sophisticated urologic tests using microtransducer catheters to simultaneously record urethral, vesical, and intraabdominal (via a vaginal catheter) pressures and electromyographic activity of the pelvic floor. Information can be obtained by subtracted urethrocystometry, urethral pressure profilometry, instrumented voiding studies, and electromyographic recordings of the urethral sphincter. Approximately 10% of patients with lower urinary tract dysfunction require urodynamic testing to elucidate their diagnosis. Referral for multichannel urodynamic testing should be made for patients with the conditions listed in Table 16.5. Women over age 65 are candidates for urodynamic testing because of the higher prevalence of detrusor instability and urethral incompetence in this group of patients.

Treatment

Stress Incontinence

Genuine stress incontinence can be approached nonsurgically in women with mild symptoms, in women who desire subsequent childbearing, or in patients who are poor surgical candidates. In postmenopausal women, topical estrogen replacement is recommended to improve the uroepithelium, submucosal vascularity, and submucosal elastic tissues. These changes, however, produce an inconsistent rise in urethral pressure, and it appears that the beneficial effects of estrogen are not solely dependent on augmentation of urethral pressures (38, 39). The usual dose of vaginal estrogen cream is 1 to 2 g three times a week for 6 to 12 weeks. Up to 70% of patients with mild to moderate incontinence have reported a favorable clinical response after initiation of estrogen therapy (39, 40).

α-Adrenergic stimulation of the urethral smooth muscle with phenylpropanolamine, 75 to 150 mg/day, may improve the symptoms of mild to moderate stress incontinence (40, 41). Many over-the-counter appetite suppressants contain phenylpropanolamine as the active ingredient. The patient must be cautioned to avoid caffeine-containing medications. Some women demonstrate better tolerance for the drug Ornade (phenylpropanolamine 75 mg plus chlorpheniramine 12 mg, traditionally used as an antihistamine).

Imipramine (Tofranil), 50 to 150 mg/day, is advantageous in treating mixed stress incontinence and detrusor instability because of its combined α-adrenergic and anticholinergic properties (42). This medication must be used judiciously in the elderly because imipramine can occasionally precipitate a dysphoric reaction at low dosages.

Kegel exercises, with or without the aid of a perineometer, and functional electrical stimulation facilitate improved urinary control in 40 to 75% of patients by contracting the pubococcygeus muscle and improving the tone of the voluntary external urethral musculature (43). The success of Kegel exercises is determined by the patient's ability to identify the correct muscle for the exercise and her commitment to perform the exercises according to the prescribed regime. Several approaches have been published in the literature, including instructing the patient to execute a series of rapid pelvic floor contractions and releases, fol-

TABLE 16.5. Indications for Multichannel Urodynamic Testing

HISTORY	EXAMINATION
Incontinent women over age 65	Neurologic abnormality
Prior anti-incontinence surgery	Postvoid residual > 100 mL
History of neurologic disease	Incontinent women with negative
Continuous urinary leakage	stress test, negative Q-tip test,
Mixed stress and urge incontinence	and/or normal cystometrogram
Suspected urethral diverticulum	Maximum bladder capacity
Suspected urethral spasm	< 350 mL or > 800 mL
Suspected low pressure urethra	

lowed by a contraction held for 3 seconds and released for 3 seconds for a total of 5 minutes of exercising, five or six times per day. Alternatively, patients may be requested to perform 10 to 20 pelvic floor contractions, each for 10 seconds three times per day. Vaginal cones (weights) can be inserted into the vagina once or twice a day to provide "biofeedback" to the pelvic muscles and an objective measure of progress for the patient. Cones should be used in women with the ability to generate a voluntary pelvic muscle contraction that is suboptimal in strength or duration.

Functional electrical stimulation provides stimulation of the pudendal nerve, which causes contractions of the pelvic floor and periurethral skeletal muscles (44). A vaginal probe is inserted for 10 to 15 min twice daily that provides an electrical current to the pelvic musculature, resulting in a type of "electronic Kegel" exercise. This technique has been adopted more readily in Europe than in the United States but is gaining popularity here. Electrical stimulation is indicated in women who are unable to generate a voluntary pelvic muscle contraction.

Vaginal devices such as tampons, pessaries, or contraceptive diaphragms have been used to alleviate the symptoms of pelvic relaxation with or without concomitant urinary incontinence. By compressing the urethra between the device and the pubic symphysis, urethral resistance is increased and the urethra and urethrovesical junction are stabilized in an appropriate anatomic position during episodes of stress. The most effective brand and type of tampon is the OB super tampon because of its position in the vagina. An appropriately fitted ring pessary may produce continence in up to 75% of women (45). This form of therapy is particularly well suited for older women with prolapse and incontinence who are poor surgical candidates. In addition, younger women who experience stress incontinence only during intense exercise (aerobics, tennis) may benefit from insertion of a pessary or diaphragm temporarily just before exercise. A recent new supportive device is the bladder neck support prosthesis (Introl, Uromed) that is designed to provide selective additional support of the urethrovesical junction. Although this device can be helpful for some patients, it is more expensive than a ring pessary. Other new devices are the urethral patch (Impress) and urethral plug (Reliance), which are disposable devices that obstruct the urethra, preventing loss of urine in women with mild stress incontinence. These devices are removed at each void and replaced. External irritation, increased prevalence of urinary tract infections, and hematuria have been reported with these devices.

Although nonsurgical approaches to stress incontinence produce beneficial results with minimal side effects, these methods are only temporary measures to restore urinary continence. Surgical options provide a more permanent chance for cure but are associated with more potential complications. Thus, surgical procedures should be reserved for women who decline or fail conservative therapies and for women who have completed childbearing.

Detrusor Instability

The treatment approaches to detrusor instability include behavioral therapy, biofeedback, medications, functional electrical stimulation, surgery, and psychological counseling, as summarized in a comprehensive review by Wall (46).

Behavioral therapy, referred to as bladder retraining, attempts to reestablish the cortical inhibition of reflex bladder emptying that is lost in patients with detrusor instability. Using the patient's pretreatment voiding diary as a guide, a regular voiding interval is chosen that is shorter than the patient's usual interval between voiding and incontinence. The patient is instructed to void regularly during the waking hours according to the present interval, whether or not she has the urge to void, and to ignore other desires to void even if it results in urinary leakage. She records her micturition times on a preprinted card. After 7 to 10 days, the number of incontinent episodes should be less, and the scheduled voiding interval can be increased by 30 minutes. This process is continued until the desired voiding interval of every 3 to 4 hours is achieved. Success depends on the motivation of the patient and physician but can approach 80% in some series (46, 47). A variation of behavioral therapy can be applied to the elderly institutionalized patient: fluid restriction, elimination of caffeine, and regular toileting or prompted voiding at 2-hour intervals.

Biofeedback facilitates the inhibition of abnormal detrusor contractions by inserting a pressure catheter into the bladder that provides an auditory or visual stimulus when bladder pressure rises. The patient is encouraged to relax her muscles to decrease the recorded signal. Weekly sessions in a motivated patient can yield a success rate of up to 50%.

Although advocates of both bladder retraining and biofeedback report excellent success rates without side effects, the time-consuming nature of these treatments makes them unacceptable for many women. Anticholinergic and antispasmodic medications provide an excellent alternative to behavioral therapy with a success rate of 60 to 80% (46, 47). Preparations that have proven to be effective are shown in Table 16.6. The drug of choice is usually either oxybutynin (Ditropan), with its improved effectiveness but significant risk of side effects, or propantheline (Pro-Banthine), which appears to be associated with less adverse reactions. Other

TABLE 16.6. Pharmacologic Management of Detrusor Instability

Drug	Dosage	Comments
Propantheline (Pro-Banthine)	15–30 mg PO TID–QID	Cure rates 60–80%, fewer side effects, variable absorption
Oxybutynin (Ditropan)	5–10 mg PO TID–QID	Cure rates 60–80%, side effects in up to 75% of patients
Dicyclomine (Bentyl)	20 mg IM QID	Effective if used parenterally
Flavoxate (Urispas)	100–200 TID–QID	Limited data on efficacy, more expensive
Imipramine (Tofranil)	25–50 mg PO BID–TID	Cure rates 60–74%, beneficial for childhood nocturnal enuresis or mixed stress and urge incontinence
Terodiline (Micturin)	12.5–25 mg PO BID	Not available in United States

more costly drugs marketed for detrusor instability do not appear to be any more efficacious. These medications are associated with typical anticholinergic side effects and are contraindicated in women with narrow-angle glaucoma. In patients who experience significant side effects from these drugs, the combination of low doses of more than one type of medication may produce an additive beneficial response while diminishing the reported side effects.

Surgical intervention is associated with significant morbidity and should be reserved only for severely affected individuals. Surgical procedures may include partial denervation of the hypogastric nerve, implantation of a sacral nerve root-stimulating device, or, in extreme cases, urinary diversion.

Urethral Diverticula

The approach to patients with a urethral diverticulum varies depending on the presenting symptoms. Some diverticula are asymptomatic and require no treatment. Acute inflammation of the diverticular sac presents as a tender suburethral swelling, and purulent material can be expressed from the urethral meatus upon massage of the anterior vaginal wall. Diagnosis is confirmed by urethroscopy or positive pressure urethrography using a Tratner or Davis balloon catheter (48). An inflamed diverticulum may be managed initially by either transvaginal aspiration of the purulent material followed by a 7- to 10-day course of antibiotics designed to cover uropathogens or by urethral dilation with transvaginal massage to express the purulent contents of the diverticular sac. Surgical procedures to repair a diverticulum are best postponed until any acute inflammation has subsided. The operative approach depends on the location of the sac in relationship to the maximum urethral pressure point, which is determined by urethral pressure profilometry. Thus, preoperative urodynamics with urethral pressure profiles are essential. Diverticula at the most distal end of the urethra may be treated with a Spence procedure in which a marsupialization of the sac is performed by opening the sac and suturing the diverticular mucosa to the vaginal mucosa with a running locked suture (49). A proximal diverticulum must be isolated surgically from the surrounding tissue of the urethrovaginal septum and excised (50). A multilayer closure with alternating directions of the suture line is recommended to repair the defect in the urethrovaginal system.

IRRITATIVE BLADDER PROBLEMS

Although urinary incontinence primarily affects women over age 35, women of all ages may suffer from conditions that produce irritative bladder complaints. Patients typically report significant urinary urgency and frequency, which may be associated with dysuria, suprapubic pressure, pain on distention of the bladder, nocturia, postvoid fullness, or dyspareunia. These symptoms may be episodic in nature or they may be chronic with acute exacerbations. Many patients are treated repetitively with only temporary relief of symptoms. The nonspecific nature of these complaints may result in misdiagnosis when recurrent symptoms are attributed to the same condition. It is essential that the physician take a careful detailed history and reevaluate each episode to explore the possibility of other causes for the patient's irritative bladder complaints. The conditions most commonly associated with irritative bladder symptoms are acute urinary tract infection, acute urethritis, chronic urethritis (urethral syndrome), interstitial cystitis, or detrusor instability. Nonurologic etiologies should also be considered, including vaginal infection, acute or chronic vulvitis, or atrophic vaginitis.

Diagnosis and Treatment

Acute Urinary Tract Infections

It has been estimated that approximately 25% of women experience an acute urinary tract infection per year, resulting in millions of office visits to primary care physicians. Women are particularly susceptible to cystitis because of their anatomically short urethra and the extensive colonization of the introitus with uropathogens from the rectal reservoir (51). The primary pathogen in community-acquired infections is *E. coli* (80%), although recent reports have indicated that 10 to 20% of acute infections in young women are due to *Staphylococcus saprophyticus* (52). Other pathogens include *Klebsiella* species (5%) and *Proteus* species (2%).

Bacteria gain access to the bladder via instrumentation or other trauma or are massaged into the bladder during sexual intercourse (53). Once bacteria are present within the bladder, it is the balance between the bacterial virulence and the host defense mechanism that determines whether an acute infection will develop. Host defense factors may be compromised by

- Infrequent voiding, which leads to poor bladder washout of uropathogens
- Anatomic obstruction or anomalies of the urinary tract
- Neutral urinary or vaginal pH
- Foreign bodies
- Stones
- Neurologic abnormalities
- Diabetes mellitus
- Hemoglobinopathies
- Immunodeficiencies
- Pregnancy

Acute urinary tract infections with bacterial inflammation of the uroepithelium produce complaints of urinary urgency, frequency, nocturia, internal dysuria, suprapubic pressure, and postvoid fullness. Occasionally, patients may experience low back pain, urinary incontinence, or hematuria. These symptoms are frequently associated with sexual activity and occur within 24 to 48 hours of coitus in 75% of patients. Diaphragm users are particularly susceptible to infections, which may be partially due to obstruction of the urethra and urethral trauma caused by the diaphragm. Recent evidence also implicates vaginal spermicides in the pathogenesis of coitally related urinary tract infections because of changes in the vaginal pH and normal bacterial flora.

In patients with an initial urinary tract infection, a presumptive diagnosis may be made in a symptomatic patient if a midstream microscopic urinalysis reveals bacteria and white blood cells or a positive nitrite test on dipstick. Treatment is initiated without results of a culture. However, in patients with repetitive symptoms, the diagnosis should be confirmed with a catheterized urine sent for culture and sensitivity. Culture results aid in selecting appropriate antibiotic therapy and can clarify the pattern of infecting organisms to determine which patients may benefit from more extensive testing.

The microscopic evaluation of an unspun urine specimen should reveal one or more bacterium per high-power field if there are more than 10^4 colony-forming units (CFU)/mL of bacteria in the urine. Pyuria is defined as more than 10 leukocytes/mL in unspun urine and should be present in nearly all women with acute urinary tract infections. Microscopic hematuria is seen in approximately 50% of women with cystitis and is rarely found in other conditions associated with dysuria.

An alternative to urine microscopy is the urine dipstick. The urinary nitrite test detects the conversion of urinary nitrate to nitrite by bacteria within the bladder. To optimize accuracy, the test should be performed on a concentrated first morning void. False-negative results may be obtained with infections due to enterococci because they do not convert nitrate to nitrite and in the presence of urinary dyes such as bilirubin, phenazopyridine (Pyridium, Uristat), or methylene blue.

Urinary cultures have long been the primary tool used to diagnose acute urinary tract infections. The traditional approach of defining a positive culture as more than 10^5 CFU/mL of urine has been questioned by several authors. Twenty to 24% of women with symptomatic infections have less than 10^5 CFU/mL of urine. Important work by Stamm et al. (54) suggests that in symptomatic women, a bacterial count of 10^2 CFU/mL on urine culture should be sufficient to establish the diagnosis of an acute urinary tract infection, and treatment should be initiated.

Cystoscopy and an intravenous pyelogram are indicated in only some patients because of their relatively low yield and potential complications (55). Women who experience persistent infections or recurrent infections with the same organism, particularly *Proteus mirabilis* due to its association with renal calculi, should undergo testings. Other indications include women with suspected renal anomalies, a history of childhood infections, or recurrent painless hematuria.

General considerations in the treatment of urinary tract infections include adequate hydration and frequent bladder emptying to improve the bladder washout phenomenon, good perineal hygiene, and the short-term use of urinary analgesics such as phenazopyridine (Pyridium, Uristat) during the initial symptomatic period. Numerous antibiotic regimes have been advocated for the treatment of bacteriuria, and there has been significant debate regarding the optimal duration of therapy for the patient with an uncomplicated infection. Currently, a significant body of literature exists supporting the use of single-dose antibiotic therapy, which is nearly as effective in treating acute infections and preventing recurrent infections as longer courses of treatment (56, 57). In contrast to the traditional 7- to 10-day treatment regimes, single-dose therapy for uncomplicated infections has the advantages of increased patient compliance, decreased side effects, lower cost, and decreased likelihood of altering the fecal flora reservoir with the development of resistant strains of organisms. Single-dose therapy can be accomplished with trimethoprim-sulfamethoxazole double strength (Bactrim DS), two tablets; sulfisoxazole (Gantrisin), 1 to 2 g; or amoxicillin (Amoxil, Polymox), 3 g. Although both nitrofurantoin (Macrodantin) and norfloxacin (Noroxin) may be effective, limited data are available on these antibiotics. Cephalosporins do not appear to be adequate to treat infections in a single dose. Fosfomycin (Monuril) was recently introduced as a single-dose medication for urinary tract infections but has a clinical efficacy of only 70%. Contraindications for single-dose therapy include pregnancy, symptoms for more than 5 days, elevated postvoid residual, urinary tract anomalies, and an indwelling urinary catheter.

Because there is debate regarding the optimum balance of adequate therapy to prevent recurrences with sufficiently short treatment duration to avoid side effects, some investigators compromised and advocated a 3-day treatment course in uncomplicated infections (58). Appropriate agents include nitrofurantoin (Macrodantin), 60 to 100 mg every 6 to 8 hours; trimethoprim-sulfamethoxazole double strength (Bactrim DS), one tablet twice daily; amoxicillin (Amoxil, Polymox), 650 mg three times a day; or cephalexin (Keflex), 250 to 500 mg every 6 hours. The recently introduced synthetic quinolone derivatives (norfloxacin [Noroxin], ciprofloxacin [Cipro], ofloxacin [Floxin]) have the advantage of an expanded antibacterial spectrum, including coverage against *Pseudomonas aeruginosa* and enterococci. However, because of their cost and the fact that these drugs provide no significant advantage in uncomplicated infections, routine use should be discouraged. Quinolone derivatives should be reserved for patients with resistant infection and/or as an alternative to parenteral antibiotics. Quinolones should not be used in pregnancy.

Patients with three or more documented recurrent infections in 1 year should be considered candidates for postcoital antibiotic prophylaxis or continuous nightly prophylaxis for 3 to 6 months using either nitrofurantoin (Macrodantin), 50 mg at bedtime, or trimethoprim-sulfamethoxazole double strength (Bactrim DS), one-half tablet at bedtime. One advantage of trimethoprim-sulfamethoxazole (Bactrim) is that it is excreted in the vaginal secretions and may eradicate vaginal colonization of uropathogens. Postmenopausal women should be prescribed estrogen vaginal cream 1 g three times per week, to create an acidic vaginal pH and prevent colonization of the introitus with enteric organisms. The use of cystoscopy or intravenous pyelography to assess women with recurrent infections is rarely indicated except in cases where cultures have revealed unusual organisms such as *Proteus* or when a urinary tract anomaly is suspected.

Urethral Syndrome

Urethral syndrome is an elusive chronic condition characterized by urinary urgency and frequency, intermittent or constant dysuria, suprapubic pressure, postvoid fullness, or dyspareunia in the absence of a positive urine culture (59). Symptoms appear worse during waking hours than at night and may be preceded by an actual acute urinary tract infection in some patients. Often the patient has been treated repetitively for several months with antibiotics for presumed recurrent cystitis, yielding only temporary relief of symptoms.

The diagnosis of urethral syndrome is suggested in women with irritative symptoms that usually have persisted for several months and are associated with a negative urine culture. A detailed history should address the possible etiologic factors listed in Table 16.7, and a thorough physical examination should exclude gynecologic sources of these symptoms. A voiding diary provides objective evidence of the severity of the patient's symptoms and should illustrate the propensity for diurnal versus nocturnal frequency in patients with urethral syndrome. Urethroscopy may reveal hypoestrogenic changes of the urethral mucosa or nonspecific erythema and exudate that may also be observed in asymptomatic women. Cystoscopy should be performed to exclude intrinsic bladder pathology, especially carcinoma in situ or bladder tumors in the older patient. Cystometry or urethral pressure profilometry may be indicated to detect the presence of low-amplitude detrusor contractions or urethral spasm (59).

The treatment of urethral syndrome is an imprecise and frustrating science be-

TABLE 16.7. Proposed Etiologic Factors in Urethral Syndrome

Periurethral gland inflammation due to infection or trauma
Hypoestrogenism
Urethral smooth and/or skeletal muscle spasm (functional obstruction)
Trauma secondary to diaphragm use, tampons, coitus
Allergic reactions due to perfumed sanitary napkins, feminine hygiene sprays, vaginal douches, contraceptive spermicides
Chlamydial urethritis
Peripheral neuropathy secondary to herpes
Urethrohymenal fusion
Psychogenic factors

cause most therapeutic options yield cure rates of only 60%, and many patients develop recurrent symptoms despite medical intervention. Treatment should begin by eliminating any potentially reversible cause of urethral syndrome (Table 16.7) and by discontinuing the ingestion of caffeinated beverages, which may aggravate the urgency symptoms. Estrogen replacement with 1 to 2 g of conjugated estrogen vaginal cream should be initiated three times per week in perimenopausal and postmenopausal women.

If urethral inflammation is suspected, urethral dilation and massage can be performed using a series of urethral dilators or sounds (60). After antiseptic preparation of the urethral meatus and using copious amounts of 2% lidocaine (Xylocaine) jelly as a urethral lubricant and topical anesthetic, a 16-Fr dilator is inserted into the urethra and gentle massage of the anterior vaginal wall over the urethral dilator is accomplished to promote drainage of infected periurethral glands. Serial dilation is continued until blanching of the external urethral meatus is observed (but only to maximum 36 Fr) or the patient experiences significant discomfort. Although this procedure is generally well tolerated, some patients require a more extensive anesthetic such as a bladder pillar block using 10 mL of 1% lidocaine injected submucosally at the cervicovaginal junction (2 and 10 o'clock). Urethral dilation may be repeated weekly or biweekly for two or three treatments and then episodically as necessary. Patients should be prescribed an antibiotic (such as nitrofurantoin [Macrodantin]) and phenazopyridine (Pyridium, Uristat) for 24 hours after treatment to prevent the risk of iatrogenic urinary tract infection and relieve discomfort.

If urethral dilation and massage fail, patients may be treated with periurethral steroid injections. With a urethral sound in place to guide the injection and the urethra visualized in cross-section as a clock, 0.25 mL of triamcinolone (Aristocort suspension), 10 mg/1 mL, is injected submucosally along the length of the urethra at the 3, 5, 7, and 9 o'clock positions using a 30-gauge needle. Using this approach, Altman (61) found 87% of his patients who were followed had relief of symptoms from 6 months to 5 years after treatment.

Pharmacologic management of urethral syndrome has been aimed at the treatment of possible chronic urethral infections with antibiotics or relief of functional urethral spasm with muscle relaxants. Empiric treatment of *Chlamydia* with 10 to 14 days of doxycycline (Vibramycin, Doryx) or erythromycin (Eryc, E-Mycin) is cost effective and may be helpful. Occasionally, patients may respond to long-term therapy (3 to 6 months) with low-dose antibiotics designed to eradicate uropathogens. Functional urethral obstruction may be due to spasm of the urethral smooth or skeletal muscle. Kaplan et al. (62) reported relief of symptoms in six women treated with diazepam (Valium) for 2 to 6 months. Recommended doses of diazepam are 2.5 to 5.0 mg three to four times a day. This drug may be used alone or in combination with a smooth muscle relaxant such as phenoxybenzamine (Dibenzyline), 10 to 40 mg/day, or prazosin (Minipress), 1 to 2 mg three times a day (63).

Other treatment modalities that have been found anecdotally to be effective are the Richardson urethrolysis, urethral cryotherapy, and hymenoplasty to correct urethrohymenal fusion (59). With any of the therapeutic approaches outlined, one of the most essential requirements for success is a caring and supportive physician.

Interstitial Cystitis

Interstitial cystitis is a debilitating chronic inflammation of the bladder wall that is estimated to affect 1 in 350 to 1 in 415 outpatients with a 10:1 predominance of women to men (64). Patients report incapacitating suprapubic pain on bladder distention that precipitates the need for frequent voids throughout the day and night.

Typically, these women experience severe pain (not simply suprapubic pressure) that is usually relieved by voiding but may be exacerbated at the end of micturition in a few patients. Urge incontinence is a rare finding encountered in the later stages of the disease. Spontaneous remissions are uncommon, and patients may become progressively more debilitated by the frequency of voiding and the persistent pain.

Multiple theories have been proposed to explain interstitial cystitis, but no hypothesis is completely accepted at present (64). Infectious, allergic, autoimmune, and neurologic causes have been implicated. One theory supports the concept of a defect in the protective glycosaminoglycan layer of the bladder mucosa, which allows toxins to penetrate into the submucosa and precipitate a chronic inflammatory reaction.

The diagnosis of interstitial cystitis is based on suggestive symptoms and may be further supported by cystoscopic findings. Because of the severe pain associated with bladder distention, general anesthesia may be required to ensure an adequate cystoscopic examination. A double distention technique is used. The initial bladder distention produces the classic submucosal changes of petechial hemorrhaging and splitting of the mucosal layer (Hunner's ulcer), leading to gross hematuria. Emptying the bladder followed by refilling of the bladder to clear the induced gross hematuria facilitates visualization of these mucosal changes (65). In the early stages of the disease, small submucosal hemorrhages may be visualized without mucosal fissures, scarring, or a reduced bladder capacity. The more severe form of interstitial cystitis is characterized by submucosal petechial hemorrhages, fissures, linear scars, and the classic Hunner's ulcers. Bladder capacity may be significantly reduced and gross hematuria encountered with bladder drainage. Bladder biopsies should confirm the findings of chronic inflammation and vasodilation of the submucosa (66). Biopsy is also indicated to exclude other pathologic conditions, including tuberculosis, radiation cystitis, and carcinoma in situ of the bladder. Other diagnostic tools that may be helpful are a voiding diary, which should reveal significant diurnal and nocturnal frequency with reduced functional bladder capacity, and a normal postvoid residual with negative urine culture. Urodynamic evaluation is rarely necessary except to eliminate other potential causes of the patient's symptoms, such as detrusor instability. A cystometrogram reveals a hypertonic bladder with decreased bladder capacity.

The therapeutic approaches to interstitial cystitis can be divided into bladder instillation therapy, surgical management, or systemic agents (64). Bladder hydrodistention can be accomplished at the time of diagnostic cystoscopy. Distention of the bladder is believed to injure the bladder submucosal nerve plexuses and destroy detrusor muscle stretch receptors, resulting in increased bladder capacity and diminished pain. To avoid the complication of bladder rupture, the bladder pressure during distention should never exceed the patient's systolic blood pressure. Using prolonged bladder distention with a Helmstein balloon for pressure monitoring, Dunn et al. (67) reported complete symptom remission in 64% of their patients. Other self-limited complications of hydrodistention are hematuria, backache, and urinary retention.

Dimethyl sulfoxide (DMSO) is the only medication approved for instillation therapy in patients with interstitial cystitis (68). Its properties include anti-inflammation, bacteriostasis, local anesthesia, cholinesterase inhibition, relaxation of skeletal and smooth muscle, and dissolution of pathologic deposits of collagen. DMSO is an extremely caustic medication and should be used with care and close monitoring for a clinical response over the first several treatments before it is used further. The initial DMSO (Rimso-50) treatment should be administered as 50 mL of a 25% solution via a urethral catheter after topical urethral anesthesia has been applied. The solution is retained for 15 minutes and then released by spontaneous voiding. Subsequent instillations should be performed on a weekly or biweekly basis using a 50% solution for a maximum of four to six treatments total. Cataracts are a contraindication to DMSO administration. Side effects include garlic taste, lethargy, headache, nausea, and potentiation of the effects of ethyl alcohol. A review of several published series found a satisfactory response rate of 53 to 90% over 6 months to 2 years (68, 69). In patients who become refractory to DMSO therapy alone, intravesical instillation of a mixed solution containing DMSO (25 to 50% strength) and hydrocortisone (100 to 150 mg) may be used to augment the anti-inflammatory response. A recent retrospective report by Ramahi and Richardson (70) found symptomatic relief in 80% of patients treated with a combination of weekly bladder pillar block (using 1% lidocaine [Xylocaine] and 40 mg of triamcinolone [Aristocort suspension]) and passive bladder distention, to no more than 500 mL, followed by instillation of 50 mL of 50% DMSO for 30 minutes.

Systemic agents with variable anecdotal effectiveness include antihistamines, azathioprine (Imuran), corticosteroids, heparin, pentosan polysulfate (Elmiron), and tricyclic antidepressants. If these measures fail, surgical therapy with a neodymium: yttrium-aluminum-garnet laser to the bladder mucosa has been found to be 65% effective in improving symptoms in an uncontrolled trial of 39 patients (71). Procedures that are reserved for the most refractory patients include selective sacral neurectomy, inferior hypogastric nerve resection, cystoplasty, cystolysis, or bladder augmentation.

Detrusor Instability

Occasionally, women with low-amplitude detrusor contractions that are insufficient to produce urge incontinence may experience significant urgency and frequency. Subthreshold detrusor contractions of less than 15 cm H_2O have been shown to cause urgency in 85% of patients (32). However, women with detrusor instability rarely suffer from dysuria or suprapubic pain. The diagnosis is relatively easily established by a cystometrogram where uninhibited detrusor contractions are observed and coincide with the patient's complaint of urgency. Treatment is outlined in the previous discussion of detrusor instability.

VOIDING ABNORMALITIES

Voiding difficulties may present with complaints related to urinary hesitancy, urinary retention, or urgency and frequency symptoms due to the patient's inability to adequately empty her bladder with each void. Urgency and frequency symptoms not associated with an elevated postvoid residual are considered to be due to irritative bladder problems and are discussed in the previous section.

Normal voiding is accomplished by initial voluntary relaxation of the urethral smooth and skeletal musculature followed by the onset of a detrusor contraction of sufficient duration and amplitude to allow complete evacuation of urine. The force generated by the detrusor to expel urine may be augmented by an increase in intra-abdominal pressure through voluntary straining. Thus, voiding may be facilitated in some patients by abdominal straining.

Urinary hesitancy with difficulty initiating a urinary stream may be due to inadequate urethral relaxation at the onset of voiding or due to failure of the bladder to develop a detrusor contraction in a timely fashion to initiate micturition. If these problems are overcome by the patient consciously attempting to relax her urethral sphincter and/or by abdominal straining, satisfactory voiding may be accomplished with negligible postvoid residual urine volume. If, however, either process remains suboptimal, acute or chronic urinary retention may develop. Acute retention is defined by

Stanton (72) as a "sudden painful or painless inability to void over a 24 hour period, requiring catheterization, which yields at least 50% of the maximum cystometric capacity." The many potential causes of acute urinary retention are listed in Table 16.8.

Chronic urinary retention may begin insidiously or as a sequelae of an episode of acute urinary retention that leads to permanent damage to the lower urinary tract. Stanton (72) defined chronic retention as an "insidious failure of bladder emptying that results in at least 50% of the maximum bladder capacity being retained." Thus, the diagnosis of chronic retention should be reserved for patients who demonstrate elevated residual urine volumes on at least two occasions, several days apart. Infrequent voiding in a woman with normal fluid intake may contribute to the development of chronic retention by gradual overdistention of the bladder, leading to damage or denervation of the detrusor muscle. Neurogenic factors that may be associated with progressive retention include

- Parasympathetic denervation due to radical pelvic surgery
- Effects of systemic diseases such as diabetes mellitus, hypothyroidism, or collagen-vascular diseases on the sensory input for bladder filling
- Lesions or trauma to the spinal cord

In some patients, detrusor function can be lost simply as a consequence of the aging process (73). Anticholinergic medications may also contribute to chronic urinary retention. Retention due to chronic urethral obstruction is rare in women. It may be encountered in women with large pelvic masses or after anti-incontinence surgery. The ultimate sequelae of retention are symptoms of urgency and frequency, overflow or stress incontinence, recurrent cystitis, and ureteral reflux.

Diagnosis

The hallmark of the diagnosis of urinary retention is an elevated postvoid residual, usually above 100 to 200 mL. It is, however, unusual to encounter overflow incontinence unless the residual volume exceeds 300 to 400 mL. The subsequent evaluation of these patients should be directed at elucidating the underlying cause for the retention and correcting it. Neurologic and pelvic examination, voiding diary, urinalysis and urine culture, and basic uroflowmetry should be performed. Most patients, especially those with overflow incontinence, also require referral for multichannel urodynamics testing, which should include urethrocystometry, urethral pressure profilometry (to detect urethral spasm), and electromyographic studies (to rule out detrusor sphincter dyssynergia). An intravenous pyelogram and cystourethroscopy may be necessary. Finally, underlying neurologic conditions may be excluded by a computed tomography or magnetic resonance imaging of the brain and spinal cord.

TABLE 16.8. Potential Causes of Acute Urinary Retention

Trauma secondary to abdominal or pelvic surgery
Labor and delivery
Epidural general anesthesia
Urethrocystitis
Herpetic vulvitis
Neurogenic disease
Psychological disorders
Urethral obstruction due to uterine fibroids, ovarian masses, malignancies, an acutely retroverted uterus, or vaginal wall masses

Treatment

Acute urinary retention should be treated by prompt urethral or suprapubic catheter drainage for 24 to 48 hours. No more than 2 L should be drained at one time to prevent an acute hemodynamic or vasovagal response. Once the underlying cause of the retention has been eliminated, "tincture of time" is the most effective and well-tolerated treatment for acute urinary retention. Cholinergic medications such as bethanechol (Urecholine) are commonly used to improve bladder emptying and have been reported to be beneficial in subjective uncontrolled trials. However, the few published blinded well-controlled series found no advantage of these medications over placebo controls (74). Clinically, there is little indication or benefit to using cholinergic agents. If pharmacologic management is desired, α-adrenergic blocking agents may be used. α-Adrenergic blockers relax the urethral smooth muscle to facilitate voiding. Phenoxybenzamine (Dibenzyline) or prazosin (Minipress), 1 mg at bedtime, have been proven to be effective in decreasing residual urine volumes (75). Skeletal muscle relaxants such as diazepam (Valium), 2 mg two to three times a day, are even more effective in promoting voiding by relaxing the voluntary pelvic and urethral striated muscles. Response should be seen within 3 to 5 days of starting treatment. These drugs may be used in combination as described in the previous section on the treatment of urethral spasm.

Chronic urinary retention due to poor detrusor function responds poorly to pharmacologic intervention. Some women with low urethral resistance may be taught to improve bladder emptying by a combination of the Credé (direct suprapubic compression or massage by hand) and Valsalva maneuvers. Alternatively, double voiding may be recommended in which the patient is asked to void once, wait on the toilet for 30 to 60 seconds, and attempt a second void with additional emptying of the bladder. This approach is not recommended for patients with ureteral reflux.

A highly effective technique for the treatment of chronic retention, especially in women who have developed overflow incontinence, is clean intermittent self-catheterization. This procedure necessitates adequate cognitive function and manual dexterity and is contraindicated in a patient with urethral strictures. Disposable plastic catheters may be purchased inexpensively and used for 1 week before being discarded. No special antiseptic preparation is required other than regular hand washing. Topical lubricant may be used as necessary. The patient can initially be instructed on how to insert the catheter using a mirror to localize the urethral meatus. However, most patients are eventually able to perform the procedure without the aid of direct visualization. Once the catheterization is completed, the catheter should be washed with soap and warm water and stored in a clean plastic bag or container. Catheterization can be performed up to four to six times per day. If ureteral reflux is not a concern, asymptomatic bacteriuria does not require treatment.

CLINICAL NOTES

Urinary Incontinence

- Urinary incontinence occurs when the pressure in the bladder exceeds the pressure in the urethra. Common causes of this include anatomic changes of the urethrovesical junction, uninhibited detrusor contractions, or neurologic disease.
- Diagnosis is made via history and physical examination, residual urine measurement with urinalysis and culture, a stress test, assessment of the urethrovesical junction mobility, use of a urolog, and a cystometrogram.

- Physical examination of the patient with incontinence must include evaluation of the sensory and motor function of the T10 to S4 nerve distribution areas. The "anal wink" reflex and bulbocavernosus reflexes should also be assessed.
- The Q-tip test is done to assess mobility of the proximal urethra and bladder base and is considered positive when a maximum straining angle of more than 30° from the horizontal axis is observed.
- The average flow rate of urine is at least 10 mL/sec with a postvoid residual of less than 50 mL.

Treatment

- Nonsurgical treatment for genuine stress incontinence includes Kegel exercises, use of an α-adrenergic stimulator (phenylpropanolamine, 75 to 150 mg/day), biofeedback with weighted vaginal cones, functional electrical nerve stimulation of the pelvic floor, the urethral patch or urethral plug, and/or topical estrogen when indicated.
- Surgery is indicated for women who decline or fail conservative therapies and who have completed childbearing.
- Detrusor instability may be treated behaviorally or pharmacologically. Surgery should be reserved for severely affected patients.
- Behavioral therapy with detrusor instability is often called bladder retraining. Biofeedback is also used.
- Anticholinergic and antispasmodic medications for the treatment of detrusor instability have a success rate of 60 to 80%. The drug of choice is either oxybutynin (Ditropan) or propantheline (Pro-Banthine). These medications are contraindicated in women with narrow-angle glaucoma. Imipramine (Tofranil) may be used to treat mixed stress incontinence and detrusor instability but must be used with caution in the elderly woman.

Irritative Bladder Problems

- The conditions most commonly associated with irritative bladder symptoms are acute urinary tract infection, acute urethritis, chronic urethritis (urethral syndrome), interstitial cystitis, and detrusor instability. Nonurologic etiologies should also be considered.
- Single-dose antibiotic therapy for an acute urinary tract infection seems to be as effective in treating and preventing infections as longer courses of treatment.
- Patients with three or more documented urinary tract infections in 1 year should be considered candidates for postcoital antibiotic prophylaxis or continuous nightly prophylaxis for 3 to 6 months with either Macrodantin, 50 mg at bedtime, or Bactrim DS, one-half tablet at bedtime.
- The diagnosis of urethral syndrome is suggested in women with irritative symptoms that have persisted for several months and are associated with a negative urine culture. Cystoscopy should be performed to exclude other pathology. Most therapeutic options for urethral syndrome, such as urethral dilation and massage, periurethral steroid injection, antibiotics to empirically treat *Chlamydia,* and/or muscle relaxants to relieve functional urethral spasm, offer cure rates of only 60%.
- The exact etiology of interstitial cystitis is unknown, although it does afflict women more than men. Its diagnosis is based on symptoms and possibly by cystoscopic findings of Hunner's ulcers. If cystoscopy is done, bladder biopsies should be taken.
- Treatment of interstitial cystitis includes bladder instillation therapy (either as hydrodistention or with DMSO), surgical management, or system agents.
- Detrusor instability may cause irritative bladder symptoms without accompanying incontinence. Therapy is the same for both instances.

Voiding Abnormalities

- Voiding difficulties include urinary hesitancy, urinary retention, or urgency and frequency symptoms due to the patient's inability to adequately empty her bladder with each void.

- Most patients with voiding difficulties, especially those with overflow incontinence, require referral for multichannel urodynamics testing.
- Evaluation includes neurologic and pelvic examinations, voiding diary, urinalysis with culture, basic uroflowmetry. Further tests, such as intravenous pyelogram, cystourethroscopy, computed tomography or magnetic resonance imaging may also be required.
- Diagnosis of urinary retention is made by postvoid residual volumes greater than 100 to 200 mL. Overflow incontinence usually occurs at greater than 300 to 400 mL
- Treatment is prompt drainage (of no more than 2 L at a time) for 24 to 48 hours. Subsequent pharmacologic treatment with α-adrenergic blockers may be helpful if the retention is not due to poor detrusor function.
- Chronic retention, especially in women with overflow incontinence, may require regular self-catheterization.

References

1. Wyman J, Hawkins S, Choi S, et al. Psychosocial impact of urinary incontinence in women. Obstet Gynecol 1987;70:378.
2. Abrams P, Blaivas JG, Stanton SL, et al. The standardisation of terminology of lower urinary tract function. The International Continence Society Committee on Standardization of Terminology. Scand J Urol Nephrol Suppl 1988;114:5–19.
3. Consensus Conference. Urinary incontinence in adults. JAMA 1989;261:2685.
4. Enhorning GE. A concept of urinary incontinence. Urol Int 1976;31:3.
5. Asmussen M, Ulmsten U. On the physiology of continence and pathophysiology of stress incontinence in the female. Contrib Gynecol Obstet 1983;10:32–50.
6. Smith AR, Hosker GL, Warrell DW. The role of pudendal nerve damage in the aetiology of genuine stress incontinence in women. Br J Obstet Gynaecol 1989;96:29–32.
7. Allen RE, Hosker GL, Smith AR, et al. Pelvic floor damage and childbirth: a neurophysiological study. Br J Obstet Gynaecol 1990;97:770–779.
8. Staskin DR. Age-related physiology and pathologic changes affecting lower urinary tract function. Clin Geriatr Med 1986;2:701.
9. Brown AD. Postmenopausal urinary problems. Clin Obstet Gynecol 1977;4:181–206.
10. Hilton P, Stanton SL. Algorithmic method of assessing urinary incontinence in elderly women. BMJ 1981;282:940.
11. Green TH. Urinary stress incontinence: differential diagnosis, pathophysiology, and management. Am J Obstet Gynecol 1975;122:368.
12. Kaufman JM. Urodynamics in stress urinary incontinence. J Urol 1979;122:778.
13. Ouslander J, Staskin D, Raz S, et al. Clinical versus urodynamic diagnosis in an incontinent geriatric female population. J Urol 1987;137:68–71.
14. Fischer-Rasmussen W, Hansen RI, et al. Predictive values of diagnostic tests in the evaluation of female urinary stress incontinence. Acta Obstet Gynaecol Scand 1986;65:291.
15. Jarvis GJ, Hall S, Millar DR, et al. An assessment of urodynamic examination in incontinent women. Br J Obstet Gynaecol 1980;87:893.
16. Cardozo LD, Stanton SL. Genuine stress incontinence and detrusor instability: a review of 200 patients. Br J Obstet Gynaecol 1980;87:184.
17. Diokno AC, Wells TW, Brink CA. Urinary incontinence in elderly women: urodynamic evaluation. J Am Geriatr Soc 1987;35:940.
18. Bryne DJ, Stewart PA, Gray BK. The role of urodynamics in female urinary stress incontinence. Br J Obstet Gynaecol 1987;59:228–229.
19. Bent AK, Richardson DA, Ostergard DR. Diagnosis of lower urinary tract disorders in postmenopausal patients. Am J Obstet Gynecol 1983;145:218.
20. Powell P, Shepherd A, Lewis P, et al. The accuracy of clinical diagnosis assessed urodynamically. International Continence Society 10th Annual Meeting, 1980.
21. Nergardh A, Boreus LO, Holme T. The inhibitory effect of coli-endotoxin on alpha-adrenergic receptor functions in the lower urinary tract. An in vitro study in cats. Scand J Urol Nephrol 1977;11:219–224.

22. Bergman A, Bhatia NN. Urodynamics: the effect of urinary tract infection on urethral and bladder functions. Obstet Gynecol 1985;66:366.

23. Crystle CD, Charme LS, Copeland WE. Q-tip test in stress urinary incontinence. Obstet Gynecol 1971;38:313–315.

24. Fantl JA, Hurt WG, Beachley MC. Bead chain cystourethrogram: an evaluation. Obstet Gynecol 1981;58:237.

25. Quinn MJ, Beynor J, Mortensen NJ, et al. Transvaginal endosonography: a new method to study the anatomy of the lower urinary tract in stress incontinence. Br J Urol 1988; 62:414.

26. Gordon D, Pearce M, Norton P, et al. Comparison of ultrasound and lateral chain urethrocystography in the determination of bladder neck descent. Am J Obstet Gynecol 1989;160:182.

27. Walters MD, Diaz K. Q-tip test: a study of continent and incontinent women. Obstet Gynecol 987;70:208.

28. Bhatia NN, Bergman A. Use of preoperative uroflowmetry and simultaneous urethrocystometry for predicting risk of prolonged post-operative bladder drainage. Urology 1986;28:440.

29. Karl C, Gerlach R, Hannappel J, et al. Uroflow measurements: their information yield in a long-term investigation of pre- and postoperative measurements. Urol Int 1986;41:270.

30. Stanton SL, Ozsoy C, Hilton P. Voiding difficulty in the female: prevalence, clinical and urodynamic review. Obstet Gynecol 1983;61:144.

31. Sutherst JR, Brown MC. Comparison of single and multichannel cystometry in diagnosing bladder instability. BMJ 1984;288:1720.

32. Coolsae BLRA, Bok C, Van Venrooij GEPM, et al. Subthreshold detrusor instability. Neurourol Urodyn 1985;4:309.

33. Gleason DM, Bottaccini MR, Reilly RJ. Comparison of cystometrograms and urethral profiles with gas and water media. Urology 1977;9:155–160.

34. Arnold EP. Cystometry-postural effects in incontinent women. Urol Int 1974;29:185.

35. Sand PK, Hill RC, Ostergard DR. Supine urethroscopic and standing cystometry as screening methods for the detection of detrusor instability. Obstet Gynecol 1987;70:57.

36. Frigerio L, Ferrari A, Candiani GB. The significance of the stop test in female urinary incontinence. Diagn Gynecol Obstet 1981;3:301.

37. Bhatia NN, Ostergard DR. Urodynamics in women with stress urinary incontinence. Obstet Gynecol 1982;60:552–559.

38. Bhatia NN, Bergmann A, Karram MM. Effects of estrogen on urethral function in women with urinary incontinence. Am J Obstet Gynecol 1989;160:176–181.

39. Hilton P, Stanton SL. The use of intravaginal estrogen cream in genuine stress incontinence. Br J Obstet Gynaecol 1983;90:940.

40. Kinn AC, Lindskog M. Estrogens and phenylpropanolamine in combination for stress urinary incontinence in postmenopausal women. Urology 1988;32:273.

41. Collste L, Lindskog M. Phenylpropanolamine in the treatment of female stress urinary incontinence. Urology 1987;30:398–403.

42. Castledan CM, George CF, Renwick AG, et al. Imipramine: a possible alternative to current therapy for urinary incontinence in the elderly. J Urol 1981;125:318.

43. Tchou DC, Adams C, Varner RE. Pelvic floor musculature exercises in treatment of anatomical stress incontinence. Phys Ther 1988;68:652.

44. Bazeed MA, Thuroff JW, Schmidt RA, et al. Effect of chronic electrostimulation on sacral roots of striated urethral sphincter. J Urol 1982;128:1357.

45. Bhatia NN, Begman A, Gunning JE. Urodynamic effect of vaginal pessary in women with stress urinary incontinence. Am J Obstet Gynecol 1983;147:876.

46. Wall LL. Diagnosis and management of urinary incontinence due to detrusor instability. Obstet Gynecol Surv 1990;45(suppl):lS.

47. Fantl JA, Hurt WG, Dunn LJ. Detrusor instability syndrome: the use of bladder retraining drills with and without anticholinergics. Am J Obstet Gynecol 1981;140:885.

48. Davis HJ, Cain LG. Positive pressure urethrography. A new diagnostic method. J Urol 1956;75:753.

49. Spence HM, Duckett JW. Diverticulum of the female urethra: chemical aspects and presentation of a single operative technique for care. J Urol 1970;104:432.

50. Tancer ML, Mooppan MM, Pierre-Louis C, et al. Suburethral diverticulum treatment by partial ablation. Obstet Gynecol 1983;62:511–513.

51. Fowler JE, Stamey TA. Studies of introital colonization in women with recurrent urinary infections. VII. The role of bacterial adherence. J Urol 1977;117:472.

52. Latham RH, Running K, Stamm WE. Urinary tract infections in young adult women caused by *Staphylococcus saprophyticus.* JAMA 1983;250:3063.

53. Buckley RM, McGuckin M, MacGregor RR. Urine bacterial counts after sexual intercourse. N Engl J Med 1978;298:321.

54. Stamm WE, Counts GW, Running KR, et al. Diagnosis of coliform infection in acutely dysuric women. N Engl J Med 1982;307:463–468.

55. Fowler JE Jr, Pulaski T. Excretory urography, cystography, and cystoscopy in the evaluation of women with urinary tract infection. N Engl J Med 1981;304:462.

56. Greenberg RN, Reilly PM, Luppen KL, et al. Randomized study of single-dose, three-day, and seven-day treatment of cystitis in women. J Infect Dis 1986;153:277.

57. Fihn SD, Stamm WE. Interpretation and comparison of treatment studies for uncomplicated urinary tract infections in women. Rev Infect Dis 1985;7:468–478.

58. Bump RC. Urinary tract infection in women: current role of single-dose therapy. J Reprod Med 1990;35:785.

59. Scotti RJ, Ostergard DR. Urethral syndrome. In: Ostergard DR, Bent AK, eds. Urogynecology and Urodynamics: Theory and Practice. 3rd ed. Baltimore: Williams & Wilkins, 1991:264.

60. Bergman A, Karram M. Bhatia N. Urethral syndrome: a comparison of different treatment modalities. J Reprod Med 1989;34:157.

61. Altman BL. Treatment of urethral syndrome with triamcinolone acetonide. J Urol 1976;116:583.

62. Kaplan WE, Firlit CF, Schoenberg HW. The female urethral syndrome: external sphincter spasm as etiology. J Urol 1980;124:48–49.

63. Raz S, Smith RB. External sphincter spasticity syndrome in female patients. J Urol 1976;115:443.

64. Bowen LW, Sand PK, Ostergard DR. Interstitial cystitis. In: Ostergard DR, Bent AK, eds. Urogynecology and Urodynamics: Theory and Practice. 3rd ed. Baltimore: Williams & Wilkins, 1991:329.

65. Messing EM, Stamey TA. Interstitial cystitis: early diagnosis, pathology and treatment. Urology 1978;12:381–392.

66. Messing EM. The diagnosis of interstitial cystitis. Urology 1987;29(suppl 4):4–7.

67. Dunn M, Ramsden PD, Roberts JB, et al. Interstitial cystitis, treated by prolonged bladder distension. Br J Urol 1977;49:641–645.

68. Sant GR. Intravesical 50% dimethyl sulfoxide (Rimso-50) in treatment of interstitial cystitis. Urology 1987;29(suppl 4):17.

69. Perez-Marrerro R, Emerson LE, Feltis JT. A controlled study of dimethyl sulfoxide in interstitial cystitis. J Urol 1988;140:36–39.

70. Ramahi AJ, Richardson DA. A practical approach to painful bladder syndrome. J Reprod Med 1990;35:805.

71. Shanberg AM, Malloy T. Treatment of interstitial cystitis with neodymium:YAG laser. Urology 1987;29(suppl 4):31–33.

72. Stanton SL. Voiding difficulty and retention. In: Stanton SL, ed. Clinical Gynecological Urology. St. Louis: CV Mosby, 1984:257.

73. Schuman JE. Some changes of aging. J Otolaryngol 1986;15:211.

74. Finkbeiner A. Is bethanechol chloride clinically effective in promoting bladder emptying? A literature review. J Urol 1985;134:443.

75. Wein AJ. Pharmacotherapy of the bladder and urethra. In: Stanton SL, Tanagho EA, eds. Surgery of Female Incontinence. 2nd ed. New York: Springer-Verlag, 1986:229–250.

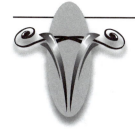

CHAPTER 17

Benign Disorders of Vulva and Vagina

MICHAEL P. HOPKINS
MELANIE K. SNYDER

Benign disorders of the vulva are a common cause for patient anxiety and visits to the primary care physician's office. Fortunately, most disorders that involve the vulva and the vagina are nonmalignant in nature. It is incumbent, however, for the examining physician to recognize those disorders that are serious and require extensive intervention from those that require only topical therapies. The gold standard for the initial management of vulvar disease is to perform a biopsy to establish a tissue diagnosis (1,2). When there is any question regarding a lesion, a biopsy must be performed. Most patients present to the office with the complaints of either pruritus or a "lump." This chapter covers the differential diagnosis of vulvar pruritus and common benign disorders affecting the vulva and vagina. A brief discussion of premalignant conditions that affect the vulva and vagina is also presented. Covered elsewhere in this textbook are chapters on infectious etiologies and human papilloma virus (HPV), which account for most vulvovaginal problems.

VULVAR PRURITUS

Pruritus of the vulva should always be considered a symptom, not a diagnosis (Table 17.1). It is a common disorder, and many patients present with this complaint (3). Chronic pruritus and/or vulvodynia may cause chronic scratching, leading to lichenification of the skin. With this increase in thickening, the skin becomes white, dry, and fissured and is susceptible to secondary infections. Burning or stinging of the vulva (vulvodynia) often accompanies vulvar pruritus. When the physical examination is normal and no etiology can be found, the initial therapy should be topical steroid therapy such as triamcinolone (Aristocort, Kenacort, Kenalog), 0.25% twice daily, for 2 months. A biopsy should be performed if this does not produce relief of symptoms. This should be done in the region of the most intense symptoms if there is no visible abnormality. The most common etiology for vulvar pruritus is yeast dermatitis, although other infectious etiologies should be considered (see Chapter 6). If the vulva is chronically exposed to urine, this can produce vulvar irritation, burning, and itching. Estrogen deficiency is a common cause of vulvar pruritus in the postmenopausal patient. The estrogen-deficient tissues are thinned, exposing the fine nerve endings. Topical estrogen therapy usually relieves the symptoms (4).

Common Causes of Vulvar Pruritus

Environmental and Dietary Causes

A search for an environmental or dietary etiology of contact dermatitis as a cause of the vulvar pruritus should be undertaken. Chemicals in deodorant soaps, bubble bath products, or perfumed feminine hygiene products can be irritating and either

417

TABLE 17.1. Common Causes of Vulvar Pruritus

Environmental/allergic reaction	Bacterial vaginosis
Contact dermatitis	Urinary tract infection
Dietary methylxanthines	Fecal incontinence
Yeast	Malignancy or premalignant changes of vulva
HPV	Parasitic infections
Vulvar dystrophy	Dermatoses
Vestibulitis	Systemic diseases (such as leukemia or
Estrogen deficiency	uremia)
(vaginal atrophy)	

cause or intensify symptoms (5). Contact dermatitis causes the skin of the vulva to be weepy and eczematoid in appearance. If it is severe, vesicles may develop. It is important to remember that a patient may have used an agent for months or years without any problem and then have an "allergy" develop. If the dermatitis is severe, a 1:20 dilution of Burrow's solution as a compress may be used for 20 to 30 minutes each day, several times during the day. Otherwise, hydrocortisone (0.5 to 1.0%) or fluorinated corticosteroids (Valisone 0.1% or Synalar 0.01%) may be used two to three times daily. The patient should also be instructed to keep the vulvar skin as dry as possible and wear only cotton underwear washed in bland detergent. Methylxanthines should be eliminated from the diet.

Human Papilloma Virus

HPV is a very common cause of vulvar pruritus or burning in the premenopausal patient. (The diagnosis is usually established by biopsy.) Treatment of HPV will often resolve the symptoms. (Further discussion of HPV is found in Chapter 9.)

Vulvar Dystrophies

Vulvar dystrophies are composed of a spectrum of atrophic and hyperplastic lesions. Lichen sclerosus et atrophicus is a slow ongoing process where homogenization of the subdermal layer takes place. The cause is unknown. The acute phase may be red to purple in appearance and have an hourglass shape involving the vulva, perineum, and perianal area. The skin is quite thin and is often described as being similar to cigarette paper. With progression, the vulvar tissues become white in appearance (5–7). This whitish change can be minimal or can involve the entire vulva. It can produce agglutination of the labium and the clitoris to the extent that the vulvar structures contract and anatomic boundaries are hard to distinguish. The turgor of the tissues is decreased and the intense pruritus is often accompanied by dysuria and dyspareunia. Treatment with topical steroidal (triamcinolone 0.25% twice daily) or testosterone cream (3% in petrolatum twice daily) is necessary and usually produces slow but satisfactory results (8). Use of an oral antihistamine at night may help alleviate some of the pruritus and decrease any scratching done while the patient is asleep.

Lichen planus is a chronic outbreak of violaceous papules that usually occurs in women over 30 and appears on the flexor surfaces, mucous membranes, and the vulva. These lesions are extremely pruritic and may be painful. The initial outbreak may follow intense emotional stress. Some women may develop a desquamative vaginitis, despite having normal estrogen levels. Treatment is with topical steroids. If severe, the patient may require oral steroids.

Hyperplastic dystrophy (lichen simplex chronicus) may also present with pruritus. It can be treated with topical steroids after a tissue diagnosis has been made (5, 8–12).

Vestibulitis

Vestibulitis is an inflammation of the vestibular glands usually located at the 4 and 6 o'clock position on the vestibule. Inflamed reddened glands that are punctate in appearance at the 4 and 6 o'clock positions are visualized and may be accompanied by focal ulcerations of the mucosa (13). When these are identified, gentle pressure with a cotton swab usually reproduces intense symptomatology consistent with the patient's symptoms. Patients often describe vestibulitis as an intense burning of the vulva or as if someone is placing a "hot poker" in the area. The etiology for this disorder is unknown. Although spontaneous remission in up to 30% of patients in 6 to 12 months has been reported, the initial treatment should be with Topicort cream or ointment. This topical steroid does not have an alcohol base, which would irritate the already inflamed area. Dietary oxalates should be avoided (chocolate, coffee, tea, spinach, peanuts). Although this only helps a small percentage of patients, the response can be dramatic. When these measures fail, perineoplasty should be considered. In this surgical procedure, the glands are excised and the vaginal mucosa advanced over the affected area.

Malignancy

Malignancy can cause pruritus. Biopsies should be liberally performed to establish the diagnosis. The etiology of vulvar malignancies is unknown, although chronic irritation is thought to be one causative agent. Therefore, any patient with persistent symptoms should be considered to be at risk. Biopsies every 1 to 2 years may be necessary to ensure nothing has changed over the time interval of observation. Vulvar intraepithelial neoplasia can be a white or pigmented lesion, and it can also be verrucous in nature. Invasive malignancies are usually ulcerative in nature, although they can be verrucous.

When there is no obvious reason for vulvar pruritus and all etiologies have been eliminated, steroidal creams should be the first therapy of choice. Amitriptyline (Elavil), 25 to 50 mg at bedtime, may be effective, and this can be tried when topical steroidal therapy fails. Surveillance with history and physical examination should be continued. Abnormalities can develop that were not obvious on initial examination (Table 17.2).

VULVAR LESIONS

Patients may discover a growth on the vulva that they often describe as a "lump." The anxiety level in this situation is usually high because the patient presumes it is malignant. Fortunately, most of these growths are benign (Table 17.2). The clinician, however, must be aware of the potential for malignancy. Usually, biopsy or complete removal of any growth is required. This can be performed in an elective fashion in the office or operating room, depending on the size and location of the lesion. Pa-

TABLE 17.2. Benign Growths of the Vulva

Epidermal inclusion cyst (sebaceous cyst)	Hidradenitis
Bartholin's duct cyst	Granular cell myoblastoma
Nevus	Schwannoma
Endometriosis	Neurofibroma
Fibroma	Hydrocele
Fibroepithelial polyp	Supernumerary mammary tissue
Lipoma	

tients with large lesions and/or lesion(s) close to the clitoris will require anesthesia. Large lesions may be very vascular and should be removed in the operating room. Smaller lesions can be removed in the office.

Benign Vulvar Lesions

The Bartholin's duct cyst is the most common cystic growth in the vulva. It commonly occurs in younger women, and treatment in young women is rendered only if the cyst is infected, it enlarges, or is producing symptoms. Although infection is the most common cause of obstruction, about 2% of patients present with an asymptomatic Bartholin's duct cyst. Cysts often rupture spontaneously, but incision and drainage may be required. If the cyst is infected, it should be marsupialized and drained or a Word catheter inserted. Appropriate antibiotic coverage, such as cefpodoxime (Vantin), 200 mg orally twice daily for 7 days, or metronidazole (Flagyl), 400 mg orally twice daily, with ampicillin, 250 mg four times a day, for 7 days should be given. Any postmenopausal patient who develops an enlarged Bartholin's gland should have it removed. These glands can be malignant, and any growth in this age group is suspicious for malignancy (14, 15).

Fibroma(s) of the vulva is the most common benign solid vulvar tumor and usually develops along the insertion of the round ligament into the labium majus. Microscopically, it is similar to a fibroid of the uterus. These benign processes should be removed because a leiomyosarcoma or sarcoma of the vulva can arise in the same area and removal is necessary to establish the diagnosis.

Lipomas are the second most common benign solid tumor of the vulva. They are superficial, commonly located in the labia majora, and their risk of malignant transformation is very low. They can involve the vulva and should be locally removed. They are usually asymptomatic.

Epidermal inclusion cysts are a common disorder usually presenting as a small hard lump and contain a white sebaceous-looking material. Epidermal inclusion cysts are more frequently found in the vagina after trauma than in the vulva. They are usually asymptomatic and do not require treatment, unless infected. If infected, incision and drainage is the mainstay of therapy. If infection(s) is recurrent or if they produce pain, they should be excised after the acute inflammation has subsided.

Nevi of the vulva are very common, and elective removal should be considered because of their malignant potential. They have a wide variety of appearances and may range in size from a few millimeters up to 2 cm. When excised, a margin of 5 to 10 mm of normal skin surrounding the nevus and the underlying dermis should be removed. This can be done at the time of an obstetric delivery or in the office with local anesthesia. Any recent changes in size, shape, color, or demonstration of friability mandate biopsy.

Hidradenomas are benign tumors arising form the apocrine glands. Most are cystic, although they can be solid. These tumors are found only in Caucasian women 30 to 70 years of age. Hidradenitis suppurativa is discussed later in the chapter.

Fibroepithelial polyps (acrochordon) are benign growths that should be removed to ensure they are not malignant.

Although rare, endometriosis can involve the vulva. This is usually characterized by a cyclical painful swelling in the vulva. Systemic therapy for endometriosis is effective for this, although excision is usually the treatment of choice.

Granular cell myoblastoma or schwannoma of the vulva is a very rare entity. It is a benign slow-growing tumor that arises in a neural sheath and is similar to schwannomas found elsewhere in the body. These are infiltrating and increase in size, which may lead to erosion through the skin surface and result in an ulcerative lesion that may be confused with cancer. Because the edges are indistinct in this lesion, wide local excision with free margins is required for treatment. Periodic reexamination of the patient should be done to detect any recurrence and allow prompt excision if detected.

Generalized neurofibromatosis and café au lait spots (von Recklinghausen's disease) rarely involves the vulva, but when it does, excision is required for diagnosis and is the treatment of choice for symptomatic tumors (16, 17).

A hydrocele or cyst of Nuck develops when loose peritoneum follows the round ligament to its insertion into the labium majus and then fills with peritoneal fluid. Rarely, a bowel loop is also present in the canal. Treatment must include ligation of the peritoneal sac at the inguinal ligament or the cyst will recur. Drainage of the cyst fluid is not effective treatment.

Supernumerary mammary tissue can involve the vulva on one or both sides. This follows the "milk line" from the breast down to the vulva. This tissue may go unnoticed until the patient is pregnant or lactating. Simple excision is all that is necessary. Rarely do these develop malignancy.

Premalignant or Malignant Changes of the Vulva

Premalignant or malignant changes occur in the vulva. Premalignant changes usually afflict women 50 to 60 years of age, although vulvar dysplasias have been occurring in younger women more frequently in recent years (18). Premalignant vulvar lesions are asymptomatic in approximately 50% of women, although when symptoms occur, the most prominent one is pruritus. Vulvar dysplasia (or vulvar intraepithelial neoplasia [VIN]) is reported as VIN I, II, or III (synonymous with carcinoma in situ). VIN is multifocal, and there is no typical appearance of the lesion(s). When suspected, colposcopy is done. Because colposcopy of the vulva is difficult to do, it should be done both with and without the green filter. The diagnosis is established by a punch biopsy. The biopsy specimen should include an area of normal-appearing skin for easier histologic diagnosis and/or grading of any dysplasia. If vulvar dysplasia is detected, colposcopic examination of the vagina and cervix should also be done. Circumscribed lesions of the vulva should be treated by wide local excision. Superficial but multifocal disease may be treated by "skinning vulvectomy" followed by split-thickness skin graft. Another acceptable treatment is CO_2 laser vaporization of the vulva. Patients treated for VIN should be followed with colposcopy every 3 to 4 months until they are disease free for 2 years; follow-up after than can occur every 6 months.

Patients with malignant lesions of the vulva often present with a mass or growth. These may or may not be painful depending on the ulcerative nature of the lesion. Patients with large vulvar cancers often have little or no discomfort because of its slow-growing nature. The most common cancer to affect the vulva is squamous cell carcinoma (Table 17.3). The diagnosis is established by a punch biopsy. Biopsy should be done where the visibly normal epithelium meets the abnormal area. This provides the pathologist a transition area in the specimen. If the punch biopsy is questionable, then complete excision is necessary. Invasive squamous cell carcinoma of the vulva usually requires radical therapy.

TABLE 17.3. Malignant Growths of the Vulva

Squamous cell carcinoma	Sarcoma
Adenocarcinoma	Melanoma

Melanoma is the second most common carcinoma involving the vulva. Approximately 5 to 10% of all malignant melanomas in women arise in the vulva, and it is thought that up to 30% of these malignancies arise from preexisting nevi. Prognosis is related to depth of invasion, and removal of any nevi is recommended. Certainly, any suspicious-appearing nevi require immediate biopsy.

Adenocarcinoma rarely affects the vulva. This often arises from a Bartholin's gland and is treated similarly to squamous cell carcinoma.

A variety of sarcomas can involve the vulva, the most common being a leiomyosarcoma. This usually arises in the round ligament in the area of its insertion into the labium majus.

Paget's disease of the vulva is a rare occurrence and appears as a velvety red lesion. Pruritus and tenderness are common symptoms. Paget's disease is an intraepithelial disease, and diagnosis is by biopsy. Because the disease often extends beyond the visualized areas, local excision should include wide margins. In about 10 to 15% of cases, Paget's disease of the vulva is associated with an underlying adenocarcinoma. Generous biopsies should be taken of any thickened area(s) to rule out adenocarcinoma. If underlying adenocarcinoma is found, radical vulvectomy with bilateral inguinal lymph node dissection is the requisite treatment. Because Paget's disease of the vulva may be associated with gastrointestinal neoplasm, an evaluation of the colon should be performed in these patients.

DERMATOLOGIC DISEASES OF THE VULVA

Dermatoses that involve other areas of the body can also affect the vulva (Table 17.4). The moisture and heat of the vulva may change the appearance of dermatologic disorders involving the vulva. Therefore, a skin inspection of the rest of the body should be done because this may reveal more classic lesions of the dermatologic disorder.

Psoriasis may involve only the vulva, although other areas of the body (scalp, extensor surfaces, and trunk) are usually affected as well. Vulvar psoriasis usually appears as red or reddish-yellow papules in the intertriginous areas. These often enlarge into distinct dull-red plaques that bleed easily. Its visual appearance may be confused with candidiasis. Initial treatment is with fluorinated corticosteroids. If these fail, referral to a dermatologist may be needed.

Hidradenitis suppurativa is a chronic refractory infection of the skin and subcutaneous tissue arising from the apocrine glands. It causes deep scarring and pits and, when advanced, leads to multiple draining abscesses and sinuses. The initial therapy is with antibiotics and topical steroids; in some cases, antiandrogens and isotretinoin are also used. Diagnosis should be confirmed by biopsy. The treatment of choice is early, aggressive, wide local excision. These patients may need referral to a specialist for long-term follow-up.

Acanthosis nigricans is a pigmented, raised, papillomatous lesion that rarely involves the vulva. It can become extensive, and excision for diagnosis and cosmetic reasons may be necessary.

Intertrigo can involve the vulva along the genitocrural folds. It results from

TABLE 17.4. Common Generalized Skin Diseases Involving the Vulva

Contact dermatitis	Seborrheic dermatitis
Neurodermatitis	Cutaneous candidiasis
Psoriasis	Lichen planus

chronic moisture and is typically seen beneath an abdominal pannus. An associated fungal or bacterial infection may be present. Efforts to promote dryness such as absorbent cotton garments can be helpful.

Vitiligo results from loss of melanin and produces a white area on the vulva.

SYSTEMIC DISEASES AFFECTING THE VULVA

Crohn's disease can affect the vulva and present as persistent, nonhealing, or poorly healing ulcers. Systemic treatment for Crohn's disease is necessary (17).

Behcet's syndrome is a rare and recurrent syndrome that produces nonhealing ulcerative lesions of the oral and genital tract. The ulcers are preceded by vesicles or papules. Ocular involvement begins as superficial inflammation that may develop into iridocyclitis and even blindness. The etiology is unknown and treatment is palliative, using oral steroids.

Lymphoma or leukemic infiltrates may involve the genital tract. Biopsy usually establishes this, and treatment is directed at the underlying disease.

VAGINAL LESIONS

Vaginal lesions are less common than vulvar lesions. Most patients do not present with a vaginal lesion, as it is not visible to them (19). When a patient presents with "a lump" in the vagina, the most common finding is a cystocele, rectocele, and/or enterocele. Treatment involves the reestablishment of normal anatomy via a mechanical device or surgery and reassurance to the patient that this is not malignant. Complaints of vaginal dryness and dyspareunia are usually related to an infectious etiology or to vaginal atrophy due to hypoestrogenism.

Benign Vaginal Lesions

Benign growths of the vagina are usually diagnosed at the time of the routine examination (Table 17.5). The entire vagina should be inspected, which requires rotating the speculum 90° throughout the examination. A vaginal lesion can be missed if it is present beneath the blades of a speculum.

Inclusion cyst is the most common cystic lesion of the vagina. They are usually found in the posterior or lateral walls of the lower one third of the vagina. They are more common in parous women and often result from birth trauma or gynecologic surgery. As a result, they are commonly found at the site of a previous episiotomy or at the vaginal cuff after hysterectomy. Most are asymptomatic. If the cyst causes dyspareunia or pain, excisional biopsy is the treatment of choice.

Fibroepithelial polyps can arise from the lateral walls of the vagina or at the vaginal cuff after hysterectomy. These are benign but require excision for diagnosis.

Gartner's duct cysts arise from Wolffian remnants and occur on the lateral sidewalls. They are usually about 1 cm in diameter and firm on palpation. These can usually be followed and do not necessarily require excision.

A Skene's gland cyst can occur in the suburethral area when these glands be-

TABLE 17.5. Benign Growths of the Vagina

Gartner duct cyst	Endometriosis
Fibroepithelial polyp	Condyloma
Skene's gland cyst	

come occluded. They are usually small and can be followed conservatively. If they enlarge significantly, they may require removal.

Endometriosis can rarely involve the upper vagina after hysterectomy. This probably results from implantation near the posterior vaginal cuff either before or during hysterectomy. This can result in cyclic or continuous bleeding. A biopsy is necessary to establish the diagnosis. Treatment can be with excision or long-term progesterone therapy such as megestrol acetate (Megace), 80 mg/day, for 3 months, decreasing to maintenance of 20 mg/day.

Condyloma or HPV can involve the vagina with a verrucous-like growth. Biopsy should be performed to establish a benign diagnosis. Treatment can be observation or removal (see Chapter 9).

Premalignant and Malignant Vaginal Lesions

Vaginal intraepithelial neoplasm (VAIN) is the terminology used to describe vaginal dysplasia. This spans the spectrum from VAIN I (mild dysplasia) to VAIN III (severe dysplasia or carcinoma in situ). Premalignant neoplasms (VAIN) are almost always asymptomatic and often detected by an abnormal Pap smear. A tissue diagnosis must be established when an abnormal cytologic smear of the vaginal cuff is obtained. Colposcopy is performed with biopsy of the most abnormal area. If there is any question of invasion, then excision under anesthesia must be undertaken. VAIN is usually multifocal, and one half to one third of patients with VAIN have been treated for similar disorder of the cervix or vulva. VAIN can be satisfactorily treated with 5-fluorouracil therapy (Efudex cream), reserving local excision for those patients who fail conservative therapy. Because VAIN is usually multifocal, follow-up should occur every 3 to 4 months with colposcopy of the entire lower genital tract for 2 years and 6 months thereafter until they have been disease free for 5 years.

Vaginal malignancy is an uncommon disorder that occurs with increasing frequency with increasing age. When these occur, they are usually located in the upper one third of the vagina (19) (Table 17.6), although patients with invasive neoplasms almost always present with bleeding. The most common type of premalignant or malignant vaginal neoplasm is a squamous cell. All patients should be counseled to continue yearly Pap smears of the vaginal cuff after a hysterectomy. Women who have undergone a total hysterectomy for a premalignant or malignant process of the cervix are more likely to develop malignancy in the vagina. The greatest risk factor for vaginal malignancy is a previous history of a vulvar or cervical malignancy.

Invasive vaginal carcinoma must be treated with either radical surgery or extended radiotherapy.

The second most common malignancy involving the vagina is melanoma. Any discolored areas of the vagina should have a biopsy specimen taken, similar to the vulva. Other, rarer malignancies can involve the vagina, including adenocarcinomas and sarcomas. Any child with a vaginal growth must have a tissue diagnosis established to rule out childhood sarcomas of the vagina. Any abnormal vaginal growth should be considered suspicious and should have a biopsy specimen taken.

Vulvovaginal disease can be a challenging and vexing problem for the clinician.

TABLE 17.6. Malignant Growths of the Vagina

Squamous carcinoma in situ	Adenocarcinoma
Squamous cell cancer	Sarcoma
Melanoma	Embryonal rhabdomyosarcoma

TABLE 17.7. Common Vulvar Disorders and Their Initial Management[a]

Disorder/Symptom	Appearance	Therapy
Pruritus	Excoriated Reddened	Steroid cream
Estrogen deficiency	Atrophic Thinned	Estrogen replacement Topical estrogen
Dystrophy Lichen sclerosus	White	Steroid cream Topical testosterone
Hypertrophic	White/red	Steroid cream
Vestibulitis	Cherry-red spots, 4 and 6 o'clock	Steroid cream
Vulvar intraepithelial neoplasia	White pigmented Verrucous	Excision
Malignancy	Ulceration Verrucous	Radical surgery
Melanoma	Brown, irregular border	Radical surgery

[a]A biopsy should be liberally used.

Many problems can arise if an accurate diagnosis is not established. The hallmark of diagnosis should be biopsy. If there is any question whatsoever, biopsy is mandatory to rule out malignancy. Once an accurate diagnosis is established, therapies can be selectively directed to the problem (Table 17.7). The problems can be chronic in nature and the clinician must remember that other problems may develop over time. Thus, constant vigilance and reexamination with rebiopsy may be necessary when following these patients. Satisfactory results can usually be achieved when an accurate diagnosis is established.

CLINICAL NOTES

- When in doubt about a vulvar lesion, perform a biopsy.
- Vulvar pruritus is a symptom, not a diagnosis. Prolonged pruritus with associated scratching may lead to thickening of vulvar skin.
- Contact dermatitis of the vulva may be treated by hydrocortisone or fluorinated corticosteroids. If severe, a dilute solution of Burrow's solution may be used in compresses.
- Lichen sclerosus, planus, and hyperplastic dystrophy are best treated with topical steroids.
- Vulvar vestibulitis may remit spontaneously in up to 30% of patients. Therapy is with topical steroids. If this fails, perineoplasty should be considered.
- Bartholin's duct cyst is the most common cystic growth in the vulva. Treatment is indicated for infection, pain, and in patients over 40 years of age (to rule out underlying adenocarcinoma).
- Fibroma of the vulva is the most common, benign, solid vulvar tumor. Treatment is excision.
- Lipoma is the second most common benign solid tumor of the vulva.
- VIN is multifocal, with no typical appearance. Treatment options include wide local excision, skinning vulvectomy, or laser therapy.
- Paget's disease of the vulva is associated with an underlying adenocarcinoma about 10 to 15% of the time.

- Psoriasis of the vulva is treated with fluorinated corticosteroids.
- Inclusion cyst is the most common cystic lesion of the vagina. They are usually found at the site of previous trauma.
- VAIN is usually multifocal, and diagnosis is most frequently made by abnormal cytology on Pap smear. Initial therapy is with use of 5-fluorouracil (Efudex) cream.

References

1. Taylor PT. Biopsy of lesions of the female genital tract. Surg Oncol Clin North Am 1995;4:121–135.
2. Kaufman RH, Gardner HL. Vulvar dystrophies. Clin Obstet Gynecol 1978;21:1081–1106.
3. Bornstein J, Pascal B, Abramovici G. The common problem of vulvar pruritus. Obstet Gynecol Surg 1993;48:111–118.
4. Friedrich EG Jr. Vulvar Disease. 2nd ed. Philadelphia: WB Saunders, 1983.
5. Friedrich EG Jr. Vulvar dystrophy. Clin Obstet Gynecol 1985;28:178–187.
6. Panet-Raymond G, Girard C. Lichen sclerosus et atrophicus. Can Med Assoc J 1972;106:1332–1334.
7. Ridley CM. Lichen sclerosus. Dermatol Clin 1992;10:309–318.
8. Soper JT, Creasman WT. Vulvar dystrophies. Clin Obstet Gynecol 1986;29:431–439.
9. O'Keefe RJ, Scurry JP, Dennerstein G, et al. Audit of 114 non-neoplastic vulvar biopsies. Br J Obstet Gynaecol 1995;102:780–786.
10. Kaufman RH. Hyperplastic dystrophy. J Reprod Med 1976;17:137–145.
11. Wilkinson EJ. Normal histology and nomenclature of the vulva, and malignant neoplasms, including VIN. Dermatol Clin 1992;10:283–296.
12. Soper DE, Patterson JW, Hurt G, et al. Lichen planus of the vulva. Obstet Gynecol 1988;72:74–76.
13. Furlonge CB, Thin RN, Evans BE, et al. Vulvar vestibulitis syndrome: a clinico-pathological study. Br J Obstet Gynaecol 1991;98:703–706.
14. Leuchter RS, Hacker NF, Voet RL, et al. Primary carcinoma of the Bartholin gland: a report of 14 cases and review of the literature. Obstet Gynecol 1982;60:361–368.
15. Dunn S. Adenoid cystic carcinoma of Bartholin's gland—a review of the literature and report of a patient. Acta Obstet Gynaecol Scand 1995;74:78–79.
16. Lewis FM, Lewis-Jones MS, Toon PG, et al. Neurofibromatosis of the vulva. Br J Dermatol 1992;127:540–541.
17. Cormen ML, Veidengeimer MC, Coller JA, et al. Perineal wound healing after proctectomy for inflammatory bowel disease. Dis Colon Rectum 1978;21:155–159.
18. Campion MJ, Franklin EW, Burrell MO, et al. Vulvar neoplasia in relation to other genital tract neoplasia: a regional disease. Colpo Gynecol Laser Surg 1988;4:111.
19. Hopkins MP. Vaginal neoplasms. In: Copeland LJ, ed. Textbook of Gynecology. 2nd ed. Philadelphia: WB Saunders, 1997.

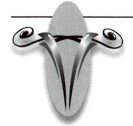

CHAPTER 18

Breast Disease

DANIEL P. GUYTON

Diseases of the breast comprise a diverse clinical spectrum. The etiologies and therapies of breast diseases remain clouded by clinical inaccuracies, social myths, and continually evolving medical controversies. Success in the battle against breast disease, and more specifically breast cancer, is markedly enhanced by the presence of a highly educated public and the widespread availability of noninvasive screening examinations. Efforts to conquer breast cancer are hindered, however, by the sheer magnitude of the problem. The American Cancer Society estimated that 181,600 new cases of breast cancer would be diagnosed in 1997 and 44,000 women would die that year from breast cancer (1).

Despite our best efforts, the crude mortality curve for breast cancer has remained remarkably flat with relatively small yearly fluctuations from 1930 to 1993. With great fanfare, a downward trend of 4.7% in the curve was recently announced. This may be a harbinger of a long-awaited improved extended outlook, hopefully as a result of earlier detection programs involving screening mammography (2).

Fortunately, most patients with breast disease in a busy clinician's practice will have one of the more common benign breast diseases and not breast cancer. From the patient's perspective, however, benign disease may be as frightening as breast cancer. The physician must recognize that fear of cancer is widespread and is often the motivating factor to seek medical attention.

All physicians who treat women must be familiar with the clinical fundamentals of benign and malignant breast disease. This chapter discusses breast anatomy, proper history and examination skills, and benign and malignant breast disease.

CLINICAL ANATOMY

A brief review of the normal breast anatomy is necessary to better understand the common pathologic conditions. The breast itself is composed of fat and parenchymal tissue that often extends well into the axilla. The parenchymal tissue is composed of microscopic ducts that drain toward the nipple. These ducts emanate from lobules consisting of secretory units or alveoli. The ducts, the lobules, and the alveoli all increase in size during pregnancy. The amount of fat and parenchyma varies with age and parity.

Most blood supply to the breast originates from the internal mammary artery, and the major lymphatic drainage is through the axillary and internal mammary chains of lymph nodes. The supraclavicular lymph nodes should not be palpable. Enlargement of this nodal group usually occurs with late-stage breast cancer but may also be noted in other disease processes. The skin overlying the breast is relatively thin compared with other regions of the body. It rarely exceeds 1.5 mm in thickness. Thus, patchy irregular thickness of the skin is abnormal and may occur with tumor infiltration, infection, or other breast and/or systemic disorders.

Ectopic glandular tissue is commonly present in the axilla, and this can proliferate during pregnancy and cause significant discomfort. Such proliferation will regress either with delivery or cessation of lactation. From a histologic perspective, this is normal breast tissue and is subject to both benign and malignant disorders. It should not be confused with a prominent axillary tail of Spence, a normal anatomic variant that may also enlarge during pregnancy. The axillary tail of Spence is usually continuous with the glandular tissue of the breast in contrast to ectopic axillary tissue, which may be totally discrete from the breast parenchyma.

DEVELOPMENTAL ABNORMALITIES

Common abnormalities of development include lack of development, underdevelopment, and premature development of breast tissue. Underdevelopment is termed hypoplasia, whereas complete lack of development is termed amastia.

Complete lack or absence of breast development is very rare. Genetic abnormalities such as Turner's syndrome (45,XO) or Klinefelter's syndrome (47,XXY) lead to stunting of breast development of variable degrees. Both chromosomal abnormalities are characterized by notable physical features involving body height and habitus, distribution of facial or body hair, and/or skeletal aberrations (3).

Poland's syndrome is characterized by congenital absence of both the breast tissue and the underlying muscle. It is always unilateral, and the lack of both the pectoralis major and minor muscles serves as distinguishing features. The major thoracic bone and cartilaginous structures may be involved, and brachysyndactyly (shortening of the digits accompanied by webbing between two or more fingers and/or toes) is also a common associated finding. Modern plastic and thoracic surgical techniques at the appropriate age are effective in correcting these complex anatomic deformities.

Premature breast development in children usually results from estrogen stimulation of an idiopathic etiology. Premature breast development should not be confused with precocious puberty in which not only breast but also labial enlargement and pubic hair growth are stimulated. See Chapter 1 for discussion of this pediatric problem.

Abnormalities of the Mammary Ridge

Supernumerary nipples and/or breast tissue may develop anywhere along the mammary ridge and are a common finding. There is an embryonic line, the mammary ridge or milk ridge, curving from the anterior axilla to the normal midclavicular nipple location to the inguinal region, ending at the labia (Fig. 18.1). These bilateral ridges originate during the fifth week of gestation and normally regress before birth. Supernumerary nipples (polythelia) with or without breast tissue may be present anywhere along the mammary ridge but may not become apparent until a woman's first pregnancy when the hormonally stimulated growth of breast parenchyma occurs. Although accessory nipples may be found anywhere along the ridge, they are usually located in the lower abdominal region.

PATIENT HISTORY

The first step in evaluating a woman with a suspected breast mass begins with a complete history. Many large series demonstrated that most breast masses are self-detected, although quoted percentages vary with the screening programs used (4, 5). The patient's emotional response to a self-detected mass is often complex. Sentiments range from panic to denial. Accompanying these often unspoken emotions may be feelings of guilt for not seeking medical attention at an earlier date, for "hiding" the mass from the woman's partner, or even fear of genetically transmitting the

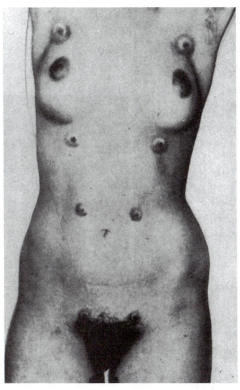

FIGURE 18.1. Supernumerary nipples may develop anywhere along the mammary ridge but are most common in the lower abdominal area. (Reprinted with permission from Mitchell GW Jr, Bassett LW. The Female Breast and Its Disorders. Baltimore: Williams & Wilkins, 1990:10.)

same problem to her daughter(s). All or none of these emotional concerns may surface during the examination. For this reason, the establishment of a physician-patient relationship is paramount during the initial history. Compassion, empathy, and support are all important qualities that cannot be replaced by preprinted forms. The clinician must regard the fear of cancer as real and must not be optimistically cavalier or, at the other extreme, leave the patient devoid of all hope upon conclusion of the encounter.

One goal of history taking is to educate the patient about any social and/or genetic risk factors she may have that may ultimately affect the decision analysis (Table 18.1). Present age, age at menarche, age at first full-term pregnancy, and age at menopause (if applicable) should all be recorded. For those patients with a self-detected breast mass, it is very important to review, in the patient's own words, exactly how she identified the problem. Did she learn of a friend with breast cancer and then performed a breast self-examination? Was she injured? Did she note a sudden pain or discomfort? Were her undergarments stained from a bloody nipple discharge? The answers to these questions and other details of the history of the mass may all serve to point the examiner in the correct direction. Lesions uncovered through screening mammography will often be nonpalpable and frequently are the most difficult for the patient to comprehend.

A careful family history focuses upon any relative with breast or ovarian cancer, especially a mother, sister, or daughter, and their approximate age at cancer diag-

TABLE 18.1. Breast Cancer Risk Factors

<12 years old at menarche
>35 years old at first term pregnancy
Multiple term pregnancies
>55 years old at menopause
Family history of breast cancer in mother, sister, or daughter; even greater risk if
   Cancer was diagnosed premenopausally
   Cancer was bilateral
   Breast cancer was present in two or more first-degree relatives
Patient or family history of ovarian or uterine cancer
Patient history of cancer in one breast (increases risk of cancer in the other)
Fibrocystic changes of the breast with proliferative changes, papillomatosis, or
   atypical epithelial hyperplasia
Living in industrialized nation (with notable exception of Japan)
Caucasian women at greater risk than non-Caucasians (in U.S.)

nosis. All of this should be recorded. Often patients will have already sought out the answers to these questions from their relatives. Genetic linkages are more significant when cancers occur in premenopausal relatives (5). Most breast cancers are sporadic and not related to any recognized genetic mutations. Nevertheless, historical questions may alert the clinician to an elevated risk in specific patients. Recently, the presence or absence of pain has been the subject of renewed debate. Pain was thought to be a rare symptom of invasive cancer because nerves that track pain are more sensitive to acute stretching than to slow growth. Hence, a cyst that enlarges very rapidly was thought to cause a greater sense of pain than a slowly growing tumor. However, several large series point out that pain is an important symptom of invasive cancer found in 5 to 22% of patients with invasive tumors (6, 7). Thus, this symptom alone should not be used to avoid or delay further evaluation.

EXAMINATION OF THE BREASTS

Proper examination of the breast is fundamental to detecting, diagnosing, and treating breast disease. A thorough breast examination requires both a visual and a physical inspection. The following sections describe a complete breast examination. The reader is also referred to Figure 18.2 for a visual display of the proper complete breast examination.

Inspection

The initial step in the breast examination is inspection. The physician should stand in front of the patient who is seated with her arms bent and her hands on her iliac crests. The patient is asked to exert pressure on her iliac crests while the physician searches for asymmetry, dimpling, or retraction of the overlying skin or any mass altering the contour of the breast. Retraction, when present, is usually not a subtle finding. Although most common with carcinoma, retraction may also be seen with fat necrosis (a benign condition discussed later in the chapter). The color of the skin should be noted because it may be altered with infection, edema, or the classic peau d'orange of carcinoma (which is due to obstruction of the dermal lymphatics). The patient is then asked to raise her arms above her head and press her hands against each other while the physician once again visually inspects the breast. This process

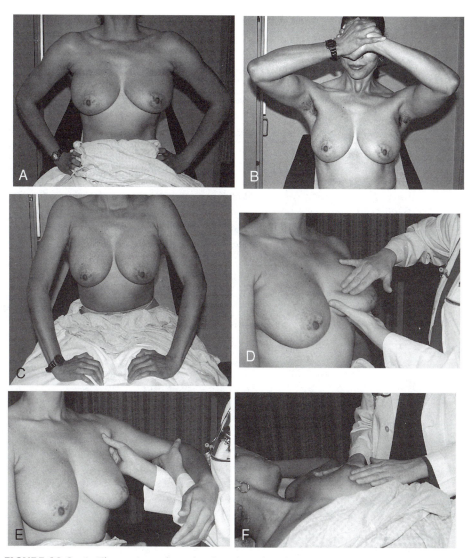

FIGURE 18.2. **A.** The patient places her hands on her iliac crests/hips and pushes on them. The breasts are inspected for symmetry, skin changes, dimpling, and/or retraction. **B.** The patient clasps her hands overhead and pushes her hands against each other. The breasts are inspected for symmetry, skin changes, dimpling, and/or retraction. **C.** The patient places her hands on her knees, leans forward slightly, and pushes her hands against her knees. The breasts are inspected for symmetry, skin changes, dimpling, and/or retraction. **D.** For larger breasts, palpation with one hand while the other supports the breast (in the sitting position) may reveal masses not otherwise felt on supine examination. **E.** The axilla are palpated while the ipsilateral arm is supported. To do a thorough examination, it is very important for the patient to relax the arm and shoulder as much as possible (i.e., the arm should be freely movable by the physician). **F.** The breast is inspected with the patient in the supine position with the ipsilateral arm slightly raised.

is repeated a third time with the patient leaning slightly forward and pushing her hands against her knees with her elbows slightly bent.

The nipple areolar complex is inspected carefully. The nipples should be everted and symmetric. On occasion, the patient will inform the examiner that one of her nipples has been inverted all her life. A physiologically inverted nipple can always be manually everted but a nipple retracted secondary to an underlying malignancy cannot. The presence of an encrustation or scaly covering may represent Paget's disease—carcinoma involving the nipple, and not infrequently the areola, but without an underlying palpable mass. In Paget's disease, the nipple may appear erythematous and inflamed and may bleed when touched.

Palpation

As with inspection, the patient is examined in both the sitting and supine position. In sequence, the supraclavicular region, the breast, and the axilla should all receive careful palpation. To best examine the axilla, it is necessary to bend the arm at the elbow and slightly abduct the entire arm. This serves to open the apex of the axilla and permit accurate examination by the examiner's hand as it slides against the rib cage in search of adenopathy. It is important for the patient to relax her arm and shoulder so that both are freely movable.

The breasts should be examined in the sitting position as part of the complete breast examination. The examiner supports the breast in the extended nondominant hand and lightly palpates the breast in a sequential fashion with the fingertips of the dominant hand. This examination is particularly helpful in women who have large pendulous breasts.

Next, the patient is asked to assume a recumbent position. If the patient has reported a mass, it may be advantageous to examine the opposite breast initially to gain an appreciation for any masses that may be symmetrical. Occasionally, it is helpful to have her rotate her upper body slightly to one side. This will elevate the breast, allowing exposure of the lateral chest wall. Using a small circular motion, the entire breast is examined in a systematic fashion. The ipsilateral arm is then raised with the hand placed behind the head and the breast examined again.

Even among experienced clinicians, it is often difficult to distinguish between simple glandular tissue and a mass requiring biopsy. Several points may be helpful. Glandular or parenchymal tissue may be sensitive to the touch at examination, whereas a malignancy may be painless upon direct palpation. This tenderness (or lack thereof) with palpation is irrespective of symptoms of *pain* reported by the patient. If a mass is identified in the upper outer quadrant of one breast, a similar mass should be found in the upper outer quadrant of the other breast if it is a benign tissue mass. Subtle distinctions in the size and prominence may be present, but larger palpatory differences may require biopsy. Asymmetric masses, whether identified on examination or by screening mammography, must be viewed with caution because this is considered one of the "soft" signs of malignancy (8). Frequently there is a ridge of fibrous tissue occupying the inframammary fold bilaterally. The tissue represents the attachment of the breasts to the underlying chest wall and is usually curvilinear in shape with a variable degree of thickness. Again, this should be a symmetric finding.

Distinction between a tense cyst and a solid mass is extremely difficult (if not impossible) by palpation alone. Both cystic and solid masses that prove histologically benign may present a smooth rounded surface. Mobility is a key feature because malignancies tend to be irregular and fixed to the adjacent tissue. Because of their infiltrative nature, malignancies, particularly those located at the periphery of the breast or below the nipple, will lead to retraction of the overlying tissue. Although these features are helpful palpatory findings in distinguishing a benign mass from a malignant one, they alone should never serve to singularly exclude biopsy.

Special Situations

This section discusses the examination of pregnant patients, the equivocal examination, patients with breast implants, and patients who have received irradiation for malignancy.

Pregnancy

During the first and second trimesters of pregnancy, ductal proliferation occurs under the influence of circulating hormones. This enlargement should be symmetric, although rare instances of massive enlargement of one breast (unilateral gigantism) have been reported. Breast examination during this period of rapid growth in pregnancy may be difficult and confusing. The best safeguard is careful examination of both breasts at the time of the initial office visit along with thorough documentation of the initial findings. A new asymmetric mass should not be followed in pregnancy; whether benign glandular tissue or a tumor, the mass will increase in size. In equivocal cases, consultation should be obtained earlier rather than later. When compared stage for stage, breast cancer occurring in pregnancy does not carry a poorer prognosis. The historical impression of pregnancy-related poorer prognosis is now attributed to delay in diagnosis, that is, these cancers were detected at a later stage (9).

Treatment for breast cancer in a pregnant patient is very individualized. If disease is localized and found in the first or second trimester, it is probably best treated with excision and radiation (just as it would be in the nonpregnant woman). Although the numbers are small, there seems to be no increase in adverse pregnancy effects for chemotherapy use after the first trimester. If the tumor is localized and found early in the third trimester, definitive treatment is indicated. Late in the third trimester, the definitive therapy may begin immediately postpartum. If the cancer is discovered while the woman is nursing, she should stop breast feeding and receive definitive therapy. In those cases of advanced incurable breast cancer, palliative therapy is offered and the desires of the mother and therapies needed dictate continuation or termination of the pregnancy.

For women with a previous history of breast cancer, most recurrences occur in the first 2 to 3 years after diagnosis so they should be counseled to avoid pregnancy in that time period. After that, there is no clear difference in survival for women who become pregnant after a history of breast cancer.

The Equivocal Examination

Little is written on this common and frequently vexing problem, that is, what should be done for the patient with an equivocal breast examination? An equivocal examination is one where no discrete mass is evident, nothing is seen radiographically, and yet after careful palpation the physician remains uncertain. Usually, findings consist of glandular prominence. They should not be confused with a "lump" or "mass" because these require histologic diagnosis. If the patient has no genetic or social risk factors and is premenopausal, then reexamination after the next menstrual cycle should be performed. Appropriate referral should not be delayed when the area in question persists through one cycle, in a patient with recognized risk factors, or when the patient is postmenopausal (irrespective of hormone replacement) because the incidence of breast cancer increases with age. In the presence of asymmetry, prompt referral is indicated.

Breast Augmentation

Implants placed for augmentation alter the *shape* of a woman's breast but should not alter the nature of the glandular tissue. It is important to determine if any breast reduction or sculpturing was performed concomitantly because excisional surgery may lead to palpatory differences. Implants can occasionally induce the formation of a fibrous capsule, resulting in breasts that are very firm. Granulomas indistinguishable by palpation from malignancy can also form in patients with silicone implants. These granulomas will be discrete, rock hard, and fixed to the surrounding tissue. They are often superficial and readily palpable; excisional biopsy is required for diagnosis. Needle aspiration of a breast mass in a patient with silicone-filled implants should be performed by an experienced clinician using ultrasound guidance to decrease risk of puncturing the implant, thus causing leakage and potential granuloma formation.

Scientific evidence supporting the development of systemic side effects after silicone implant insertion is lacking. The development of connective tissue disorders in patients with silicone-filled implants was thought to be a cause and effect relationship, presumably arising from "leaking" prostheses (10). The Nurses Health Study directed by the Harvard School of Public Health compared 1183 women with silicone implants and no evidence of connective tissue disorder with 516 women without implants but definitively diagnosed with connective tissue disorders (11). Careful analysis of the two groups failed to identify any association between silicone breast implants and connective tissue diseases. It is not necessary to remove silicone implants unless specific problems directly attributable to the implants arise.

Postirradiation

Radiation therapy is often given after excision of small invasive breast cancers to reduce the incidence of recurrence within the tumor bed. The examination of the patient who has completed a course of postoperative irradiation should follow the same procedure as outlined above with one caveat. The physician must carefully examine the incision for tumor recurrence that will present as a firm raised lesion within or adjacent to the surgical incision. Mammography represents an important adjunct in this situation.

Palpatory changes secondary to irradiation are actually unusual, and the overall incidence of late skin changes or fibrosis is small. The treated breast may appear slightly smaller and may have a slight generalized firmness in the previous tumor bed. Subtle changes may be more difficult to detect postirradiation.

RADIOGRAPHIC EVALUATION OF THE BREAST

Radiographic evaluation of breast disease plays a critical role in optimal patient care. Screening mammography programs appear effective in early detection of tumors and at earlier stages, consequently improving survival. Radiographic-assisted alternatives to open biopsy are evolving and hold much promise for providing accurate pathologic diagnoses without surgery in many women.

Screening Mammography

The guidelines for routine screening mammography are controversial. Intuitively, this is a program that makes good common sense for all women. When analyzing a large statistical study, key questions must be addressed to avoid unintentional extrapolation of benefits. Did the study prove a reduction in breast cancer mortality was due to early screening? Do such programs actually detect cancer at an early (i.e., more curable) stage or are they merely detecting more cancers? Can the benefits of mortality reduction be applied to women of all age groups? What are the limitations of screening mammography? And, finally, how well do national or organizational policy screening recommendations intended for huge populations at risk translate into the one-on-one advice given by a physician to her or his patient? Because screening mammography plays such an essential role in the care of the individual patient, issues regarding the current screening policy are summarized.

Overall, in randomized trials involving wide age groups of women, there appears to be a reduction of approximately 25% in breast cancer mortality resulting from screening programs (12–14). The benefit of screening women 50 to 69 years old is clear. Their breasts have less glandular tissue and more fatty replacement, making it less likely for a tumor to be hidden by dense breast parenchyma. This allows a greater sensitivity of the screening mammogram.

In 1992, the Canadian National Breast Screening Study reported an actual increase in breast cancer deaths in women 40 to 49 years old who were identified during the national screening program (15). This alarming finding has been debated by numerous authors and recently refuted (16). Eight randomized trials studied the efficacy of screening programs specifically in this younger age group and, in sharp contrast to the Canadian study, reported a 24% reduction in mortality among women 40 to 49 years old in these screening programs. Tumors tended to be identified at an earlier stage, and the subsequent reduction in mortality is thought to be due, at least indirectly, to earlier treatment.

The radiographic characteristics considered highly suggestive of breast cancer include architectural distortion of the adjacent tissue, sharply irregular borders, spiculation, or a mass associated with clustered microcalcifications. The most reliable indicator for malignancy is the nature of the tumor margin. Another important feature of malignancy is peripheral spiculation around the tumor. Mammography provides a more accurate estimate of the actual tumor size than does physical examination. Malignancy often induces edema and a desmoplastic response in the tissue around the tumor, thus making the malignancy feel larger than it is.

The radiographic characteristics of various benign breast disorders are reviewed in Table 18.2. Screening mammography has several well-recognized limitations. Specific histologic forms of breast cancer (medullary, mucinous, and cystosarcoma phyllodes) may, in fact, appear as well-circumscribed masses. In women with very radiographically dense breasts, small cancers within the breast are difficult to detect irrespective of the age of the patient. Metastases to the breast from extramammary malignancies are usually well circumscribed and may appear benign on mammogram.

Several authors stressed that a clear distinction must be made between detection of a mammographic abnormality and the radiographic description of its physical features. Nearly every mammographically detected lesion that demonstrates benign characteristics may still harbor a malignancy. The lobulated and well-circumscribed lesions seen on mammogram and ultrasound study in Figure 18.3 were interpreted as fibroadenoma. Biopsy proved both to represent invasive cancer. Thus, a "negative" mammogram should not delay biopsy if a dominant or clinically suspicious mass is present. It may *reinforce* a clinical impression. Mammography currently has a 10 to 15% false-negative rate and a 6 to 10% false-positive rate.

One retrospective study found misinterpretation to be a slightly more common cause of error than simply overlooking the lesion (17). The shape of the lesion, although helpful, may be unreliable.

When the abnormal area is indeterminate or only vaguely abnormal, a shortened interval follow-up, usually 6 months, is recommended. This is valuable for assessing any change in the radiographic appearance of the lesion. Additional views

TABLE 18.2. Radiographic Findings in Benign Breast Disorders

Benign Breast Disorders	Mammographic Characteristics
Cysts	Frequently multiple Smooth, sharp border May have thin radiolucent halo
Intramammary lymph node	Upper outer quadrant, near chest wall Usually < 1 cm Kidney bean-shaped with smooth outline May be partially replaced by fat
Mole	Well-circumscribed
Fibroadenoma	Sometimes multiple Lobulated, but with a small margin May have thin radiolucent halo If hyalinized, may have coarse calcifications
Surgical scar	May have radial spiculations if recent Follow-up mammogram shows decreasing size/prominence
Lipoma	May be difficult to detect on mammography
Sclerosing adenosis	Most common benign disorder that mimics malignancy on mammogram; it falls in the spectrum of breast changes in fibrocystic breast disease May appear as ill-defined, mottled, or nodular process May appear as homogenous soft tissue density with indistinct margins
Breast abscess	May appear similar to inflammatory carcinoma (primarily diagnosed on aspiration or biopsy)
Traumatic fat necrosis	Variable mammographic features May be confused with carcinoma

(magnified or cone down) can also be very helpful in sorting out a true mass from vague abnormalities secondary to tissue superimposition. Masses that are less than or equal to 1 to 1.5 cm and have smooth margins and no calcifications are almost always benign. Such lesions can be followed with repeat mammography in 3 to 6 months initially and then yearly for a minimum of 2.5 to 3 years (18).

Patients are often uncomfortable with waiting, and careful clinical judgment individualized for each patient is required. To a woman with an increased risk for breast cancer (e.g., she has a first-degree relative with breast cancer), watchful waiting may be unacceptable. Stereotactic biopsy, described below, may offer an acceptable alternative in the case of indeterminate patterns. Radiographically indeterminate lesions require histologic diagnosis in the presence of clinical suspicion or high patient anxiety.

Microcalcifications

As the use of screening mammography increases, an increase in the detection of microcalcifications is likely to follow suit. The significance of microcalcifications is that they may represent one of the earliest signs of detectable malignant disease in situ. There may or may not be an associated mass evident. Typically, malignant calcifications are small, linear, and branched or tightly clustered or in a compact irregular

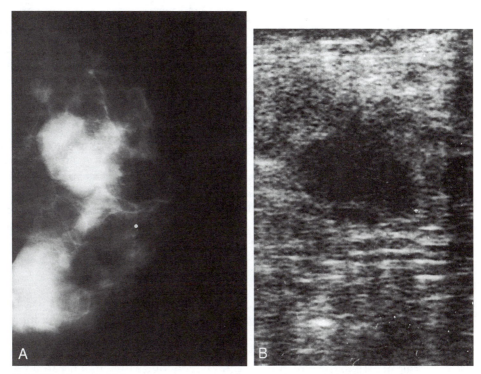

FIGURE 18.3. A. This mammogram was interpreted as probable fibroadenoma. **B.** Sonographically, it was also interpreted as probably fibroadenoma. Histologically, the mass proved to be invasive cancer.

pattern. They are pleomorphic and numerous. Clustering alone is an indeterminate sign because it may be found with both benign and malignant disease.

The microcalcifications of benign lesions are usually larger, rounder, fewer, and vary less in size than the microcalcifications of malignancy. Some benign disorders like sclerosing adenosis, fat necrosis, and apocrine metaplasia may have microcalcifications similar to those of carcinoma(s). Cancerous microcalcifications usually follow a ductal pattern because most cancers arise from the ducts. The absolute number of calcifications does not correlate with either benign or malignant disease, but benign calcifications tend to be scattered throughout the entire breast and are of similar size and shape.

Ultrasonography

Ultrasound, easily done in the office, is most commonly used to help identify palpable cystic and solid masses, but correlation between a lesion seen mammographically and its appearance on ultrasound requires expertise. An advantage to ultrasound evaluation is its complete absence of irradiation (preferable for the pregnant patient). Also, because no compression of the surrounding breast tissue is required, it is a nearly painless procedure. Ultrasound is an important adjunct for diagnosing breast disease in younger women. Their breasts are less fatty and are more dense and fibrous. On ultrasound, there is a large amount of homogenous echoes, making detection of sonolucent masses easier. In contrast, fat transmits sound poorly, and isolated fat masses may appear as sonolucent masses. The sensitivity and specificity of ultrasound are too low, however, to allow for its use as a screening tool for malignancy.

Breast tissue is very heterogenous so abnormalities near the surface of the breast may be distorted or missed in the near fields of the transducer. To adequately perform breast ultrasound, a fluid offset must be located between the breast and the transducer. A water-filled plastic bag or commercially available offset pad is used if the transducer does not have a built-in fluid offset. For breast imaging, the transducer should be 5 MHz or greater and the depth of focus should not exceed 2 cm.

Ultrasound is ideal for evaluation and follow-up of patients with multiple breast cysts. It can detect breast cysts as small as 2 mm. The most reliable diagnostic feature of a cyst in ultrasound is an anechoic interior. With compression, cysts usually flatten. Simple cysts demonstrate a clear fluid-filled space between the anterior and posterior wall. These are almost always benign. Complex cysts appear with echogenic structures between the anterior and posterior border and may be septated. Further discussion on cysts follows in the section on benign breast conditions.

Ultrasound-guided biopsy or aspiration may be performed on solid and cystic lesions (19, 20). In skilled hands this is technically simple, straightforward, and associated with a high degree of accuracy.

Magnetic Resonance Imaging

Magnetic resonance imaging (MRI) using gadolinium contrast is a newer radiographic tool. The label accumulates around tissue composed of a high degree of vascularity such as that seen with invasive cancer. Although cysts may be reliably detected by MRI, ultrasonography is less expensive and more accessible. The clinical role of MRI in the screening, diagnosis, and/or treatment of breast disease is being researched (21). Presently, MRI has no role in clinical screening for breast carcinoma and is not a useful adjunct to mammography because MRI findings have no bearing on the selection of appropriate treatment strategies.

Stereotactic-Guided Biopsy

Stereotactic-guided biopsy is a relatively new technique using geometric concepts to target a nonpalpable lesion. A single-view mammogram is taken from two opposing angles and a computer then calculates the x, y, and z axes, thus determining the exact location of the lesion in the breast. Digitalized equipment now permits near real-time visualization of the biopsy procedure. It may be used on women with breast implants.

Currently there are two different systems on the market; they differ primarily in the amount of tissue removed at biopsy. One system uses a fine needle for biopsy, whereas the other is a stereotactic core biopsy, commonly using a 14-gauge needle. If a core sample exhibits ductal carcinoma in situ (DCIS), open biopsy is necessary because 30% of the cases of DCIS are associated with an invasive carcinoma (22–24).

Initial reports are very promising in terms of accuracy and patient acceptance as well for reducing the need for operative biopsy. One study of 2988 cases reported 94.6% sensitivity and 99.8% specificity for the procedure (25). The average cost of stereotactic-guided biopsy in 1995 was $1200 including the radiologist's fee. The average cost savings from this procedure compared with immediate excisional biopsy was estimated at $1700 in one study (26). Mammographic findings that are suspicious or highly suggestive of malignancy in a woman with a high level of anxiety are indications for stereotactic biopsy.

FINE-NEEDLE ASPIRATION OF A MASS

Fine-needle aspiration is a technique for obtaining a tissue sample of a palpable (or with ultrasound guidance, a nonpalpable) mass using a fine-gauge needle. It can be diagnostic when malignant cells are recovered and therapeutic when used to aspirate a cyst. Its usefulness is limited by the need for a skilled cytopathologist, a high rate of insufficient samples, and an inability to differentiate between in situ and invasive carcinoma.

For accuracy, the mass must be discrete and not simply glandular parenchyma of the breast. The patient should be informed that this technique is typically not painful and her preference for use of no, topical, or local anesthetic should be followed. After preparation of the skin with alcohol, the mass is aspirated using a 20- or 22-gauge syringe (Fig. 18.4). Aspiration is not begun until the mass is entered, and four or five passes in a very short time period are necessary for an adequate specimen. If a long time is taken in obtaining the biopsy, the specimen will be contaminated with blood or blood clots. Frank blood obscures the cellular pattern so the procedure should be

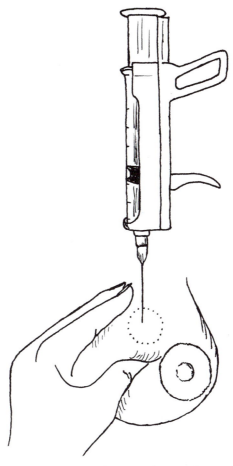

FIGURE 18.4. Fine-needle aspiration technique. The needle is placed in the mass and withdrawn at different angles and different areas at the mass at least five times. This should be done in a minimum of time to avoid contamination of the specimen. Suction must be maintained throughout the biopsy process but is discontinued with the entry of biopsy material into the needle hub. The needle is then withdrawn, the syringe removed, and 5 to 10 mL of air drawn into the syringe. The needle is reattached and the air used to place the cytologic specimen onto the slide. If adequate material is not obtained, the aspiration can be repeated but must be entered on a separate track.

repeated. It is usually possible to tell when the needle has entered the mass because of differences in its consistency compared with the surrounding tissue. The aspirated contents are then deposited upon a glass slide, smeared, and fixed immediately using a commercially available fixative such as that used for a Pap smear.

Several points regarding the interpretation of fine-needle aspiration material bear emphasis. With any patient, the decision to perform this aspiration should not be regarded as an end point in the evaluation of a discrete mass. Rather, it represents only an initial component of the entire evaluative process. Although false positives are unusual, false negatives range from 5 to 25%, with an average of 8% in multiple series. Clinicians should view a negative report as nondiagnostic. The actual false-positive rate probably depends on the skill levels of both the clinician and the cytopathologist. Fine-needle aspiration cannot differentiate between in situ and invasive cancer so further excision is required in most cases. Both a small tumor size and an aspirate containing a sparse number of cells may lead to diagnostic difficulties (27).

Complications from fine-needle aspiration are relatively few, with the most frequent being hematoma formation. If this occurs, it is readily apparent and should be treated with gentle direct compression until expansion of the underlying tissue is no longer noted. If mammography is performed soon after a hematoma, the original mass may be obscured; therefore, mammography should be performed before attempting aspiration or no less than 2 weeks after the aspiration. A more unusual complication with fine-needle aspiration is pneumothorax. This is more prone to occur when the lesion lies in close proximity to the chest wall, but the risk can be diminished by manipulating the mass over a rib when possible. The patient usually becomes quickly dyspneic. Immediate chest radiograph followed by reexpansion with a small suction catheter is the treatment of choice. Infection after fine-needle aspiration is extremely rare.

EVALUATION OF NIPPLE DISCHARGE

Nipple discharge may present in women of all age groups. The patient will find discoloration on her undergarments or night clothes or may notice the discharge during performance of breast self-examination. In taking the history and performing the examination, several things should be noted: nature of the discharge, factors that elicit the discharge (spontaneous or requiring pressure), relation to menses, presence or absence of a mass, unilateral or bilateral, and single or multiple ducts involved. The physician should also ask about conditions of overstimulation of the nipple. These might include tight clothes, inadequate support while exercising, and constant examination of the breasts for discharge. Medical illnesses and medications may also cause nipple discharge (Table 18.3). Nipple discharge due to oral contraceptives is usually from multiple ducts, is usually more evident just before menses, and resolves upon stopping the medication.

In a patient who is not breast-feeding, the most common causes of nipple discharge are breast cancer, intraductal papilloma, and mammary dysplasia. Most nipple discharge is secondary to a benign etiology, with only 6 to 15% of cases associated with cancer. The color of the discharge may range from a clear serous drainage to green or brownish to frank blood. The most common cause of bloody nipple discharge is an intraductal papilloma, a benign lesion involving the ductal system in proximity to the nipple. A mass may or may not be present. The involved duct(s) should be identified. This is usually accomplished by exerting pressure at different sites around the nipple at the margin of the areola. Cytologic examination of the discharge should be done, bearing in mind that a negative result does not rule out cancer (28, 29).

TABLE 18.3. Causes of Nipple Discharge

IDIOPATHIC

DRUG INDUCED
Phenothiazines, butyrophenones, reserpine, methyldopa, imipramine, amphetamine, metoclopramide, sulpiride, pimozide, oral contraceptive agents

BREAST LESIONS
Intraductal papilloma, ductal ectasia, fibrocystic changes, carcinoma, breast abscess

CENTRAL NERVOUS SYSTEM LESIONS
Pituitary adenoma, empty sella, hypothalamic tumor, head trauma

MEDICAL CONDITIONS
Chronic renal failure, sarcoidosis, Schuller-Christian disease, Cushing's disease, hepatic cirrhosis, hypothyroidism

CHEST WALL LESIONS
Thoracotomy, herpes zoster

Before the examination, slides should be readily available for a cytologic preparation using a fixative such as that used for a Pap smear. The clinician should mentally divide the areola into quadrants and first feel for the presence of an underlying mass. If identified, the mass is gently compressed while watching for any discharge to appear. If no mass is identified and no discharge is noted after the initial examination, palpation is repeated. Occult blood in a discharge may be identified using stool guaiac cards. Occasionally, neither the physician nor the patient are able to replicate the discharge, and a return office visit is required. Application of a small amount of benzoin to the nipple, temporarily blocking the duct drainage, 48 hours before the office visit is said to be an effective aid in the identification of discharge. If unilateral discharge persists for more than 1 month, even without localization of the duct(s) or a tumor, exploration or follow-up at intervals of 1 to 3 months is necessary. A mammogram should be done as well. If the discharge is chronic and unilateral, and particularly if it is bloody, this is an indication to resect the involved duct(s).

Bilateral milky discharge may be an expression of a pituitary tumor and a prolactin level should be checked; prolactin levels can be falsely elevated, however, immediately after a breast examination. Mammography is indicated for the nonlactating woman complaining of unilateral breast discharge. Ductography is also helpful to outline the offending duct and visualize any intraluminal lesion. However, if a palpable mass is identified, ductography is probably not necessary and the entire mass should be promptly excised.

BENIGN CONDITIONS

Cysts

Cysts are very common, occurring in as many as 50% of all women at some point in their lives. Most cysts are multiple and are only a few millimeters in diameter, although some may grow to be 4 cm in size. The common clinical presentation is a newly discovered breast mass that may be located in any quadrant of the breast. It may occur suddenly, demonstrating a rapid increase in size; these are often associated with significant pain and discomfort. Cysts may reach such large size that they actually result in asymmetry on inspection of the breasts. Palpable cysts are usually smooth, rounded, and relatively mobile, but occasionally they may blend into the underlying tissue because of associated fibrosis. They often create a "shotty" consistency in the breast. Some cysts are exceptionally firm and nontender; in this situation, it is very difficult to distinguish cystic from solid lesions on the basis of physical examination alone.

Mammographically, cysts appear as smooth rounded densities and are often multiple and widely scattered throughout either one or both breasts (30). The increasing availability of high-resolution ultrasonography has greatly simplified the management of these lesions. As discussed in an above section, cysts can be classified as simple or complex, single or clustered. A limitation of ultrasound is its inability to detect very small (less than 5 mm) lesions. Radiographically, simple cysts (free from any septation) may be aspirated if palpable or they may be observed. Aspiration is often performed in the case of a palpable cyst so as not to interfere with breast examination by either the patient or physician. For those cysts causing discomfort, aspiration provides immediate symptomatic relief. Histologically, simple cysts occasionally possess an epithelial lining and contain fluid that is characteristically clear with a yellow-green or brown tint (24).

Complex or clustered cysts should be aspirated and the fluid sent for cytologic analysis because ductal obstruction can be caused by microscopic tumor growth. After aspiration, the underlying breast tissue should always be repalpated for the presence of a mass. If a mass is found, excisional biopsy is required because a small carcinoma may have occluded the duct, leading to cyst formation. Other indications for cyst excision are early recurrence (less than 6 weeks after complete aspiration) and recurrence of the same cyst after two aspirations. Recurrence may be indicative of persistent ductal obstruction.

Fibroadenomas

Fibroadenomas are the most common benign breast tumors, occurring most frequently in young women. Classically, a fibroadenoma presents as a firm discrete solid mass detected by the patient. These are generally painless and tend to occur in women 20 to 40 years of age but may also be identified in teenage girls. They are more frequent and occur at an earlier age in women of African-American heritage. Data support observation of breast masses cytologically diagnosed as fibroadenomas.

On examination of the mass, the surface feels smooth and is occasionally lobulated. These are not infiltrative lesions so they are typically highly mobile. They are firm, discrete, and nontender masses and usually measure 1 to 5 cm in diameter, although they can grow to be quite large (the "giant" fibroadenoma). Multiple lesions occur in one or both breasts in as many as 10 to 15% of patients. The etiology of fibroadenoma is thought to be estrogen related. It is noteworthy that estrogen replacement therapy may lead to fibroadenoma development and growth in postmenopausal women (31).

Fibroadenomas usually decrease in size in the later reproductive years. They may eventually calcify and form a characteristic "popcorn" pattern of microcalcifications on mammogram (Fig. 18.5). This may occur when a large fibroadenoma degenerates. Coarse microcalcifications seen with fibroadenomas are generally quite different from the coarse microcalcifications associated with ductal carcinoma.

Histologically, fibroadenomas demonstrate an increased cellularity with large numbers of regularly shaped epithelial cells. As might be expected, they are estrogen receptor positive. The four generally accepted indications for removal of a fibroadenoma are

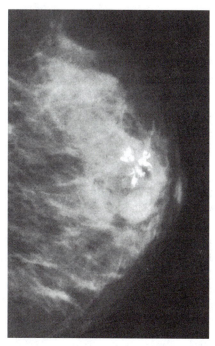

FIGURE 18.5. Mammogram with two fibroadenomas. The upper mass has typical popcorn-like calcifications. The lower lesion, although uncalcified, has a typical smooth margin with sufficient surrounding fat to make it visible. (Reprinted with permission from Mitchell GW Jr, Bassett LW. The Female Breast and Its Disorders. Baltimore: Williams & Wilkins, 1990:134.)

- Inability to differentiate between benign and malignant processes
- Recent enlargement
- Periareolar location
- Patient concern

The natural history of fibroadenomas is only now beginning to be delineated. In a small series of only 20 fibroadenomas, 40% decreased in size or spontaneously resolved, one third enlarged, and the remainder remained unchanged (32). Some authorities believe selected fibroadenomas, particularly those occurring in young women where the incidence of malignancy is low, may be carefully observed (33). The reported incidence of carcinoma arising in association with a fibroadenoma is quite low (34, 35). For those that are nonpalpable, histologic identification using stereotactic-guided biopsy or excision may be an attractive alternative. When the diagnosis is in question, biopsy represents the safest course for most women of all ages. For reasons that are unclear, the overall risk for the development of breast cancer may be elevated in women who undergo excisional biopsy for these fibroadenomas (36).

Whatever course is selected, patients should be clearly reminded that any new lesion requires complete evaluation and should not be assumed to be "merely another fibroadenoma."

Fat Necrosis

Fat necrosis is a pathologic and clinical term descriptive of lesions that, on palpation, may readily be confused with malignancy. A careful history may disclose a traumatic incident preceding the examination by several weeks to months. Lack of a recalled traumatic event does not, however, preclude the diagnosis. Trauma in automobile accidents may occur directly or from the safety belt shoulder strap. Events ranging from toddlers bouncing upon a woman's chest to a direct blow from a golf ball have all been implicated. Regardless of the mechanism of injury, the patient will notice a painful hematoma that will slowly resolve. Only about 50% of patients are able to recall a history of trauma or injury to the breast. It is common to see fat necrosis after radiation therapy and/or segmental resection of the breast.

On examination, the mass is usually discrete, fixed to the underlying breast tissue, and may be very hard. This lesion occasionally leads to retraction of the overlying skin that is indistinguishable from that seen with carcinoma; mammographic findings can also resemble those of carcinoma. Unless the patient is seen in the acute state of trauma recovery, there will not be any associated tenderness.

If the history is clear and the mass follows a well-documented trauma, a short period of observation may be indicated to await resolution. The clinical dilemma that arises is the presence of such a mass without any external evidence of trauma. Fine-needle aspiration may yield a small amount of fluid with an oily consistency. If the mass does not appreciably decrease in size, excisional biopsy is usually required to rule out malignancy. Histologic examination shows only the presence of chronic inflammation with a predominance of lymphocytes. This lesion is not associated with an increased risk of breast cancer.

Sclerosing Adenosis

Sclerosing adenosis may present as a hard, fixed, nontender mass indistinguishable from cancer. Pain may or may not be an associated clinical feature. Mammographically, it may also mimic invasive cancer. It is uncommon before the age of 30. Excisional biopsy is required to differentiate this lesion from invasive cancer. Women with this entity are thought to have a slightly greater risk of developing breast cancer over their lifetime.

Cystosarcoma Phyllodes

This is an uncommon tumor that usually affects women beyond the age of 30. They have a tendency to recur, although nodal and distant metastasis are rare. The patient presents with a well-defined but rapidly growing mass. They average 5 to 8 cm in diameter, are firm, and are often lobulated. After excision, it may histologically be classified as either benign or malignant, although there is no uniformly accepted standard of histologic division between these types. Both types, therefore, should be considered as potentially aggressive tumors.

"Fibrocystic Disease"

Historically, the clinical diagnosis "fibrocystic disease" or "mammary dysplasia" was given to women who had prominent areas of glandular tissue ("lumpy breasts") but who had no histologic evaluation performed. This term is often applied to explain the normal physiologic changes, which may be painful or uncomfortable, that are associated with cyclic production of estrogen and progesterone in the premenopausal woman. To label this as a disease is incorrect. This entity is common among women 30 to 50 years of age and is rare in the postmenopausal woman.

The patient may notice either a "lump" or pain in her breast that initiates an office visit. The pain is not necessarily related to the menstrual cycle. On physical examination, palpable glandular changes vary widely. Some women have a small relatively discrete but tender mass, whereas other women demonstrate large glandular areas with bilateral involvement of entire quadrants. The degree of tenderness may be marked with even gentle palpation. Serial examinations throughout the course of one menstrual cycle usually clarify the situation because the involvement will tend to fluctuate in size and tenderness. Mammographically, the involved regions appear as indistinct densities. These radiographic changes should be apparent bilaterally.

If biopsy is required, the histologic changes that may be found represent a full spectrum of microscopic cysts, adenosis, fibrosis, and apocrine changes. Pathologic reports should conform to widely accepted guidelines and report the changes as proliferative or nonproliferative for risk assessment. When fibrocystic changes are accompanied by proliferative changes, papillomatosis, or atypical epithelial hyperplasia, there is an increased risk of cancer.

Acute Infection and Abscesses

Lactational breast abscesses occur in the postpartum period and result from a progression of mastitis. The patient is usually nursing her infant and suddenly develops an acutely painful, red, and swollen breast. The infection is thought to arise from a mechanical obstruction of a duct, leading quickly to infection by a skin organism, commonly *Staphylococcus aureus*. The infection should be treated immediately with antibiotics (oxacillin or dicloxacillin [Dynapen]), and breast feeding (or pumping) should continue in the hope of opening up the plugged duct and permitting drainage. If the lesion progresses and forms a localized mass with signs of infection, an abscess is present that must be drained, and nursing should be discontinued.

Clinicians are now also seeing older nonlactating women with subareolar abscesses. The etiology is unclear but may involve carcinoma or even tuberculosis. Fistula formation from a duct to the areola has also been identified. The causative bacteria involve a much wider spectrum, including *Escherichia coli* and *Bacteroides* species (37, 38). This type of infection is usually centrally located and may be refractory to antibiotics. If incision and drainage are required, an incisional biopsy of the involved lactiferous duct(s) at the nipple base is usually also performed because this type of infection may (rarely) be associated with carcinoma. These types of abscesses carry a significantly higher incidence of recurrence, and reexcision of the entire involved ductal system may be necessary for cure. These should be treated by a surgeon with expertise in breast disease.

Mastodynia

Mastodynia is a poorly understood yet frequently encountered clinical entity. It has been the subject of many anecdotal lay articles purporting a better understanding and promising revolutionary treatments. When interacting with a patient with this complaint, a wise physician will be empathetic but truthful about the limitations of current understanding of this condition. The physician should always remember that pain may be associated with breast cancer, as discussed in the section on history taking above.

Mastodynia, or the broader term mastalgia, describes the complaint of breast pain. The pain is real, not imagined, and not caused by neurosis but often very difficult to treat. Numerous psychological studies of women with mastalgia have been completed, but all have failed to document any significant difference in the psychological profiles of women with this symptom compared with asymptomatic control subjects (39). The etiology of the pain in this condition remains unclear.

The pain is often described by the patient as having a burning or searing quality and may radiate from the nipple areola complex directly into the axilla. The patient may actually be able to trace the pain pathway with her fingers. The severity of the pain is variable. It occasionally is of such degree that the patient is unable to lie on her stomach to sleep and any type of external pressure accentuates her discomfort. Physical examination usually reveals nodularity or simply a diffuse area of tenderness that may be very impressive.

The treatment plan must first recognize the patient's pain. Reassurance and support are essential measures. A search for underlying pathologies that may mimic the syndrome of myalgia, such as muscular strain or blunt trauma, should be undertaken. Mammography is advised to exclude any nonpalpable cause such as a cyst deep within the glandular structures or, rarely, a malignancy. This is particularly important in a postmenopausal woman where cyclic mastalgia is not normally encountered. Surgery, unless to exclude the above pathologic causes, is rarely advisable because excision of the painful tissue has not been proven effective.

Treatment based on hormonal therapy using bromocriptine (Parlodel), danazol (Danocrine), or more recently tamoxifen (Nolvadex) have all demonstrated encouraging results, with success ranging from 66 to 75% (40). All have significant potential side effects, and the decision to institute pharmacologic therapy should be carefully undertaken. Abstinence from caffeine, or more broadly from methylxanthines, has not been shown to effectively improve symptomatology. Other widely used therapies include evening primrose oil and vitamin E supplements. Evening primrose oil is a natural substance composed of linoleic and linolenic essential fatty acids. Therapy is based on a hypothesis that mastalgia arises from an abnormality in prostaglandin metabolism. It is usually given as one tablespoon at bedtime. Because evening primrose is without reported side effects, there has been great hope that it may prove an acceptable alternative to drug therapy (41). In clinical studies, vitamin E (tocopherol) has not demonstrated any improvement in the symptoms of mastalgia.

MALIGNANT CONDITIONS

Although the overall incidence of breast cancer *appears* to be increasing, the higher rates can almost all be attributed to an increase in the number of tumors identified that are less than 2 cm in size (12). This is probably secondary to the increasingly widespread use of screening mammography that aids in the detection of nonpalpable (i.e., clinically occult) masses. As the tumor size at detection decreases, the proportion of self-detected cancers decreases.

There are numerous histologic types of breast cancer (Table 18.4). The histologic subtypes such as scirrhous, tubular, or medullary are morphologic distinctions among the various patterns of infiltrating (invasive) ductal carcinoma.

In Situ Breast Cancer

Traditionally, this type of cancer has been divided into two distinct patterns: lobular carcinoma in situ (LCIS) originating from the lobules, and DCIS, originating from the ducts themselves. This distinction is made more on the histologic appearance than site of origin.

Lobular Carcinoma in Situ

Patients with LCIS are generally symptom free (i.e., no palpable mass or pain), and the tumor is identified on a biopsy specimen usually performed for another reason. In contrast to other types of tumors, there are no characteristic mammographic findings specific for LCIS. LCIS does not metastasize, and most lesions occur during the reproductive years.

For these reasons and as our understanding of this lesion has increased, many clinicians now consider LCIS representative of a marker for the development of invasive

TABLE 18.4. Histologic Types of Breast Cancer

DUCTAL ADENOCARCINOMA
In situ
  Intracystic, Paget's disease
Infiltrative
  Medullary, colloid (mucinous), tubular, papillary, inflammatory (clinical, not
    histologic, subtype), Paget's disease, apocrine duct, not otherwise specified
    with desmoplasia

LOBULAR ADENOCARCINOMA
Noninvasive
  Intraductal, in situ
Infiltrating
  Signet-ring cell variant

RARE VARIANTS
Juvenile (secretory), adenoid cystic, epidermoid, carcinoid, squamous cell, lipid-rich,
  spindle cell (pseudosarcomatous), carcinoma with osseous or chondromatous
  metaplasia

SARCOMA AND CARCINOSARCOMA
Cystosarcoma phyllodes (malignant), angiosarcoma, leiomyosarcoma,
  neurosarcoma, malignant lymphoma, carcinosarcoma, mixed tumors

cancer and not a true malignancy per se (42). The estimated incidence of future malignancy ranges between 10 and 30%. Importantly, the risk for invasive cancer affects both breasts and not just the one that was biopsy positive. The clinical conundrum we currently face is that the two treatment options are at opposite ends of the spectrum: close observation versus prophylactic bilateral simple mastectomy, usually in conjunction with reconstruction. As the treatment recommendations for LCIS are evolving, these patients are best served by careful counseling by an experienced clinician.

Ductal Carcinoma in Situ

DCIS is frequently associated with microcalcifications identified mammographically. It is also seen in association with invasive cancer. Although not generally palpable on physical examination, the mass may be identified grossly in an excisional biopsy specimen. Most cases are diagnosed on mammogram or other imaging studies. Approximately 33% of patients have more than one focus of DCIS, although it is rarely bilateral. Treatment options include wide local excision with clear margins (usually requiring needle localization) or simple mastectomy.

Current debate centers on the need for postoperative irradiation after local excision, although, with few exceptions (microscopic tumor size being one), postoperative irradiation is advised to decrease the risk of local recurrence. It is estimated that approximately 50% of patients with postsurgical residual DCIS will develop an infiltrative carcinoma of the same breast within 10 years. Axillary lymphadenectomy is not necessary for most DCIS lesions. As with LCIS, these patients are more prone to development of invasive cancer. The risk is estimated to be approximately 10% and, in contrast to LCIS, involves the ipsilateral breast alone (42). For a summary of current clinical data and clinical recommendations, the reader is referred to the 1995 review by Barth et al. (43).

Invasive Breast Cancer

To reiterate a theme prominent in this chapter, any solid discrete mass requires precise histologic identification. The most common breast cancer in the United States is infiltrating ductal carcinoma, accounting for 60 to 70% of breast cancers. False-negative mammograms occur, particularly in young women.

The preoperative evaluation for a small tumor with no palpable nodes includes bilateral mammography, chest radiograph, complete blood count, and screening blood chemistries. If symptoms or laboratory tests suggest bone or liver metastasis, a bone scan and/or liver scan should be done. The treatment of invasive cancer is evolving. Options include modified radical mastectomy, segmental mastectomy with axillary node dissection followed by radiotherapy, and modified mastectomy with immediate reconstruction. The procedure selected primarily depends on tumor size in relation to the size of the affected breast, patient preference, and (to a lesser degree) the histologic tumor type. In this regard, the role of the surgeon is to advise the patient on the most appropriate treatment for her as an individual with cancer.

Trials are now in progress to determine the efficacy of sentinel axillary node excision as a staging replacement for complete axillary lymphadenectomy. The tumor bed is marked either using a radiolabel or a nonabsorbable dye, and the axilla is then explored with the sentinel node identified as the most proximate to the demonstrated path of tumor drainage (44).

The prognosis of invasive breast cancer depends on the stage of the disease. This remains at present the single best determinant of survival. Different pathologic or histologic patterns have little, if any, impact on survival. For small invasive cancers localized to the breast that are estrogen receptor positive and well differentiated, the cure rate is approximately 80 to 90% at 5 years. Once axillary metastases have occurred, this figure declines to approximately 40% at 5 years and probably to less than 25% at 10 years. Long-term follow-up is necessary for patients with invasive cancer. Hence, clinical trials should report follow-up of 10 years or greater to be meaningful.

SPECIAL CLINICAL SITUATIONS

Four common clinical scenarios will raise questions between patients and clinicians:

- Link between estrogen replacement therapy and development of breast cancer
- Presence of the BRCA gene or breast cancer occurring on a hereditary or genetic basis
- Importance of breast self-examination
- Medicolegal aspects surrounding breast cancer litigation

Hormone Replacement Therapy and Breast Cancer

Although it is clear that some breast carcinomas demonstrate nuclear receptor positivity toward estrogen, it is much more difficult to prove a cause and effect relationship between exogenous estrogen administration and the transformation of a benign breast cell into a malignant tumor. Published retrospective studies are conflicting and demonstrate an increased risk, no elevation of risk, and in some even a reduction in risk for breast cancer development when exogenous estrogen is used. The studies differ in their statistical methodologies, patient populations (younger versus older women), dosage and types of estrogen, and duration of replacement therapy (45). The recognized beneficial effects of estrogen replacement therapy include a reduction in the demineralization of the large bones of the skeleton and a reduction in mortality from acute myocardial infarction. The results from prospective studies are clearly needed for the ultimate resolution of this controversy (46).

Probably the wisest course is for the clinician and patient to recognize the complete answer is not yet fully known and to *individualize* estrogen replacement recommendations. As an example of one of several individual issues, estrogen replacement may not be contributory to a hypothetical reduction in death from myocardial infarction in an otherwise healthy woman without cardiac risk factors and who exercises regularly. Similarly, the decision to administer estrogen in patients with strong family history for breast cancer must be carefully weighed.

Hereditary Breast Cancer

As noted previously (Table 18.1), women with a first-degree relative (mother, sister, or daughter) with breast cancer carry an increased risk for a similar fate over their lifetime. Reported relative risks are 2.3 for one first-degree relative, 2.7 for one first-degree relative diagnosed before menopause, and 13.6 if both the mother and a sister had breast cancer (47).

A thorough discussion of hereditary breast cancer, including a discussion of the BRCA cancer susceptibility genes, appears in Chapter 19.

Breast Self-Examination

Because most breast cancers are still self-detected (although this proportion has been changing with the regular use of screening mammography), education of patients on the importance of regular breast self-examination should represent a central role for the physician (48, 49). This habit should be encouraged in all women in their late 20s and older. The self-examination should follow the same fundamental principles as used in the clinician's examination. The first step is inspection in front of a mirror looking for changes first with the hands pressed to the hips and then with the arms extended. The second step is palpation of the breast and the axillary tissue. Palpation may be done with the breast wet or dry in the recumbent, sitting, or standing position. It is best done approximately 1 week after the cessation of the menstrual period. Women who are not menstruating should be advised to perform their self-examination on the same date each month. Although debate centers about the differentiation between a discrete lump and simply glandular tissue, it is probably far better for the woman to report to her physician any change that persists in the way her breasts feel rather than to become too focused on the medical definition of a lump.

Malpractice Issues

A recent careful analysis of breast cancer litigation in the United States has been published (50). These authors found that breast cancer litigation is the second most common cause of indemnity payments nationwide. Contained within this report was a review of 118 recently filed malpractice cases. Gynecologists were named 47% of the time and radiologists only 13% of the time. The most common complaint was a delay in diagnosis with an average delay of 14 months from the time the patient herself detected an abnormality. The average age of the plaintiff was 44 years of age. A further study analyzed the difficulties in breast cancer detection in these younger women. The authors noted the inability to detect breast cancer was inversely proportional to the age of the patient, ranging from 36% at age 40 to 9% by age 75 (51).

SUMMARY

Most diseases of the breast are benign conditions. Our current level of knowledge permits risk evaluation for each woman. Progress must continue to ensure improved and ongoing access to screening programs. These, coupled with innovative methods of diagnosis and improved therapy, may in turn lead to a continued reduction in mortality from carcinoma of the breast.

CLINICAL NOTES

- Ectopic glandular tissue and the normal tail of Spence may enlarge during pregnancy.
- Supernumerary nipples may be with or without breast tissue and are common findings.
- Elicit the history in the patient's own words, taking care to recognize the emotional concerns that may be present.
- Examination of the breast is visual and palpatory in both the sitting and supine positions.
- Ask the patient to demonstrate any mass she may have noted.
- Any new mass should be evaluated, regardless of pregnancy state.
- Implants alter the shape of a woman's breasts but not the nature of the glandular tissue. If reduction or sculpting was done, palpatory differences may be noted.
- With silicone implants, granulomas may form that are indistinguishable from malignancy. Excisional biopsy is required for diagnosis.
- There are no data to support any causal link between silicone implants and connective tissue disease. There is evidence to refute it. Unless the implants are causing problems, there is no need to replace silicone implants with saline ones.
- When examining a breast that has been irradiated, carefully examine the incision for any tumor recurrence. Palpatory changes secondary to irradiation are unusual.
- Mammography results in earlier detection of occult malignancy. It should never serve to replace further evaluation of a breast mass with histologic examination.
- Ultrasound is helpful to distinguish between solid and cystic masses. It is also helpful as an adjunct evaluation tool in young women with dense breasts and in whom mammography is difficult to interpret. It is not sensitive or specific enough to replace mammography as a screening tool.
- Stereotactic biopsy holds great promise as an alternative to open biopsy.
- If DCIS is found on stereotactic biopsy, open biopsy is necessary because of the high incidence of associated invasive carcinomas.
- Fine-needle aspiration is helpful when positive. Negative results are to be viewed as non-diagnostic.
- Mammography should be done either before fine-needle aspiration or no sooner than 2 weeks afterward.
- Only 6 to 15% of cases of nipple discharge are associated with cancer. Other causes such as medications, stimulation, intraductal papilloma, and mammary dysplasia need to be ruled out.
- Breast cysts are quite common. Complex or clustered cysts should be aspirated and fluid sent for analysis to rule out the presence of a microscopic tumor growth.
- Cysts should be excised if a mass is noted after aspiration, the cyst recurs less than 6 weeks after aspiration, or it recurs after two aspirations.
- Fibroadenomas may develop and grow in response to estrogen replacement therapy in older women.
- Fibroadenomas should be removed in the event of recent enlargement, patient concern, periareolar location, or when they are unable to be distinguished from a malignant process.
- Fat necrosis may mimic malignancy on examination. Usually, the patient is unable to recall any history of trauma.
- Mastitis is treated with oxacillin or dicloxacillin and continued breast feeding. If a breast abscess develops, then breast feeding is discontinued and surgical intervention is required.
- Mastodynia is often difficult to treat. Available therapies include the use of bromocriptine, danazol, or tamoxifen. Evening primrose oil has also been found to be helpful. Avoidance of caffeine and use of vitamin E have not proven to be reliable and effective therapies.

- LCIS is a marker for the development of invasive cancer for both breasts. Controversy surrounds the best treatment modality.
- DCIS is usually treated with wide local excision or simple mastectomy. There is an increased incidence of invasive carcinoma in the affected breast.
- Postoperative radiation is advised for most cases of DCIS to decrease the risk of local recurrence.
- The most common breast cancer in the United States is infiltrating ductal carcinoma. Treatment depends on tumor size, patient presence, and histologic tumor type.
- No definitive evidence exists proving that estrogen replacement therapy, either alone or in conjunction with progesterone, causes breast cancer.

References

1. Parker Sl, Tong T, Bolden S, et al. Cancer statistics. CA Cancer J Clin 1997;47:5–27.
2. Wingo PA, Ries LA, Rosenberg HM, et al. Cancer incidence and mortality, 1973–1995: a report card for the U.S. Cancer 1998;82:1197–1207.
3. Keller-Wood M, Bland KI. Breast physiology in normal, lactating and diseased states in the breast. In: Bland KI, Copeland EM, eds. The Breast: Comprehensive Management of Benign and Malignant Diseases. 1st ed. Philadelphia: WB Saunders, 1991:36–45.
4. Haggenson CD. Disease of the Breast. Philadelphia: WB Saunders, 1986:502.
5. Henderson IC. Risk factors for breast cancer development. Cancer 1993;71:2127–2140.
6. Preece PE, Baum M, Mansel RE, et al. Importance of mastalgia in operable breast cancer. Br Med J (Clin Res Ed) 1982;284:1299–1300.
7. River, L, Silverstein I, Grant J, et al. Carcinoma of the breast: the diagnostic significance of pain. Am J Surg 1951;82:733–735.
8. Sickles EA. Mammographic features of 300 consecutive non palpable breast cancer. Am J Radiol 1986;146:661–663.
9. Petrak JA. Pregnancy associated breast cancer. J Surg Oncol 1991;7:306–310.
10. Sanchez-Guerrero J, Colditz GA, Karlson EW, et al. Silicone breast implants and the risk of connective-tissue diseases and symptoms. N Engl J Med 1995;332:1666–1670.
11. Nurses Health Study database. Cambridge, MA: Harvard School of Public Health, 1998.
12. Harris JR, Lippman DE, Veronesi V, et al. Breast cancer (first of three parts). N Engl J Med 1992;327:319–328.
13. Nystrom C, Rutqvist LE, Wall S, et al. Breast cancer screening with mammography: overview of Swedish randomized trials. Lancet 1993;341:973–978.
14. Faulk RM, Sickles EA, Sollitto RA, et al. Clinical efficacy of mammographic screening with elderly. Radiology 1995;194:193–197.
15. Miller AB, Baines CJ, To T, Wall C. Canadian National Breast Screening Study: 1. Breast cancer detection and death rates among women aged 40 to 49 years. Can Med Assoc J 1992;147:1459–1476.
16. Smart CR, Hendrick RE, Rutledge JH III, et al. Benefit of mammography screening in women ages 40–49 years: current evidence from randomized controlled trials. Cancer 1995;75:1616–626.
17. Bird RE, Wallace TW, Yankaskas BC. Analysis of cancers missed at screening mammography. Radiology 1992;184:613–617.
18. Homer MJ. Imaging features and management of characteristically benign and probably benign breast lesions. Radiol Clin North Am 1982;25:939–951.
19. Jokich PM, Monticciolo DL, Adler HT. Breast ultrasonography. Radiol Clin North Am 1992;30:993–1009.
20. Meyer JE, Christian RE, Frenna TH, et al. Image guided aspiration of solitary occult breast "cysts." Arch Surg 1992;127:433–435.
21. Weinreb JC, Newstead G. MR imaging of the breast. Radiology 1995;196:593–610.
22. Porter SH. Percutaneous large core breast biopsy. Cancer (Suppl) 1994;74:256–262.
23. Schmidt RA. Stereotactic breast biopsy. CA Cancer J Clin 1994;44:172–191.

24. Hernandez CE, Connelly PT, Strickler SA, et al. Are stereotaxic breast biopsies adequate? Surgery 1994;116:610–615.

25. Mitnick JS, Vazquez MF, Pressman PJ, et al. Stereotactic fine-needle aspiration biopsy for the evaluation of nonpalpable breast lesions: report of an experience based on 2,988 cases. Am Surg Oncol 1996;3:185–191.

26. Cross MJ, Evans WP, Peters GN, et al. Stereotactic breast biopsy as an alternative to open excisional biopsy. Ann Surg Oncol 1995;2:195–200.

27. O'Malley F, Casey TT, Winfried AC, et al. Clinical correlates of false negative fine needle aspiration of the breast in a consecutive survey of 1005 patients. Surg Gynecol Obstet 1993;176:360–364.

28. Tabar L, Dean PB, Penteck Z. Galactography: the diagnostic procedure of choice for nipple discharge. Radiology 1983;149:31–38.

29. Philip J, Harris WG. The role of ductography in the management of patients with nipple discharge. Br J Clin Pract 1984;38:293–297.

30. Hughes LE, Bundred NJ. Breast macrocysts. World J Surg 1989;13:711–714.

31. Kutten F, Fournier S, Durand JC, et al. Estradiol and progesterone receptors in human breast fibroadenomas. J Clin Endocrinol Metab 1981;52:1225–1229.

32. Dent DM, Cart PJ. Fibroadenoma. World J Surg 1989;13:706–710.

33. Hindle WH, Alonzo LJ. Conservative management of breast fibroadenoma. Am J Obstet Gynecol 1991;164:1647–1651.

34. Pick PW, Iossitedes FA. Occurrence of breast carcinoma within a fibroadenoma. A review. Arch Pathol Lab Med 1984;108:590–594.

35. Ozella LU, Gump FE. The management of patients with carcinoma in fibroadenomatous tumors of the breast. Surg Gynecol Obstet 1985;160:99–104.

36. Dupont WD, Page DL, Parl FF, et al. Long term risk of breast cancer in women with fibroadenoma. N Engl J Med 1994;331:10–15.

37. Bland KF. Inflammatory infections and metabolic disorders of the mammal. In: Bland KF, Copeland EM, eds. The Breast: Comprehensive Management of Benign and Malignant Diseases. 1st ed. Philadelphia: WB Saunders, 1991:87–112.

38. Dixon JM. Outpatient treatment of non lactational breast abscesses. Br J Surg 1992;79:56–57.

39. Preece PE, Mansel RE, Bolton PM, et al. Clinical syndromes of mastalgia. Lancet 1976;2:670–673.

40. Souba WW. Evaluation and treatment of benign breast disorders. In: Bland KI, Copeland EM, eds. The Breast: Comprehensive Management of Benign and Malignant Diseases. 1st ed. Philadelphia: WB Saunders, 1991:715–729.

41. Gateley CA, Miers M, Mansel RE, et al. Drug treatment for mastalgia: 17 years experience in the Cardiff Mastalgia Clinic. J R Soc Med 1992;85:12–15.

42. Bland KI, Fryberg FR. Selective management of in situ carcinoma of the breast. Breast Dis 1992;3:11–22.

43. Barth A, Brenner RJ, Giuliano AE. Current management of ductal carcinoma in situ. West J Med 1995;163:360–366.

44. Giuliano AE, Kirgan DM, Guenther JM, et al. Lymphatic mapping and sentinel lymphadenectomy for breast cancer. Ann Surg 1994;220:391–398.

45. Colditz GA, Harkinson SE, Hunter DT, et al. The use of estrogen and progestin and the risk of breast cancer in post menopausal women. N Engl J Med 1995;332:1589–1592.

46. Henrich JB. The postmenopausal estrogen breast cancer controversy. JAMA 1992;268:1900–1902.

47. Sattin RW, Rubin GL, Webster LA, et al. Family history and the risk of breast cancer. JAMA 1985;235:1908.

48. Champion V. The role of breast self-examination in breast cancer screening. Cancer 1996;69:1985–1991.

49. Fletcher SW, O'Malley MS, Earp JC, et al. How to teach women breast self-examination. Ann Intern Med 1993;112:772–779.

50. Dietrick JC, Vasques MF, Kronouet S, et al. Malpractice litigation involving patients with carcinoma of the breast. J Am Coll Surg 1995;181:315–321.
51. Lannin DR, Harris RP, Swanson FH, et al. Difficulties in diagnosis of carcinoma of the breast in patients less than fifty years of age. Surg Gynecol Obstet 1993;177:457–462.

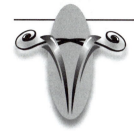

C H A P T E R   1 9

Hereditary Cancer Diagnosis and Management

MICHAEL CARNEY
ANDREW BERCHUCK

Of the nearly 270 million people living in the United States today, 100 million will develop an invasive cancer at some point in their lives. Close to 600,000 Americans will die of cancer this year alone (1). Most of these cancers are sporadic cases unlinked genetically to other family members, but as many as 10% of certain cancer types can be traced through family lines.

Long before we knew anything about DNA or molecular genetics, some families were described as being "full of cancer." A grandmother might have had breast cancer, a mother ovarian cancer, and two sisters breast cancer. In other families, every generation was observed to have had at least one case of colon cancer that arose at surprisingly young ages. Individuals in these families believed they were predestined to get cancer. The first description in the medical literature of such a "cancer family" was by Warthin in 1913 (2), when he described a "family G" in which there were many cases of gastrointestinal and uterine cancer. He followed this family for many years and found that 17 of 48 descendants died of cancer or had been operated on for cancer (3).

Subsequently, numerous other large families in which cancer is extremely common have been reported (4). For many years we were unable to explain this phenomenon. It was thought that perhaps some dietary or environmental carcinogen might be at fault. Although substances in the environment, hormones, and individual behaviors play a role in the genesis of many cancers, the question of why some families were predisposed to certain cancers remained a mystery. Now, more recently, it has been convincingly demonstrated that most familial cancers have a hereditary basis.

Malignancies of the colon, breast, and ovary are the most common hereditary cancers in women, and it is thought that 5 to 10% of these cancers have a hereditary basis (5). It is estimated that more than 15,000 people this year will develop hereditary colorectal cancer. In addition, 2000 to 3000 women will be diagnosed with a hereditary form of ovarian cancer and 10,000 to 20,000 women will suffer from a familial type of breast cancer. The recent identification of autosomal dominant cancer susceptibility genes represents a milestone in the management of hereditary cancer syndromes. With the availability of genetic testing, it is hoped that cancer prevention and early detection efforts can be focused on mutation carriers, whereas noncarriers in these families can be reassured that they are not at increased risk. The ability to reassure those with negative tests is limited somewhat by the possible existence of other as yet undiscovered genes, however. Because the benefits of genetic testing remain unproven, it is important that women receive educational material and counseling before deciding to undergo testing. In addition, posttest counseling and follow-up is crucial to help women work through various issues, including decisions regarding prophylactic surgery and other interventions designed to decrease cancer mortality.

BASIC CANCER GENETICS

It is now known that cancer is a disease in which there is loss of growth regulatory controls. Proliferation of cells normally is regulated by a complex series of molecular pathways that contain numerous checks and balances. The proteins that comprise these pathways are encoded by genes within the cellular DNA. Oncogenes encode proteins that stimulate proliferation, whereas tumor suppressor genes encode proteins that inhibit proliferation (Table 19.1). In each organ there is a carefully programmed balance between these opposing classes of gene products. In some organs, such as the bone marrow, the genetic program allows constant proliferation, whereas in others, such as the brain, proliferation rarely occurs. In addition, these same genes are involved in regulating differentiation and apoptosis (programmed cell death), which are processes that also serve to control the population of cells within an organ.

It has been convincingly demonstrated that alterations in the genes that control cellular growth can cause malignant transformation. Oncogenes can be activated by several mechanisms. In some types of cancers, amplification of oncogenes (e.g., c-*myc*, HER-2/*neu*) has been noted. Instead of two copies of one of these growth-stimulatory genes, there may be as many as 40 copies. Some oncogenes may become overactive if affected by point mutations (e.g., K-*ras*). Finally, oncogenes may be translocated from one chromosomal location to another, and they may come under the influence of promoter sequences that cause overexpression of the gene (e.g., a*bl*). Loss of tumor suppressor gene function can also result in overactive proliferation and outgrowth of a tumor. This usually involves a two-step process in which both copies of a given tumor suppressor gene are inactivated. In most cases, mutation of one copy of a tumor suppressor gene occurs along with complete loss of the other copy of the gene because of deletion of a large segment of the chromosome where the gene resides.

TABLE 19.1. Characteristics of Oncogenes and Tumor Suppressor Genes

	Oncogene	Tumor Suppressor Gene
NORMAL CELLS		
Effect on proliferation	Stimulation	Inhibition
Examples	K-*ras*, HER-2/*neu*, c-*myc*	p53, BRCA1, BRCA2, APC
CANCER CELLS		
Required alterations	1	2
Types of alterations	Point mutation, amplification, rearrangement	Point mutation, deletion
Role of alterations	Gain of function ("dominant")	Loss of function ("recessive")
Germ-line inheritance	Rare	Yes
Somatic mutations	Yes	Yes

More recently, it has been appreciated that DNA repair genes play an important role in preventing the development of human cancers. Each time a cell divides, the DNA is copied so that both cells receive a complete set of the genetic code. Although DNA synthesis occurs with high fidelity, it is estimated that spontaneous errors (mutations) occur about once every million bases. In addition, in nondividing cells, mutations may arise because of endogenous processes such as methylation and deamination and because of exposure to mutagens such as those in tobacco smoke. The cellular DNA repair systems are able to repair much of this genetic damage, but some mutations elude this surveillance system. In general, cancer occurs only after damage to several growth regulatory oncogenes and tumor suppressor genes. The rate at which critical mutations occur in cells may be accelerated if the DNA repair genes themselves have undergone inactivating mutations.

Alterations in oncogenes, tumor suppressor genes, and/or DNA repair genes have been implicated in the development of essentially every type of human cancer. It is thought that most nonhereditary cancers increase with aging because the longer one is alive, the higher the likelihood of acquiring sufficient genetic damage to result in outgrowth of a clinically recognizable cancer. Cervical cancer is a notable exception, but the incidence of this cancer peaks at an earlier age because of the critical etiologic role of the sexually transmitted human papilloma virus. Inherited mutations in tumor suppressor and DNA repair genes, and rarely oncogenes, appear to be responsible for most hereditary cancers (Table 19.2).

TABLE 19.2. Hereditary Cancer Syndromes

Syndrome	Gene	Chromosome	Predominant Cancers
Familial breast/	BRCA1	17q21	Breast, ovarian
ovarian cancer	BRCA2	13q12	
Ataxia-telangiectasia	AT	11q22	Breast
Hereditary nonpolyposis	MSH2	2p16	Colon, endometrial,
colon cancer	MLH1	3p21	ovarian, others
	PMS1	2q31	
	PMS2	7p22	
Familial polyposis coli	APC	5q21	Colon, colonic polyps
Li-Fraumeni	p53	17p13	Sarcomas, leukemias, breast, brain, others
Wilms' tumor	WT1	11p13	Kidney
von Hippel-Lindau	VHL	3p25	Kidney, others
Neurofibromatosis	NF1	17q11	Neurofibromas
	NF2	22q12	
Retinoblastoma	Rb	13q14	Retinoblastoma sarcomas
Familial melanoma	MLM	9p21	Melanoma
Multiple endocrine neoplasia type 2	*ret*[a]	10q11	Thyroid, adrenal, parathyroid
Hereditary papillary renal carcinoma	*met*[a]	7q31	Papillary kidney

[a]Oncogenes.

Persons who inherit a mutation in a cancer-causing gene have a strikingly increased lifetime risk of developing one or more cancers. These cancers often develop at a younger age than would be expected. In addition, many cancers that occur in young children, such as retinoblastoma and Wilms' tumor, have been shown to arise because of inherited mutations in tumor suppressor genes. Although carriers have the mutation in every cell of their body, most cells do not undergo malignant transformation. Paradoxically, organs that normally express high levels of a given tumor suppressor gene product often are not prone to develop cancers when a mutation in that gene is inherited.

PRINCIPLES OF CANCER GENETIC COUNSELING

Obtaining a thorough cancer history from the patient and/or the family is a vital first step in caring for families with hereditary cancer. The seemingly simple act of gathering information forms the foundation on which the rest of the process is based. The importance of careful documentation of family history, including review of clinical materials from other cancer cases in the family, has been stressed for many years by Henry T. Lynch, one of the pioneers of hereditary cancer genetics. His own compulsively assembled pedigrees allowed him to define two familial cancer syndromes: Lynch I (colon cancer) and Lynch II (colon cancer and other cancers). In fact, Warthin's "family G" turned out to be consistent with Lynch II syndrome.

Unfortunately, most clinicians are not compulsive enough in gathering a family history. Lynch et al. (6) reviewed the charts of 200 consecutive patients previously evaluated by another oncologist. They discovered that glaring omissions in the cancer family history were frequent. In most of the charts, the family history was either entirely omitted or described as negative when in many cases familial clusters of cancer actually were present. In another study, David and Steiner-Grossman (7) surveyed the recording of family cancer history in the records of 64 New York hospitals and found that only 4 of 64 actually had a place to record such a history in the record.

A complete family cancer history should begin by ascertaining cancer information of all first-degree relatives, including mother, father, siblings, and children. Data on second-degree relatives, including grandparents, aunts, and uncles, also should be obtained. If more extended family history is available, it should also be recorded. In addition, family members without cancer should not be overlooked because their unaffected status can provide clues to the inheritance pattern. A family cancer history should ideally be obtained from more than one individual in families where there is a suspicion of a hereditary syndrome (8). This information can be depicted diagrammatically in a pedigree (Fig. 19.1). To make a pedigree as accurate as possible, it is ideal to obtain pathologic records and medical summaries of affected relatives, although this can be quite cumbersome.

The pedigree can convey concisely a large amount of information, including the presenting cancer case (proband), others who have been diagnosed with cancer, those who have died, and those at risk. Important additional information recorded includes the age at onset of cancers, second cancers, bilaterality of a cancer, stage of the cancer, and metastatic location. In addition, cancer histology, age of unaffected individuals, exposure to carcinogenic agents, suspected extended family history of cancers, and the pattern of cancer occurrence among generations is recorded (9). Likewise, if there is a known genetic disorder in the family, this should be noted because some syndromes predispose individuals to certain cancers (e.g., Fanconi's anemia, xeroderma pigmentosa, Bloom's syndrome, and ataxia-telangiectasia). Finally, a complete history of potential modifying factors

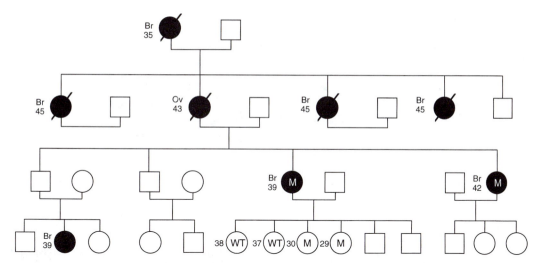

FIGURE 19.1. Familial ovarian cancer pedigree with BRCA1 mutation. The age of family members and type of cancers are noted. *Slashes* denote individuals who have died of cancer. Individuals denoted *M* have the 5382insC mutation in BRCA1, whereas individuals denoted *WT* have normal BRCA1. □, males; ○, females; ■, affected males; ●, affected females.

should be obtained, including hormone use, birth control pill use, menopausal status, diet, parity, breast-feeding history, and concomitant medical conditions (Table 19.3).

Once a family is suspected of having a hereditary cancer syndrome, genetic counselors should be involved in all phases of the genetic testing process because they are specifically trained in the process of educating patients about inherited diseases (10). If it is thought that there is a sufficiently high likelihood that a family may carry a mutation in a cancer-causing gene, extensive nondirective counseling and education is essential before genetic testing. Individuals should understand the risk of testing positive, potential benefits of the test, and the social and psychological implications of testing. Even those who receive negative test results can have significant deleterious effects, including survivor guilt. A patient should be required to sign a written consent form confirming that they have been fully educated and informed about the test and its potential repercussions and benefits. About three fourths of the candidates who seek counseling elect to undergo cancer genetic testing.

Test results should be conveyed in a setting in which multidisciplinary input from genetic counselors, oncologists and others is available. Additional psychological support and encouragement is also offered at this juncture. The lifetime cancer risk and the options for prevention should be reviewed. Because cancer genetic testing is relatively new, the optimal strategy for decreasing cancer incidence and mortality in carriers remains uncertain. Referral to cancer genetic clinics will facilitate research in this area that hopefully will lead to evidence-based clinical guidelines in the future. One of the most difficult problems in cancer genetic counseling is the family with a strong history in which a mutation in a cancer susceptibility gene cannot be found. Hopefully, referral of these families to institutions with expertise in cancer genetics will lead to the identification of other as yet undiscovered cancer-causing genes.

TABLE 19.3. Assessment of Hereditary Cancer Risk

Obtain personal and family history of cancer
Confirm precise cancer diagnosis in affected individuals
Estimate risk of hereditary cancer syndrome
Education and informed consent
Genetic testing
Posttest counseling and follow-up

HEREDITARY BREAST AND OVARIAN CANCER

It has been estimated that about 5 to 10% of breast and ovarian cancers are due to autosomal dominant hereditary syndromes. Recently, several breast and/or ovarian cancer susceptibility genes have been identified. Germ-line mutations in BRCA1 and BRCA2 appear to account for most hereditary ovarian cancer cases and at least half of hereditary breast cancers.

BRCA1

Hall et al. (11) demonstrated in 1990 that a fraction of familial breast cancer was linked to a locus on chromosome 17q. The following year, Narod et al. (12) reported that families with both breast and ovarian cancer also showed linkage to 17q. The responsible gene (BRCA1) was identified on 17q21 in 1994, and it was demonstrated that mutations in this gene segregate with breast and ovarian cancer in affected families (13).

The BRCA1 gene encodes a protein of 1863 amino acids whose exact cellular function remains unknown. The report of a normal woman who inherited two mutant copies of this gene indicates that BRCA1 probably is not requisite for normal growth and development (14). It is thought that BRCA1 is a tumor suppressor, because the normal copy of BRCA1 is invariably deleted in breast and ovarian cancers that arise in women who inherit a mutant BRCA1 gene (15). Loss of BRCA1 function probably represents an initial event that facilitates the development of other genetic alterations that culminate in the development of a clinically recognizable cancer. In this regard, characterization of breast and ovarian cancers in BRCA1 carriers has revealed the presence of loss of heterozygosity at other loci and mutations in the p53 gene (16).

Initial studies in families selected on the basis of strong family history and early age of onset suggested that germ-line mutations in BRCA1 were responsible for about 50% of hereditary breast cancers and 90% of hereditary ovarian cancers (17). In families with BRCA1 mutations, the lifetime risk of developing breast cancer was about 80 to 90%, whereas the risk of ovarian cancer was about 30 to 60% (18). The increased risk begins to be manifest earlier for breast cancer than for ovarian cancer (19). Carriers have an increase in breast cancer risk in their 20s, whereas ovarian cancer risk does not rise appreciably until the mid-30s. More recently it has been suggested that initial estimates of both the fraction of hereditary cancers accounted for by BRCA1 and its penetrance may have been too high because of ascertainment bias as a result of the high fraction of initial study families with large numbers of breast and ovarian cancer cases (20–23). Population-based studies are now underway that will better define the frequency of germ-line BRCA1 mutations and their penetrance.

It also has been noted that various BRCA1 mutations may differ in the extent to which they predispose to breast or ovarian cancer. It has been suggested that mutations in the carboxy terminus of the gene may result in a higher frequency of breast cancer relative to ovarian cancer (24, 25). Conversely, mutations in the proximal amino end of the gene result in a higher likelihood of developing ovarian cancer. As the molecular function of BRCA1 becomes known, perhaps it will be found that different parts of the molecule are functionally important in the breast and ovary.

Differences in penetrance also have been noted among families with identical BRCA1 mutations. Two hypotheses, both of which may be relevant, have been proposed to explain variable penetrance. First, it has been suggested that other genes may modify the penetrance of BRCA1. Alternatively, it is possible that gene-environment interactions may modify risk. For example, it has been shown that pregnancy and oral contraceptive pill use decrease the risk of ovarian cancer in the general population. It is thought that this protective effect is due to inhibition of ovulation. It is possible that reproductive risk factors such as pill use that affect breast and ovarian cancer incidence in the general population may also modify risk in BRCA1 carriers (26).

The incidence of prostate and colon cancers was found to be increased by approximately three- and fourfold, respectively, in one study of BRCA1 carriers (19). A more recent study of Ashkenazi Jewish carriers confirmed the increased risk of prostate cancer, but colon cancer risk was not increased (27). The tissue specificity of malignancies in BRCA1 carriers is intriguing, because significant expression of this gene is seen in a number of other tissues, including thymus and testis (13).

It has been reported that BRCA1-associated breast cancers are characterized by higher grade, medullary features, aneuploidy, and high proliferation index relative to sporadic breast cancers (28–30). Despite these poor prognostic features, BRCA1-associated breast cancers presented at lower stage and had relatively favorable outcomes in one study (29). The histologic features of ovarian cancers in BRCA1 carriers do not differ strikingly from sporadic cancers. Most cases are advanced-stage moderate to poorly differentiated serous cancers (31, 32), but Rubin et al. (32) found that survival of BRCA1 carriers with ovarian cancer was better than that of a control group of sporadic cases that was matched for age, stage, and other prognostic factors.

BRCA2

A significant fraction of breast cancer families that do not have BRCA1 mutations were found to be linked to chromosome 13q12 in 1994 (33). In 1995, this second breast cancer susceptibility gene (BRCA2) was identified (34). Notable attributes of BRCA2 families include early age of onset and the occurrence of male breast cancer (35, 36). Ovarian cancer is a less-prominent feature of these families, and there are about 10 female breast cancer cases and one male breast cancer case for each ovarian cancer case in BRCA2 families.

Similar to BRCA1, the structure of BRCA2 is not related to other known genes, and its role in normal breast and ovarian epithelium remains unclear. Like BRCA1, however, expression of BRCA2 is low in quiescent cells and increases dramatically as cells enter the S phase (37, 38).

Initial studies estimated that BRCA2 is responsible for approximately 40% of hereditary breast cancers and 5 to 10% of hereditary ovarian cancers. In these studies, the lifetime risk of developing breast cancer in BRCA2 carriers was 80 to 90%, whereas the risk of developing ovarian cancer was only about 10%. As noted for BRCA1, these initial penetrance estimates may have been artifactually high because of ascertainment bias (20, 21). Studies are underway that will determine the carrier frequency and penetrance in the general population. As is the case for BRCA1, a genotype-phenotype correlation has been noted with BRCA2. It appears that ovarian cancer is most often observed in families with mutations in the large exon 11 (39).

The clinicopathologic characteristics of breast cancers that occur in BRCA2 carriers appear similar to those of sporadic cases, but there is the suggestion that BRCA2-

associated cases are less often tubular and are of higher grade (30). Because ovarian cancer is less frequent in BRCA2 carriers, large series that examine the clinicopathologic features of BRCA2-associated ovarian cancers have not yet been reported.

Genetic Testing for Hereditary Breast and/or Ovarian Cancer

Mutations have been observed throughout the large BRCA1 and 2 genes, and approximately 80 to 90% of the mutations predict truncated protein products (40). Missense mutations that encode a full-length protein product in which a single amino acid is altered occur in about 10 to 15% of hereditary cases. In some families it may be difficult to distinguish disease-causing mutations from insignificant rare polymorphisms (13). Segregation of a missense alteration with breast and ovarian cancer in a family suggests, but does not prove, its significance. In small families and families in which some individuals decline testing, segregation analysis may not be possible.

Because mutations in BRCA1 and 2 occur throughout these large genes, the most reliable method of detecting mutations is to sequence the entire coding region. If sequencing is performed using genomic DNA from a blood sample, intronic splice sites, which occasionally may be the target of mutations, also can be examined. Studies that define the sensitivity and specificity of automated sequencing have not yet been reported, but the false-negative rate is estimated to be very low. Because automated DNA sequencing is highly labor intensive, other methods also have been used for mutational screening. Reliance on methods other than DNA sequencing probably lowers sensitivity for detecting mutations to about 70 to 90%, however. Although automated DNA sequencing is labor intensive and costly, it remains the gold standard for mutational testing. New technologies that allow rapid and less-expensive mutational testing may be on the horizon (Fig. 19.2).

Because testing for mutations in BRCA1 and 2 is relatively new and trials have not yet been performed to prove that genetic testing reduces cancer mortality, it has been suggested that perhaps testing should be confined to research protocols. On the other hand, it can be argued that the appropriate role of health care providers is to provide access to information and nondirective counseling and that individuals should decide for themselves whether or not to undergo testing.

Normal

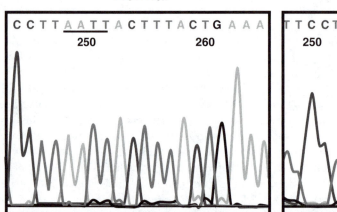

Mutant

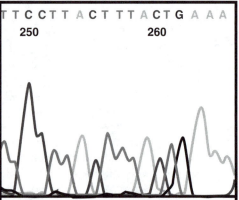

FIGURE 19.2. Automated DNA sequencing of BRCA2 mutation in exon 11 (6872delAATT): *left,* normal wild-type BRCA2 sequence; *right,* cancer demonstrating deletion of bases AATT.

Although mutations in BRCA1 and 2 have been noted in some women in the absence of a family history of breast or ovarian cancer, the incidence is low and cost considerations prohibit mutational screening in the general population. The probability of finding a BRCA1 or 2 mutation in a woman over age 50 who is the only individual in her family with ovarian or breast cancer is less than 3%. At the other extreme, in families with two cases of breast cancer and two cases of ovarian cancer, the probability of finding a mutation may be as high as 80 to 90% (Table 19.4) (24). Those who believe that it is reasonable to test "high-risk" individuals generally advocate testing when the family history suggests at least a 10 to 20% probability of finding a mutation. In practical terms, this translates into two first-degree relatives with either ovarian cancer at any age or breast cancer before age 50. It is preferable to test affected individuals in a high-risk family first, because a negative test in an unaffected individual may reflect failure to inherit the mutant allele even though others in the family carry a mutation. In cases in which affected individuals have died or are unwilling to be tested, unaffected individuals may be tested first. Another option is to retrieve tissue blocks from deceased individuals, which can then be tested. Once a specific mutation is identified in an affected individual, other individuals in the family can be tested much more rapidly and inexpensively.

One significantly underemphasized opportunity in familial cancer clinics is to reassure women who do not have a strong family history or who have a negative BRCA1/2 test that they probably are not at high risk of developing ovarian or breast cancer. This reassurance must be tempered with the realization that other undiscovered breast/ovarian cancer susceptibility genes may exist. Although it appears that most hereditary ovarian cancer is due to BRCA1 and 2, only about half of familial breast cancers may be attributable to mutations in these two genes.

Because the benefits of genetic testing remain hypothetical, it is important that women receive educational material and counseling explaining the postulated risks and benefits before deciding to undergo testing. In addition, posttest counseling and follow-up is crucial to help women work through various issues, including decisions regarding prophylactic surgery and other interventions designed to decrease cancer mortality. Testing can raise conflicts in families when some individuals do not wish to share information regarding test results. The psychological sequelae of testing also may be significant regardless of whether one receives a positive or negative test result.

Confidentiality remains a critical issue in cancer susceptibility testing. Misuse of genetic information potentially could have devastating consequences, including difficulty in securing employment and life, health, or disability insurance (41). Some

TABLE 19.4. Clinical Characteristics of BRCA1 and BRCA2 Carriers

PRIMARY FACTORS INCREASING LIKELIHOOD OF FINDING BRCA1 OR BRCA2
Two or more first-degree relatives with breast or ovarian cancer
Early onset of breast cancer (20–40 years old)
Early onset of ovarian cancer (30–50 years old)
Male breast cancer (BRCA2 only)
Ashkenazi Jewish heritage

CANCERS THAT INCREASE LIKELIHOOD OF FINDING BRCA1 OR BRCA2
Prostate cancer (BRCA1 only)
Colon cancer (BRCA1 only)
Pancreatic cancer (BRCA2 only)

individuals may ask their insurance company to pay for BRCA1/2 testing and may be willing to have this information recorded in their medical records. In the current climate in which it remains unclear whether legislation that protects mutation carriers will be enacted, many elect to pursue testing privately either through a research study or by paying for commercial testing themselves. In this setting, it is often difficult for health care providers to decide what should be documented in medical records. If it is noted that a patient has a high risk of carrying a mutation and should consider genetic testing, one could be accused of failing to respect confidentiality. Conversely, vague notes designed to protect confidentiality leave one open to the accusation of having failed to adequately inform an individual of the possibility that they may carry a mutation in a cancer susceptibility gene. Resolution of these and other social, ethical, and legal issues that surround genetic susceptibility testing represent significant challenges for the next decade.

With the discovery of BRCA1 and 2, only some cases of familial ovarian cancer should be managed as we have in the past, by simply recommending prophylactic oophorectomy on the basis of a strong family history (42–44). Although the penetrance of various mutations is still somewhat uncertain, it is clear that carriers have a strikingly increased risk of ovarian cancer relative to the general population. Annual screening with CA-125 and/or ultrasound is reasonable, but of unproven efficacy, in women during the reproductive years. Fortunately, the incidence of ovarian cancer in carriers does not begin to rise appreciably until the late 30s when most women have completed their family. In view of this, prophylactic oophorectomy probably is a reasonable approach to decreasing ovarian cancer mortality in mutation carriers.

Prophylactic oophorectomy is an attractive option in mutation carriers for several reasons. First, this procedure can now be performed laparoscopically in an outpatient setting. In addition, most women do not view removal of the ovaries as cosmetically mutilating, and oophorectomy causes only modest changes in body image and self-esteem. Finally, estrogen replacement can be administered either orally or transdermally, thereby avoiding the deleterious side effects of premature menopause. Although there is some concern that estrogen replacement might increase the risk of breast cancer in these women, this risk already is exceedingly high.

One concern regarding prophylactic oophorectomy is the observation that a small fraction of women subsequently developed intraperitoneal carcinomatosis that was indistinguishable from ovarian cancer. This rarely occurs, however, and it is thought that oophorectomy should be greater than 90% protective. Another strategy that has been suggested to decrease risk of ovarian cancer in women with mutations is use of oral contraceptives, which decreases the risk of ovarian cancer in the general population by as much as 60%. Oral contraceptives might be a particularly attractive alternative for young women who have not yet completed childbearing, but it has not yet been proven that the protective effect observed in the general population pertains to mutation carriers. Finally, as with estrogen replacement, there is some concern that oral contraceptive pills might increase the risk of breast cancer.

Prevention of breast cancer mortality in BRCA1 and BRCA2 carriers presents different issues because these cancers are much more readily detected at an early stage than ovarian cancers. As a result, breast cancer 5-year survival in the United States is approximately 70% compared with only 30% for ovarian cancer. Furthermore, unlike oophorectomy, mastectomy causes marked alterations in self-esteem and body image, even when breast reconstruction is performed. Many prophylactic mastectomies performed in the past have been subcutaneous mastectomies in which most of the breast tissue is removed but the nipple is preserved. Advocates of prophylactic mastectomy today generally recommend total mastectomy because malignancy can potentially form in the nipple if it is not removed. Even if a total mastectomy is performed, there is no guarantee that all breast tissue will be successfully excised.

Although some women continue to choose mastectomy, close surveillance with mammography and breast self-examination may prove equally effective in reducing mortality in view of the good prognosis for women with early breast cancer. In this regard, Lynch (45) found that whereas 76% of BRCA1 mutation carriers accepted prophylactic oophorectomy, only 35% considered mastectomy a reasonable option. Beginning between the ages of 25 and 35, biannual mammography and clinical breast examinations are recommended for individuals choosing intensive screening (46). Chemoprophylaxis of breast cancer using antiestrogens such as tamoxifen is another unproved strategy being considered to reduce the incidence of breast cancer in carriers. See Table 19.5 for an overview of the management options for BRCA1/2 carriers.

Founder Mutations

Although the frequency of mutations in the general population is estimated to be about 1 in 800 for BRCA1 and somewhat less for BRCA2, it is apparent that this frequency varies significantly between ethnic groups. In addition, "founder mutations" that presumably arose in a single ancestor have been identified repetitively in many ethnic groups (47). The most common founder mutations described thus far are the BRCA1 185delAG and BRCA2 6174delT mutations that occur in about 1.0 and 1.4% of Ashkenazi Jews, respectively (48, 49). The high frequency of these three mutations implies that they likely arose about 100 generations ago. A third less-common founder mutation (BRCA1 5382insC) also has been noted in Ashkenazi populations. Since 1 in 40 Ashkenazi individuals carry one of these three specific mutations, it would be relatively easy and inexpensive to test the entire Ashkenazi population for these mutations. It may be premature to consider such a strategy until it has been proven that testing translates into a decrease in breast and ovarian cancer mortality.

In one Israeli study, it was found that about half of women with ovarian cancer and one third of women with breast cancer had one of three Ashkenazi founder mutations (50). This contrasts sharply with the estimate that BRCA1 and 2 mutations account for only 5 to 10% of breast and ovarian cancer cases in other Caucasian populations. The high frequency of germ-line BRCA1 and 2 mutations in Israeli women with breast or ovarian cancer is somewhat surprising, because the incidence of these cancers is not strikingly higher than that observed in other ethnic groups.

Several studies examined the penetrance of the Ashkenazi founder mutations. One Israeli study that examined extended families of women with breast or ovarian

TABLE 19.5. Management Options for BRCA1 or BRCA2 Carriers

TO DECREASE RISK OF FUTURE OVARIAN CANCER
Oral contraceptive use until after childbearing years
Encourage breast feeding
Prophylactic oophorectomy after childbearing complete
Annual transvaginal ultrasound, CA-125 level, and physical/pelvic exam in
   individuals choosing not to have oophorectomy or in untested high-risk individuals

TO DECREASE RISK OF FUTURE BREAST CANCER
Prophylactic bilateral total mastectomy
Biannual mammography and clinical exam plus monthly breast self-exam beginning
   at 25 years old for individuals choosing not to undergo mastectomy or for
   untested high-risk individuals

cancer who carried BRCA1 185delAG mutations concluded that carriers had a 70% lifetime risk of breast or ovarian cancer (51). A study of Ashkenazi Jews in the District of Columbia area found that mutation carriers had a 56% lifetime risk of breast cancer and a 16% risk of ovarian cancer (27).

HEREDITARY COLON CANCER

Colon cancer represents the third most common cause of cancer mortality in American women behind breast and lung cancer. The incidence of colon cancer is increased in populations in which dietary fat intake is high. Colon cancer develops in a stepwise progression from normal mucosa; to hyperplasia and polyp; and finally to dysplasia, cancer in situ, and invasive cancer (8). Because this disease has a well-defined clinically recognizable precancerous phase, colon cancer mortality can be decreased in populations in which screening programs are instituted (52). Effective screening methods include fecal occult blood testing and sigmoidoscopy. When a positive screening result is obtained, colonoscopy and/or barium enema is performed to search for polyps and cancers. Unfortunately, available screening tests are underused, and half of patients with colon cancer die of their disease.

Most colon cancers are thought to arise because of sporadic mutations that accumulate over a lifetime, but some cases are the result of a hereditary predisposition. Among the 70,000 women diagnosed with a colorectal cancer this year in the United States, about 15% will have a first-degree relative with colon cancer. Individuals who have a first-degree relative with colon cancer are twice as likely to develop colon cancer compared with the general population (53). The risk is substantially greater if the relative was under 45 years old at diagnosis.

Familial Adenomatous Polyposis

First characterized in the early 1970s, the familial adenomatous polyposis coli syndrome (abbreviated APC or FAP) is inherited as an autosomal dominant trait with penetrance of at least 90% (54, 55). The condition is infrequent and affects only 1 in 7000 persons, accounting for about 1% of all colon cancers. Virtually all individuals who inherit this syndrome develop hundreds of polyps throughout the colon and invasive colon cancer at a young age (56). Each polyp is thought to have the same chance of malignant transformation as a sporadic polyp. The sheer number of polyps in the inherited syndrome makes the combined risk for malignant transformation at multiple sites substantial. Patients with this syndrome also may develop gastric, periampullary, and duodenal polyps and are at risk for cancers in these areas too.

In 1991, Bodmer et al. (57) localized the gene causing familial polyposis to chromosome 5q21. It was subsequently cloned and found to encode a 300-kDa cytoplasmic protein. In addition to being responsible for familial polyposis syndrome, the FAP gene frequently is mutated in the course of sporadic colon cancer development (58). Most mutations in the FAP gene are frameshift or nonsense changes that cause early termination of the protein product. The exact function of the FAP protein remains unclear but is thought to act as a tumor suppressor. There is some evidence that the protein may be involved in signal transduction, cellular adhesion, and microtubule function (59). Unlike most tumor suppressor genes in which inactivation of both copies of the gene usually occurs, mutation of only one copy of the FAP gene is required for polyp formation (60). Progression to a fully invasive cancer is accompanied by alterations in other genes, such as p53, DCC (deleted in colon cancer), and K-*ras* that also are involved in the development of sporadic colon cancers (61).

Although FAP syndrome is relatively rare, recently a polymorphism in this gene has been identified that occurs in 6% of Ashkenazi Jews (T to A in codon 1307). Although the polymorphism does not affect the function of the APC protein, it creates a stretch of eight adenine bases that is highly susceptible to inactivating mutations. Affected individuals appear to have about a 20% lifetime risk of colorectal cancer. Although the penetrance of this APC polymorphism is lower than that of clearly deleterious APC mutations, because the polymorphism is much more frequent, it probably is estimated to be responsible for about 28% of familial colorectal cancer in the Ashkenazi population (62).

Hereditary Nonpolyposis Colon Cancer

The most common form of hereditary colon cancer is a hereditary nonpolyposis colorectal cancer (HNPCC) that accounts for about 5 to 10% of colorectal cancers. HNPCC was originally described as the Lynch syndromes type I and II. The Lynch type I syndrome described families with predominantly large bowel cancers, whereas the Lynch type II syndrome included large bowel cancers and cancers in other abdominal organs.

Clinically, the HNPCC syndrome is characterized by early age at onset (median age, 46 years), proximal colon cancers (70%), and a high rate of metachronous cancers. Colonic cancers in individuals with HNPCC usually are proximal to the splenic flexure, diploid, and have a more favorable prognosis than sporadic colon cancers. Patients treated with subtotal colectomy have a 45% chance of developing another colon cancer in the remaining colon (63). Patients with the Lynch type II variety of this syndrome also have a propensity for developing a number of other cancers. Endometrial cancer is the second most common malignancy in women with HNPCC. In addition, HNPCC carriers have an increased risk of ovarian, small bowel, stomach, pancreatic, ureteral, and renal cancers (Table 19.6). Patients with HNPCC generally form premalignant, widely based, sessile colonic adenomas rather than polyps.

In 1991, the International Collaborative Group on Hereditary Nonpolyposis Colorectal Cancer met and established the Amsterdam criteria for the diagnosis of the syndrome (64):

1. Histologically verified colorectal cancer in three or more relatives, one of whom is a first-degree relative of the other two
2. Colorectal cancer involving at least two successive generations
3. At least one family member who has developed colorectal cancer by age 50

TABLE 19.6. Clinical Characteristics of HNPCC

PATIENT CHARACTERISTICS
Early onset of colorectal cancer
Proximal tumor localization
Multiple primary colorectal cancers
Extracolonic cancers: endometrium, stomach, small intestine, upper urologic tract, ovaries, skin

FAMILY CHARACTERISTICS
Histologically confirmed colorectal cancer in at least three relatives, one of whom is a first-degree relative of the other two
Occurrence of disease in at least two successive generations
At least one family member with colon cancer before age 50
Autosomal dominant inheritance
High penetrance (90%)

It is now known that HNPCC syndrome occurs because of inherited mutations in one of a family of genes involved in DNA mismatch repair. The first of these genes to be identified was MSH2 on chromosome 2p (65, 66). Subsequently, the MLH1 gene on chromosome 3p was noted to be responsible for other HNPCC families. Mutations in these two genes appear to account for most HNPCC families in which mutations can be identified, but other DNA repair genes, including PMS1 and PMS2, have been implicated in some cases. The function of the DNA repair genes is well known from older studies in yeast and bacteria. Mutations of these genes in these species lead to the accumulation of mutations, particularly in areas of the DNA that have repetitive sequences (e.g., CACACA). These repetitive sequences, called microsatellites, are dispersed throughout all the chromosomes and are a frequent site of mutations in humans who inherit mutations in one of the DNA repair genes. Although some microsatellites are within the coding sequence of genes, most reside in the intervening noncoding regions. Microsatellite mutations within growth regulatory genes may contribute to malignant transformation, but it is unclear whether microsatellite mutations outside of the genes are important in carcinogenesis or merely a symptom of the underlying problem.

Genetic Testing for Hereditary Colon Cancer

With the identification of genes responsible for hereditary colon cancer, families suspected of having familial colon cancer can now undergo genetic testing. Many issues that were discussed with regard to BRCA1 and 2 testing in families with breast and ovarian cancer apply to genetic testing for hereditary colon cancer. Pedigrees should be thoroughly documented, and the other critical steps in the genetic counseling process must occur. The previously described Amsterdam criteria requiring at least one family member with a diagnosis of colon cancer at an early age and at least three affected individuals in two contiguous generations serves as a reasonable guideline for selecting candidates for genetic testing.

When screening for HNPCC, often the tumor first is analyzed for mutations in microsatellite DNA sequences because these are present in most colon cancers that arise in individuals who inherit mutations in the DNA repair genes. If microsatellite mutations are found, the DNA repair genes are then screened for mutations. As is the case for BRCA1 and 2, this is a highly labor-intensive process. There is no apparent correlation between clinical presentation (e.g., Lynch I versus Lynch II) and involvement of a specific DNA repair gene. Because MSH2 and MLH1 are responsible for most HNPCC families, these genes should be examined first. Genetic testing is more straightforward in individuals who present with familial polyposis, because this disorder is caused by a single gene (APC).

Once a mutation is detected, testing can be offered to all family members. In view of the high penetrance of these mutations (approximately 90%), every effort should be made to identify all carriers within a family. It has been demonstrated that colon carcinomas and resulting mortality are reduced in cohorts in which mutations have been identified (59). There is evidence to suggest that patients with HNPCC can develop invasive lesions from adenomas in as little as 2 years. This is in contrast to the general population, where this transition is thought to require 8 to 10 years. For this reason, screening and surveillance must be performed frequently.

Current recommendations for colon cancer surveillance in HNPCC patients begin with genetic counseling at age 20. A full colonoscopy should be performed every 2 years until age 35 and then annually thereafter. Colonoscopy rather than sigmoidoscopy is appropriate because most colon cancers in this syndrome are right sided (59). If cancer is found, at least a subtotal colectomy is indicated. Patients found to have an adenoma on colonoscopic screening are advised to undergo surgery because colonoscopic polyp resection is often inadequate with these broad-based lesions. In addition, patients who develop adenomas have a substantial risk of recurrent polyps and cancer formation (Table 19.7).

It is well accepted that individuals who carry APC mutations should undergo prophylactic total colectomy. Half of these patients develop colon cancer by 40, and all develop cancer by age 70 (63). In addition, some experts believe that prophylactic colectomy with ileorectal anastomosis also is a reasonable option for asymptomatic HNPCC mutation carriers. The choice between close surveillance and prophylactic surgery is one that each carrier must decide for themselves after nondirective counseling.

In view of the increased risk of endometrial cancer, yearly endometrial sampling is suggested beginning at age 30 (67, 68). In addition, the uterus and ovaries should be removed prophylactically in patients undergoing colectomy. Although pelvic ultrasound and serum CA-125 levels have been advocated for ovarian cancer screening in HNPCC families, the utility of these techniques for diagnosing ovarian cancer while it is still confined to the ovaries is unproved.

A low-fat high-fiber diet with lots of fruits and vegetables is associated with a decreased incidence of colorectal cancer in the general population. It is not known whether dietary interventions would decrease the incidence of cancer in HNPCC families, however. There is some evidence that chemoprevention with sulindac reduces adenoma development in some APC carriers (69). Additionally, data have linked aspirin intake to a reduction in colon cancer risk, but it is not known if this affects the incidence of hereditary colon cancers (70).

GENETICS OF OTHER GYNECOLOGIC CANCERS

Like other human cancers, endometrial, cervical, vaginal, and vulvar cancers appear to arise because of alterations in cancer-causing genes. Alterations in these genes generally are acquired, however, and there is little evidence that inherited mutations in dominant cancer susceptibility genes play a significant role in the development of these cancers. The most prominent exception is cases of endometrial cancer that occur in association with a strong family history of colon cancer, in which case a diagnosis of HNPCC should be considered.

There is now evidence to suggest that more subtle weakly penetrant genetic effects may contribute to cancer susceptibility, however. A number of genetic polymorphisms that change a single amino acid of protein may alter their function sufficiently to either increase or decrease cancer risk. In some cases, the effect on cancer susceptibility of these polymorphisms may depend on dietary and environmental exposures. These less-dramatic genetic effects may explain why all morbidly obese women do not develop endometrial cancer and why all women infected with oncogenic types of human papilloma virus do not develop cervical cancer.

TABLE 19.7. Guidelines for Surveillance of Mutation Carriers in HNPCC

Test	Age at Initiation (yr)	Frequency
ColonOscopy[a]	20–25	Every 2 yr until 35 years old; annually thereafter
Endometrial curettage	30	Annually
Transvaginal ultrasound, CA-125 level	30	Annually

[a]Subtotal colectomy is indicated when a polyp or cancer is found.

The genetic alterations that underlie gestational trophoblastic disease have been elucidated to a great extent (71). The predominant genetic alteration is an imbalance of parental chromosomes. In the case of partial moles, this involves an extra haploid copy of one set of paternal chromosomes, whereas complete moles generally are characterized by two complete haploid sets of paternal chromosomes and an absence of maternal chromosomes. Although the risk of repeat molar pregnancy is only about 1%, women who have had two molar pregnancies have about a 25% risk of developing another mole. Although this suggests a hereditary defect that affects gametogenesis, this remains speculative. Thus far, there is no evidence that mutations in specific genes contribute to the development of gestational trophoblastic disease.

CLINICAL NOTES

- Up to 10% of certain cancer types can be traced through family lines.
- Cancer of the colon, breast, and ovary are the most common hereditary cancers in women; it is thought that 5 to 10% of these cancers have a hereditary basis.
- Cancer results from loss of growth regulatory controls. Oncogenes encode proteins that stimulate proliferation, whereas tumor suppressor genes encode for proteins that inhibit proliferation.
- In caring for a patient or family with hereditary cancer, a thorough cancer history is absolutely essential. Data on all first- and second-degree relatives must be obtained. Other extended family history should be recorded if available.
- Five to 10% of breast and ovarian cancers are due to autosomal dominant hereditary syndromes. Most hereditary ovarian cancer cases are due to germ-line mutations in BRCA1 and BRCA2. At least half of hereditary breast cancers are due to germ-line mutations in BRCA1 and BRCA2.
- In families with BRCA1 mutations, the lifetime risk of breast cancer is about 80 to 90% and the lifetime risk of ovarian cancer is 30 to 60%. The incidence of prostate and colon cancers is also increased.
- In families with BRCA2 mutations, the lifetime risk of breast cancer is about 80 to 90% and the lifetime risk of ovarian cancer is 10%.
- The probability of finding a BRCA1 or 2 mutation in a woman over age 50 who is the only individual in her family with ovarian or breast cancer is less than 3%.
- Testing for BRCA1 or 2 mutations is generally reserved for a patient with two first-degree relatives with either ovarian cancer at any age or breast cancer before age 50.
- The benefits of genetic testing remain hypothetical. Women must receive adequate educational materials and counseling explaining the postulated risks and benefits before deciding to undergo testing. Confidentiality remains a critical issue in cancer susceptibility testing.
- Prophylactic oophorectomy for carriers of BRCA1 or 2 mutations is an attractive option because it can be done laparoscopically, usually only causes modest changes in body image or self-esteem, and estrogen replacement is available. It does not guarantee that malignancy such as intraperitoneal carcinomatosis will not develop, although this rarely occurs.
- Prevention of breast cancer in BRCA1 and 2 carriers is more complex. Mastectomy causes marked alterations in body image and self-esteem, even with breast reconstruction. Total mastectomy is recommended because cancer may form in the nipple if it is not removed. There is still no guarantee with total mastectomy that all breast tissue will be excised.
- Close surveillance with mammography and breast examination may prove equally effective in reducing mortality. Biannual mammography and breast examinations are recommended to begin between ages 25 and 35 for those affected individuals.
- Colon cancer is the third most common cause of cancer mortality in American women, behind lung and breast cancer.
- Familial APC syndrome is an autosomal dominant trait and accounts for about 1% of all

colon cancers. Individuals with APC mutations should undergo prophylactic total colectomy because half of these patients will develop colon cancer by age 40 and all develop cancer by age 70.

- A polymorphism in the gene associated with FAP affects approximately 6% of Ashkenazi Jews. Affected individuals have a 20% lifetime risk of colon cancer.
- The most common form of hereditary colon cancer is HNPCC, which accounts for about 5 to 10% of colorectal cancers. There are three criteria for this diagnosis: colorectal cancer in three or more relatives with one being a first-degree relative of the other two, colorectal cancer in two successive generations or more, and one family member who developed colorectal cancer by age 50.
- Patients with mutations in MLH1 or MSH2 genes are at risk for HNPCC. They should undergo genetic counseling at age 20, and a full colonoscopy should be done every 2 years until age 35 and the annually thereafter.

References

1. Parker SL, Tong T, Bolden S, et al. Cancer statistics. CA Cancer J Clin 1997;47:5–27.
2. Warthin AS. Heredity with reference to carcinoma. Arch Intern Med 1913;12:546–555.
3. Warthin AS. The further study of a cancer family. J Cancer Res 1925;9:279–286.
4. Lynch HT, Albano WA, Lynch JF, et al. Recognition of the cancer family syndrome. Gastroenterology 1983;84:672–673.
5. Hardcastle JD. Colorectal cancer. CA Cancer J Clin 1997;47:66–68.
6. Lynch HT, Follett KL, Lynch PM, et al. Family history in an oncology clinic. Implications for cancer genetics. JAMA 1979;242:1268–1272.
7. David KL, Steiner-Grossman P. The potential use of tumor registry data in the recognition and prevention of hereditary and familial cancer. NY State J Med 1991;91:150–152.
8. Muto T, Bussey HJ, Morson BC. The evolution of cancer of the colon and rectum. Cancer 1975;36:2251–2270.
9. Lynch HT, Lynch JS. Breast cancer genetics: family history, heterogeneity, molecular genetic diagnosis and genetic counseling. Curr Probl Cancer 1996;20:331–365.
10. Lynch HT, Fusaro RM, Lemon SJ, et al. Survey of cancer genetics: genetic testing implications. Cancer 1997;80:523–532.
11. Hall J, Lee M, Newman B, et al. Linkage of early onset familial breast cancer to chromosome 17q21. Science 1990;250:1684–1689.
12. Narod SA, Feunteun J, Lynch HT, et al. Familial breast-ovarian cancer locus on chromosome 17q12-q23. Lancet 1991;338:82–83.
13. Miki Y, Swensen J, Shattuck-Eidens D, et al. A strong candidate for the breast and ovarian cancer susceptibility gene BRCA1. Science 1994;266:66–71.
14. Boyd M, Harris F, McFarlane R, et al. A human BRCA1 gene knockout. Nature 1995;375:541–542.
15. Smith SA, Easton DF, Evans DG, et al. Allele losses in the region 17q12–21 in familial breast and ovarian cancer involve the wild-type chromosome. Nat Genet 1992;2:128–131.
16. Tirkkonen M, Johannsson O, Agnarsson BA, et al. Distinct somatic genetic changes associated with tumor progression in carriers of BRCA1 and BRCA2 germ-line mutations. Cancer Res 1997;57:1222–1227.
17. Ford D, Easton DF. The genetics of breast and ovarian cancer. Br J Cancer 1995;72:805–812.
18. Easton DF, Ford D, Bishop DT. Breast and ovarian cancer incidence in BRCA1-mutation carriers. Breast Cancer Linkage Consortium. Am J Hum Genet 1995;56:265–271.
19. Ford D, Easton DF, Bishop DT, et al. Risks of cancer in BRCA1-mutation carriers. Breast Cancer Linkage Consortium. Lancet 1994;343:692–695.
20. Rebbeck TR, Couch FJ, Calzone K, et al. Genetic heterogeneity in hereditary breast cancer: Role of BRCA1 and BRCA2. Am J Hum Genet 1996;59:547–553.
21. Serova OM, Mazoyer S, Puget N, et al. Mutations in BRCA1 and BRCA2 in breast cancer families: are there more breast cancer susceptibility genes? Am J Hum Genet 1997;60:486–495.

22. Couch FJ, DeShand ML, Blackwood A, et al. BRCA1 mutations in women attending clinics that evaluate the risk of breast cancer. N Engl J Med 1997;336:1409–1415.

23. Langston AA, Malone KE, Thompson JD, et al. BRCA1 mutations in a population-based sample of young women with breast cancer. N Engl J Med 1996;334:137–142.

24. Shattuck-Eidens D, McClure M, Simard J, et al. A collaborative survey of 80 mutations in the BRCA1 breast and ovarian cancer susceptibility gene. Implications for presymptomatic testing and screening. JAMA 1995;273:535–541.

25. Gayther SA, Warren W, Mazoyer S, et al. Germline mutations of the BRCA1 gene in breast and ovarian cancer families provide evidence for genotype-phenotype correlation. Nat Genet 1995;11:428–433.

26. Narod S, Goldgar D, Cannon-Albright L, et al. Risk modifiers in carriers of BRCA1 mutations. Int J Cancer 1995;64:394–398.

27. Struewing JP, Hartge P, Wacholder S, et al. The risk of cancer associated with specific mutations of BRCA1 and BRCA2 among Ashkenazi Jews. N Engl J Med 1997;336:1401–1408.

28. Eisinger F, Stoppa-Lyonnet D, Longy M, et al. Germ line mutation at BRCA1 affects the histoprognostic grade in hereditary breast cancer. Cancer Res 1996;56:471–474.

29. Marcus JN, Watson P, Page DL, et al. Hereditary breast cancer: pathobiology, prognosis, and BRCA1 and BRCA2 gene linkage. Cancer 1996;77:697–709.

30. Breast Cancer Linkage Consortium. Pathology of familial breast cancer: Differences between breast cancers in carriers of BRCA1 or BRCA2 mutations and sporadic cases. Lancet 1997;359:1505–1510.

31. Stratton JF, Gayther SA, Russell P, et al. Contribution of BRCA1 mutations to ovarian cancer. N Engl J Med 1997;336:1125–1130.

32. Rubin SC, Benjamin I, Behbakht K, et al. Clinical and pathological features of ovarian cancer in women with germ-line mutations of BRCA1. N Engl J Med 1996;335:1413–1416.

33. Wooster R, Neuhausen SL, Mangion J, et al. Localization of a breast cancer susceptibility gene, BRCA2, to chromosome 13q12–13. Science 1994;265:2088–2090.

34. Wooster R, Bignell G, Lancaster J, et al. Identification of the breast cancer susceptibility gene BRCA2. Nature 1995;378:789–791.

35. Phelan CM, Lancaster JM, Cumbs C, et al. Mutation analysis of the BRCA2 gene in 49 site-specific breast cancer families. Nat Genet 1996;13:120–122.

36. Lancaster JM, Wooster R, Mangion J, et al. BRCA2 mutations in primary breast and ovarian cancers. Nat Genet 1996;13:1–5.

37. Vaughn JP, Cirisano FD, Huper G, et al. Cell cycle control of BRCA2. Cancer Res 1996;56:4590–4594.

38. Rajan JV, Wang M, Marquis ST, et al. BRCA2 is coordinately regulated with BRCA1 during proliferation and differentiation in mammary epithelial cells. Proc Natl Acad Sci USA 1996;93:13078–13083.

39. Gayther SA, Mangion J, Russell P, et al. Variation of risks of breast and ovarian cancer associated with different germline mutations of the BRCA2 gene. Nat Genet 1997;15:103–105.

40. Couch FJ, Weber BL. Mutations and polymorphisms in the familial early-onset breast cancer (BRCA1) gene. Hum Mutat 1996;8:8–18.

41. Genetic testing and insurance. The Ad Hoc Committee on Genetic Testing/Insurance Issues. Am J Hum Genet 1995;56:327–331.

42. Wilson CA, Payton MN, Elliott GS, et al. Differential subcellular localization, expression and biological toxicity of BRCA1 and the splice variant BRCA1–11b. Oncogene 1997;14:1–16.

43. Friedman LS, Ostermeyer EA, Szabo CI, et al. Confirmation of BRCA1 by analysis of germline mutations linked to breast and ovarian cancer in ten families. Nat Genet 1994;8:399–404.

44. Castilla LH, Couch FJ, Erdos MR, et al. Mutations in the BRCA1 gene in families with early-onset breast and ovarian cancer. Nat Genet 1994;8:387–391.

45. Lynch HT. Many at risk consider prophylactic oophorectomy. OB/GYN News, July 1, 1997.

46. Hoskins KF, Stopfer JE, Calzone KA, et al. Assessment and counseling for women with a family history of breast cancer. JAMA 1995;273:577–585.

47. Szabo CI, King MC. Population genetics of BRCA1 and BRCA2 (editorial). Am J Hum Genet 1997;60:1013–1020.

48. Struewing JP, Abeliovich D, Peretz T, et al. The carrier frequency of the BRCA1 185delAG mutation is approximately 1 percent in Ashkenazi Jewish individuals. Nat Genet 1995;11:198–200.

49. Oddoux C, Struewing JP, Clayton CM, et al. The carrier frequency of the BRCA2 6174delT mutation among Ashkenazi Jewish individuals is approximately 1%. Nat Genet 1996;14:188–190.

50. Abeliovich D, Kaduri L, Lerer I, et al. The founder mutations 185delAG and 5382insC in BRCA1 and 6174delT in BRCA2 appear in 60% of ovarian cancer and 30% of early-onset breast cancer patients among Ashkenazi women. Am J Hum Genet 1997;60:505–514.

51. Levy-Lahad E, Catane R, Eisenberg S, et al. Founder BRCA1 and BRCA2 mutations in Ashkenazi Jews in Israel: frequency and differential penetrance in ovarian cancer and in breast-ovarian cancer families. Am J Hum Genet 1997;60:1059–1067.

52. Winawer SJ, Zauber AG, Ho MN, et al. Prevention of colorectal cancer by colonoscopic polypectomy. N Engl J Med 1993;329:1977–1981.

53. St. John DJ, McDermott FT, Hopper JL, et al. Cancer risk in relatives of patients with common colorectal cancer. Ann Intern Med 1993;118:785– 790.

54. Bussey HJ. Gastrointestinal polyposis. Gut 1970;11:970–978.

55. Bussey HJ. Familial polyposis coli. Pathol Annu 1979;14:61–81.

56. Lipkin M, Sherlock P, DeCoose JJ. Risk factors and preventative measures in the control of cancer of the large intestine. Curr Prob Cancer 1980;4:1–57.

57. Bodmer WF, Bailey CJ, Bodmer J, et al. Localization of the gene for familial adenomatous polyposis on chromosome 5. Nature 1987;328:614–616.

58. Solomon E, Voss R, Hall V, et al. Chromosome 5 allele loss in human colorectal carcinomas. Nature 1987;328:616–619.

59. Parsons R. Molecular genetics and hereditary cancer: hereditary nonpolyposis colorectal carcinoma as a model. Cancer 1997;80:533–536.

60. Fearon ER. Molecular abnormalities in colon and rectal cancer: In: Mendelsohn J, Howley PM, Israel MA, et al., eds. The Molecular Basis of Cancer. Philadelphia: WB Saunders, 1995:340.

61. Fearon ER, Vogelstein B. A genetic model for colorectal tumorigenesis. Cell 1990;61: 759–767.

62. Laken SJ, Petersen GM, Gruber SB, et al. Familial colorectal cancer in Ashkenazim due to a hypermutable tract in APC. Nat Genet 1997;17:79–83.

63. Lynch HT, Lynch J. Genetic counseling for hereditary cancer. Oncology 1996;10:27–34.

64. Vasen HF, Mecklin JP, Khan PM, et al. The International Collaborative Group on Hereditary Non-Polyposis Colorectal Cancer (ICG-HNPCC). Dis Colon Rectum 1991;34:424–425.

65. Leach FS, Nicolaides NC, Papadopoulos N, et al. Mutations of a MutS homolog in hereditary nonpolyposis colorectal cancer. Cell 1993;75:1215–1225.

66. Lescoe MK, Rao MRS, Copeland NG, et al. The human mutator gene homolog MSH2 and its association with hereditary nonpolyposis colon cancer. Cell 1993;75:1027–1038.

67. Menko FH, Wijnen J, Khan PM, et al. Genetic counseling in hereditary nonpolyposis colorectal cancer. Oncology 1996;10:71–76.

68. Burke W, Daly M, Garber J, et al. Recommendations for follow-up care of individuals with an inherited predisposition to cancer. I. Hereditary Nonpolyposis Colon Cancer. JAMA 1997;227:915–919.

69. Giardiello FM, Hamilton SR, Krush AJ, et al. Treatment of colonic and rectal adenomas with sulindac in familial adenomatous polyposis. N Engl J Med 1993;328:1313–1316.

70. Thun MJ, Namboodiri MM, Heath CW Jr. Aspirin use and reduced risk of fatal colon cancer. N Engl J Med 1991;325:1593–1596.

71. Mutter GL. Gestational trophoblastic disease. In: Langdon SP, Miller WR, Berchuck A, eds. Biology of Female Cancers. New York: CRC Press, 1997.

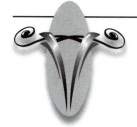

CHAPTER 20

Domestic Violence

ABBEY B. BERENSON

Domestic violence is any act between intimate partners that is intended or perceived to be intended to cause physical or psychological harm (1). Although violence may be perpetrated against men or in same-sex relationships, most studies on domestic violence focused on violence perpetrated by men against women partners. In its least severe form, domestic violence includes verbal or psychological abuse, threats of violence, throwing an object, pushing, grabbing, slapping, or spanking. More severe domestic violence includes kicking, hitting, sexual assault, threatening with a weapon, or using a weapon (2). Progressive social isolation, intimidation, and deprivation of food, clothing, money, and transportation are also examples of domestic violence (3).

Most studies on the incidence of this crime indicate that domestic violence has reached epidemic proportions in the United States. In fact, women who reside in this country are more likely to be assaulted and injured, raped, or killed by a current or ex-male partner than by all other types of perpetrators combined (4). Between 8 and 12% of married or cohabiting women in the United States experience domestic violence each year, whereas severe violence is experienced by 2 to 4% (5–8). Overall, approximately two million American women report being victims of domestic violence each year (9, 10).

As alarming as these figures are, most experts agree that data obtained by national surveys probably underestimate the frequency of this crime for a variety of reasons. First, victims frequently do not report domestic violence even when questioned because of shame, guilt, or fear of the perpetrator. Many surveys focus on only married and cohabiting women and thus fail to consider abuse by boyfriends who did not live with their partner (2). Furthermore, national samples often do not include women who do not speak English, who are homeless, or who are incarcerated, hospitalized, or institutionalized. Overall, the true prevalence of domestic violence in the United States has been estimated to be double that reported, or four million women per year (4). Thus, as many as 21 to 30% of all U.S. women experience violence at the hands of an intimate partner at least once in their lives and up to 9% experience severe violence (2, 9).

In addition, women abused by an intimate partner are far more likely than those attacked by a stranger to be assaulted multiple times within a 12-month period. In one study, 50% of women who reported domestic violence described more than one incident in the past year (7). Straus and Gelles (6) observed in their study on domestic violence that victims experienced a mean of six incidents in a 12-month period.

In contrast to the popularly held myth that domestic violence occurs only in minorities or among those who live in poverty (11–13), women of any age, race, educational level, geographic location, or socioeconomic status may fall victim to this tragedy (Table 20.1). Research suggests that the higher prevalence reported among minorities and women of low socioeconomic status may be related to the use by these women of the public health care system, where violence is more likely to be reported. Nonminorities and women of higher economic status are more likely to use private health care services where reporting is less frequent (12).

TABLE 20.1. Myths and Facts About Battered Women

Myth Battered women are always from lower socioeconomic groups.

Fact Domestic violence is primarily reported in lower socioeconomic groups because they use emergency facilities (which report such incidents) more often than they see private practitioners (who generally do not). Most studies, however, show that abuse occurs regardless of race, religion, or socioeconomic category.

Myth Battered women must enjoy the abuse; otherwise they would leave.

Fact All studies have shown that battered women are not masochists. The reasons for their remaining in an abusive relationship are complex and multiple, but their lives are chaotic, frightening, violent, and often isolated socially.

Myth A women who is beaten probably provoked her partner.

Fact A victim of abuse may believe that she deserves the battering, but the responsibility for the violence resides with the batterer. The woman may accept responsibility for the violence as a means of maintaining control over her situation. Believing that her actions may allow her to control the batterer and prevent a future incident misleads her into a false sense of security.

Myth The battered woman who is serious about solving the problem have the batterer arrested and put in jail.

Fact Women will not routinely resort to arrest of the batterer for reasons that include loss of income, fear of retaliation, and the realization that the court system will probably play down her accusations and perhaps quickly release the batterer. Many jurisdictions and law enforcement officers tend to minimize the significance of domestic violence, whereas similar episodes of violence between unrelated individuals are not treated as lightly.

Myth If a battered woman remarries, she usually chooses another violent man.

Fact Some abused women remain single after leaving an abusive relationship, whereas many who do marry make a conscious effort not to marry a batterer. Because many women who have been abused leave such a relationship and subsequently seek and find a safer one, a history of abuse in a patient does not necessarily indicate that her current relationship is abusive.

Reprinted with permission from Domestic violence. Tech Bull 1995;209:1–9. © American College of Obstetricians and Gynecologists.

The costs to society that result from domestic violence are immense. These include both emergency and long-term care for victims, costs for maintaining shelter and housing for victims and their children, and the expense of intervention by police and the judicial and social services systems. The cost of domestic violence to U.S. business in terms of lost work time, increased health care costs, high turnover, and lower productivity is estimated at $3 billion to $5 billion annually (11). Moreover, children who witness domestic violence in the home are more likely to develop emotional or behavioral problems that include physical aggression, adjustment complications, academic problems, developmental delay, lower levels of social competence, or depressive symptoms (14). Additionally, studies show that children who witness battering of their mothers in their homes are likely to be abused as well (15–18) and more likely to be a partner in a violent relationship when they reach adulthood (14, 16, 19).

CYCLE OF VIOLENCE

Researchers report that violence in an intimate relationship is characterized by three phases that escalate in frequency and intensity over time (16). During the first phase, tension accumulates. The batterer expresses anger and hostility but not in an explosive form (12). Abusive acts, such as name calling, use of intimidating remarks, acts of deliberate meanness, and mild physical abuse, such as pushing, are common. In response to these acts, the woman attempts to alter her behavior in the hope that this will please the batterer and the abuse will subside. These attempts to calm the batterer's behavior may be successful for a time, an effect that reinforces the woman's belief that she is responsible for the abuse. As time passes, however, she finds it more and more difficult to pacify the batterer. She may withdraw, fearful that she will inadvertently provoke him. This withdrawal may be the signal for the perpetrator to become more hostile (12).

In the second phase, the perpetrator explodes and battering occurs. There is a discharge of the tension that had built up during the first phase. Physical abuse occurs that may result in severe injury (20). Often, the abusive event is accompanied by heavy drinking that the victim may mistakenly identify as the cause of the battering.

After the abuse, however, the abuser becomes apologetic and promises it will not happen again. He may shower the victim with gifts and flowers. During this third phase, he is remorseful, attentive, and kind, leading the victim to believe that the problem has passed. As the cycle continues, the batterer learns that he can control, intimidate, and manipulate the victim. Consequently, the first phase of each cycle lasts for a longer period of time, the expression of violence becomes more severe, and the third phase lasts for a shorter period (12, 21). This abusive cycle leaves many women demoralized and lacking the self-esteem necessary to leave the situation.

CHARACTERISTICS OF THE PERPETRATOR

Most male batterers grew up in an abusive home themselves, suggesting that domestic violence is a learned behavior (22). In fact, clinical studies of male batterers demonstrate that 75% were either physically abused as a child or observed physical violence between their parents. Furthermore, those who were physically abused as children tend to abuse their partner more frequently than batterers who were not abused themselves (23).

Both antisocial and borderline personality disorders have been observed more often among men who batter than among nonviolent control subjects (24). In addition, batterers are more likely to demonstrate low self-esteem and intense feelings of inadequacy (11). They have a strong fear of abandonment and thus often exhibit extreme jealousy. As a result of these feelings, they have a strong need to control every aspect of their environment. They often treat their partner as chattel, expecting them to report in frequently and obtain permission for almost every action. Stereotypic role expectations are enforced. To demonstrate her love and devotion, the wife may be forced to care for her husband in ways his mother did. Any independence or autonomy exhibited by the victim is perceived as a threat. These feelings are especially heightened if the victim intends to end the relationship.

When confronted with his behavior, the typical batterer will refuse to take responsibility for his actions and may even blame the victim for his behavior. He frequently minimizes the abuse and fails to characterize his behavior as harmful. In fact, he may accuse the victim of reporting the violence to others to gain legal or economic advantage or to take revenge. He is likely to be supported in these beliefs by his male friends, because male friends of the batterer are more likely to approve of violence against a spouse than are male friends of nonabusive husbands (25).

Up to 50% of batterers have a serious alcohol problem. In about 40% of assaults, the perpetrator is acutely intoxicated (26). Domestic violence is especially common in marriages where the man is an alcoholic. Over half of alcoholics report hitting their partner in the year before entering treatment for their drinking problem (27).

BARRIERS TO LEAVING AN ABUSIVE ENVIRONMENT

Physicians and other health care workers may feel frustrated when encountering the victim of domestic violence because they cannot comprehend why a woman stays in an abusive environment. However, the belief that a woman can easily leave this environment reflects a misunderstanding of the complexity of the problem. The average victim attempts to leave the home two to five times before she is able to successfully terminate the relationship (28). A number of psychological and practical barriers exist.

Fear

Women attempting to leave an abusive relationship often report threats of harm to themselves, the children, and other family members. Some women may feel that by staying in the relationship they are protecting other family members from violence.

In many cases, the abuse does not stop even if they leave the home. Men who batter are motivated by a need to exercise power and control over the victim. The abuser may begin stalking the victim. If children are involved, divorce proceedings, custody battles, and visitation rights may be used to gain access to and exercise control over the victim (11). Moreover, women attempting to leave an abusive environment are at increased risk of homicide (29). A recent study of 38,648 female homicides occurring from 1976 to 1987 reports that 61% were committed by a male partner (30, 31).

Social Isolation

As the cycle of battering continues, the batterer exercises more and more control over the victim. As a result, many women become progressively isolated from friends, family, and community. In an effort to appease the batterer, the woman tries to conform to rigid rules of behavior. The batterer may restrict access to friends, family, telephone, car, and community (30). She may have no privacy because the batterer accompanies her to the doctor's office, grocery store, and so on. In doing so, the batterer controls virtually every aspect of the woman's life. As a result, the victim becomes more and more dependent on the batterer for social, emotional, and financial support (32).

Financial Dependence

Many battered women do not have access to bank accounts, credit cards, or cash. This makes the process of leaving extremely difficult. Without financial resources, it is nearly impossible for women to obtain food and shelter for themselves and their children. The need to hide from the abuser may make it difficult to obtain or continue employment. In addition, many victims are unable to obtain work because they lack job skills and prior work experience. Thus, the victim may choose to stay in an abusive environment because she fears becoming homeless.

Inadequate Social Support

Social support for victims of domestic violence is severely lacking. Nationally, only two of five victims are able to gain timely admittance to a shelter (33). Many shelters are full at almost all times. In addition, the facility may restrict whom it admits. For example, some shelters are unable to accommodate women with a large number of children or those with a male child over the age of 12 years (16). Victims of domestic violence who abuse alcohol or drugs may also be denied admittance (34, 35). If a woman does gain admission, she is usually restricted to a stay of 2 to 6 weeks. Consequently, many women return to an abusive home after a stay in a shelter because they have no alternative place to stay.

Social services may also fail the abused woman by causing her to fear that she will lose custody of her children (17). Approximately 40% (11) of men who batter their wives also beat their children. Thus, children of battered women are more likely to be removed from the home by child protective services than children of nonbattered women (16).

Inability of the Police and Justice System to Provide Safety

Historically, police and the justice system have viewed violence within the context of the family as outside their jurisdiction. Violent acts perpetrated by strangers are subject to criminal prosecution, whereas the same acts committed in the context of an intimate relationship may be treated as minor transgressions or dismissed entirely. Until recently, few laws existed to address violence occurring in the family.

Cultural views have perpetuated the belief that a man has a right to exercise control within the family. The expression "rule of thumb" originated in English common law that states that a man is not permitted to beat his wife with an object wider than his thumb (36). Persistence of these views impedes the courts and police from providing adequate protection for victims of domestic violence.

Consequently, women perceive the legal system as ineffective (30, 37, 38). Protective and restraining orders are valuable only if the batterer respects the order and if the police are willing to enforce it. When these measures fail, many women attempt to live in hiding, a choice that interferes with employment, keeping children in school, and maintaining a normal social and home environment (30). Mandatory reporting laws, which were passed to protect the domestic violence victim, may actually increase the risk of violence because perpetrators are usually jailed for only a few days.

ROLE OF HEALTH CARE PROVIDERS

Clearly, a multidisciplinary approach that includes health care workers, social services, the police, and the legal system is necessary to resolve this problem. Physicians and other health care workers, however, are in an excellent position to identify victims and provide them with information and alternatives.

Recognition of the Victim

The medical community may encounter the domestic violence victim in a variety of settings. The victim of recent abuse, especially if severe, frequently presents for care at an emergency center. It has been estimated, in fact, that approximately 12% of emergency room visits by women with partners are for injuries or stress resulting from domestic violence (39). Among pregnant women, as many as one third who present with trauma have an injury that was inflicted intentionally (40). However, the cause of these injuries frequently goes undetected by emergency room personnel. In one study, only 13% of victims stated that they were asked about domestic violence or reported its occurrence to the doctor or nurse (39). Furthermore, domestic violence was recorded in the medical record in only 2% of those cases in which it was the reason for the emergency room visit.

To detect domestic violence, clinicians must have a high index of suspicion when women present to the emergency room with injuries. One reason to suspect violence is an injury to the head, face, or neck, because victims of domestic violence are 12 times more likely to be injured in this region than those experiencing trauma from other causes. Overall, injuries that occur as a result of domestic violence occur on the central region of the body such as the head, face, neck, chest, breasts, or abdomen, in contrast to accidental injuries, which tend to be peripheral (41). In addition, multiple injury sites in different stages of healing are suggestive of ongoing violence.

Time of arrival to the emergency center may also suggest the possibility of abuse, because victims of domestic violence are more likely to present between 11:00 pm and 7:00 am (42). Furthermore, a delay between the time of injury and arrival for care is strongly suggestive of domestic violence because victims often delay seeking care for their injuries (32).

Most visits to physicians by the domestic violence victim, however, do not take place in the emergency room but in the private practitioner's office. Victims of abuse make more visits to the doctor than nonvictims for somatic complaints such as choking sensation, hyperventilation, chest pain, gastrointestinal symptoms, headaches, and chronic back, abdominal, or pelvic pain. Functional bowel disease is reported twice as often by battered as nonbattered women (43). Reports of insomnia, anxiety, depression, eating disorders, or panic symptoms are also common (15, 32, 35, 44, 45). Usually, no etiology for these somatic complaints can be determined if domestic violence is not considered (20).

Violence During Pregnancy

Prior studies document that between 6 and 8% of pregnant women in the United States experience domestic violence (46–48). Furthermore, between 12 and 88% of these women reported experiencing violence for the first time while pregnant (46–48). Adolescents are at especially high risk of physical abuse during pregnancy because they are vulnerable to assault from a parent and from a boyfriend or spouse. A woman whose partner is unhappy about the pregnancy or for whom the pregnancy is not planned also is more likely to experience violence than one whose partner desires the pregnancy (49). Other factors associated with violence include depression, inadequate emotional support, and heavy use of alcohol and drugs during the pregnancy (46).

Violence during pregnancy may have severe consequences for the infant and the mother. If the mother is struck in the abdomen, the fetus may experience a direct injury. Morey et al. (50) reported a case of fetal bruising and intraventricular hemorrhage after a blow to the abdomen. Unhealthy behaviors associated with domestic violence also may adversely affect the fetus. For example, abused women are more likely than those without a history of abuse to delay seeking prenatal care until the third trimester (51). In addition, victims of violence are more likely than nonvictims to use multiple illicit substances during pregnancy and to continue to use drugs throughout the gestation (52).

Two controlled studies observed that victims of domestic violence are more likely to deliver a low-birth-weight (less than 2500 g) infant (51, 53), whereas one study demonstrated a higher risk of premature delivery (53). In addition, abuse during pregnancy has been associated with low maternal weight gain, anemia, and infections (51). Studies have yet to document whether these effects are due to a direct or indirect mechanism.

Victims may be at even higher risk of abuse during the postpartum period than during the pregnancy itself. In a study of 36 women abused during pregnancy, victims reported being hit more frequently during the 3 months after delivery than during the pregnancy or preconception period (54). An increase in abuse during this period may be related, in part, to the numerous stresses that accompany new parenthood, such as sleep deprivation, lack of privacy, and increased expenses. Thus, it is important to screen women for physical violence at their postpartum visit and before and during pregnancy. The safety of all children residing in an abusive home should also be determined.

Children of Abuse Victims

Children are frequently witnesses or victims of domestic violence. Relative to the general population, households where domestic violence occurs are more likely to have children and more likely to have children under 5 years of age (55). As many as 1 in 10 calls to the police regarding domestic violence is made by a child (55). Children may also be victims of physical abuse; in fact, assault on a child is 15 times more likely to occur in a home where domestic violence is present (16). In one study, 53% of men who battered their wives also reported hitting their children, and 28% of the wives admitted they had abused their offspring (56).

Children who are not victims of physical assault may still develop emotional or behavioral problems as a result of witnessing the abuse. Children who reside in a violent household frequently exhibit feelings of guilt, shame, lack of trust, poor self-esteem, helplessness, and hopelessness (57). Girls may identify with the mother and learn passivity, whereas boys often learn that bullying and inflicting violence on others is acceptable. Children may also develop academic problems, developmental delays, preoccupation with physical aggression, difficulty with social skills, and depression (14). Play therapy has been demonstrated to help children work through their feelings in the immediate posttrauma period (12). Individual therapy may also be a useful adjunct. Without intervention, children are likely to carry into their own adult lives the abusive behaviors they learned while growing up.

One of the most difficult areas for the provider is how to respond if it is suspected that the child and the spouse are being physically abused. Mandatory reporting may result in removal of the child from the mother's care, which may be harmful to both victims. In these cases, physicians may find it useful to consult with their ethics committee, risk management, and battered women's advocates for advice on how to enhance the safety of the mother and child and work with state agencies to ensure the best outcome for both (58).

Screening and Intervention

Although it is important to identify victims of abuse at the time of an acute injury, screening should not be limited to emergency centers. To increase the detection of domestic violence so that women at risk may be identified before injury occurs, both the American Medical Association (AMA) and the American College of Obstetricians and Gynecologists (ACOG) have recommended that universal screening is implemented in office-based practices. Domestic violence advocates have developed simple protocols that help a physician to incorporate screening and intervention into their practice. One of the most popular, RADAR, uses a simple mnemonic to help the physician remember the screening steps (Fig. 20.1) (32).

R—Remember to Ask

Universal screening of all patients communicates your willingness to listen and provide help. It also educates unaffected patients that violence may occur in an intimate relationship. Both male and female patients should be screened for intimate violence because this phenomenon may also occur against husbands and also in lesbian and homosexual relationships.

Questions about violence in intimate relationships may be awkward at first. However, most practitioners easily adapt questioning about violence to their own practice style. Many physicians begin with the statement "Because violence is so common in

Remember to ask

Ask directly

Document findings

Assess safety

Review options and refer

FIGURE 20.1. The mnemonic "RADAR" is intended to help the physician in the screening of patients for domestic violence.

many women's lives, I have begun to ask about it routinely." To detect the verbal abuse characteristic of battering in its earliest stage, many practitioners ask "Does your partner threaten you, call you names, or yell at you?" (59). This should be followed with direct screening questions such as "Are you in a relationship in which you have been physically hurt or threatened?" "Have you ever been hit, kicked, or punched by your partner?" This wording is more effective than asking if she has been physically or sexually abused, because women may not identify themselves as victims of abuse.

It is important to establish an environment that encourages women to disclose their victimization. The manner in which screening questions are asked and the perceived safety of the setting have an impact on how a woman will respond (60). Physicians, who are taught to be decisive and authoritative in treating patients, may inadvertently reinforce the idea that one must complacently accept another's controlling behavior (61). The managed care environment of today's medical practice requires that physicians make rapid assessments, diagnoses, and treatment recommendations (61). This methodology, however, disempowers the patient. For the victim of domestic violence, this may only reinforce the idea that she is incapable of making decisions and must accept that others control her environment.

Women who report satisfaction with their clinician declare the most helpful response is to listen, be sympathetic, and offer appropriate options (15). Therefore, a patient who responds positively to direct questioning should be encouraged to elaborate. As she discusses her abuse, assure her that she does not deserve to be a victim of violence and is not to blame for the situation. Let her know that there are resources available to help her. Providing a woman with information and options that help her escape the abuse restores a sense of control over her life. The physician should avoid instructing the patient to leave but instead should establish a willingness to help when she is able to make that decision. If the victim does not want to further discuss the problem during the visit, ask her at a follow-up visit if she wishes to discuss it at that time.

A—Ask Directly

Some practitioners screen patients for a history of current or past abuse using a self-reported health information questionnaire. Although this is certainly better than not screening at all, most experts agree that direct questioning during the routine medical inquiry is a more effective way to elicit sensitive information (62). Use of a structured interviewing tool, such as the Abuse Assessment Screen (Fig. 20.2), has

Abuse Assessment Screen

1. **Have you ever been emotionally or physically abused by your partner or someone important to you?**
   Yes   No

2. **Within the last year, have you been hit, slapped, kicked, or otherwise physically hurt by someone?**
   Yes   No
   If yes, by whom (circle all that apply)
   Husband   Ex-husband   Boyfriend   Stranger   Other   Multiple
   Number of Times:_____

3. **Since you've been pregnant, have you been hit, slapped, kicked, or otherwise physically hurt by someone?**
   Yes   No
   If yes, by whom (circle all that apply)
   Husband   Ex-husband   Boyfriend   Stranger   Other   Multiple
   Number of Times:_____

   - Mark area of injury(ies) on a body map
   - Score the most severe incident according to the following scale:

     1 threats of abuse, including threat of using a weapon

     2 slapping, pushing; no injuries and/or lasting pain

     3 punching, kicking, bruises, cuts, and/or continuing pain

     4 beating, severe contusions, burns, broken bones

     5 head, internal, and/or permanent injury

     6 use of a weapon, wound from a weapon

4. **Within the past year, has anyone forced you to have sexual activities?**
   Yes   No
   If yes, by whom (circle all that apply)
   Husband   Ex-husband   Boyfriend   Stranger   Other   Multiple
   Number of times:_____

5. **Are you afraid of your partner or anyone you listed above?**
   Yes   No

FIGURE 20.2. Use of a structured abuse assessment screen has been demonstrated to result in higher rates of detection of domestic violence. (Reprinted with permission from Norton LB, Peipert JF, Zierler S, et al. Battering in pregnancy: an assessment of two screening methods. Obstet Gynecol 1995;85:321–325. © American College of Obstetricians and Gynecologists.)

been demonstrated to result in higher rates of detection than an interview that does not use a structured screen (63).

It is important to provide a confidential setting in which to inquire about intimate violence. In an effort to control the victim and prevent disclosure, many batterers accompany their partner to the emergency room or doctor's office. In fact, many batterers will complete medical history forms or answer medical history questions for their partner, never allowing the victim to respond (64). If this is the case, some means must be developed to separate the victim from the batterer. One effective strategy is to require the batterer to go to the reception area to complete forms. Another tactic is to request that the victim provide a urine sample or complete some other laboratory test. The nurse may accompany her to another area to complete this task and administer screening questions at this time. Once the interviewer and patient are alone, the woman must be reassured that the interview is confidential and that her answers will not be discussed with others without her permission. If confidentiality is not ensured, many women will not disclose battering because it is simply too dangerous for them to admit that violence is a problem.

D—Document Findings

Accurate documentation in the medical record of injuries resulting from domestic violence will greatly assist the victim if she initiates court proceedings. Include in the record the date and location of the attack, the name and relationship of the alleged perpetrator, and the patient's description of how the injury occurred. Medical descriptions of the injury may be included but should not replace the victim's own words. For example, record "My boyfriend hit me in the lip" rather than "Patient sustained injury to lip" (58). Inconsistencies between the appearance of the injury and the patient's explanation of how it occurred should also be recorded. Although it is important that documentation be precise, it should not be excessive. Too much detail should be avoided because inconsistencies between the medical record and the police report may be damaging to the victim (58).

All injuries observed should be described in the medical record and marked on a body map (Fig. 20.3). If old injuries are apparent, these should be marked on a second body map. Color photographs of newly acquired injuries should be taken after obtaining written consent. A Polaroid camera has the advantage of immediate availability of the photographs, which can then be placed in the medical record. A card with the patient's name and hospital or patient number and the date and time should be included with each photograph. If available, a data back camera will record the patient's name and identifying number directly on the photograph. The back of each photograph should be legibly marked with the photographer's name. Other physical evidence of abuse, such as torn or bloody clothing, should also be labeled and stored. If sexual abuse has occurred, the evidence should be properly collected using a forensic rape kit, labeled, and given to authorities after obtaining informed consent (58).

Good legible documentation often avoids the necessity of the physician testifying in court. If the physician does have to testify, a carefully recorded medical chart can be useful to refresh his or her memory. Good documentation may also help the victim obtain a protective order, retain custody of her children, or eliminate the need for her to testify in court. The value of good documentation cannot be underestimated. If the case later comes to trial, the medical record may be the only evidence that abuse occurred besides the victim's report.

Body Map

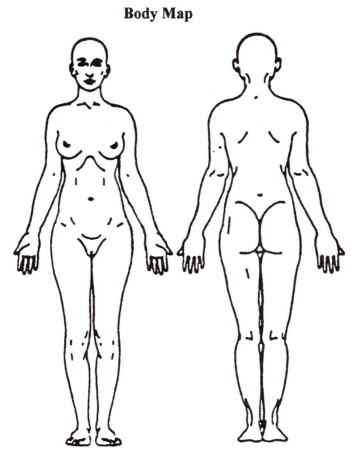

FIGURE 20.3. A body map is useful for documenting injuries for the medical record. If old injuries are apparent, these should be marked on a second body map. (Courtesy of Med-Law, P.O. Box 9953, Conroe, TX 77387. From Sexual Assault Evidence Kit.)

A—Assess Safety

Assess the severity of the violence by asking the victim if she is afraid to go home and if there are guns or other weapons in the house. Assess the safety of children by asking if there have been threats to them as well. If the patient is in eminent danger, help her determine if there is someone with whom she can stay. Allow her the opportunity of making a private phone call. If she needs access to a shelter, a referral should be made to one with immediate availability, if possible.

R—Review Options and Refer

Physicians who are knowledgeable about the resources in their community are best equipped to assist the victim of domestic violence. Information on resources may be directly given to the patient and displayed in private areas of the clinic, such as the women's room, where victims can review it away from the perpetrator.

Legal assistance may be available through legal aid programs for low-income women, legal adjuncts of shelters or other domestic violence agencies, bar association referral services, criminal justice advocacy units, and immigration assistance organizations (58). Local domestic violence programs and state domestic violence coalitions are often aware of resources in their particular community. The local Young Women's Christian Association often also has information on resources.

Working with the battered woman to develop an exit plan is also important (Table 20.2). The victim should be prepared to leave quickly if she perceives that she is in danger. Victims also should be advised to memorize the national shelter hotline number (1-800-799-SAFE). This 24-hour hotline directs victims to the nearest shelter from any location in the United States. Multilingual counselors also offer crisis counseling. This service can also provide clinicians with brochures, information packets, and shelter locations in their area.

In many cases, the woman may not be ready to leave the abusive situation. Although the physician has an obligation to counsel and refer the patient to appropriate agencies and shelters, the patient must be the one to determine when it is safe to change her life situation (38). Disallowing the right to a choice may only further disempower the victim, who may feel betrayed both by the abusive partner and the system that is supposed to offer protection.

BARRIERS TO SCREENING FOR DOMESTIC VIOLENCE

Despite the recommendations by national medical organizations, many physicians have not incorporated universal screening into their office-based practices. Barriers that prevent the widespread implementation of these recommendations by physicians include lack of training, prejudices, lack of understanding, time constraints, frustration at being unable to help the victim, fear of offending the patient, and, in some cases, reticence because of a personal history of abuse.

Lack of Training

In a survey of ACOG fellows, lack of training was the most common reason cited for failing to incorporate universal screening in their practices. Thirty-four percent stated that they had received no training in this area, and 49% agreed that they felt inadequate in dealing with abuse victims because of inadequate training. A study of primary care physicians demonstrated that 57% believed that their medical training had not taught them how to deal with domestic violence victims (65). Education had a direct impact on clinical practice. The physicians who had received training in domestic violence were more likely to screen than those who had received no instruction (66).

Although some medical schools and residencies have initiated programs to incorporate domestic violence training in their curricula, such programs have been

---

TABLE 20.2. Advice for Patients: Preparing an Exit Plan

Open a savings and/or credit card in your own name to establish or increase your independence.

Leave money, an extra set of keys, copies of important documents, extra medicines, and clothes with someone you trust.

Determine who would be able to let you stay with them for a while or lend you some money.

Keep the shelter or hotline phone number close at hand and keep some change or a calling card with you at all times for emergency phone calls.

Review your safety plan often to ensure the safest way to leave your batterer.

Remember: leaving your abuser is the most dangerous time.

slow to develop. A survey of medical schools demonstrated that 53% do not offer instruction in domestic violence (67). Sixty percent of residency programs in obstetrics and gynecology reported dissatisfaction with their training in this area (68). Even as schools and training programs improve their domestic violence curricula, also needed are efforts to provide continuing education regarding domestic violence to physicians who have completed training. Thus, physicians must seek out educational courses or obtain written resources to enhance their skills and knowledge.

Cultural, Socioeconomic, and Gender Prejudice

A significant barrier to screening is that health care providers frequently regard domestic violence as a problem limited to poor or minority patients. In one study, health care providers from five different communities stated that most cases of family violence occur in Latino, African-American, Native American, or Southeast Asian communities and occur primarily in indigent families. In fact, almost one half of obstetrician/gynecologists surveyed reported that they do not screen for domestic violence because they do not perceive this to be a problem among their private patients (66). When violence is detected among patients of higher socioeconomic groups, physicians are less likely to report these cases to protective services or the criminal justice agencies (13). Physicians are also less likely to recognize that abuse can occur in homosexual relationships or among the elderly.

Time Constraints

Another reason commonly cited by physicians for not screening for domestic violence is a lack of time (66, 69). The recent pressure to increase patient volume within a managed care setting has exacerbated this problem. However, screening for domestic violence requires only a few minutes of the physicians' time in most cases (69). For example, screening may consist of a single question, such as "At any time has a partner ever hit you, kicked you, or otherwise physically hurt you?" If time constraints prevent verbal questioning, written questionnaires may be used. In fact, the inclusion of a single written question on the medical history form of all patients has been demonstrated to be more effective in detecting prior abuse than the use of discretionary screening, even when verbal, with a few selected patients (62).

Frustration at Inability to Help Victims

Approximately one third of gynecologists surveyed stated that they do not screen because, when abuse is detected, they are unable to help the victim. This perception is inaccurate because the screening process itself helps the victim by conveying a sense that others care about her situation. In addition, the physician can distribute educational brochures, make referrals, and document the abuse in the medical record for future court proceedings.

Fear of Offending Patients

Often, clinicians fear that patients will be offended by questions on abuse (59, 62). However, there is no scientific evidence to support this claim. In a recent study on men and women seen in a primary care practice, 80% reported that they favored universal screening for assault (70). Moreover, many patients expressed gratitude at being asked these questions (69).

History of Abuse

Physicians may also be reluctant to ask about domestic violence because of their own prior experiences. In one study, 13% of physicians cited a personal history of abuse as a barrier to screening (66). Women who have witnessed or experienced abuse in their own lives may be fearful that discussing domestic violence will evoke their own painful memories and make it difficult for them to maintain a professional demeanor (61).

In addition, the abusive nature of medical training may hinder the physician's ability to recognize domestic violence. Students and house officers often report feeling controlled and humiliated. Anxiety, depression, and exhaustion are common. Women may experience sexual harassment and gender discrimination. When physicians fail to recognize their own experiences as abusive, it is harder for them to empathize with a woman in an abusive relationship (61).

ELDER ABUSE

Between 4 and 10% of elders in the United States suffer from neglect or physical, sexual, or psychological abuse (71). This number continues to increase, with approximately 100,000 additional cases reported each year since 1981 (72). Individuals over the age of 75 years are especially at risk, as well as those who are institutionalized or physically or mentally impaired (73). In one study, 36% of staff reported that they had observed physical abuse of residents in their institution (73).

It is estimated that only 7 to 20% of elder abuse cases are actually reported (74). This may be due, in part, to a lack of consistency among state laws regarding definitions of abuse, reportable age, or the agency to which it is reported. More frequently, elders do not report abuse because they fear retaliation or are ashamed and embarrassed. Despite a recommendation by the AMA that physicians routinely screen elders for abuse, doctors infrequently detect or report this type of abuse. In fact, physicians account for only 2% of reported cases (74).

Routine screening for abuse should be incorporated into the medical history of all elderly patients. Recommended questions include "Are you afraid of anyone at home?" "Has anyone at home ever hurt you?" "Have you ever signed any documents that you didn't understand?" "Has anyone ever failed to help you take care of yourself when you needed help?" (73). Physicians should also be suspicious of abuse if the patient gives vague or inappropriate explanations of how injuries occurred, if the caregiver answers questions on behalf of the patient, if the elder appears afraid of the caregiver or overly compliant, or if conflicting histories regarding how an injury occurred are obtained from the patient and caregiver (71). Injuries to several areas of the body, fractures, and delays in reporting injuries are also suggestive of abuse. Lacerations or abrasions to the lips or gums may indicate forced feeding. Neglect should be considered when soiled clothes or bedding, malnutrition, anemia, dehydration, hypothermia, pressure sores, and subtherapeutic levels of medication are detected.

All but four states mandate reporting of elder abuse when detected (72). If a physician is uncertain about how to follow-up or refer, he or she may contact the elder protection agency in the area. This agency can frequently advise the physician what action should be taken, based on the facts presented.

LEGAL ISSUES

Informed Consent

Informed consent must be obtained for the medical evaluation and treatment in all nonemergency conditions. The process includes the taking of photographs or radiographs of injuries resulting from domestic violence and referrals. All patients have the right to refuse such interventions. If the victim is under 18 years of age, parental consent is usually required. If, however, the parent is the suspected perpetrator, the physician may provide emergency treatment without parental consent. Permission to render nonemergency treatment may be obtained by court order or a court-appointed guardian. Some states also permit the taking of photographs and radiographs without parental consent in cases of suspected child abuse (75).

Protocol and Education Requirements

Hospitals and medical schools should be aware of education and protocol requirements relating to domestic violence. For example, the Joint Commission on Accreditation of Healthcare Organizations requires that policies are established to identify victims of domestic violence, obtain informed consent, collect evidence, document findings, and educate providers (58). Some states mandate education in domestic violence or sexual abuse for health care providers or require that protocols be developed for screening and intervention. Legislation has also been proposed to give preferential federal funding to professional schools that require training in domestic violence.

Mandatory Reporting

Forty-five states and the District of Columbia have laws that require health care providers to report cases of domestic violence to a government agency. Most states have laws that require reporting any violence involving a weapon. Some states require reporting any injury that results from a crime, act of violence, or nonaccidental act (38). As awareness about domestic violence increases, these laws are being applied more frequently to cases of suspected spousal abuse. In addition, several states have mandatory reporting laws that specifically address domestic violence. For example, health care providers in California must inform the police if they render treatment to anyone with a physical injury caused by "assaultive or abusive conduct." In Kentucky, all cases of suspected abuse, neglect, or exploitation must be reported to the Cabinet for Human Resources (38).

It is important for the practitioner to be aware of reporting laws specific to his or her state, because laws vary by jurisdiction. Regardless of the jurisdiction, the decision to make a report is a difficult one. Many reporting laws include vague terms, such as "grave injury," "assaultive or abusive conduct," and "reasonable cause" that are not clearly defined. The lack of clear definitions requires the practitioner to make a judgment about what incidents should be reported.

The decision on whether to report may be further complicated when the victim does not want a report filed. Concern over a violation of provider-patient confidentiality may prevent a practitioner from making a report. Case law exists where practitioners have been held liable for a breach of confidentiality if a report was made that was not required by law (38). However, recent court cases have established that provider-patient confidentiality does not apply when law mandates that a report be made (38). Furthermore, some states do not require a victim's consent when filing a report.

Failure to report when required by law may result in a small ($10) or large ($1000) fine or even a jail sentence (38, 58). Precedence has been established where providers have been held liable for failure to diagnose and report child abuse (38); so far, these precedents have not included domestic violence.

Mandatory reporting laws were originally passed to enhance patient safety, improve the response of the health care system to domestic violence, and hold perpetrators accountable (38). These laws, however, may not be effective in accomplishing these goals. Simply filing a report does not guarantee effective intervention for victims if a coordinated response by health care workers, social service agencies, and law enforcement does not ensue. Although victims of child abuse may be referred to Child Protective Services, no agency exists that has responsibility for coordinating cases and ensuring intervention for domestic violence victims. Shelters and safe houses are available in some communities, but they are limited in number and capacity. In addition, most are severely underfunded and understaffed. Police and the criminal justice system are often reluctant to intervene and prosecute cases of domestic violence (38, 76). Moreover, cases that are prosecuted may not result in favorable outcomes for women. Findings from a recent study indicate that the judge who hears a domestic violence case may have more influence on the outcome of the case than is reasonably allowed by law (77). In fact, it has been reported that some judges often rule in favor of perpetrators or dismiss domestic violence cases entirely (77).

In addition, mandatory reporting may interfere with the health care of the victim. If providers are required to report suspected domestic violence, women may be reluctant to seek care when injured or perpetrators may prevent victims from seeing a doctor. Physicians may perceive that their obligations have been met when they report violence, and they may fail to offer counseling or appropriate referrals. If the physician perceives mandatory reporting as harmful, he or she may choose not to screen, which serves to isolate the victim further.

The most serious problem with mandatory reporting, however, is that it may place the victim in serious danger. Studies show that up to 50% of batterers threaten retaliation if the woman attempts to leave or seeks help (78–80), and more than 30% of batterers may inflict further harm during prosecution (80). The victim may have already observed that calling the police causes the violence to escalate. If she requests that the violence not be reported to the state authorities, it is ethically questionable to override her wishes on the grounds that reporting is in her best interests (38). When a report is filed, the physician should discuss with the patient the legal obligation to report and conscientiously address the risk of reprisal and possible need for shelter or a protective order (38).

Testifying in Court

In certain cases, physicians may be asked to testify in court regarding statements in the medical record or their findings during an examination. Usually, the medical record may be brought into the courtroom to refresh the physician's memory. Provider-patient testimonial privileges, however, may prevent the physician from revealing confidential information without the patient's consent. In such cases, physicians may require legal advice regarding confidentiality laws in their state (58).

Insurance Discrimination

Battered women may have difficulty in obtaining health, life, or other types of insurance coverage because several carriers have deemed victims of abuse to be an excessive risk. Unfortunately, this action may further deter victims from seeking health care. State and federal legislation has been passed or is pending to forbid this type of discrimination (58). Health providers can assist their patients by supporting such legislation and combating insurance company policies that impede effective medical intervention (58).

RESOURCES FOR HEALTH CARE PROVIDERS

Domestic violence resources are available to health care providers at minimal or no cost from a variety of sources (Table 20.3). Patient education materials should be

TABLE 20.3. Domestic Violence Resources for Patients and Health Care Providers

Source	Available Materials	Phone Number
Family Violence Prevention Fund	Bumper stickers, brochures, posters (10 of each free)	800-END-ABUSE
National Resource Center on Domestic Violence	Information and technical assistance on training, program development	888-RXABUSE
American Medical Association	Booklets: "Diagnostic and Treatment Guidelines on Domestic Violence," "Domestic Violence: A Directory of Protocols for Health Care Providers"	800-621-8335
American College of Obstetricians and Gynecologists	Patient education pamphlet: "The Abused Woman" (order no. AP083) Speaker's package: "Domestic Violence: The Role of the Physician in Identification, Intervention, and Prevention" (order no. AA223)	800-762-2264, ext. 197

made available in both public and private settings. Women's bathrooms have been used to distribute information to women who do not have privacy elsewhere in the facility. The National Resource Center on domestic violence provides free brochures on what to do during an explosive incident and how to obtain a protective order. The Family Violence Prevention Fund (1-800-END-ABUSE) provides bumper stickers, brochures, flyers, and posters. A patient education pamphlet entitled "The Abused Woman" is available from ACOG.

ACOG and the AMA have also developed materials to educate physicians in the detection and treatment of domestic violence victims. A technical bulletin entitled "The Battered Woman" (No. 124) was mailed to all fellows in 1989 and is available upon request. A brochure on diagnostic and treatment guidelines on domestic violence and a directory of protocols used for domestic violence is available from the AMA. In addition, ACOG has a speaker's package on domestic violence to assist physicians who wish to speak on this topic in their community.

Numerous resources are also available for both physicians and patients on the Internet. Over 300,000 entries provide information on hotlines, available resources, pending legislation, and statistics.

CONCLUSION

Admittedly, the physician cannot single-handedly solve the problem of domestic violence nor force patients into making lifestyle changes. Rather, the physician's role should be to screen patients, document findings, validate circumstances, and refer patients to sources of help (32, 59). Health care workers should remain current on legal issues surrounding domestic violence so they can advise the patient of her rights and fulfill their own responsibilities. Overall, the physician should remain caring and supportive of the victim, even if she chooses not to leave the abusive situation.

Optimally, communities will work together to assist the abused woman. Collaboration between the legal system, medical community, domestic violence advocacy community, and child protective services is critical to provide both a support structure and a referral system for the victim of domestic violence (61).

CLINICAL NOTES

Domestic Violence

- U.S. women are more likely to be assaulted, injured, raped, or killed by a current or ex-male partner than by all other types of perpetrators combined.
- Women of all ages, races, educational levels, geographic locations, and socioeconomic status are affected (Table 20.1).

Cycle of Violence

- There are three phases that escalate in frequency and intensity over time.
- In phase 1, tension accumulates, the batterer is deliberately mean and may be mildly physically abusive, and the woman tries to pacify her abuser.
- In phase 2, the perpetrator explodes and battering occurs. Alcohol is often involved but is not the *cause* of the abuse.
- In phase 3, the abuser becomes apologetic and promises it will never happen again.

Characteristics of the Perpetrator

- Seventy-five percent of male batterers grew up witnessing or experiencing domestic violence.
- Antisocial borderline personality disorders are more common compared with nonbattering men.
- The batterer does not take responsibility for abusive actions and blames the victim(s).
- Up to 50% have a serious alcohol problem.

Barriers to Leaving an Abusive Environment

- Women fear further violence to themselves, their children, and other family members.
- Social isolation, financial dependence, and inadequate social services may hinder women.
- Police and justice system are unable to provide adequate protection.

Role of Health Care Providers

- Women should be screened for domestic violence at office visits and in emergency rooms (Fig. 20.1). In addition to the signs of trauma seen on physical examination, victims of abuse complain more frequently of somatic complaints for which no etiology can be determined if domestic violence is not considered.
- Prenatal care visits are an excellent time to ask screening questions. Six to 8% of U.S. pregnant women experience domestic violence, putting them at increased risk for premature delivery and low-birth-weight infants. Victims may be at even higher risk of abuse during the postpartum period.
- When children are also involved, either as witnesses or victims, the physician's response is even more critical because removing the child from the mother's care may be harmful to both victims.

Barriers to Screening for Domestic Violence

- Physicians should consider and try to overcome their own potential barriers to finding and reporting domestic violence: lack of training, cultural/socioeconomic/gender prejudices, time constraints, frustration at inability to hep victims, fear of offending patients, or a personal history of abuse.

Elder Abuse

- The elderly should also be screened at office visits and in the emergency room.
- There are mandatory reporting laws for elder abuse in 46 states.

Legal Issues

- You must obtain informed consent for taking photographs or radiographs to document domestic violence in nonemergent situations; exceptions exist when the consent would have to be obtained from the alleged perpetrator.
- Forty-five states and the District of Columbia have mandatory reporting laws for domestic violence, but these laws may interfere with the health care of the victim or actually place the victim in further danger. When a report is filed, the physician should discuss it with the patient and address the issues of reprisal, shelter, and protective orders.

Resources for Health Care Providers

- Resources are available to the clinician to help victims of domestic violence (Table 20.3).

References

1. Ward RD. Doris Ann Suciu, MD. A leader in the fight against domestic violence. Mich Med 1994;93:26–27.
2. Wilt S, Olson S. Prevalence of domestic violence in the United States. JAMA 1996;51:77–82.
3. American Medical Association. Diagnostic and Treatment Guidelines on Domestic Violence. Chicago: American Medical Association, 1992.
4. Council on Scientific Affairs, American Medical Association. Violence against women. JAMA 1992;267:3184–3189.
5. Straus MA, Gelles RJ, Steinmetz SK. Behind Closed Doors: Violence in the American Family. New York: Anchor Books, 1980.
6. Straus MA, Gelles RJ. Physical Violence in American Families. New Brunswick, NJ: Transaction Publishers, 1990.
7. Schulman MA. Survey of Spousal Violence Against Women in Kentucky. Washington, DC: U.S. Government Printing Office, 1979.
8. Plichta SB, Weisman CS. Spouse or partner abuse, use of health services, and unmet need for medical care in U.S. women. J Womens Health 1995;4:45–54.
9. Novello AC, Rosenberg M, Saltzman L, et al. From the Surgeon General, U.S. Public Health Service. A medical response to domestic violence. JAMA 1992;267:3132.
10. McCauley J, Kern DE, Kolodner K, et al. The battering syndrome: prevalence and clinical characteristics of domestic violence in primary care internal medicine practices. Ann Intern Med 1995;123:734–746.
11. Hoffman AC. Advances in domestic violence shelters. Med Law 1996;15:467–478.
12. Domestic violence. ACOG Tech Bull 1995;209:1–9.
13. Cohen S, De Vos E, Newberger E. Barriers to physician identification and treatment of family violence: lessons from five communities. Acad Med 1997;72:S19–S25.
14. Attala JM, Bauza K, Pratt H, et al. Integrative review of effects on children of witnessing domestic violence. Issues Compr Pediatr Nurs 1995;18:163–172.
15. Richardson J, Feder G. Domestic violence: a hidden problem for general practice. Br J Gen Pract 1996;46:239–242.
16. McKay MM. The link between domestic violence and child abuse: assessment and treatment considerations. Child Welfare 1994;73:29–39.
17. Barkan SE, Gary LT. Woman abuse and pediatrics: expanding the web of detection. J Am Med Womens Assoc 1996;51:96–100.
18. Rosenberg ML, Fenley MA, Johnson D, et al. Bridging prevention and practice: public health and family violence. Acad Med 1997;72:S13–S18.

19. Kornblit AL. Domestic violence—an emerging health issue. Soc Sci Med 1994;39: 1181–1188.

20. McLeer SV, Anwar RA. The role of the emergency physician in the prevention of domestic violence. Ann Emerg Med 1987;16:1155–1161.

21. Walker LE. The Battered Woman. New York: Harper & Row, 1979.

22. Hattendorf J, Tollerud TR. Domestic violence: counseling strategies that minimize the impact of secondary victimization. Perspect Psychiatr Care 1997;33:14–23.

23. Murphy CM. Treating perpetrators of adult domestic violence. Md Med J 1994;43: 877–883.

24. Else LT, Wonderlich SA, Beatty WW, et al. Personality characteristics of men who physically abuse women. Hosp Commun Psych 1993;44:54–58.

25. Smith M. Male peer support of wife abuse. J Interpers Violence 1991;6:512–519.

26. Leonard KE. Drinking patterns and intoxication in marital violence: review, critique and future directions for research to U.S. Department of Health and Human Services. In: Alcohol and Interpersonal Violence: Fostering Multidisciplinary Perspectives. Rockville, MD: National Institutes of Health, 1992:253–280. [Research Monograph 24, NIH Publication No. 93–3496.]

27. Murphy CM, O'Farrell TJ. Factors associated with marital aggression in male alcoholics. J Fam Psychol 1994;8:321–325.

28. Chescheir N. Violence against women: response from clinicians. Ann Emerg Med 1996;27:766–768.

29. Carpenito LJ. Domestic violence: why do they stay? Nurs Forum 1996;31:3–4.

30. Browne A. Violence against women by male partners. Am Psychol 1993;48:1077–1087.

31. Browne A, Williams KR. Gender, intimacy, and lethal violence: trends from 1976 through 1987. Gender Soc 1993;7:78–98.

32. Alpert EJ. Violence in intimate relationships and the practicing internist: new "disease" or new agenda? Ann Intern Med 1995;123:774–781.

33. Gremillion DH, Kanof EP. Overcoming barriers to physician involvement in identifying and referring victims of domestic violence. Ann Emerg Med 1996;27:769–773.

34. Galbraith S, Rubinstein G. Alcohol, drugs, and domestic violence: confronting barriers to changing practice and policy. J Am Med Womens Assoc 1996;51:115–117.

35. Goldberg ME. Substance-abusing women: false stereotypes and real needs. Soc Work 1995;40:189–798.

36. Jones III RF. Domestic violence—an epidemic. Int J Gynaecol Obstet 1993;41:131–133.

37. Easley M. Domestic violence. Ann Emerg Med 1996;27:762–763.

38. Hyman A, Schillinger D, Lo B. Laws mandating reporting of domestic violence. JAMA 1995;273:1781–1787.

39. Abbott J, Johnson R, Koziol-McLain J, et al. Domestic violence against women. JAMA 1995;273:1763–1767.

40. Poole GV, Martin JN Jr, Perry KG Jr, et al. Trauma in pregnancy: the role of interpersonal violence. Am J Obstet Gynecol 1996;174:1873–1878.

41. McCoy M. Domestic violence: clues to victimization. Ann Emerg Med 1996;27:764–765.

42. Olson L, Anctil C, Fullerton L, et al. Increasing emergency physician recognition of domestic violence. Ann Emerg Med 1996;27:741–745.

43. Drossman DA, Leserman J, Nachman G, et al. Sexual and physical abuse in women with functional or organic gastrointestinal disorders. Ann Intern Med 1990;113:828–833.

44. Swett C. High rates of alcohol problems and history of physical and sexual abuse among women inpatients. Am J Drug Alcohol Abuse 1994;20:263–272.

45. Koss MP, Heslet L. Somatic consequences of violence against women. Arch Fam Med 1992;1:53–59.

46. Amaro H, Fried LE, Cabral H, et al. Violence during pregnancy and substance use. Am J Public Health 1990;80:575–579.

47. Stewart DE, Cecutti A. Physical abuse in pregnancy. Can Med Assoc J 1993;149:1257–1263.

48. Helton AS, McFarlane J, Anderson ET. Battered and pregnant: a prevalence study. Am J Public Health 1987;77:1337–1339.

49. Ballard TJ, Saltzman LE, Gazmararian JA, et al. Violence during pregnancy: measurement issues. Am J Public Health 1998;88:274–276.

50. Morey MA, Begleiter ML, Harris DJ. Profile of a battered fetus. Lancet 1981;2:1294–1295.

51. Parker B, McFarlane J, Soeken K. Abuse during pregnancy: effects on maternal complications and birth weight in adult and teenage women. Obstet Gynecol 1994;84:323–328.

52. Martin SL, English KT, Clark KA, et al. Violence and substance use among North Carolina pregnant women. Am J Public Health 1996;86:991–998.

53. Bullock LF, McFarlane J. The birth-weight/battering connection. Am J Nurs 1989; 89:1153–1155.

54. Stewart DE. Incidence of postpartum abuse in women with a history of abuse during pregnancy. Can Med Assoc J 1994;151:1601–1604.

55. Fantuzzo J, Boruch R, Beriama A, et al. Domestic violence and children: prevalence and risk in five major U.S. cities. J Am Acad Child Adolesc Psychiatry 1997;36:116–122.

56. Walker LE. The Battered Woman Syndrome. New York: Springer, 1984.

57. Thormaehlen DJ, Bass-Feld ER. Children: the secondary victims of domestic violence. Md Med J 1994;43:355–359.

58. Hyman A. Domestic violence: legal issues for health care practitioners and institutions. J Am Med Womens Assoc 1996;51:101–105.

59. Chez RA, Jones RF III. The battered woman. Am J Obstet Gynecol 1995;173:677–679.

60. Warshaw C. Intimate partner abuse: developing a framework for change in medical education. Acad Med 1977;72:S26–S37.

61. Warshaw C. Domestic violence: changing theory, changing practice. J Am Med Womens Assoc 1996;51:87–91.

62. Freund KM, Bak SM, Blackhall L. Identifying domestic violence in primary care practice. J Gen Intern Med 1996;11:44–46.

63. Norton LB, Peipert JF, Zierler S, et al. Battering in pregnancy: an assessment of two screening methods. Obstet Gynecol 1995;85:321–325.

64. Shadigian E. Domestic violence: identification and management for the clinician. Compr Ther 1996;22:424–428.

65. Reid SA, Glasser M. Primary care physicians' recognition of an attitudes toward domestic violence. Acad Med 1997;72:51–53.

66. Parsons LH, Zaccaro D, Wells B, et al. Methods of and attitudes toward screening obstetrics and gynecology patients for domestic violence. Am J Obstet Gynecol 1995;173: 381–387.

67. Education about adult domestic violence in U.S. and Canadian medical schools, 1987–1988. MMWR Morb Mortal Wkly Rep 1989;38:17–19.

68. Chambliss LR, Bay RC, Jones RF III. Domestic violence: an education imperative? Am J Obstet Gynecol 1995;172:1035–1038.

69. Dialogues on domestic abuse. Interviewer: Ronald A. Chez, MD. Guest experts: Richard F. Jones III, MD, Evan Stark, PhD, MSW, and Carole Warshaw, MD. Women battering: it can happen anywhere. Contemp Ob/Gyn 1997;42:78–88.

70. Friedman LS, Samet JH, Roberts MS, et al. Inquiry about victimization experiences. Arch Intern Med 1992;152:1186–1190.

71. Costa AJ. Elder abuse. Prim Care 1993;20:375–389.

72. Jones JS. Elder abuse and neglect: responding to a national problem. Ann Emerg Med 1994;23:845–848.

73. Periodic Health Examination, 1994 Update. 4. Secondary prevention of elder abuse and mistreatment. Canadian Task Force on the Periodic Health Examination. Can Med Assoc J 1994;151:1413–1420.

74. Rosenblatt DE, Cho KH, Durance P. Reporting mistreatment of older adults: the role of physicians. J Am Geriatr Soc 1996;44:65–70.

75. Clarke OW. Report of the Council on Ethical and Judicial Affairs. Physicians and family violence: ethical considerations. JAMA 1992;267:3190–3193.

76. Kinports K, Fisher K. Orders of protection in domestic violence cases: an empirical assessment of the impact of the reform statutes. Tex J Womens Law 1993;2:163–276.

77. Ford J, Rompf EL, Faragher T, et al. Case outcomes in domestic violence court: influence of judges. Psychol Rep 1995;77:587–594.
78. Bureau of Justice Statistics. Report to the Nation on Crime and Justice: The Data. Publication NCJ-87068. Washington, DC: Bureau of Justice Statistics, U.S. Department of Justice, October 1983.
79. Hart BJ. State codes on domestic violence: analysis, commentary, and recommendations. Juvenile Fam Court J 1992;43:79.
80. Hart BJ. Battered women and the criminal justice system. Am Behav Sci 1993;36:624–638.

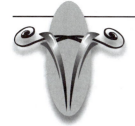

C H A P T E R   2 1

Sex Counseling in the Office

GRETCHEN GROSS

For many reasons physicians commonly avoid the issue of sexual functioning with their patients (1). They may believe it not relevant to their specialty or patient population, they may be embarrassed or fear embarrassing their patients, or they may believe that a lack of formal training precludes them from discussing, diagnosing, or treating sexual disorders. The physician who wants to avoid the topic can unconsciously create an atmosphere that prevents the patient from raising the subject.

Research shows, however, that women identify their doctor as the most likely professional to turn to for help in the areas of sexual health and functioning (1–7). The clinical question then is not *whether* to ask a patient about sexual health and functioning but *how* to ask without causing levels of embarrassment on the part of either the patient or the physician. If the physician is too embarrassed, ashamed, or uninformed to take an adequate sexual history, sexual dysfunction will go undiagnosed and untreated.

Physicians who are open to counseling patients on sexual dysfunction will find a substantial percentage of their patients have sexually related questions or problems. Reports on the prevalence of sexual dysfunctions in the general population range from 25 to 50% (1, 2). Among "normal" couples (who reported that their marital and sexual relations were happy and satisfying), 40% of men reported erectile or ejaculatory dysfunction and 63% of women reported arousal or orgasmic dysfunction. Fifty percent of men and 77% of women reported difficulties such as lack of interest or inability to relax. These couples were responding to a question about any sexual problems occurring in their marriage at that particular time (8). One survey in a family practice setting found that 56% of the patients reported having one or more sexual problems (1). Research from gynecologic practices shows that when left entirely up to the patient, only 3% of women initiated discussions about their sexual problems. When physician asked about sexual problems, 16% of women acknowledged problems (1).

Current understanding of sexual functioning rests largely on the work of William Masters and Virginia Johnson. The sexual response cycle as they described it is composed of four phases: excitement, plateau, orgasmic, and resolution. Each phase is associated with specific physiologic changes. During the excitement phase, the woman experiences lubrication of the vagina, enlargement of the clitoris and labia majora, nipple erection, breast swelling, and a ballooning of the vaginal apex and walls. The man experiences enlargement of the penis and an increase in its length. Both men and women experience tachycardia and an increase in blood pressure.

The distinction between the excitement phase and plateau phase is imprecise. The woman has some further enlargement of the upper vagina, uterus, and clitoris, whereas the lower one third of the vagina may narrow slightly because of the continued swelling of the outer tissues. The man may experience the release of a few drops of fluid from the bulbourethral or Cowper's glands; that minimum of fluid contains large numbers of active sperm. Additionally, the testes increase in size by almost 50%. Both men and women experience intensification of the increases in respiratory rate, heart rate, muscle tone, and blood pressure.

The orgasmic phase in women is accompanied by a series of rhythmic muscular contractions beginning in the uterus and extending to the cervix, or possibly to the vagina. In men, these contractions occur in the muscles of the perineal floor. The semen is discharged from the seminal vesicles into the bulbous urethra and at the same time the prostate contracts, releasing prostatic fluid into the bulbous urethra. The semen is then ejaculated through the urethra.

The resolution phase involves the return to normal size of the engorged female or male genital structures. The total time to resolution in women varies. Men have a refractory period during their resolution phase in which they are unable to become aroused again. The length of this refractory period varies but lengthens with age. Women do not experience a true refractory phase and so may have multiple orgasms (9).

The work of Masters and Johnson contributed greatly to our understanding of the sexual response cycle in human beings. Their work, however, focused almost solely on the physical responses and did not address the individual's overall sexual functioning. There is little explanation or exploration of emotional, psychosocial, and cultural aspects of sexual arousal, expectations, and response (10, 11). An individual's sexual experience and functioning involves eroticism, desire, and personal meaning and the physiologic components of excitement and response. Clinicians who focus primarily on earlier sexual data are more likely to approach sexual functioning from a technical perspective where the emphasis is on intercourse and orgasm. This approach overlooks the complex interplay of physiology and emotion.

When sexual functioning is seen primarily from an organic perspective, technique is usually emphasized as a remedy for dysfunction. This approach often neglects the role of emotional and mental health in healthy sexual functioning. Patients have concerns that go beyond the mechanics of intercourse and orgasm, including changes in levels of sexual interest and desire, "normal" versus "abnormal" functioning, postoperative sexual functioning, and the impact of acute or chronic illness in their sexual functioning (12). If a patient's questions about her sexual functioning are not approached from a global health perspective, concomitant emotional states such as depression, anger, sexual anxiety, or rejection may be missed. The three primary sources of sexual anxiety that can lead to dysfunction are fear of failure, performance anxiety, and excessive need to please one's partner (13).

An individual's ability to be sexually intimate, to be "sexually related" to a significant partner, can effect the level of emotional intimacy and connection to that partner. Therefore, sexual difficulties have to be examined in the context of the patient's relationship to their partner (14). When diagnosing sexual dysfunction, it is necessary to ask a patient about her partner's sexual functioning because her dysfunction(s) may be in direct response to his. For example, a woman's decreased sexual desire or interest might be a response to her partner's inability to maintain an erection. Decreased self-esteem and increased anxiety for both partners are components of nearly all sexual dysfunctions.

By the time a woman seeks advice for a sexual problem or dysfunction, she and her partner have probably been troubled by it for some time. When she does seek professional help, she will most likely talk first to her primary care physician or obstetrician/gynecologist (1–7, 14). The response she receives from that caregiver sets the stage for her willingness to engage in further treatment. A patient who feels embarrassed or ashamed when talking about her sexual health and has these feelings reinforced by a care provider will continue to feel isolated and "damaged." She may not ask for help again. In these cases, a dysfunction that might otherwise have a good chance at resolution will become deeply entrenched.

TAKING A SEXUAL HISTORY

The most effective way to integrate sexual functioning into patients' global health status is by routinely taking a sexual functioning history. Although the scope of the history remains a debated topic, one source claims that up to 95% of sexual problems can be detected when sexual histories are routinely taken (15). In a study where physicians asked the patients only two specific questions regarding sexual functioning, "Are you sexually active?" and "Are you having any sexual difficulties or problems at this time?," 16% of the patients cited sexual difficulties, the most common being dyspareunia (48%) and decreased sexual desire (21%) (1). See Table 21.1 for questions to include in a brief sexual history.

Physicians' interest in taking a sexual history appears linked to their attitudes toward sexual functioning and their knowledge levels. Those physicians who do not take sexual histories underestimate the prevalence of sexual dysfunction in their practices. Over 66% of physicians who routinely inquire about sexual problems identify significant concerns in at least 50% of their patients, whereas over 75% of physicians who do not inquire estimate that less than 10% of their patients have sexual dysfunction (16). Therefore, physicians who state that they do not see sexual dysfunction in their clinical populations are not looking hard enough or are avoiding the topic altogether.

A brief history comprised of four salient questions has been shown to uncover sexual dysfunctions equally as effectively as a more lengthy and complex questionnaire (17):

• Are you sexually active?
• Are there any problems?
• What do you think might be causing the problem?
• Do you have any pain with intercourse?

These questions elicit enough information from patients to allow the physician to initiate further discussion and evaluation. The physician may then continue the workup or refer the individual or couple to a specialist who will provide the patient with information to help resolve the dysfunction (17).

SEXUAL DYSFUNCTIONS IN WOMEN

Dyspareunia and inhibited sexual desire are the most common sexual dysfunctions for which women seek help (1, 3, 17–19). Table 21.2 lists causes of these and other sexual dysfunctions. A complete history provides an understanding of the impact of

TABLE 21.1. Sample Questions for a Brief Sexual History

How frequently do you have intercourse or sex play (including masturbation)?
Are you sexually active with men, women, or both?
Are you satisfied with the current frequency of sexual activity?
  Is your partner satisfied with this frequency?
Do you have difficulty becoming sexually aroused?
  If so, do you have this problem with a partner and while masturbating?
  Does your partner have difficulty becoming aroused?
Do you have problems reaching orgasm?
  If, so do you have problems both with a partner and while masturbating?
Do you and your partner have similar levels of sexual interest?
Is intercourse ever painful?
  If so, when does the pain occur?

TABLE 21.2. Sexual Dysfunctions and Their Causes in Women

DYSPAREUNIA
Organic Causes

With Thrusting: Endometriosis, varices of the broad ligament, scars or adhesions, ovary adhering to cul-de-sac, adnexal masses, pelvic inflammatory disease, rectal problems, cystitis, orthopedic problems

At Orgasm: Endometriosis, scars, varices of broad ligament

Others: Urinary tract infections, urethritis, hymenal strands, bacterial vaginitis, postmenopausal or postsurgical vaginal atrophy, fourchette irritation, vulvar vestibulitis, vestibular adenitis, atrophic vulvovaginitis, obstetric trauma, mediolateral episotomy, significant pelvic relaxation, leiomyomas, advanced pelvic carcinoma

Functional Causes

Inadequate foreplay or arousal, lack of communication between partners regarding levels of arousal and excitement

Psychological Causes

Current depressive episode, somatization or conversion disorder, phobic or panic disorder, history of chronic pelvic pain, history of sexual abuse or rape, substance abuse or chemical dependency, major anxiety-based sexual conflicts, hostility toward partner, general sexual aversion, entrenched negative sexual expectations inhibiting sexual responsiveness, fear of pregnancy or sexually transmitted diseases, lack of resolution of previous pregnancy loss or termination, low desire, nongenital chronic pain syndromes

INHIBITED SEXUAL DESIRE
Organic Causes

Chronic illness (e.g., diabetes), endocrine alterations (endocrinopathy, physiologic fluctuations, panhypopituitarism, ovariectomy, adrenalectomy, use of oral contraceptives), neurologic illness or trauma (multiple sclerosis, spinal cord injury), fatigue, medications, drug and/ or alcohol abuse, pregnancy

Psychological Causes

History of sexual assault, current depressive episode, premenstrual syndrome or premenstrual dysphoric disorder

VAGINISMUS
Organic Causes

Vaginitis, vaginal strictures after posterior colporrhaphy, scarring from mediolateral episiotomies

Psychological Causes

Response to past painful vaginal penetration, orthodox religious background, history of rape or sexual abuse

ANORGASMIA
Functional Causes

Premature ejaculation in partner, erectile dysfunction in partner, insufficient stimulation, lack of knowledge about orgasms

Psychological Causes

Cultural or religious restrictions, inability to relax, feelings of guilt

VULVODYNIA (ALSO SEE CHAPTER 6)
Organic Causes

Persistent infections (especially human papilloma or *Candida*), vulvar papillomatosis, vulvar dermatoses,

cyclic vulvitis, vulvar vestibulitis, irritant contact dermatitis, steroid-induced "periorificial" dermatitis

the dysfunction on the individual's emotional state and their ability to fully participate in the relationship. It also includes a review of the individual's and couple's attempts to resolve the dysfunction (19). It is important to establish the timing, situation, and duration of the disorder. The patient usually comes with her own theories
of what might be affecting her functioning, and she can provide important information that might not be otherwise discovered. A complete physical evaluation to
rule out the presence of organic factors is necessary.

Dyspareunia

There are four degrees of dyspareunia: complete, situational, primary, and secondary. The diagnosis of complete dyspareunia can be made when the patient's pain
occurs with each and every attempt at vaginal penetration, both with her current
partner(s) and during penetration with masturbation. It need not have occurred in
all prior sexual encounters but is present with all current partners. Situational dyspareunia occurs in some situations or with some partners but not necessarily with all
current partners. Primary dyspareunia involves vaginal pain that has been present
from the woman's very first attempt at vaginal penetration and need not be limited
to penetration with a penis. The pain does not come and go with each attempt or
with each situation or partner.

Finally, secondary dyspareunia interrupts an otherwise uncomplicated history of
penetration. This is often seen when there has been a change in the woman's physical or mental health status, such as in the aftermath of rape or sexual abuse, or after any number of gynecologic surgeries, illnesses, or events, including childbirth
(20). A complete assessment of dyspareunia documents the history of the dyspareunia and attempts to determine the type of dyspareunia present (Table 21.3).

With the exception of vaginismus, most cases of dyspareunia have an organic
cause (Table 21.2). In long-standing cases of dyspareunia, organic causes are present in up to one third of cases (19). The impact of dyspareunia is not limited solely
to the presenting patient; coital pain can result in further sexual dysfunction for
both partners. The fear of pain with intercourse infringes on a couple's desire for
sexual intimacy. A man's erectile and ejaculatory functioning can be affected by his
fear of causing his partner pain (21). Repeatedly painful sexual experiences can set
up an expectation of future pain, reinforcing avoidant behaviors. The operant con-
ditioning model explains the role that random painful or negative experiences play
in the establishment of persistent and dysfunctional behaviors (19, 22).

It is important to rule out anxiety and depressive disorders in the dyspareunic patient. Untreated depressive or anxiety disorders can inhibit a woman's ability to emotionally engage in a sexual experience, resulting in inadequate lubrication and pain
with intercourse. Women who have had an experience of coital pain may become focused on only their physiologic state during sex. This is called "spectatoring," the com-
pulsion to judge or evaluate one's performance during sex. It is a cognitive process that
virtually ensures inadequate emotional involvement and relaxation during sex.

If a patient's dyspareunia is found to be physiologic in etiology, it remains important to consider that the individual and couple may still experience some emo-

TABLE 21.3. Assessment of Dysparuenia

What is the chronology of the discomfort?
What is the impact of the pain on the patient?
What is the impact of the pain on the patient's relationship with her partner?
How has the patient attempted to resolve the dyspareunia before consulting her
    physician?

tional sequelae, such as negative responses to intercourse, avoidance of sexual intimacy, fear of inadequacy, or a heightened level of self- or other-blame. It is fairly common to see sexual dysfunctions develop in the partner in response to the initial problem, frequently making medical treatment of the dyspareunia itself insufficient (23). In these situations, both partners will benefit from couples' counseling to help stop the cycle of primary and secondary sexual dysfunction.

If it appears that coital pain is due to insufficient excitation and lubrication before intercourse because of insufficient foreplay, treatment options include the use of copious amounts of lubricants and encouraging the woman to determine the moment and depth of penile entry. In addition, there are some excellent books that patients and their partners can read to increase their understanding of sexual excitement and response. Barry and Emily McCarthy have authored a series of books on sexual awareness and satisfaction in men, women, and couples; these books have been well received by patients (23–25). Barbach's book, *For Yourself: The Fulfillment of Female Sexuality,* on sexual functioning and awareness in women is well known and respected among clinicians and patients as well (26).

Inhibited Sexual Desire

Inhibited sexual desire is a complex dysfunction. Normally, sexual interest levels fluctuate because of any number of factors, including physical, emotional, financial, and sociologic stressors. When any couple is trying to coordinate their libidos to have mutually desired and gratifying sex, problems may arise. A couple who finds it difficult to match the timing of their desire does not meet diagnostic criteria for inhibited sexual desire (20). However, if one or both partners feel a diminished or absent ability to achieve sexual arousal or if they lack sexual interest, then a desire phase dysfunction should be considered (27).

Organic factors that can inhibit sexual desire in women include chronic physical or emotional illness, pregnancy, menopause, and use of certain medications (Table 21.4). Psychosocial factors, such as a lack of interest in the current partner, unresolved relationship issues, hostility or anger, infidelity, or other breach of trust, and changes in family dynamics, such as having a baby, all may contribute to inhibited sexual desire. Other issues, like financial stressors, drug or alcohol abuse, and situational or chronic depression in either partner, may also play an important role in the development of inhibited sexual desire.

Sexual dysfunctions often present as a symptom of a mood disorder. Depression decreases the libido, but some people attempt to improve a depressed mood by increasing sexual activity. Hypersexuality is a behavior often found in the manic state. The diagnosis of inhibited sexual desire requires symptoms specific to sexual desire rather than general symptoms of psychological functioning of the individual. If the person is describing inhibited sexual desire symptoms but also reports changes in sleep and eating patterns, emotional lability, and lack of overall energy, it is likely that the primary diagnosis is depression rather than inhibited sexual desire. It is important to note that pharmacologic agents in the treatment of depression frequently have decreased libido as a side effect. Virtually every antidepressant currently available has some side effect that negatively affects sexual functioning and satisfaction (28–30). There is a higher incidence of sexual side effects seen with selective serotonin uptake inhibitors than was reported in initial studies of drugs in this class. Sertraline (Zoloft), fluoxetine (Prozac), and paroxetine (Paxil) have all been associated with total or partial anorgasmia, decreased libido, or delayed orgasm (31–34). Physicians play an important role in educating patients about the sexual side effects of these medications and monitoring patients for changes in sexual function. Switch-

TABLE 21.4. Common Medications That Can Cause Sexual Dysfunction

	Decreased Desire	Increased Desire	Erectile Disorder	Ejaculatory Disorder	Orgasmic Disorder	Decreased Lubrication or Responsiveness	Gynecomastia	Priapism	Painful Clitoral Tumescence	Hormonal Alterations
ANTIHYPERTENSIVES										
Atenolol (Tenormin)			X							
Clonidine (Catapres)	X		X	X	W					
Enalapril (Vasotec)			X							
Methyldopa (Aldomet)	X		X	X	W					
Propanolol (Inderal)	X		X							
Reserpine (Serpasil)	M		X	X						
Spironolactone (Aldactone)	X		X			X	X			
PSYCHOTROPICS										
Alprazolam (Xanax)	X				X					
Barbiturates	X		X	X						
Bupropion (Wellbutrin)	X		X							
Buspirone (BuSpar)	X		X	X				X		
Clomipramine (Anafranil)	X		X	X	X					
Clonazepm (Klonopin)	X		X		X					
Diazepam (Valium)	X			X	X					
Doxepin (Adapin, Sinequan)				X						
Fluoxetine (Prozac)	X			X	X					
Imipramine (Tofranil)			X	X	W					

Continued

TABLE 21.4 (continued). **Common Medications That Can Cause Sexual Dysfunction**

	Decreased Desire	Increased Desire	Erectile Disorder	Ejaculatory Disorder	Orgasmic Disorder	Decreased Lubrication or Responsiveness	Gynecomastia	Priapism	Painful Clitoral Tumescence	Hormonal Alterations
Lorazepam (Ativan)	X									
Nortriptyline (Pamelor)	X		X		X					
Oxazepam (Serax)	X									
Paroxetine (Paxil)			X	X	X					
Phenelzine (Nardil)				X	X					
Prochlorperazine (Compazine)	X	X	X	X		W		X		
Sertraline (Zoloft)					X					
Trazodone (Desyrel)		X						X		
Venlafaxine (Effexor)			X	X	X					
OTHERS										
Benztropine (Cogentin)			X							
Bromocriptine (Parlodel)			X					X		
Carbamazepine (Tegretol)	X		X							
Cimetidine (Tagamet)			X				X			
Danazol (Danocrine)	X	X								
Disulfiram (Antabuse)			X							
Diphenhydramine (Benadryl)	X		X							
Famotidine (Pepcid)			X							

Continued

TABLE 21.4 (continued). Common Medications That Can Cause Sexual Dysfunction

	Decreased Desire	Increased Desire	Erectile Disorder	Ejaculatory Disorder	Orgasmic Disorder	Decreased Lubrication or Responsiveness	Gynecomastia	Priapism	Painful Clitoral Tumescence	Hormonal Alterations
Heparin								X		
Hydroxyzine (Atarax, Vistaril)	X		X							
Isotretinoin (Acutane)				X						
Meclizine (Antivert)			X							
Medroxyprogesterone (Provera, Depo-Provera)	X		X							
Naproxen (Aleve, Anaprox, Naprosyn)	X									
Nizatidine (Axid)			X							
Phenytoin (Dilantin)	X		X							
Ranitidine (Zantac)	X		X							
DRUGS OF ABUSE										
Alcohol, acute	X		X	X						
Alcohol, chronic	X		X							
Marijuana	X									X

M, known effect in men; W, known effect in women; X, effect reported in both sexes or sex not specified.

ing medications or suggesting a drug holiday can significantly decrease the sexual dysfunction side effects and improve patient compliance.

For many women, sexual functioning and substance abuse have a complex interrelationship. Alcohol and drug abuse affects the libido, and sexual dysfunction is a commonly seen side effect of alcoholism in women (27, 35). Alcoholism, sexual abuse/assault history, and sexual dysfunction are now a well-recognized triumvirate. These complex issues should be carefully addressed when the patient requests treatment for any one of these three problems. Careful collaboration among the patient's physician, counselor, and other health care providers is central to the development and implementation of a sound treatment plan.

Many women experience more emotional discomfort after they stop drinking or using the medications that previously left them emotionally numb. If the patient is not prepared for an increase in flashbacks, anxiety, and depressive symptoms during this treatment phase, she may very well relapse to avoid this dysphoric time. Therefore, it is central to the patient's recovery that she work with a professional who is well aware of the complex interrelationship between addictions, sexual dysfunction, and a history of abuse and/or assault.

Vaginismus

Vaginismus involves the *involuntary* spasm of the pelvic muscles that surround the vagina, specifically the perineal and levator ani muscles. These contracted muscles prevent penetration of the vagina or allow penetration only with a great deal of pain. These involuntary contractions may be strong enough to cause pain alone or may be painful only if penetration is attempted. As with other sexual dysfunctions, there are variations in severity, duration, and onset. Unfortunately, women who experience an initial episode of vaginismus often repeatedly attempt intercourse, which strengthens the psychological connection between intercourse and pain. These repeated experiences of pain and failure reinforce sexual dysfunction. Organic causes of vaginismus, including vaginitis, vaginal strictures after posterior colporrhaphy, or scarring from mediolateral episiotomies, are frequently ruled out early in the workup. More often, vaginismus is a phobic response to a painful stimuli, in this case painful vaginal penetration. It is directly related to fear, anxiety, or guilt (19, 36). The most common etiologic factor in cases of vaginismus is an orthodox religious background (37–39), but it is not uncommon for women who have vaginismus to be victims of sexual abuse or rape. Diagnosis can help lead a woman into counseling where she can begin to resolve this response to prior trauma.

Treatment of vaginismus hinges on helping the patient break her behavioral response to negative stimuli and to relearn vaginal muscle control. It is important for the woman to be in control of each phase of treatment of vaginismus. If she feels out of control or forced to proceed faster than she desires, it is likely that her behavioral response (anxiety, muscle contractions, sexual aversion) will be reinforced. She should be taught Kegel exercises for control of vaginal muscles. Vaginal dilation exercises can also be practiced in private in a relaxed and nonsexual setting; these exercises promote understanding of anatomy and being comfortable with the sensations resulting from touch. Either dilators or fingers can be used in this exercise, depending on the patient's preference and comfort level. Dilators come in four graduated sizes; the woman starts with the smallest one, covers it with lubricant, places it in her vagina, and leaves it in place for 10 to 15 minutes. The next larger size is lubricated and placed intravaginally for another 10 to 15 minutes. Gradually, the woman works up to being able to place the largest dilator intravaginally without difficulty. Steege (19) suggests that women who use their fingers rather than dilators establish a role as active participants rather than passive recipients in treatment.

The partner becomes active in the vaginal dilation exercises only when the patient is emotionally and physically ready and after the anxiety of being touched is extinguished. At that point, specific instructions direct the experiences temporarily away from the initial goal of intercourse. Introducing the partner prematurely is counterproductive to treatment. Some women feel pressured to hurry their partner's participation as an indicator to him that things are moving along rapidly. It is appropriate for the health care provider to tell the patient that she is moving too rapidly and may be risking a setback in the process.

After ruling out organic causes of vaginismus, it is important to not make the only focus of treatment the patient's physiologic responses. Patients may be instructed in the use of vaginal dilators, but this is not productive if little attention is paid to the emotional sequelae of the dysfunction on both partners. It is important to understand the impact of vaginismus on both the patient and the couple. Referring them to a counselor who collaborates with their physician is a good treatment plan. If left unattended, a couple's lack of accurate sexual knowledge and/or impaired communication skills will likely cause many levels of dysfunction in their marriage.

Anorgasmia

Anorgasmia is the inability to reach orgasm. Orgasmic problems are very common, with 8 to 10% of women in the United States never achieving orgasm. A woman may have primary orgasmic problems (she has never experienced orgasm) or she may suffer secondary orgasmic problems (she previously has had orgasms but currently does not). For some women, the ability to reach orgasm is situational; for example, some women achieve orgasm only through fantasy or with oral stimulation but not with penile stimulation.

The diagnosis of anorgasmia is based on history. Treatment depends on the type of anorgasmia and its etiology. Primary may be easier to treat than secondary, where the underlying issues must be defined and resolved. Situational anorgasmia may be resolved through the use of a bridging technique, combining an act known to allow achievement of orgasm with the technique the woman would like to use to achieve orgasm.

Orgasm is a learned response and can be voluntarily inhibited. Factors that may contribute to anorgasmia include cultural or religious restrictions, premature ejaculation or erectile disorders in one's partner, an inability to relax and enjoy the sexual experience without guilt, and ignorance of the basic physiology of a woman's body. A woman with primary anorgasmia may need to learn what an orgasm feels like. For some women, education on the need for sufficient clitoral stimulation, adequate communication with her partner, and "self-permission" to be sexual is necessary. Self-stimulation is also recommended as a way of learning what is arousing and what ultimately leads to orgasm. Some women may prefer to masturbate alone at first, allowing the partner to become involved later, because learning to be orgasmic alone is easier. The final step is becoming orgasmic with a partner, and the individual woman needs to learn the most effective means for her to achieve this.

SEXUAL DYSFUNCTIONS IN SPECIFIC POPULATIONS OF WOMEN

Lesbians

Lesbians often report feeling uncomfortable in heterosexually oriented clinics where there is bias and ignorance. It is discomforting to be repeatedly questioned about the need for birth control when it is not necessary or when fear of a judgment-laden response inhibits asking questions about donor insemination. Questions about sexual functioning arise throughout a woman's life cycle, and lesbian women are no exception. A lack of information and resources can lead to ongoing dysfunction that might otherwise be relatively easy to treat.

Our culture is replete with myths about lesbians. One myth suggests that because both partners are female and have matching genitalia, they will enjoy the same approaches to lovemaking, have matching levels of desire, will be expert at pleasing one another, and therefore do not need to communicate individual likes and dislike to one another (40). As with heterosexuals, lack of communication between partners may result in sexual dysfunction. Lesbian psychosocial development includes a meshing phase, at which point the partners overidentify with one another, tending to overlook any individual aspects (40). As an increased awareness of each partner's individuality grows, individual sexual appetites and preferences will also emerge.

Although most lesbians report satisfaction with their sex lives (41, 42), there is a substantial minority who report dissatisfaction or some form of sexual dysfunction. The most commonly reported dissatisfaction reported by lesbians occurs in areas of frequency and levels of sexual desire (43–45). Blumstein and Schwartz (43) found that over time, lesbian couples have less frequent sex than do heterosexuals. There are conflicting data on whether or not lesbians in general are comfortable with this decrease in frequency (41, 43). A physician can, by sharing accurate information about patterns in lesbian couples' sexual functioning, alleviate concerns of "abnormality." A lesbian who is unaware of the trend toward decreased sexual frequency over time in long-term relationships may find this information useful because this suggests a normal pattern rather than a pathology.

Breast and Gynecologic Cancer Patients

Breast and gynecologic cancer patients experience changes in their sexual functioning for several reasons. If surgery is needed, there may be a decline in self-esteem because of the loss of reproductive organs or a change in appearance. Some women report a change in the nature of their orgasms because of the loss of their cervix or uterus, which rhythmically contracts during orgasm (46). Surgical scars may result in coital pain. Treatment may result in disfigurement, physical and emotional fatigue, and a profoundly lowered self-esteem.

It is not uncommon that women who have undergone treatment for breast and gynecologic cancers present in counseling offices with many issues, including questions about their femininity, body image, and sexual desirability. If a patient has had surgery or radiation treatment, she may have problems with vaginal lubrication or stenosis, leading to dyspareunia. If dyspareunia develops, one should consider a concomitant sexual dysfunction in her partner. Partners can develop a sexual dysfunction or aversion secondary to their fear of causing physical pain or in response to anatomic or emotional changes in their partners. Partners of women who experience coital pain frequently develop erectile difficulties (21).

The woman's age at the time of diagnosis and treatment has an impact on her emotional experience and functioning. A 32-year-old patient who must have a hysterectomy to prevent the spread of cancer will face issues of infertility, self-image, and sexual attractiveness differently than will a 68-year-old woman undergoing the same treatment. Although the issues of sexual attractiveness, desirability, and functioning are universal, in the case of the younger woman, the additional experience of surgical infertility complicates an already traumatic diagnosis and treatment plan.

Both partners usually have questions beyond the scope of the immediate diagnosis and treatment plan but hesitate to ask the physician. A woman who wants to ask her physician about possible changes in orgasmic functioning, physical sensations, and desire level yet feels her physician is only concerned with the cancer may not ask these relevant questions. Partners may feel a need to alter their sexual patterns, fearing they might hurt their partner. Physicians can help a patient and her partner by simply leaving time for ancillary questions. Open-ended question are useful, such as "At some point, many people have important questions about how the disease (or surgery, radiation, chemotherapy) will effect their sexual functioning. What are your concerns at this point?" Asking these questions at various stages of treatment regardless of the woman's age is important. The woman who initially had no questions may find that she has questions 4 months postoperatively. Encouraging direct and open communication between the physician, the patient, and her partner decreases misunderstandings about the immediate and long-term impact of cancer and its treatment on their lives.

Cancer patients may be hesitant to express anger or sadness about changes in sexual function or relationships. The patient may report "I'm alive. I beat cancer. So I feel petty to be angry that I have pain when my husband and I try to make love. But our sex life has been so important to us that I feel such a loss now that it's changed." The physician should hear her concerns and offer appropriate treatment. The dyspareunia can be addressed by telling the patient about over-the-counter lubrication gel and the relationship between adhesions and discomfort. Discussing the woman's need to experience sexual intimacy as a celebration of her life and her marriage, both of which outlasted the cancer, conveys empathy and helps the woman with feelings of guilt she may be experiencing over her anger.

Many women report that a return to their precancer level of sexual desirability and functioning is an integral part of their recovery process. Despite a good recovery and a positive prognosis, women are still vulnerable to developing reactive depressions secondary to the profound impact of cancer on their lives, changes in their sexual self-image and functioning, their perceived desirability, or their surgically or medically induced infertility. Physician awareness of these concerns and potential responses to cancer diagnosis and treatment will support the patient's need to deal with many facets of a cancer diagnosis.

Infertility Patients

By the time a couple is seen in an infertility clinic they have usually endured at least 12 months of trying, and failing, to become pregnant. Each unsuccessful month leaves them with a greater sense of concern, anxiety, guilt, blame, or anger at not becoming pregnant. After establishing a relationship with a specialist, it is possible that there will be several more months of evaluations and pharmacologic or surgical interventions. In the course of this process, the couple might learn more about the nature of their infertility, and their diagnosis may lessen their hopes of pregnancy.

Because of the invasive nature of an infertility workup and treatment regimen, intimate sexual behavior comes under the scrutiny and direction of strangers. Couples are told when to have sex and when to abstain. Men are asked to produce semen samples for analysis, and postcoital mucus may be examined. As conception becomes more strongly linked to attendance at the infertility clinic than to lovemaking, many couples experience diminished sexual desire and increased problems with arousal and orgasmic functioning (46, 47). The emphasis on timed intercourse can eventually result in decreased sexual activity during nonfertile periods (48–50). Patients report that the changes in their sexual relationships that become established during infertility treatment linger long after the treatment itself has ended, irrespective of the outcome (46, 51).

Further, there is a population of patients who are infertile because of their sexual dysfunctions, such as anejaculation. It is possible for some men to ejaculate with masturbation but not while having intercourse with their partners. Although these couples may become pregnant as a result of insemination, the problem itself has not been addressed and may actually be aggravated by treatment. Artificial insemination in this population may makes it easier for the couple to resist psychotherapy, which would direct treatment at the root of the dysfunction (52). Because infertility due to sexual dysfunctions can be successfully treated in one half to two thirds of cases by brief therapy with the couple, this offers an opportunity for the couple to experience full sexual functioning and, possibly, pregnancy without clinical intervention (53).

Infertility patients are a population particularly vulnerable to sexual dysfunction, both iatrogenic and preexisting. Taking an accurate sexual history before, during, and after treatment and educating the couple on the impact of treatment on their sexual functioning may prompt a couple to seek help relatively rapidly if symptoms of dysfunction develop.

Sexual Abuse and Rape Victims

Physicians encounter sexual assault victims in many different settings in the course of their practice. They meet them in the emergency room soon after the assault when the injuries and experience are raw, in well-woman clinics, during routine obstetric care, and in delivery rooms. The women may be forthcoming and fully aware of the extent of the abuse or they may only be aware of strong visceral responses to internal or breast examinations. They may present with panic disorder, depression, or substance abuse. They may be hypersexual or, conversely, avoidant of sex altogether. This might appear as conscious or subconscious avoidance behaviors, as in the case of vaginismus. The most frequently cited symptom of childhood sexual abuse in adult women is depression (54–57). Adults abused in childhood generally experience chronic sexual problems in adulthood, including fear and avoidance of intimate emotional or sexual relationships, aversion to sexual contact, dysfunctions of desire and arousal, and primary or secondary anorgasmia (56). These patients are equally likely to appear as sexually promiscuous women needing repeated treatment for sexually transmitted diseases and unwanted pregnancies, as they are avoidant of gynecologic care and sexual behavior altogether.

Incest survivors and rape victims often experience "flashback" memories triggered by seemingly benign situations and individuals. Because of the nature of the gynecologic or obstetric visit, the medical setting is ripe for intrusive memory flooding. Triggers can be as minute as words used, being in an unfamiliar place, body position reminiscent of the abuse position, being physically moved or touched by someone, feeling sexually aroused, or feeling similar physical responses to touch, hair color, facial features, or caring gestures (58).

Sexual abuse and assault survivors still struggle with the stigma placed on them in our society. For this reason, women may not be initially forthcoming about their trauma, fearing judgmental responses by physicians and others. They may continue to carry their own sense of guilt and blame for the assault. This often prevents them from telling their stories to helping professionals. Adults who were molested as young children may have taken the blame for the abuse; this defense fits a child's developmental vulnerability to assume responsibility for events out of their control. Many predators also instruct their child victims that the child wanted the abuse or liked the special attention. Thus, when a woman tells a physician, who is a relative stranger, about her abuse history, the physician should be aware that his or her response to this information is integral to the patient's recovery process. This woman may not have told anyone else about her history or she may be quite comfortable telling her story; compassion and respect are always warranted.

Alcohol and drug abuse is frequently seen in this patient population. Women use medications and alcohol to numb their emotional pain and to suppress conscious memories and flashbacks. Some medicate themselves in an attempt to help themselves be sexually active without being emotionally present. Whether the substance abuse predated the assault or was adopted as a dysfunctional coping mechanism in the wake of the trauma, treatment must include the complex relationship between the assault, the patient's sexual dysfunction, and her abuse of or dependence on medications or alcohol.

Maintaining boundaries with these patients is essential; lack of boundaries and role clarity makes victims feel vulnerable. Ongoing communication between physician and patient before and during examinations is frequently welcomed by the patient. It decreases the likelihood of intrusive memory flooding by keeping the woman in the present.

Abused women may access counseling at various stages in their lives. Each developmental phase may raise more issues relating back to the trauma. If the physician recognizes symptoms such as sexual dysfunctions of various degrees, avoidance of basic health care, repeatedly avoiding visits, or drug-seeking behaviors, she or he should not hesitate to support the patient by referring her to counseling.

SEXUAL DYSFUNCTIONS IN MEN

Sexual dysfunction is not limited to women. Men suffer from a variety of dysfunctions (Table 21.5), and, like women, some have organic causes, physiologic causes, or may result from specific medications (Table 21.4).

Premature Ejaculation

Premature ejaculation occurs when men pass rapidly from the excitement phase of the sexual response to the orgasmic phase with little, if any, time spent in the plateau state. It is a misconception that premature ejaculation is not as bothersome to men as it is to

TABLE 21.5. Sexual Dysfunctions and Their Causes in Men

ERECTILE DYSFUNCTION (IMPOTENCE)

Organic Causes	*Psychological Causes*
Peyronie's disease of the penis, prostatic surgical procedures, testicular failure, seminal vesiculitis, hypospadias, endocrine alterations (Addison's disease, acromegaly, pituitary insufficiency, low androgen level), chronic illnesses/conditions (diabetes, liver disease, adrenal neoplasms, obesity, fatigue), use/abuse of substances (alcohol, narcotics, estrogenic, or parasympatholytic medications), neurologic diseases (multiple sclerosis, amyotrophic lateral sclerosis, transection of the spinal cord, parkinsonism, peripheral neuropathies, lesions of the hypothalamus/limbic system/spinal cord, spina bifida)	Depression, marital discord, guilt associated with sexuality, sexual phobias, performance anxiety (fear of failure, pressure of sexual demands, inability to abandon self to sexual feelings)

PREMATURE EJACULATION

Organic Causes (should be ruled out in men with prior history of good ejaculatory control)	*Psychological Causes*
Prostatitis, neurologic disorders	Repetition of acquired patterns of rapid ejaculation, anxiety, low sensitivity threshold

RETARDED EJACULATION (INCLUDING ANEJACULATION)

Organic Causes	*Psychological Causes*
Neurologic injury or illness, use/abuse of alcohol	History of traumatic sexual events (sexual abuse, partner's infidelity, being discovered while masturbating as a youth), sexual guilt, suppressed anger, ambivalence toward partner, anxiety

women. Men may complain of limited gratification, feelings of frustration or anxiety, and may suffer from performance anxiety, ultimately leading to erectile problems.

To effectively treat this disorder, it is helpful to understand the physiology of ejaculation, which occurs in two phases. In the first phase, the terminal vas deferens, seminal vesicles, and prostate contract while the bladder sphincter closes. The bolus of semen is forced into the prostatic urethra at this time. The second phase is manifested in the rhythmic contractions of the perineal muscles, forcing the semen out of the urethra in spurts. Once the first phase of ejaculation has begun, ejaculation cannot be consciously stopped.

Therapy for premature ejaculation is behavioral. The man must learn to differentiate between a high level of excitement and impending orgasm. The squeeze technique may be used as a means of interrupting the response cycle at the excitement phase, allowing the man to better learn his body response and enabling him to create a plateau state. The squeeze technique consists of the woman placing her thumbs over the frenulum of the penis, her index fingers on top of the glans penis, and her middle fingers just behind (proximal) to the corona, applying pressure for 10–15 seconds. All of this is done when the man feels he is very close to orgasm. Ordinarily this prevents the man from ejaculating and causes him to lose some of his erection. This pressure does not hurt the erect penis. Stimulation of the penis ensues again, and the squeeze technique is used for a second time. The third time, the man is allowed to ejaculate (59).

In addition to learning how to create a plateau state, it is important to note that sufficient frequency of ejaculation may also enable the man to lengthen the time to orgasm. Allowing the male partner more opportunities to attempt to postpone ejaculation is more successful than decreasing ejaculatory frequency.

Erectile Dysfunction

Erectile dysfunction is the inability to obtain an erection sufficient to penetrate the vagina or to maintain an erection until ejaculation. Although it is tempting to classify erectile disorders into either psychogenic or organic etiologies, there is enormous overlay between the two. A man may have had erectile difficulties initially because of an organic cause and then later develop a psychogenic component as well. The presence of one cause does not preclude the presence of another.

It is common for erectile dysfunctions associated with psychogenic causes to appear with a sudden onset and to occur intermittently. Erectile disorders with an organic basis often present with gradual onset and are persistent or progressive. One commonly used test to distinguish psychogenic from organic erectile dysfunction is nocturnal penile tumescence monitoring. Nocturnal erections occur in healthy males ages 3 to 79 years approximately every 90 to 100 minutes during sleep. These last an average of 20 to 40 minutes per episode, commonly accompany rapid eye movements states of sleep, and decrease in quantity and quality as men age (60). One commonly used clinical technique to prove the absence of nocturnal erections is to place an intact ring of postage stamps around the flaccid penis. The pressure of even a partial erection is sufficient to cause visible breakage in the perforations between the stamps. Nocturnal penile tumescence can be measured in a sleep study in a formal sleep laboratory or with a "RigiScan" instrument (Bard Instruments).

If a man is not depressed and has normal nocturnal penile tumescence for his age, his erectile dysfunction is considered to have a psychogenic etiology. If there are no nocturnal erections, only partial nocturnal erections, or if sufficient rigidity is not achieved, the etiology is more likely organic. If the cause is not organic, appropriate individual and/or couples counseling is the therapy of choice.

The major organic causes of erectile dysfunction include vascular disorders, neurologic disorders, medications, endocrinologic disorders, or surgical etiologies (Table 21.5). For patients with vascular, neurologic, or surgical causes, penile implants or the use of vasoactive agents injected into the cavernosa are treatment options. The patient should be assessed for these potential therapies by a qualified urologist. Medications that are commonly associated with the onset of erectile disorders include antihypertensives, antidepressants, central nervous system sedatives or anxiolytics, H_2-blockers, alcohol, and antipsychotics (Table 21.4). Changing the medication, altering the dose or dosing schedule, or taking a drug holiday may alleviate the dysfunction.

SUMMARY

There are many opportunities to recognize sexual dysfunction in a medical practice specializing in women's reproductive health. Prevalence rates of sexual dysfunction in a general population range from between 25 and 50%. The challenge for most physicians lies in establishing a comfort level with the subject matter and gaining the necessary sensitivity and interpersonal communication skills needed when discussing sexual functioning. Approaching sexual health as an integral part of a patient's overall health helps practitioners decrease their own hesitancy and embarrassment when talking about sex with patients. This increases awareness, diagnosis, and treatment, enabling the patient to return to an optimal level of sexual function.

Managed care has ensured the role of family practitioners and gynecologists as gatekeepers and primary providers for women's health care. To do justice to their patients, physicians must consider the emotional and physical well-being of their patients. However, the physician cannot be expected to provide counseling or ongoing therapy in areas in which they have no specific training. The physician's duty to his or her patients is to inquire, listen, and integrate care for her physical and her emotional well being, referring to a counselor when appropriate. It is hoped that physicians who recognize their own professional limitations will willingly refer patients to trained experts who will work collaboratively with the physician for the best interests of the woman's health.

CASE STUDY

Vaginismus (An Unconsummated Marriage)

Susan and Mark, both 25 years old, never consummated their marriage. They were referred for counseling by Susan's primary care physician after she was diagnosed with vaginismus. In the process of taking a sexual and psychosocial history, this couple revealed important information that affected their treatment plan. Susan and Mark both came from strict fundamentalist religious families where sex was never discussed. Before marriage, neither partner had experienced extensive sexual foreplay, individual or mutual masturbation, or sexual intercourse. Neither partner had much accurate information about sexual excitement, behavior, and responsiveness. Susan had never experienced vaginal penetration of any kind, including tampon use.

Just before her marriage, Susan had an appointment with a gynecologist for her first pelvic examination. Susan went to the examination with significant anxiety and tension. She remained anxious during the examination, and as the physician inserted a speculum, Susan felt pain that stayed with her for several hours after.

Susan and Mark's attempts at intercourse on their honeymoon night were unsuccessful. Intercourse was impossible, and their repeated attempts were both physically and emotionally painful for both partners. Because neither were comfortable talking about sex, they did not communicate their concerns and questions, and the dysfunction escalated. Their repeated attempts at intercourse merely reinforced the behavioral response. Approximately 1 month after their honeymoon, they stopped being sexual altogether. Fearing additional frustration and fear, Susan withdrew physically from Mark. Because of their lack of information and experience, neither partner knew to introduce alternative modes of sexual intimacy. Their marriage was suffering and Susan developed a reactive depression.

Treatment Plan

The couple needed to be educated about sexual excitement, response, positions, and techniques. Several books were suggested, taking into account their religious beliefs. Mark and Susan were told that their problems would take some time to resolve, and they were given suggestions for alternative ways to convey their love to each other. They were advised to refrain from any further attempts at intercourse for a limited period. Couples are often relieved to have a temporary moratorium placed on intercourse, fearful that further attempts will result in more failure and pain. This timeout period often reignites their interest in one another sexually, replacing anxiety with anticipation, interest, and emotional excitement.

Over several sessions, Susan was given exercises focusing on graduated levels of touch and sensate focus. She began with exploration of her labia minora and majora, clitoris, and vaginal opening. She then moved on to exploring her vagina. First, she inserted one well-lubricated finger, then two, into her vagina. Successful pain-free insertion of a junior-size tampon represented a significant triumph, as Susan began to believe that she could have a foreign body inserted into her vagina without pain. Susan continued to develop the two skills most beneficial in healthy sexual functioning: tactile awareness and verbal communication.

She and Mark began to talk together about sexual feelings and to share information that each was learning about their own sexual responses and interests. Gradually, Susan wanted Mark to begin inserting his fingers into her vagina as her interest in him as a sex partner was reemerging. She talked with her physician about possible use of dilators but preferred to see what progress she and Mark might make together. Susan's depression was lifting as she experienced success with her treatment program and relief of her intense self-blaming.

Mark was also learning about his body and sexual functioning. He had many inaccurate expectations of sexual performance for both Susan and himself. Reading *Male Sexuality* (61) opened Mark's eyes and led to many interesting conversations with Susan. By including Mark in the treatment process, the blaming of Susan as the "one with the problem" eased. They both realized that communication was central to their resolution of difficulties. Susan and Mark were changing their experience of sex from one of fear, obligation, and revulsion to one of enjoyment, interest, and curiosity about their bodies.

The treatment process took several months of weekly counseling. Five months after they left counseling, Susan called with a concern. They were considering pregnancy but she remained fearful of the pelvic examinations. Susan returned to counseling to learn progressive relaxation exercises that she later used before her gynecologic examination. She communicated her history and concerns with her new obstetrician before the examination. She requested that the physician tell her what she was doing at each point of the examination and to stop at any time if Susan expressed high levels of anxiety. Susan was able to have a successful pelvic examination and has since had a successful pregnancy and vaginal delivery.

CLINICAL NOTES

Taking a Sexual History

- Women want to be able to discuss sexual questions and problems with their primary care physicians and obstetrician/gynecologists.
- Sexual dysfunction diagnoses are often missed because key questions are not asked.

Sexual Dysfunctions in Women

- Dyspareunia may be complete, situational, primary, or secondary; it has many organic, functional, and psychological causes.
- Inhibited sexual desire also has many causes, but it is important to rule out depression or other mood disorders as the primary problem.
- Vaginismus can often be overcome with Kegel and vaginal dilation exercises in addition to counseling,
- Anorgasmia may be primary, secondary, or situational. Behavioral treatment techniques are available.

Sexual Dysfunctions in Specific Populations of Women

- Lesbians are just as susceptible to sexual dysfunctions as heterosexuals but may be even more hesitant to ask their physicians questions.
- Breast and gynecologic cancer patients and their partners have sexual dysfunction sequelae from both their diseases and their treatments.
- Infertility patients have a tendency to develop new sexual dysfunctions because of the regimentation of intercourse that is part of their treatment.
- Sexual abuse and assault victims may be sexually promiscuous or sexually avoidant; remember, you may be the first person who has asked them about their prior traumas.

Sexual Dysfunctions in Men

- Premature ejaculation can be treated with behavioral techniques.
- Erectile dysfunction may be differentiated into organic or psychogenic based on nocturnal penile tumescence testing.

References

1. Bachmann GA, Leiblum SR, Grill J. Brief sexual inquiry in gynecologic practice. Obstet Gynecol 1989;73:425–427.
2. Ende J, Rockwell S, Glasgow M. The sexual history in general medical practice. Arch Intern Med 1984;144:558–561.
3. Frenken J, Van Tol P. Sexual problems in gynaecological practice. J Psychosom Obstet Gynaecol 1987;6:143–155.
4. Ketting E. Gynaecology—duty or service? J Psychosom Obstet Gynaecol 1984;3:107–114.
5. Lewis CE. Sexual practices: are physicians addressing the issues? J Gen Intern Med 1990;5(suppl):78–81.
6. Nease DE, Liese BS. Perceptions and treatment of sexual problems. Fam Med 1987;19:468–470.
7. Hansen JP, Bobula J, Meyer D, et al. Treat or refer: patients' interest in family physician involvement in their psychosocial problems. J Fam Pract 1987;24:499–503.
8. Frank E, Anderson C, Rubinstein D. Frequency of sexual dysfunction in "normal" couples. N Engl J Med 1978;299:111–115.

9. Masters WH, Johnson VE. Human Sexual Response. Boston: Little, Brown, and Co., 1966.

10. LoPiccolo L, Heiman JR. Sexual assessment and history interview. In: LoPiccolo J, LoPiccolo L, eds. Handbook of Sex Therapy. New York: Plenum Press, 1978.

11. Schnarch DM. Constructing the Sexual Crucible: An Integration of Sexual and Marital Therapy. New York: WW Norton, 1991.

12. Reamy K. Sexual counseling for the nontherapist. Clin Obstet Gynecol 1984;27:781–788.

13. Kaplan HS. The New Sex Therapy. New York: Brunner/Mazel, 1974.

14. Baker M. A GP's view of sexual dysfunction and its treatment. Med J Aust 1991;155: 612–614.

15. Kolodny RC, Masters WH, Johnson VE. Textbook of Sexual Medicine. Boston: Little, Brown, and Co., 1979.

16. Burnap DW, Golden JS. Sexual problems in medical practice. Med Educ 1967;42:673–680.

17. Plouffe L. Screening for sexual problems through a simple questionnaire. Am J Obstet Gynecol 1985;151:166–169.

18. Hammond DC. Screening for sexual dysfunction. Clin Obstet Gynecol 1984;27:232–237.

19. Steege JF. Dyspareunia and vaginismus. Clin Obstet Gynecol 1984;27:750–759.

20. American Psychiatric Association. Diagnostic and Statistical Manual of Mental Disorders. 4th ed. Washington, DC: American Psychiatric Association, 1994:493–538.

21. Sarrel PM. Sex problems after menopause: a study of fifty married couples in a sex counseling programme. Maturitas 1981;4:231–237.

22. Fink P. Dyspareunia: current concepts. Med Aspects Human Sex 1972;6:28–47.

23. McCarthy B, McCarthy E. Male Sexual Awareness. New York: Carroll & Graf, 1989.

24. McCarthy B, McCarthy E. Female Sexual Awareness. New York: Carroll & Graf, 1989.

25. McCarthy B, McCarthy E. Couple Sexual Awareness. New York: Carroll & Graf, 1990.

26. Barbach LG. For Yourself: The Fulfillment of Female Sexuality. New York: Doubleday, 1975.

27. LaFerla JJ. Inhibited sexual desire and orgasmic dysfunction in women. Clin Obstet Gynecol 1984;27:738–749.

28. Finger WW, Lund M, Slagle MA. Medications that may contribute to sexual disorders: a guide to assessment and treatment in Family Practice. J Fam Pract 1997;44:33–43.

29. Segraves RT. Antidepressant-induced orgasm disorder. J Sex Marital Ther 1995;21: 192–201.

30. Margolese HC, Assalian P. Sexual side effects of antidepressants: a review. J Sex Marital Ther 1996;22:209–217.

31. Shen WW, Hsu JH. Female sexual side effects associated with selective serotonin reuptake inhibitors: a descriptive clinical study of 33 patients. Int J Psychiatry Med 1995;25:239–248.

32. Rothschild AJ. Selective serotonin reuptake inhibitors-induced sexual dysfunction: efficacy of a drug holiday. Am J Psychiatry 1995;152:1514–1516.

33. Ayd FJ Jr. Pertinent medical intelligence: fluoxetine's impact on sexual function. Md Med J 1995;44:526–527.

34. Dorevitch A, Davis H. Fluvoxamine-associated sexual dysfunction. Ann Pharmacother 1994;28:872–874.

35. Murphy WD, Coleman E, Hoon E, et al. Sexual dysfunctions and treatment in alcoholics. Sex Disabil 1980;3:240–245.

36. LoPiccolo J, Lobitz WC. The role of masturbation in the treatment of orgasmic dysfunction. In: LoPiccolo J, LoPiccolo L, eds. Handbook of Sex Therapy. New York: Plenum Press, 1978.

37. Schover LR, Montague DK, Youngs DD. Multidisciplinary treatment of an unconsummated marriage with organic factors in both spouses. Cleve Clin J Med 1993;60: 72–74.

38. Branley HM, Brown J, Draper KC, et al. Non-consummation of marriage treated by members of the Institute of Psychosexual Medicine: a prospective study. Br J Obstet Gynaecol 1983;90:908–913.

39. Scholl GM. Prognostic variables in treating vaginismus. Obstet Gynecol 1988;72:231–235.

40. Falco KL. Psychotherapy with Lesbian Clients: Theory into Practice. New York: Brunner/Mazel, 1991.

41. Rosenzweig JM, Lebow WC. Femme in the streets, butch in the sheets? Lesbian sex-roles, dyadic adjustment, and sexual satisfaction. J Homosex 1992;23:1–20.

42. Loulan J. Lesbian Passion: Loving Ourselves and Each Other. San Francisco: Spinsters/Aunt Lute, 1987.

43. Blumstein P, Schwartz P. American Couples. New York: William Morrow, 1983.

44. Nichols, M. The treatment of inhibited sexual desire (ISD) in lesbian couples. Women Ther 1982;1:49–66.

45. Hall M. Sex therapy with lesbian couples: a four stage approach. J Homosex 1987;14:137–156.

46. Keye WR. Psychosexual responses to infertility. Clin Obstet Gynecol 1984;27:760–766.

47. Gervaise PA. The psychosexual impact of infertility and its treatment. Can J Human Sex 1993;2:141–149.

48. Burns LH. Infertility as boundary ambiguity: One theoretical perspective. Fam Process 1987;26:359–372.

49. Reading A. Sexual aspects of Infertility. Infertil Reprod Clin North Am 1993;2:559–564.

50. Bain J. Sexuality and infertility in the male. Can J Hum Sex 1993;2:157–160.

51. Baram D, Tourtelot T, Muechler E, et al. Psychological adjustment following unsuccessful in vitro fertilization. J Psychosom Obstet Gynaecol 1988;9:181–190.

52. Barwin NB. Sexual problems resulting in the need for homologous artificial insemination (AIH) as a treatment for infertility: psychotherapeutic considerations. Can J Hum Sex 1993;2:179–182.

53. Delafontaine D. Artificial insemination: definition, indications, technique and results. Contracept Fertil Sex 1993;21:511–516.

54. Bachmann GA, Moeller TP, Bennett J. Childhood sexual abuse and the consequences in adult women. Obstet Gynecol 1988;71:631–642.

55. Tsai M, Feldman-Summers S, Edgar M. Childhood molestation: variables related to differential impacts on psychosexual functioning in adult women. J Abnorm Psychol 1979;88:407–417.

56. Becker JV, Skinner LJ, Abel GG, et al. Incidence and types of sexual dysfunction in rape and incest victims. J Sex Marital Ther 1982;8:65–74.

57. Finkelhor D, Browne A. The traumatic impact of child sexual abuse. Am J Orthopsychiatry 1985;55:530–541.

58. Maltz W, Holman B. Incest and Sexuality. Lexington, MA: Lexington Books, 1987.

59. Lowe JC, Mikulas WL. Use of written material in learning self control of premature ejaculation. In: LoPiccolo J, LoPiccolo L, eds. Handbook of Sex Therapy. New York: Plenum Press, 1978.

60. Karacan I. Advances in the psychophysiological evaluation of male erectile impotence. In: LoPiccolo J, LoPiccolo L, eds. Handbook of Sex Therapy. New York: Plenum Press, 1978.

61. Zilbergeld B. Male Sexuality: A Guide to Sexual Fulfillment. Boston: Little, Brown, 1978.

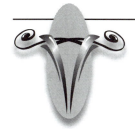

C H A P T E R 22

Psychopharmacology for Office Gynecology

MOSHE S. TOREM

It is well known that patients with psychological conditions such as conversion disorders, hypochondriasis, somatization disorders, anxiety, and depression may initially present to a medical doctor with somatic physical symptoms. Clinical prevalence studies have shown case rates of psychiatric conditions in a gynecology clinic to be as high as 53% (1). A more recent study reported psychiatric morbidity prevalence rates in a gynecology clinic of 46% (2). Both studies used a standardized questionnaire to screen for psychiatric disorders. High scores were associated with pelvic pain, younger age with no children, divorce, separation, and widowhood.

On the other hand, some medical conditions and pharmacologic adverse effects may present in a psychiatric disguise. Noncompliance with prescribed treatment and maladaptive responses to loss and other life changes pose further challenges of a psychological nature to the office practitioner.

Some psychiatric conditions may produce serious complications, including risk to the patient's life. It is incumbent on the primary care practitioner to be educated and knowledgeable in the skills of recognition and management of such patients and to know when and how to refer them for a psychiatric consultation and further psychiatric treatment. This chapter reviews the most commonly encountered disorders of anxiety, depressed mood, and sleep.

ANXIETY

Anxiety is defined by the American Psychiatric Association glossary as "apprehension, tension, or uneasiness from anticipation of danger, the source of which is largely unknown or unrecognized, primarily of intrapsychic origin. This is in distinction to *fear,* which is the emotional response to a *consciously* recognized and usually external threat or danger. It may be regarded as pathologic when it interferes with effectiveness in living, achievement of desired goals or satisfaction, or reasonable emotional comfort" (3).

The fourth edition of *Diagnostic and Statistical Manual of Mental Disorders* (DSM-IV) lists the following anxiety disorders: panic disorder (with and without agoraphobia), agoraphobia without a history of panic disorder, specific and social phobias, obsessive-compulsive disorder, posttraumatic stress disorder, acute stress disorder, generalized anxiety disorder, anxiety disorder due to a general medical condition, substance-induced anxiety disorder, and anxiety disorder not otherwise specified, including mixed anxiety-depressive disorder (4). In this section we focus on the anxiety disorders commonly seen and treated by primary care physicians.

Anxiety is a very common experience in the life of every normal human being. A patient with anxiety may be recognized by both emotional and physical signs and symptoms. The patient may exhibit or note internal tension, irritability, insomnia, a sense of impending disaster, an inability to concentrate, sadness, and difficulty

519

falling asleep. Common complaints include increased muscle tension producing headaches, general aches and pains in muscles, abdominal pain, pelvic pain, and low back pain. Other physical manifestations include tremor, muscle twitching, restlessness and a need to move around, fatigue, paresthesia, and a variety of symptoms due to hyperactivity of the autonomic nervous system. The patient may report poor appetite, chest pain, and a general sense of fatigue and low energy.

Diagnosis

To diagnose an anxiety disorder, physical illness must be considered (Table 22.1). If a physical illness is present, it should not be sufficient to explain the patient's wide range of symptoms or lack of response to treatment if an anxiety disorder is to be diagnosed. Drug intoxication (amphetamines, anticholinergics, cocaine, hallucinogens, marijuana, nicotine, methylxanthines) and drug withdrawal (from alcohol, antihypertensives, opioids, sedative-hypnotics) must also be excluded. Use of caffeine or corticosteroids may simulate anxiety disorders, as may deficiencies of thiamine, pyridoxine, folate, or iron. Diagnosis also requires that the patient's symptoms cause clinically significant distress or impairment in social, occupational, or other areas of functioning.

In assessing the patient's ability to perform the activities of daily living, one should ask about the following items and whether the patient's functioning in these areas has become impaired or less effective since the symptoms of anxiety began:

- Ability to function and complete routine daily tasks regarding personal hygiene (taking a shower regularly, brushing teeth, shampooing hair, etc.)
- Effective completion of tasks on the job
- Effective completion of personal tasks
- Effective and routine completion of tasks regarding financial matters such as balancing a checkbook and paying the bills on time
- Interpersonal relationships with family members, friends, and in the work place

A formal assessment tool that is very helpful in screening for anxiety symptoms is the Zung Self-Rating Anxiety Scale (Table 22.2). This scale consists of 20 items, is self-administered by the patient, and is very easy to score (5).

Panic Disorder

Panic disorder is characterized by the occurrence of spontaneous panic attacks. Panic *attacks* (not a codable disorder) are discrete periods of intense fear or dis-

---

TABLE 22.1. Medical Conditions That May Present with Anxiety Symptoms

ENDOCRINE
Addison's disease, Cushing's syndrome, pheochromocytoma, diabetes mellitus, carcinoid syndrome, hyperthyroidism, hypoparathyroidism, hypoglycemia, menopause, premenstrual symptoms

CARDIOVASCULAR
Angina, myocardial infarction, congestive heart failure, hypertension, mitral valve prolapse, paradoxical atrial tachycardia, pericarditis, anemia

PULMONARY
Asthma, pulmonary embolus, hyperventilation, chronic obstructive pulmonary disease

NEUROLOGIC
Tumor, transient ischemic attack, cerebrovascular disease, epilepsy, multiple sclerosis, Huntington's disease, infection, migraine

TABLE 22.2. Self-Rating Anxiety Scale[a]

During the Past Week . . .	Rarely or None of the Time (<1 Day)	Some of the Time (1–2 Days)	A Good Part of the Time (3–4 Days)	Most or All of the Time (5–7 days)
1. I've felt more nervous and anxious than usual				
2. I've felt afraid for no reason at all				
3. I've gotten upset easily or felt panicky				
4. I've felt like I'm falling apart and going to pieces				
5. I've felt that everything is all right and nothing bad will happen				
6. My arms and legs shook and trembled				
7. I was bothered by head-aches, neck pain, or back pain				
8. I felt weak and tired easily				
9. I felt calm and could sit still easily				
10. I could feel my heart beating fast				
11. I was bothered by dizzy spells				
12. I had fainting spells or felt like I would faint				
13. I could breathe in and out easily				
14. I got feelings of numbness and tingling in my fingers or toes				
15. I was bothered by stomachaches or indigestion				
16. I had to empty my bladder often				
17. My hands were dry and warm				
18. My face got hot and blushed				
19. I fell asleep easily and got a good night's rest				
20. I had nightmares				

Continued

TABLE 22.2 (continued). Self-Rating Anxiety Scale[a]

During the Past Week . . .	Rarely or None of the Time (<1 Day)	Some of the Time (1–2 Days)	A Good Part of the Time (3–4 Days)	Most or All of the Time (5–7 days)
Scoring for questions 1–4, 6–8, 10–12, 14–16, 18, 20	1	2	3	4
Scoring for questions 5, 9, 13, 17, 19	4	3	2	1

Reprinted with permission from Zung WW. A rating instrument for anxiety disorders. Psychosomatics 1971;12:371–379.
[a]The patient should be asked to answer these 20 questions (without seeing the scoring key on the last two lines) as they pertain to symptoms experienced in the past week. The total raw score may be divided by 80 (the maximum score), and the value is then multiplied by 100 to yield the SAS index. An SAS index below 45 is within normal range; no anxiety is present. An SAS index between 45 and 59 indicates the presence of minimal to moderate anxiety. An SAS index between 60 and 74 indicates the presence of marked to severe anxiety. An SAS index of 75 and over indicates the presence of most extreme anxiety.

comfort in which 4 or more of 13 recognized symptoms (Table 22.3) develop abruptly and reach a peak within 10 minutes. DSM-IV diagnosis of panic *disorder* requires recurrent unexpected panic attacks, at least one of which was followed by a month or more of persistent concern about having additional attacks; worry about the implication of the attack or its consequences; and a significant change in behavior related to the attacks (Table 22.4). Agoraphobia is not required for the diagnosis of panic disorder but it is a common comorbidity, as is major depressive disorder. Prevalence rates of panic disorder have been found to be significantly higher in women than men in 10 countries surveyed (6).

The patient should be evaluated for thyroid, parathyroid, adrenal, and substance-related causes of panic attacks. If chest pain or pressure is a symptom, the level of cardiac workup should be dictated by the presence of cardiovascular risk factors and the physician's clinical suspicion. Important psychiatric disorders to rule out include depression, schizophrenia, specific phobias, malingering, and hypochondriasis. Remember that the hallmark of panic disorder is spontaneous panic attacks; panic attacks that are situationally related generally indicate a different condition.

Generalized Anxiety Disorder

In the DSM, 3rd edition, revised (DSM-III), this diagnostic category was a "catch-all" for anxious patients who did not meet criteria for other diagnoses. In DSM-IV, generalized anxiety disorder is defined as excessive and pervasive worry accompanied by a variety of somatic symptoms (Table 22.5). In addition to pursuing medical or substance-related causes suspected from the patient's history and physical, the initial workup should include the standard chemistries, thyroid tests, and an electrocardiogram. It can be difficult to distinguish generalized anxiety disorder from major depressive disorder and dysthymic disorder, and these conditions can coexist. Other psychiatric diagnoses to rule out include hypochondriasis, somatization disorder, and personality disorders (especially avoidant, dependent, and obsessive-compulsive personality disorders).

Anxiety Due to a General Medical Condition

The diagnostic feature of the DSM-IV diagnosis of anxiety due to a general medical condition is significant anxiety in the absence of delirium that develops as a direct

TABLE 22.3. DSM-IV Diagnostic Criteria for Panic Attack[a]

Four or more of the following are required for diagnosis:
- (1) Palpitations, pounding heart, or accelerated heart rate
- (2) Sweating
- (3) Trembling or shaking
- (4) Sensations of shortness of breath or smothering
- (5) Feeling of choking
- (6) Chest pain or discomfort
- (7) Nausea or abdominal distress
- (8) Feeling dizzy, unsteady, lightheaded, or faint
- (9) Derealization or depersonalization
- (10) Fear of losing control or going crazy
- (11) Fear of dying
- (12) Paresthesias
- (13) Chills or hot flashes

Modified from American Psychiatric Association. Diagnostic and Statistical Manual of Mental Disorders. 4th ed. Washington, DC: American Psychiatric Association, 1994.
[a]These symptoms develop abruptly and reach a peak within 10 minutes. They are associated with a discrete period of intense fear or discomfort.

TABLE 22.4. DSM-IV Diagnostic Criteria for Panic Disorder (with or without Agoraphobia)

A. Both 1 and 2:
- (1) Recurrent unexpected panic attacks (Table 23.3)
- (2) ≥1 of the attacks has been followed by ≥1 month of the following:
   - a. Persistent concern about having additional attacks
   - b. Worry about the implications of the attack or its consequences
   - c. A significant change in behavior related to the attacks

B. Presence or absence of agoraphobia should be noted in the diagnostic modifier

C. The panic attacks are not due to the direct physiologic effects of a substance or a general medical condition

D. The panic attacks are not better accounted for by another mental disorder, such as social phobia, specific phobia, obsessive-compulsive disorder, posttraumatic stress disorder, or separation anxiety disorder

Modified from American Psychiatric Association. Diagnostic and Statistical Manual of Mental Disorders. 4th ed. Washington, DC: American Psychiatric Association, 1994.

physiologic effect of a general medical condition. This diagnosis can be modified with generalized anxiety, with panic attacks, or with obsessive-compulsive symptoms. Table 22.1 lists many of the medical illnesses that are associated with symptoms of anxiety. Although treatment of the underlying disorder is key, these patients may benefit from the use of anxiolytic medications in some cases.

Treatment

Jerome Frank once said, "attempts to enhance a person's feeling of well being are usually labeled treatment." The physician's approach to the patient who is suffering from anxiety is most effective when it is done in an atmosphere of calmness and when the physician is not pressed for time. The most effective treatments for patients with anxiety disorders are multimodal in nature. It makes sense to begin with the simple intervention techniques first and, when they are not successful, move on to more complex interventions. A discussion of some interventions that are easy to learn and implement in an outpatient setting follows.

TABLE 22.5. DSM-IV Diagnostic Criteria for Generalized Anxiety Disorder

A. Excessive anxiety and worry (apprehensive expectation), occurring more days than not for ≥6 months, about a number of events or activities
B. The person finds it difficult to control the worry
C. The anxiety and worry are associated with ≥3 of the following 6 symptoms (with at least some symptoms present for more days that not for the past 6 months)
   (1) Restlessness or feeling keyed up or on edge
   (2) Being easily fatigued
   (3) Difficulty concentrating or mind going blank
   (4) Irritability
   (5) Muscle tension
   (6) Sleep disturbance
D. The focus of the anxiety and worry is not confined to features of an Axis I (psychiatric) disorder, e.g., the anxiety or worry is not about having a panic attack (as in panic disorder), being embarrassed in public (as in social phobia), being contaminated (as in obsessive-compulsive disorder), being away from home or close relatives (as in separation anxiety disorder), gaining weight (as in anorexia nervosa), having multiple physical complaints (as in somatization disorder), or having a serious illness (as in hypochondriasis), and the anxiety and worry do not occur exclusively during posttraumatic stress disorder
E. The anxiety, worry, or physical symptoms cause clinically significant distress or impairment in social, occupational, or other important areas of functioning
F. The disturbance is not due to the direct physiologic effects of a substance (drug of abuse or prescribed medication) or a general medical condition and does not occur exclusively during a mood disorder, psychotic disorder, or a pervasive developmental disorder

Modified from American Psychiatric Association. Diagnostic and Statistical Manual of Mental Disorders. 4th ed. Washington, DC: American Psychiatric Association, 1994.

For panic disorder, psychoeducational and relaxation therapies may be very helpful, especially in combination with pharmacotherapy. Benzodiazepines are effective and commonly used, but symptoms frequently recur once the medication is stopped. This is true even when benzodiazepines are slowly tapered. The selective serotonin reuptake inhibitors (discussed in Depression, below) and some of the tricyclic antidepressants have been found useful in panic disorder. The treatment of panic disorder, once effective, should continue for 8 to 12 months. Although some patients may remain panic free off medications, it is common for panic disorder to have a more relapsing chronic natural history, requiring even longer term medication and psychotherapy (7).

For generalized anxiety disorder, psychoeducational intervention teaching skills in managing the symptoms of anxiety (cognitive and somatic) can be very effective. Because this is usually a chronic problem, the potential for tolerance and relapse limits the usefulness of benzodiazepines. Buspirone (BuSpar), despite its slow onset of action, is an appropriate first-line therapy. Patients with prior use of a benzodiazepine may be more compliant with buspirone therapy if a benzodiazepine is added to the regimen in the first 7 to 10 days of therapy. If benzodiazepines are chosen for this disorder, the treatment should usually last 2 to 6 weeks and then the medication tapered over 1 to 2 weeks. If buspirone is chosen, it may be used for the duration of therapy. The chronicity of this disorder necessitates emphasizing nonpharmacologic modalities. Therapy for a first instance should last 6 to 9 months but may need to be lifelong if recurrent (7).

Reassurance and Therapeutic Communication

Reassurance and suggestions are best communicated with the use of affirmative language. For example, in communicating to the patient the results of a variety of laboratory tests, many physicians say, "I've completed all of the blood tests, urine tests, and x-rays, and I found nothing wrong with you." Patients with anxiety typically focus on the word "wrong" and perceive that the physician does not believe that they are really suffering but rather that everything is "just emotional." Patients perceive this as a trivialization of their experience.

Instead, the physician may choose to say, "We have completed the blood tests, urine tests, and x-rays, and I have good news. Everything came back within the normal range. What this means is that your lungs are healthy, your heart is functioning well, and all the blood and urine tests are normal. I believe that your condition is produced by an anxiety disorder. How do you feel about this news?" This mode of communication focuses on the positive and gives the patient a specific diagnostic entity and then allows the patient to talk about his or her feelings regarding this news.

In providing reassurance to the patient with anxiety, it is important to remember that these patients are highly suggestible. Even well-intentioned physicians must be fully aware of how to communicate with such patients so that their verbal communication and actions are not contradictory in nature because this may create more anxiety in the patient. For example, suppose a patient is told as described in the paragraph above that there is no evidence of an underlying physical disease but then the physician proceeds to order more laboratory tests. This would allow the patient to perceive "something *must* be physically wrong with me or the doctor wouldn't order more tests."

After discussing the patient's diagnosis, some physicians may try to be reassuring by saying "don't worry." Patients with anxiety focus on the word "worry." Instead, physicians would be better served to communicate, "stay calm, this condition can be treated and you are going to feel much better."

Relaxation Exercises

Patients with anxiety are responsive to relaxation exercises. A practitioner who has taken a course in relaxation therapy can then teach these relaxation exercises to patients. Such an exercise may take 5 to 15 minutes and uses guided imagery and visualization. Some physicians produce an audio tape, give it to the patient to listen to, and instruct the patient to practice the exercises at home. An example of guided imagery and visualization that I have found extremely helpful in patients with anxiety disorders is found in Appendix 22.1. Practitioners who are uncomfortable providing such a service may consider referring the patient to a psychiatrist or psychologist who does provide such services.

Psychoeducational Interventions

Viktor Frankl said that "suffering ceases to be suffering in some way at the moment it finds a meaning." Free-floating anxiety causes a great deal of discomfort to patients because the patient does not understand where it comes from or what it means. In addition, the patient's attempts to control the symptoms have failed, which further increases the patient's worry and anxiety. The psychoeducational approach provides the patient with an explanation and a meaning to the anxiety. The psychoeducational approach provides the patient with a defense mechanism (intellectualization) that binds the feeling of anxiety by giving it meaning and structure. This approach begins with explaining to the patient the source of her symptoms.

For example, a patient experiencing paresthesias around her mouth or in her fingers experiences these symptoms as a result of relative ionic hypocalcemia produced from hyperventilation. Explaining this to the patient who is intellectually inclined can help relieve her anxiety. Another example is that of a patient suffering from tension headaches. Simply asking the patient to make a tight fist and hold it demonstrates how pain can originate from muscle tension. This allows the patient to understand that tension created in the muscles of the head and neck is perceived as a headache, or more specifically a tension headache. The physician may proceed by handing the patient a pamphlet that explains the symptoms of anxiety and how it can best be managed. In addition, patients may be referred to self-help books that address anxiety disorders and how to best master them.

Pharmacologic Interventions

Benzodiazepines.   Benzodiazepines are relatively safe anxiolytic medications. They can be classified into three major subgroups: short acting, intermediate acting, and long acting (Table 22.6). Two benzodiazepines in the short-acting group, midazolam (Versed) and triazolam (Halcion), are to be avoided in treating anxiety. The intermediate-acting drugs more commonly and safely used for treating anxiety are lorazepam (Ativan), alprazolam (Xanax), and oxazepam (Serax). From the long-acting group, the most commonly used drugs have been diazepam (Valium), chlordiazepoxide (Librium), and clorazepate (Tranxene). Flurazepam (Dalmane), quazepam (Doral), temazepam (Restoril), and triazolam (Halcion) are not recommended for the treatment of anxiety. These medications have utility in the treatment of some patients with insomnia and are discussed in the section below on sleep disorders. The usual doses of selected benzodiazepines are listed in Table 22.6.

Benzodiazepines are well absorbed from the intestines after oral administration, and no significant correlation has been found between plasma levels and the clinical results in reducing anxiety. The major metabolic breakdown of these medications occurs in the liver through microsomal oxidation and demethylation. Patients with liver disease or those taking estrogen, cimetidine (Tagamet), or propoxyphene (Darvon) may need dose reduction.

Generally speaking, these medications are well tolerated and have few side effects. Side effects that do occur tend to disappear with dose adjustment. The most common adverse effects are oversedation, fatigue, drowsiness, nystagmus, amnesia (most likely to happen with high-potency agents), confusion, and disorientation (most likely to occur in elderly patients). These adverse effects would be increased with concomitant alcohol, barbiturate, or sedating antihistamine use. In some patients, paradoxical agitation manifests in the form of insomnia, hallucinations, nightmares, and/or rage reactions. This is more likely to occur in patients with a prior history of aggressive behavior, and the medication should be stopped immediately.

Benzodiazepines should be administered with extreme caution to patients who perform hazardous tasks requiring mental alertness and proper motor coordination. In general, benzodiazepines lower the tolerance to alcohol and may produce a mental confusion similar to alcohol intoxication. Physical and psychological dependence, as well as tolerance and withdrawal symptoms, may be produced by all benzodiazepines. These are correlated with the dose and the duration of use. Practitioners must be aware that abrupt withdrawal of benzodiazepines after prolonged use may produce a withdrawal syndrome that may include delirium and seizures. For other points of importance regarding this drug class, please see Table 22.7.

TABLE 22.6. Benzodiazepines: Dose, Speed of Onset, and Duration of Action

	Dose (PO mg)	Speed of Onset	Duration of Action
Alprazolam (Xanax)	Start 0.25–0.5 TID; max 4 mg/day	Rapid	Intermediate
Chlordiazepoxide (Librium)	5–25 TID–QID	Intermediate	Long acting
Clonazepam (Klonopin)	Start 0.5 TID, max 20 mg/day	Intermediate	Long acting
Clorazepate (Tranxene)	7.5–15 QHS–BID	Rapid	Long acting
Diazepam (Valium)	2–10 TID–QID	Rapid	Long acting
Estazolam (ProSom)	1 QHS	Rapid	Intermediate
Flurazepam (Dalmane)	15–30 QHS	Rapid	Long acting
Halazepam (Paxipam)	20–40 TID–QID	Rapid	Intermediate
Lorazepam (Ativan)	0.5–2.0 TID–QID	Intermediate	Intermediate
Midazolam (Versed)	Not available PO	Rapid	Short acting
Oxazepam (Serax)	10–15 TID–QID	Slow	Intermediate
Prazepam (Centrax)	10 TID	Slow	Long acting
Quazepam (Doral)	15 QHS	Rapid	Long acting
Temazepam (Restoril)	15–30 QHS	Slow	Intermediate
Triazolam (Halcion)	0.125–0.5 QHS	Rapid	Short acting

TABLE 22.7. Patient Counseling Points for Benzodiazepines

The dose should be maintained as prescribed. Do not increase without consulting your physician.
Use of caffeine may counteract the therapeutic effects.
Driving a car or operating other machinery should be avoided until a clear response to the medication is determined.
Avoid the use of alcohol or sedating antihistamines.
Do not abruptly stop taking this medication.

Overdose with benzodiazepines is rarely fatal if taken alone. However, an overdose with benzodiazepines may be lethal when taken in combination with other substances such as alcohol, barbiturates, antihistamines, neuroleptics, or antidepressants. Benzodiazepines freely cross the placenta and may accumulate in the fetus. Data regarding the issue of teratogenicity of benzodiazepines in newborn babies are inconclusive.

Buspirone (BuSpar). A relatively new selective antianxiety medication is buspirone (BuSpar). It is not a benzodiazepine or a muscle relaxant and has no anticonvulsive activity. It works on the central nervous system by decreasing the noradrenergic and dopaminergic activity. Buspirone does not induce any tolerance or habituation as benzodiazepines do. Patients with a history of alcohol and substance abuse are more suited for treatment with buspirone for control of anxiety symptoms.

The starting dose of buspirone is 5 mg two times per day, and the usual effective daily dose is 10 mg three times per day. The maximum dose is 60 to 80 mg/day. The patient can expect results within 1 to 2 weeks of administering the usual dose of 30 mg/day. The maximum effect is usually reached within 3 to 4 weeks from the start of use. Elimination half-life is 1 to 11 hours, and buspirone has no active metabolite.

Headaches, light-headedness, fatigue, numbness, and upset stomach have been reported with the use of buspirone. No withdrawal side effects have been reported with this medication, and there is no cross-tolerance with benzodiazepines, barbiturates, or alcohol. Toxic effects in cases of overdose include dizziness, nausea, and vomiting. The mortality rate in cases of overdosing with buspirone alone is extremely low.

At the present time there are no adequate well-controlled studies on pregnant women and the use of buspirone. Therefore, it should be used with caution and only if the potential benefits outweigh the risks. The effect on labor and delivery in pregnant women is also unknown. In breast-feeding women, buspirone should be avoided because its excretion rate in human milk is still unknown.

Drug interactions have been noted with monoamine oxidase inhibitors (phenelzine [Nardil] and tranylcypromine [Parnate]), propranolol (Inderal), phenytoin (Dilantin), phenobarbital (Luminal), and digoxin (Lanoxin). It is recommended that buspirone is avoided when the patient is taking any of these medications.

Sedating Antihistamines.   Two antihistamines with sedative side effects have shown efficacy in the treatment of patients with anxiety: hydroxyzine (Atarax, Vistaril) and diphenhydramine (Benadryl). The starting dose for hydroxyzine is 10 mg up to three times per day, with the usual dose being 25 mg three or four times per day. The maximum dose ever used is 400 mg/day, but in office practice the dose should not exceed 150 mg/day. When used for longer periods of time, the sedation effect dissipates as patients develop tolerance to the medication, making this medication useful only for short-term treatment of anxiety symptoms.

Diphenhydramine is available over the counter in the United States and is available alone and in combination with cough syrups and decongestants. Even though diphenhydramine reduces anxiety, it also depresses rapid-eye-movement sleep in doses of 50 mg and higher. For the treatment of anxiety, the starting dose is 25 mg two to three times per day, with the usual dose being 25 mg taken two to four times per day. The maximum dose is 500 mg/day, but in office practice it should not exceed 200 mg/day.

These sedating antihistamines may produce anticholinergic side effects, such as dry mouth and, at higher doses, urinary retention. These medications should be avoided in patients with bronchial asthma, glaucoma, emphysema, and chronic pulmonary disease. Alcohol should be avoided because it may increase drowsiness.

β-Blockers.   β-Blockers have been effectively used in the treatment of the autonomic system symptoms of anxiety. The mechanism of action involves blocking the β-adrenergic receptor sites and hence preventing the actions of norepinephrine and epinephrine. This class of drugs has been used since the 1960s and has been especially successful in the treatment of anticipatory anxiety such as performance anxiety, before important examinations or public speeches, and other situational anxiety disorders. The most commonly used beta-blocker in this scenario has been propranolol (Inderal). The starting dose is usually 10 mg three times per day, and the typical effective dose is 20 mg three times per day. However, this medication can be used in higher doses if clinically indicated and well tolerated by the patient. It is important to note that the U.S. Food and Drug Administration (FDA) has not approved propranolol for this specific purpose. The common side effects include bradycardia, hypotension, dizziness, light-headedness, and occasionally excessive sedation. It may also cause depressive symptoms.

Consultation with a Psychiatrist

In the practice of office gynecology, the issues of when to consult specialists are not uncommon. When treating a patient with anxiety, the following guidelines may be helpful in deciding when to consult with a psychiatrist:

- The patient has a history of a previous psychiatric hospitalization and/or outpatient treatment by a psychiatrist.
- The patient has a history of suicide attempts.
- The patient has a history of alcoholism and/or substance abuse.
- The patient shows no response to pharmacotherapy for the anxiety within 2 to 3 weeks.
- The patient has a family history (parents, siblings) of a psychiatric disorder.
- The patient requests a referral for counseling.
- The practitioner is either untrained or uncomfortable in handling the treatment of a patient with anxiety disorder.
- The practitioner suspects a more complicated anxiety disorder, such as posttraumatic stress disorder in a rape victim or obsessive-compulsive disorder in a patient who reports excessively repetitive thoughts or actions.

Even though much progress has been made in reducing the stigma associated with psychiatric illness and treatment, there is still a level of discomfort associated with a referral for consultation or treatment with a psychiatrist. The following guidelines may be helpful. Communicate to the patient that it is you, the health care provider, who is asking for the opinion of an expert in the field of psychiatric medicine to confirm the diagnosis and recommend treatment. Explain to the patient that a diagnosis of an anxiety disorder has been made and that you are not well trained and/or comfortable in the therapeutic management of this condition. Be clear that you will continue to be the patient's physician and that the consulting psychiatrist will be helping you to best manage your patient's condition. You are not dismissing the patient or transferring her care as a whole to another doctor. Communicate to the patient your positive attitude and confidence in the specialist to whom you are referring. If you have worked with this consultant in the past, tell the patient of previous favorable experiences with similar patients. Finally, make sure you allow the patient time to ask questions and clarify any issues regarding the consultation.

DEPRESSION

It is important to clarify that the word "depression" may be used by the lay person to describe feelings of sadness, pain, helplessness, and discouragement. The American Psychiatric Association's glossary of terms emphasizes that depression may be a normal feeling in response to a loss and in the process of grief and mourning (3). It may also accompany a variety of medical conditions. It is important to distinguish depression as an emotional state or mood within the normal range of feelings in healthy people from depression as a clinical illness.

A recent survey of Fellows of the American College of Obstetricians and Gynecologists found an average of four new cases of depression diagnosed per month. Eighty percent of respondents reported receiving no residency training on the treatment of clinical depression (8). Knowing and using the DSM-IV diagnostic criteria may help the nonpsychiatrist avoid under- or overdiagnosing and treating the depressive disorders.

The DSM-IV lists the following mood disorders: major depressive disorder, bipolar I and II disorders, dysthymic disorder, cyclothymic disorder, depressive disorder not otherwise specified (including minor depressive disorder, recurrent brief depressive disorder, and premenstrual dysphoric disorder), bipolar disorder not otherwise specified, mood disorder due to a general medical condition, substance-induced mood disorder, and mood disorder not otherwise specified. In this chapter we focus on the common mood disorders with depressive symptoms, because those with manic traits (bipolar I and II, cyclothymia) need to be referred to a specialist.

Depression may encompass a wide array of signs and symptoms. There is often a general state of sadness, sense of hopelessness, and lack of interest in life. Common symptoms are feelings of guilt, slowed thinking, difficulty concentrating, loss of the ability to experience pleasure (anhedonia), low energy, and, at other times, high agitation. In addition, these patients commonly have thoughts about death and the desire to die as a way of stopping the emotional pain. A wide range of physical manifestations can be present, including insomnia or hypersomnia and weight loss or gain.

The lifetime prevalence of depression disorders in the U.S. population is estimated at 17%, with women affected twice as often as men (9). Despite the sex difference in the prevalence of major depression, there are few differences in the course of this illness. Specifically, women are not more prone to a chronic course of depression (10).

Depression may ultimately manifest itself as suicide. Suicide is the eighth leading cause of death in the United States (11). Some say this is an underestimate and that many more patients die as a result of suicide disguised in the form of an accident. Suicide attempts are even more common than completed suicide and are also more common in women (although men are more commonly "successful" at completing suicide). A study conducted in primary care clinics used a questionnaire to screen all patients for suicidal ideation within the month before the office visit. The authors reported a 2.4% prevalence of "feeling suicidal," with 58.2% of these patients receiving no mental health care during that time (12). The primary care physician must ask about suicidal ideation and plan whenever a depressive disorder is suspected.

Diagnosis

As with all DSM-IV diagnoses, it is important in the mood disorders to rule out substance abuse, medications (Table 22.8), and general medical conditions (Table 22.9) as causes of depressive symptoms. Also, the symptoms experienced must cause clinically significant distress or impairment in social, occupational, or other important areas of functioning. Questions you might ask to assess the patient's ability to perform the activities of daily living are noted under Diagnosis in the Anxiety Disorder section above.

A helpful way to screen for the symptoms of depression is the use of a standardized self-administered scale such as the Zung Self-Rating Depression Scale (13), the Beck Depression Inventory (14), or the Center for Epidemiologic Studies Depression Scale (CES-D) (15). Table 22.10 reproduces the CES-D scale in a format you may photocopy and use. Although these tools are helpful, they are not diagnostic instruments. They are quite sensitive and can be used to rule out depression in patients who score below the cutoff point.

Major Depressive Disorder

The hallmark of this diagnosis is the major depressive episode (Table 22.11), which is recognized by the presence of five or more of nine symptoms being present during a 2-week period. The major depressive episode also requires insufficient manic symptoms (e.g., inflated self-esteem or grandiosity, decreased need for sleep, pressure of speech, racing thoughts, distractibility, an increase in goal-directed activity, and excessive involvement in pleasurable activities such as shopping or sexual activities) to diagnose a mixed disorder. And, as noted above, the symptoms must be causing significant problems for the patient, and substance abuse and general medical conditions must be ruled out.

TABLE 22.8. Drugs That May Cause Depressed Mood

HORMONES AND STEROIDS
Oral contraceptives, progesterones, danazol (Danocrine), corticosteroids (both oral and inhaled)

NEUROLOGIC AGENTS
Parkinsonian agents, some anticonvulsants, meclizine (Antivert), methysergide (Sansert)

PSYCHIATRIC AGENTS
Sedative-hypnotics (benzodiazepines, barbiturates), stimulants and appetite suppressants, ethanol, disulfiram (Antabuse)

ANTI-IMFLAMMATORIES
Some nonsteroidal anti-inflammatories, opiates, pentazocine (Talwin)

ANTIMICROBIALS
Ampicillin (Principen, Omnipen), tetracycline (Achromycin), metronidazole (Flagyl), nitrofurantoin (Macrodantin), streptomycin, sulfonamides, some antifungals, some antituberculars, nalidixic acid (NegGram)

CARDIAC
Centrally acting antiadrenergics (clonidine [Catapres], methyldopa [Aldomet]), peripherally acting antiadrenergics (guanethidine [Ismelin], prazosin [Minipress], reserpine [Serpasil]), β-blockers (propranolol [Inderal]), digoxin (Lanoxin), procainamide (Procan SR, Pronestyl-SR), lidocaine (Xylocaine), acetazolamide (Diamox), hydralazine (Apresoline)

OTHERS
Some antineoplastics, anticholinesterases, cimetidine (Tagamet)

TABLE 22.9. Medical Conditions That May Present with Depressive Symptoms

ENDOCRINE
Addison's disease, Cushing's syndrome, hyperaldosteronism, hyperthyroidism or hypothyroidism, hyperparathyroidism or hypoparathyroidism, hypopituitarism, diabetes mellitus, pregnancy, menopause

NEUROLOGIC
Tumor, cerebrovascular disease, epilepsy, multiple sclerosis, Huntington's disease, Parkinson's disease, infection, trauma, dementia

AUTOIMMUNE
Systemic lupus erythematosus, rheumatoid arthritis, temporal arteritis, Sjögren's syndrome, pernicious anemia

OTHER
Infection (mononucleosis, tuberculosis, others), myasthenia gravis, cardiopulmonary disease, renal disease and uremia, acquired immunodeficiency syndrome, pancreatic cancer, lung cancer, other neoplasms

TABLE 22.10. Center for Epidemiologic Studies Depression Scale[a]

During the Past Week . . .	Rarely or None of the Time (<1 Day)	Some of the Time (1–2 Days)	A Good Part of the Time (3–4 Days)	Most or All of the Time (5–7 days)
1. I was bothered by things that don't usually bother me				
2. I did not feel like eating; my appetite was poor				
3. I felt that I could not shake off the blues, even with the help of family or friends				
4. I felt that I was just as good as other people				
5. I had trouble keeping my mind on what I was doing				
6. I felt depressed				
7. I felt everything I did was an effort				
8. I felt hopeful about my future				
9. I thought my life had been a failure				
10. I felt fearful				
11. My sleep was restless				
12. I was happy				
13. I talked less than usual				
14. I felt lonely				
15. People were unfriendly				
16. I enjoyed life				
17. I had crying spells				
18. I felt sad				
19. I felt that people disliked me				
20. I could not get "going"				
Scoring for questions 1–3, 5–7, 9–11, 13–15, 17–20	0	1	2	3
Scoring for questions 4, 8, 12, 16	3	2	1	0

Reprinted with permission from Radloff LS. The CES-D Scale: a self-report depression scale for research in the general population. Appl Psychol Meas 1977;1:385–401.
[a]The patient should be asked to answer these 20 questions (without seeing the scoring key on the last two lines) as they pertain to symptoms experienced in the past week. A total score of 22 or higher is indicative of depression when this scale is used in primary care.

If this is your patient's first episode and she has never had a manic, mixed, or hypomanic episode, the DSM-IV diagnosis will be major depressive disorder, single episode. This distinction is made because one cannot know if this problem will recur or develop into a bipolar disorder. If your patient reports two or more such episodes

TABLE 22.11. DSM-IV Criteria for Major Depressive Episode

≥5 of the following symptoms present during the same 2-week period and representing a change from previous functioning. Either (1) or (2) *must* be present.
  (1) Depressed mood most of the day, nearly every day, as indicated by either subjective report or observation by others
  (2) Markedly diminished interest or pleasure in all, or almost all, activities most of the day, nearly every day (subjective or observational)
  (3) Significant weight loss when not dieting or weight gain (>5% body weight in 1 month) or decrease or increase in appetite nearly every day
  (4) Insomnia or hypersomnia nearly every day
  (5) Psychomotor agitation or retardation nearly every day
  (6) Fatigue or loss of energy nearly every day
  (7) Feelings of worthlessness or excessive or inappropriate guilt nearly every day (not merely self-reproach about being sick)
  (8) Diminished ability to think or concentrate, or indecisiveness, nearly every day (subjective or observational)
  (9) Recurrent thoughts of death (not fear of dying), recurrent suicidal ideation with or without a specific plan, or a suicide attempt

Modified from American Psychiatric Association. Diagnostic and Statistical Manual of Mental Disorders. 4th ed. Washington, DC: American Psychiatric Association, 1994.

with an interval of at least 2 consecutive months without sufficient symptoms to meet major depressive episode diagnosis and she has never had a manic, mixed, or hypomanic episode, the DMS-IV diagnosis will be Major Depressive Disorder, Recurrent.

Dysthymic Disorder

Dysthymic disorder is not merely a mild form of major depressive disorder. Although the symptoms are usually milder forms of those found in major depression, what distinguishes dysthymic disorder is its chronicity. The depressed mood of dysthymia must have been present for more days than not for a minimum of 2 years. Table 22.12 lists the DSM-IV criteria for this diagnosis. Complicating the diagnosis, dysthymic disorder frequently coexists with other psychiatric disorders, including major depressive disorder, anxiety disorders, and substance abuse. These patients can often be sarcastic, brooding, demanding, and noncompliant, making it difficult for the clinician to work with them.

Mood Disorder Due to a General Medical Condition

It is not uncommon for depressed mood to be the major presenting symptom of an underlying physical disease. Table 22.9 lists medical conditions that may present with depression as the dominant symptom. Whereas treatment must be aimed at the underlying medical condition, patients with depressed mood may also be helped by medications and psychotherapy. In fact, depressive symptoms may persist for weeks or months even after the successful treatment of an underlying illness. It must also be remembered that these patients are at increased risk for suicide because of their depressed mood.

Treatment

The question of whether the physician should treat a patient with depression depends on the practitioner having the knowledge, interest, and skills in treating these problems. A patient without a history of suicide attempt(s), no current suicidal ideation, and in whom the depression is mild-to-moderate may be treated in a routine office practice if the patient is comfortable receiving treatment from a nonpsychiatric prac-

TABLE 22.12. DSM-IV Criteria for Dysthymic Disorder

A. Depressed mood for most of the day, for more days than not (subjective account or observed by others) for ≥2 years
B. Presence, while depressed, of ≥2 of the following
   (1) Poor appetite or overeating
   (2) Insomnia or hypersomnia
   (3) Low energy of fatigue
   (4) Low self-esteem
   (5) Poor concentration or difficulty making decisions
   (6) Feelings of hopelessness
C. During the 2-year period, patient has never been without symptoms in A and B >2 months at a time
D. The disturbance is not better accounted for by major depressive disorder
E. No manic, mixed, or hypomanic episode in history
F. Disturbance does not occur exclusively during a chronic psychotic disorder (e.g., schizophrenia)
G. Symptoms are not due to direct effects of a substance or medical condition
H. Symptoms cause clinically significant distress or impairment in social, occupational, or other important areas of functioning

Modified from American Psychiatric Association. Diagnostic and Statistical Manual of Mental Disorders. 4th ed. Washington, DC: American Psychiatric Association, 1994.

titioner. Most patients who suffer from depression respond to multimodal forms of therapy that include pharmacologic and nonpharmacologic interventions. This is true for major depressive disorder, dysthymic disorder, or depressive symptoms secondary to an underlying medical condition that is being addressed concurrently.

Nonpharmacologic Interventions

The nonpharmacologic interventions that have shown the greatest promise are the ones emphasizing cognitive restructuring and reframing (16–18). Reinforcing the fact that depression is an illness and can be treated is important. This approach reinforces the patient's defense mechanism of intellectualization. Appendix 22.2 lists informational resources for patients. In his book *Breaking the Patterns of Depression*, Yapko (19) emphasizes the importance of not only changing the patient's thinking about her condition but lists guidelines that he has found helpful for patients suffering from depression. An abbreviated version of these guidelines is listed in Table 22.13.

Encourage the patient to learn the skill of managing stress effectively in day to day living by maintaining a healthy balance between working, resting, learning, and having fun. The patient should be encouraged to develop effective problem-solving skills that are vital to managing one's life in an effective manner. The patient should be encouraged to act and behave in a way consistent with her personal integrity, her needs and values, and which is respectful of others as well. Realizing this in day to day living cannot be overstated as an important foundation for positive self-esteem. Encourage the patient to build her life around factors that are within her control whenever possible.

Pharmacologic Interventions

Antidepressant medications have been found extremely effective in the treatment of patients with depression. There are many different antidepressants from which to choose. Some basic guidelines that are helpful in selecting an antidepressant medication for a patient with depression are outlined below (20).

TABLE 22.13. Suggestions for the Patient with Depression

1. *Do not dwell on the past.* The past cannot be changed and the emphasis must be on what is happening now in the patient's life and making changes by learning new skills and implementing them in day to day living.
2. *Do not compare yourself to others.* There will always be people who are a little better than you and some are a little worse. The patient's most important task is to develop themselves to their fullest extent possible. The patient should be encouraged to believe in the uniqueness of herself and to strive to be the best person she can be.
3. *Don't create and dwell on negative possibilities.* Dwelling on the negative possibilities is one common cognitive distortions found in patients with depression. The patient should be encouraged to focus on the positive goal(s) she wants to achieve and reframe the negative(s) in a rational response.
4. *Don't leave important things unsaid or undefined.* The patient identifies the most important things in her life; for most people these are relationships, health, and work. Focusing on learning and practicing the skills that it takes to maintain healthy relationships in the family and friends, leading a lifestyle that maintains good health, and skillfully managing the activities of day to day living and responsibilities on the job are to be the patient's focus.
5. *Don't reject basic parts of yourself.* Everyone has certain traits or behaviors that they don't like. Labeling these traits as "bad" only reinforces an internal war that contributes to a feeling of incompetence, low self-esteem, and depression. Instead, the patient's focus should be realizing that each part of herself has some degree of value.
6. *Don't ignore your own needs.* The patient should identify her basic needs and make sure they are met. Trying too hard to please others in order to be liked creates an imbalance that leads to disappointment and depression.
7. *Don't ignore reality in order to blindly follow your own wishes and desires.* The patient should test her own feelings against reality. She should make it a habit to discuss her desires with friends and balance those views with her own feelings.
8. *Don't give up.* Determination and perseverance are vital.
9. *Don't leave time unstructured.* Typically, patients with depression get worse in an unstructured environment. Patients are guided to structure their day to day living by creating a balance between working, resting, learning, and having fun. Scheduling daily activities with the abovementioned balance is a natural and highly effective antidepressant.
10. *Don't stop working to improve yourself when your depression lifts.* Even when depression lifts, it is important for the patient to continue maintaining a lifestyle of activities that are designed to prevent future depressions.

Adapted from Yapko MD. Breaking the Patterns of Depression. New York: Doubleday, 1997.

It is generally recommended that primary care physicians use antidepressants from the selective serotonin reuptake inhibitor group or bupropion (Wellbutrin) because these are relatively safe in cases of overdose and have significantly fewer side effects than the tricyclic antidepressants and the monoamine oxidase inhibitors. Starting, usual, and maximum recommended doses for commonly used antidepressants are listed in Table 22.14. Selective serotonin reuptake inhibitors currently approved for use in the United States are fluoxetine (Prozac), fluvoxamine (Luvox), paroxetine (Paxil), and sertraline (Zoloft). The medications astemizole (Hismanal) and cisapride (Propulsid) are to be avoided in patients using drugs from this class, and theophylline (Slo-Phyllin, Uniphyl, Theo-Dur) should be avoided with fluvoxamine.

TABLE 22.14. Dosing for Commonly Used Oral Antidepressants

	Starting Dose (mg)	Usual Dose (mg/day Unless Noted)	Maximum Dose (mg/day)
Amitriptyline (Elavil)	25–75 QHS	150–300	300
Bupropion (Wellbutrin)	100 BID; increase to TID after 4–7 days	300–450	450
Doxepin (Sinequan)	75 QHS	150–300	300
Fluoxetine (Prozac)	20 QAM	20–40	80
Fluvoxamine (Luvox)	50 QHS	50–150	300
Imipramine (Tofranil)	25–75 QHS	150–300	300
Mirtazapine (Remeron)	15 QHS	15–45	60
Nefazodone (Serzone)	100 BID	150–300 mg BID	600
Nortriptyline (Pamelor)	25–50 QHS	50–150	150
Paroxetine (Paxil)	20 QD	20–50	50
Sertraline (Zoloft)	50 QD	50–200	200
Trazodone (Desyrel)	50 QHS	200–300 mg BID	600
Venlafaxine (Effexor)	75 BID	75–100 mg BID	300

A common mistake in treating depressive disorders is to use inadequate doses for short trials. Patients may be more compliant if they are warned that it is normal for 2 to 3 weeks to pass before the therapeutic benefits of antidepressants are noticeable. For major depressive disorder, medications should be used at the maximum dose the patient can tolerate for at least 4 weeks before being declared unsuccessful. This should be in conjunction with nonpharmacologic modalities. For dysthymic disorder, the trial period should be extended to 8 weeks. In the case of intolerable side effects, it may be helpful to try another selective serotonin reuptake inhibitor. If after an adequate trial the patient's symptoms have not improved, the primary care physician may consider trying a different class of medication (such as bupropion [Wellbutrin] or a tricyclic antidepressant) or referring to a specialist. The physician also needs to reconsider the possibility of an underlying medical condition causing the depressed mood.

Pharmacologic intervention should be continued at the minimum successful dose for at least 6 months for major depressive disorder (single episode). For recurrent major depressive disorder, therapy may need to be continued for up to 12 months. It is more difficult to determine when to discontinue antidepressants in the patient with dysthymic disorder or depression secondary to a general medical condition. Periodically reducing the dose to the point of discontinuation may be attempted.

Safety.   It is of paramount importance to emphasize the fact that some depressed patients may be very impulsive and self-destructive. A patient with major depressive disorder may be at greatest risk shortly after an antidepressant medication begins working, because it is then that she finally has the energy to commit suicide. A medication's safety profile and consideration of the potential for overdose is important when prescribing an antidepressant. The wider the gap between the therapeutic dose and the toxic lethal dose, the safer the medication.

In that sense, the tricyclic antidepressants and the monoamine oxidase inhibitors are the least safe, whereas the newer generation of antidepressants that are selective for serotonin are the safest. Atypical antidepressant medications like trazodone (Desyrel) and bupropion (Wellbutrin) are significantly safer than the tricyclics but not as safe as the selective serotonin reuptake inhibitors.

Symptom Profile. Some patients who have depression may slow down and withdraw emotionally and physically. They exhibit hypersomnia, hyperphagia, generalized fatigue, and low energy level. This subgroup of patients responds well to antidepressant medications that not only alleviate the patient's mood but also have an energizing effect by suppressing the appetite and decreasing the patient's need to sleep. Medications that belong to this group include fluoxetine (Prozac), bupropion (Wellbutrin), protriptyline (Vivactil), and, to a lesser extent, desipramine (Norpramin) and tranylcypromine (Parnate).

On the other hand, there is another subgroup of patients whose depression is associated with psychomotor agitation and restlessness. Such patients experience insomnia, anxiety, poor appetite (at times associated with weight loss), and a feeling of aimless energy. These patients respond better to antidepressants that have a sedating effect, improving their sleep and reducing their level of anxiety and agitation. The following medications belong to this group: trazodone (Desyrel), paroxetine (Paxil), sertraline (Zoloft), amitriptyline (Elavil), doxepin (Sinequan), trimipramine (Surmontil), and maprotiline (Ludiomil).

Side-Effect Profile. Some patients are particularly sensitive to anticholinergic side effects such as dry mouth, blurred vision, constipation, and urinary retention:

- More anticholinergic effects: amitriptyline (Elavil), clomipramine (Anafranil), doxepin (Sinequan), maprotiline (Ludiomil), amoxapine (Asendin)
- Less anticholinergic effects: desipramine (Norpramin), nortriptyline (Pamelor), trazodone (Desyrel), fluoxetine (Prozac), sertraline (Zoloft), paroxetine (Paxil)

Cardiovascular side effects such as orthostatic hypotension, dizziness, tachycardia, and cardiac arrhythmias are not uncommon with antidepressant medications:

- More cardiovascular effects: amitriptyline (Elavil), clomipramine (Anafranil), imipramine (Tofranil)
- Less cardiovascular effects: fluoxetine (Prozac), sertraline (Zoloft), paroxetine (Paxil), nortriptyline (Pamelor)

Amoxapine (Asendin) is the antidepressant most commonly associated with extrapyramidal side effects because of a metabolite resembling the neuroleptic drugs. Epileptic seizures have been reported in maprotiline (Ludiomil) in doses above 225 mg/day and in bupropion (Wellbutrin) in doses of 450 mg/day and higher.

The issue of weight gain is extremely sensitive in our culture. Many patients will not cooperate in taking certain medications if it is associated with weight gain:

- Associated with a weight gain of 10 pounds or more: amitriptyline (Elavil), doxepin (Sinequan), maprotiline (Ludiomil)
- Less associated with weight gain: fluoxetine (Prozac), sertraline (Zoloft), paroxetine (Paxil), bupropion (Wellbutrin), protriptyline (Vivactil), tranylcypromine (Parnate)

The relative sedative, anticholinergic, and hypotensive effects of many commonly prescribed antidepressants are detailed in Table 22.15. The selective serotonin reuptake inhibitors are minimally, if at all, associated with these side effects and thus are not included in the table.

Coexisting Medical Conditions. When considering the adverse effect profile of a medication, you must also consider interactions with coexisting medical illnesses. For example, a patient with narrow-angle glaucoma would not do well on a medication with strong anticholinergic effects. A type II diabetic would be more likely to maintain glycemic control if not prescribed a medication associated with weight gain.

TABLE 22.15. Relative Side Effects of Commonly Used Antidepressants

	Sedative Effects	Anticholinergic Effects	Hypotensive Effects
Amitriptyline (Elavil)	High	High	High
Amoxapine (Asendin)	Moderate	Minimal	Minimal
Bupropion (Wellbutrin)	Minimal	Minimal	Minimal
Clomipramine (Anafranil)	Minimal	Minimal	Moderate
Desipramine (Norpramine)	Minimal	Minimal	Moderate
Doxepin (Sinequan)	High	Moderate	Moderate
Imipramine (Tofranil)	Moderate	Moderate	High
Maprotiline (Ludiomil)	Minimal	Minimal	Minimal
Mirtazapine (Remeron)	High	Minimal	Minimal
Nefazodone (Serzone)	Moderate	Minimal	Minimal
Nortriptyline (Pamelor)	Minimal	Moderate	Moderate
Phenelzine (Nardil)	Minimal	Minimal	High
Protriptyline (Vivactil)	Minimal	High	Moderate
Tranylcypromine (Parnate)	Minimal	Minimal	High
Trazodone (Desyrel)	Moderate	Minimal	Moderate
Trimipramine (Surmontil)	High	Moderate	Moderate
Venlafaxine (Effexor)	Minimal	Minimal	Minimal

Previous Experience with a Certain Antidepressant.   Patients who had a positive previous experience with a certain antidepressant prefer to use it again if faced with the choice of taking one. The opposite of that is also true—a negative experience with a certain antidepressant diminishes the chances of its efficacy, even if everything else is compatible. Prescribing clinicians should be sensitive to this issue and inquire as to the patient's previous experience with certain antidepressants.

Previous Familiarity with a Certain Antidepressant.   Some patients are familiar with certain antidepressants based on their positive efficacy with a family member, friend, or from their own reading about it. Such information should be elicited from the patient because it potentiates the placebo effect and improves the chances of a positive therapeutic outcome providing the rest is compatible and there is no contraindication.

Timing and Patient Choice.   Many antidepressants can be given in one dose that will be sufficient for 24 hours. Most patients with insomnia benefit from a daily dose given at bedtime, because it may promote improved sleep in addition to the antidepressant effects. In this case, bedtime dosing also increases the patient's compliance in using the medication. Some patients detest being controlled and dictated to by the medical profession or any other authority figures. It is extremely important to incorporate the patient's need for empowerment and mastery into the prescribing skills of the doctor. Providing all else is equal, ask the patient to choose their own time when they wish to take their medication, whether it is before meals or after meals, in a once-a-day dose or in divided doses. This increases the patient's sense of partnership in the decision process and improves the likelihood of compliance.

Age.   Elderly patients are more sensitive to the hypotensive side effects of any medications, including antidepressants. Therefore, they should be given antidepressants with the least hypotensive side effects and should be educated regarding measures to prevent orthostatic hypotension.

Cost.   If the cost of an antidepressant is beyond the patient's economic affordability, the likelihood of compliance is reduced. Physicians should be sensitive to the issue of cost and inquire about the financial impact a specific medication may have on the patient's weekly and monthly budget. This issue should be discussed before choosing a specific antidepressant.

Consultation with a Psychiatrist

A referral for psychiatric evaluation and treatment is appropriate when

- The patient has suicidal ideation or has made a suicide attempt in the past.
- The patient has a history of previous psychiatric hospitalizations.
- The patient has a family history of depression.
- The patient has coexisting alcohol or other substance abuse.
- The patient's severity of depression is moderate or higher.
- The patient is not comfortable receiving treatment for depression from the primary care provider.
- The patient has not responded to treatment within 4 weeks of initiation of treatment.
- The patient develops complications or intolerable side effects from antidepressant medications.
- The patient requires a mood stabilizer (lithium [Eskalith, Lithane], divalproex [Depakote], valproic acid [Depakene], carbamazepine [Tegretol]) and thus needs monitoring.
- The patient is psychotic, suffering from hallucinations or delusions.

Questions Frequently Asked About Depressive Disorders

The following are frequently asked questions by patients who are diagnosed with depression.

"Doctor, what do I have?" or *"Doctor, what's wrong with me?"* This question should be answered with a straightforward statement from the physician. For example, "You have been diagnosed as suffering from depression. This disease is produced by certain biochemical changes in the function of the brain. Some people describe it as a chemical imbalance in the brain." Many patients with anxiety or depression feel responsible for their condition and perceive it as a sign of personal weakness. They should be reassured that their disorder is as much of a disease as diabetes or hypertension. As with these medical illnesses, they cannot "help" that they have the condition, but they can participate in their own recovery and maintenance.

"Will I get better?" The best straightforward response to this is "Most depressions are self-limiting." Some patients may get better on their own even without any specific treatment. However, the use of medications and psychotherapy significantly improves the chances that this will happen faster and the patient will not have to suffer as much. The patient should be repeatedly encouraged that things will get better, that they will recover from the clinical depression, and that it usually takes a couple of weeks to begin feeling better. Some patients even report feeling better within the first week of beginning the treatment with antidepressant medications. This response is very important because it helps the patient regain a sense of hope, and so many patients with depression are suffering from a sense of hopelessness and futurelessness.

"What will it take to get better?" The patient should be told that the best chances for getting well are taking antidepressant medications and engaging in active counseling and psychotherapy. The psychotherapy should focus on a multimodal approach using cognitive restructuring, include specific assignments in the form of activities and exercises, and develop, or continue to maintain, skills to improve self-esteem.

"Are there any things that I should not be doing?" Encourage the patient to avoid the

use of alcohol, because alcohol interferes with the efficacy of antidepressant medications. If the patient states that "A drink or two a day helps me stay calm," suggest the use of relaxation exercises and the possibility of adding a small amount of a benzodiazepine (on a temporary basis) until the antidepressant medication becomes therapeutic. The patient should be encouraged not to make any major life decisions while in treatment and recovering from depression.

"*Will this depression happen to me again?*" The patient should be told that she has a 50/50 chance of never having another depressive episode. Emphasize that even though recurrence may happen, there are additional therapies that can be used, such as mood stabilizers and referral to a psychiatrist. The patient should be told that about 60 to 70% of patients do respond to the first choice of an antidepressant medication. Of the 30 to 40% who do not respond, most will respond to the second antidepressant medication, bringing the overall likelihood of response to 80 to 90%.

"*Will I need to take this medication for the rest of my life?*" The need for a fairly lengthy (minimum of 6 months for major depressive disorder) treatment period should be explained to the patient at the initiation of therapy. This up-front explanation should prevent false expectations of a speedy cure.

"*Why did this thing happen to me?*" No one really knows why someone becomes ill with a clinical depression. However, we do know that clinical depression runs in families and we suspect there is a genetic component to this disease. This answer emphasizes the fact that the patient is not to blame for becoming ill.

SLEEP DISORDERS

Sleep disorders are a common problem in the outpatient clinic. It is estimated that one in seven U.S. adults have a chronic sleep-wake disorder. The estimated prevalence of insomnia is 30% per year, with one third of these reporting a severe problem (21). When a patient complains of problems sleeping, the symptoms usually can be classified as insomnia, hypersomnia, sleep-wake cycle disturbances, and/or parasomnias. Insomnia (difficulty falling or staying asleep) and hypersomnia (excessive amounts of sleep or daytime sleepiness) are the most common complaints. Sometimes a patient complaining of insomnia or hypersomnia will be found on careful history to have a sleep-wake schedule disturbance or circadian rhythm sleep disorder. This involves a misalignment between the desired sleep schedule and that allowed by travel ("jet lag"), shift work, or other external and internal forces. Parasomnias include nightmare disorder and sleepwalking and are not commonly seen by generalist physicians.

These symptoms may be primary in nature or secondary to a wide variety of medical and psychiatric conditions. Many substances, including prescription and over-the-counter medications, alcohol, and illicit drugs, may also cause sleep disorders.

Insomnia

The effects of insomnia fall along a broad continuum with the most common effect being daytime sleepiness. Studies done in laboratory animals show that lack of sleep may produce severe behavioral and physical impairment to the point of death of the animal. Insomnia may be transient or persistent. Transient insomnia is commonly seen before anxiety-provoking experiences and with life changes and grief. Persistent insomnia usually involves difficulty initiating sleep (rather than staying asleep) and often has a component of conditioned associative response.

Diagnosis

The DSM-IV diagnosis of primary insomnia may be made when the patient complains of difficulty initiating and/or maintaining sleep for at least 1 month (4). The difficulty sleeping and/or daytime sleepiness must be causing clinically significant distress in social or occupational functioning, and all reasonable medical, psychiatric, and substance causes should be ruled out to make this diagnosis.

Insomnia is a common symptom in many physical ailments, especially those that are painful or uncomfortable. Menopause or pregnancy should be considered, as should infection, cancer, endocrine disorders, and central nervous system lesions. Insomnia is also a very common presenting symptom in patients with anxiety, depression, dementia, schizophrenia, posttraumatic stress disorder, adjustment disorders, bipolar mood disorder and manic states, and a variety of personality disorders. Alcohol, caffeine, theophylline (Slo-Phyllin, Uniphyl, Theo-Dur), nicotine, amphetamines, methylphenidate, thyroid hormones, bronchodilators, steroids, antineoplastic agents, monoamine oxidase inhibitors (phenelzine [Nardil], tranylcypromine [Parnate]), pseudoephedrine (Sudafed), and many other pharmacologic agents may cause insomnia. Excessive daytime sleepiness may be promoted by use of alcohol, antipsychotic-neuroleptic agents, some tricyclic antidepressants (amitriptyline [Elavil], doxepin [Sinequan], trimipramine [Surmontil]), and opioids and other narcotic analgesic agents.

Treatment

Patients with insomnia should be offered a psychoeducational approach focusing on improving habits of sleep hygiene. Table 22.16 details suggestions for patients for promoting healthy sleep. In patients with insomnia secondary to a medical condition, the focus of treatment should be on controlling that disorder or the pain that it is causing. For patients with underlying mental health conditions, treatment may include the use of medications (e.g., antidepressants) with sedative side effects when possible. Medications causing sleep disturbances should be changed or discontinued if possible.

Benzodiazepines should be avoided in patients with persistent or primary insomnia. The focus instead should be on antidepressant medications with sedative effects to be taken about an hour before bedtime. Trazodone (Desyrel) can be given in one dose about an hour before sleep; this should be started at 50 mg at bedtime

TABLE 22.16. Suggestions for the Patient with Insomnia

Arise at the same time every day, regardless of your plans for the day.

Limit daily in-bed time to the amount before developing insomnia. For example, if you used to sleep 7 hours and awake refreshed, do not spend more than 7 hours in bed per 24 hours. Avoid daytime naps.

Develop a regular routine of daytime purposeful activity.

Gradually work up to and maintain a regular daytime exercise regimen appropriate for your age and physical condition. Nighttime exercise has variable effects and does not support healthy sleep hygiene.

Stick to regular mealtimes and avoid heavy meals for supper.

Plan relaxing evening activities such as meditation techniques, progressive muscle relaxation, a warm bathtub soak, or self-hypnosis and guided imagery. Avoid overstimulating television programs in favor of music or relaxing reading.

Develop and maintain a nighttime routine before going to bed (emptying the bladder, brushing and flossing teeth, changing to nightclothes) to prepare yourself for sleep.

Devote the bed and bedroom for sleep and/or sexual activity only. Avoid other activities in bed such as eating, writing, or doing homework.

Do not use alcohol, caffeine, nicotine, nasal decongestants, or any other medications that may interrupt healthy sleep.

but can be increased as high as 300 mg at bedtime. Under some circumstances, benzodiazepines, such as flurazepam (Dalmane) or temazepam (Restoril) 15 to 30 mg 30 to 60 minutes before bedtime, can be used for a few weeks (e.g., when the patient is under severe but time-limited stress).

Zolpidem (Ambien) has been approved by the FDA for the short-term treatment of insomnia. Even though chemically it looks different from the benzodiazepines, it does bind the benzodiazepine type I receptor. It is less addictive and less habituating than the classic benzodiazepines. It is rapidly absorbed through the gastrointestinal tract and is therefore excellent for sleep induction. Because its metabolic half-life is only about 2.5 hours, there are very few carry-over symptoms when the patient wakes up in the morning. The typical starting dose is 5 mg at bedtime and can be increased up to 10 to 20 mg 30 minutes before bedtime. Zolpidem should not be used for more than 1 or 2 months without the patient having a more thorough assessment of the nature of the chronic insomnia.

If insomnia persists despite treatment, the patient should have a polysomnogram done at a sleep laboratory to thoroughly assess the nature of the patient's insomnia and to rule out sleep disorders such as obstructive sleep apnea, nocturnal myoclonus, restless leg syndrome, sleep walking, and others. When any of the above are diagnosed, they necessitate treatment by a specialist in sleep disorders.

Hypersomnia

Hypersomnia may present as excessive amounts of sleep or daytime sleepiness or both. Its most extreme form manifests in the narcoleptic. On the other hand, it should not be diagnosed in the person who is merely a "long sleeper," preferring 9 to 10 hours of sleep most nights but not having difficulty functioning in the day.

Diagnosis

The DSM-IV diagnosis of primary hypersomnia requires excessive sleepiness (either prolonged sleep episodes or daytime sleep episodes) for at least 1 month or, if recurrent, lasting at least 3 days and occurring several times a year for at least 2 years. The excessive sleepiness must be causing clinically significant distress in social or occupational functioning, and all reasonable medical, psychiatric, and substance causes should be ruled out to make this diagnosis. Also, the excessive sleepiness must not be better accounted for by insomnia, another sleep disorder (e.g., narcolepsy, sleep apnea), or by inadequate amounts of sleep. Some people with major depressive disorder present with hypersomnia.

A common cause of secondary hypersomnia is sleep apnea (obstructive being more common than central), which is diagnosed by referring the patient to a sleep laboratory for polysomnogram. The prevalence of sleep apnea syndromes is estimated to be 1 to 3% of the total population. In obstructive sleep apnea, upper airway closure takes place as a result of collapse of the pharyngeal walls during deep sleep. This produces cyclical hypercarbia, acidosis, and hypoxia to the brain. It may also result in certain cardiac arrhythmias. When the patient wakes up to take a deep breath the upper airway obstruction is resolved and normal breathing resumes until another cycle begins. The awakening (which can occur up to 200 times per night) prevents the normal progression of the sleep cycle through its stages, making the sleep less restorative.

Obstructive sleep apnea may be recognized by the following symptoms:

- Heavy snoring
- Daytime sleepiness and fatigue with poor concentration

- Patient wakes up tired, feeling like she has not slept all night
- Prolonged pauses in breathing during sleep. This is usually confirmed by the patient's spouse or significant other

Other causes of secondary hypersomnia are metabolic, endocrine, and encephalitic conditions; use of alcohol or other depressants; and withdrawal from stimulants.

Treatment

Underlying causes of hypersomnia should be addressed. Nonsedating selective serotonin reuptake inhibitors (such as fluoxetine [Prozac]) may be helpful in patients with concomitant depressive symptoms. Treatment of obstructive sleep apnea usually involves the use of a continuous positive airway pressure machine to keep the patient's airway open during sleep. Weight loss may also be helpful in these patients. Recalcitrance to or refusal of these modalities may necessitate referral to an ear, nose, and throat specialist for evaluation of the appropriateness of surgical excision of a portion of the uvula and soft palate (uvulopalatectomy). Primary hypersomnia, like narcolepsy, can be treated with stimulants such as amphetamines but may be best referred to a specialist.

CLINICAL NOTES

- To diagnose an anxiety disorder, physical illness must be considered. If a physical illness is present, it should not be sufficient to explain the symptoms and/or lack of response if the diagnosis of anxiety disorder is to be made. The Zung Self-Rating Anxiety Scale is an effective screening tool for anxiety symptoms.
- Panic attacks are discrete periods of intense fear or discomfort with 4 or more of 13 recognized symptoms that occur abruptly and peak within 10 minutes. Panic disorder is present when there are recurrent panic attacks, with at least one of these attacks being followed by a month or more of persistent concern about recurrent attacks, the implication of the attack(s), and a significant change in behavior related to the attacks. Panic disorder is more common in women than in men. The hallmark of panic disorder is spontaneous panic attacks.
- Psychoeducational and relaxation therapies for panic disorder are helpful, especially in combination with pharmacotherapy. Benzodiazepines are effective but symptoms frequently recur with cessation of the medication even with slow tapering of use. Selective serotonin reuptake inhibitors and tricyclic antidepressants are useful. Treatment should continue for 8 to 12 months. It is common for panic disorder to have a chronic relapsing nature.
- Generalized anxiety disorder is excessive and pervasive worry accompanied by a variety of somatic symptoms. This may be difficult to distinguish from major depressive disorder or dysthymic disorder. Other psychiatric disorders must be ruled out as well. Psychoeducational intervention teaching skills can be effective for this. Because this is a chronic problem, the usefulness of benzodiazepines is limited. Buspirone (BuSpar) is appropriate first-line therapy. Therapy should last 6 to 9 months but may need to be lifelong if this problem is recurrent.
- Anxiety due to a general medical condition is significant anxiety in the absence of delirium that develops as a direct physiologic effect of a general medical condition. Although treatment of the underlying disorder is key, the patient may benefit from use of anxiolytic medications in some instances.
- Patients with anxiety are highly suggestible. Communication should involve the use of positive words and phrases and avoid those involving negative overtones, such as "don't

worry." Relaxation exercises and psychoeducational interventions are also important treatment modalities.
- Pharmacologic interventions for anxiety disorders include the use of benzodiazepines, buspirone (BuSpar), sedating antihistamines, and beta-blockers.
- There are guidelines for referral of a patient with anxiety to a psychiatrist.
- The lifetime prevalence of depression disorders in the U.S. population is approximately 17%, with women being affected twice as often as men. The ultimate manifestation of depression is suicide. Suicide is the eighth leading cause of death in the United States. If a depressive disorder is suspected, the health care provider must ask the patient about suicidal ideation and planning.
- Substance abuse, medications, and general medical conditions may be causes of depressive symptoms and must be ruled out as the cause before the diagnosis of major depressive disorder is made.
- The CES-D is one of many tools to screen patients for symptoms of depression.
- The hallmark of the major depressive episode is the presence of five of nine well-defined symptoms being present during a 2-week period in the absence of manic symptoms.
- Dysthymic disorder is distinct from major depressive disorder by its chronicity. For a minimum of 2 years, the depressed mood of dysthymia must have been present for more days than not. This disorder frequently coexists with other psychiatric disorders.
- Depressed mood may be the major presenting symptom of an underlying physical disease. Whereas treatment is aimed at the underlying condition, the use of medications and psychotherapy may also be quite helpful.
- A patient without a history of suicide attempt(s), no current suicidal ideation, and in whom the depression is mild to moderate may be treated in a routine office practice if the patient and practitioner are comfortable with this. Further guidelines for referral are available.
- The nonpharmacologic interventions with the greatest promise for depression emphasize cognitive restructuring and reframing. They reinforce the defense mechanism of intellectualization.
- Antidepressant medication therapy can be extremely helpful. Nonpsychiatric practitioners are recommended to choose antidepressants from the selective serotonin reuptake inhibitor groups or to use bupropion (Wellbutrin) because they have a good safety profile and few side effects.
- A common mistake in medical therapy for depression is to use inadequate doses for short trials. It may be 2 to 3 weeks before therapeutic benefits of antidepressants are noticed.
- For major depressive disorder, medications should be used at the maximum dose the patient can tolerate for at least 4 weeks before being declared unsuccessful. For dysthymic disorder, the trial period should be 8 weeks.
- If the patient does not improve after an adequate trial, a different class of medication should be tried or the patient should be referred to a psychiatrist.
- Medical intervention should continue at the minimum successful dose for at least 6 months for Major Depressive Disorder, Single Episode. For recurrent major depressive disorder, therapy may need to continue for up to 1 year.
- Medical intervention for depression should be used in conjunction with nonpharmacologic modalities. It should never be the sole therapy for depression.
- Patients with major depressive disorder may be at greatest risk for suicide shortly after an antidepressant begins working because they may finally have the energy to commit suicide.
- The antidepressant chosen must be one that will treat the symptom profile of the patient's depression. In addition, the side-effect profile of the medication and potential effect(s) on existing medical conditions must be considered before recommended use.
- An estimated one in seven U.S. adults has a chronic sleep-wake disorder. The estimated prevalence of insomnia is 30% per year, with one third of patients classifying it as a severe problem.
- Primary insomnia is present when the patient complains of difficulty initiating and/or

maintaining sleep for at least 1 month. Treatment involves a psychoeducational approach that focuses on improving habits of sleep hygiene. If the insomnia is secondary to a medical condition, treatment is focused on controlling the disorder or pain the condition is causing. For patients with mental health conditions and insomnia, treatment may include the use of sedating medications.

- Benzodiazepines should be avoided in patients with persistent or primary insomnia. Antidepressant medications with sedating side effects should be offered instead.
- Zolpidem (Ambien) is FDA-approved for the short-term treatment of insomnia. Starting dose is 5 mg at bedtime and can be increased up to 10 to 20 mg 30 minutes before bedtime. It should not be used for more than 1 to 2 months without a thorough assessment of the nature of the chronic insomnia.
- Patients with insomnia that persists despite treatment should have a polysomnogram to rule out sleep disorders.
- Primary hypersomnia exists if excessive sleepiness has been present for at least 1 month or, if recurrent, lasts at least 3 days and occurs several times a year for at least 2 years. The sleepiness must cause significant social or occupational dysfunction. Other causes, including another sleep disorder, must be ruled out.
- A common cause of secondary hypersomnia is sleep apnea, with obstructive being more common than central. The patient suspected of having sleep apnea should be referred to a sleep laboratory for a polysomnogram.
- Treatment for obstructive sleep apnea may include a continuous positive airway pressure machine, weight loss, or even surgery.

An Example of Guided Imagery and Visualization for Patients with Anxiety Disorders

Now that you have entered into a state of self-hypnotic trance, if you wish, open a new channel of concentration whereby you may visualize yourself being at your favorite ocean beach . . . that's right. Look at the sky. It is clear: A June day. The skies are blue and clear; maybe compare it with the color of the ocean. Notice where there is a similarity and a difference. Notice how the ocean and the sky blend together, meeting each other at the horizon. Now, look at the ocean again, and notice the waves coming onto the beach, one after the other, in rhythm. White and foamy. That's right . . . look at the sand. Is it white? Is it yellow? Or is it gray, or maybe a blend of all three? Look at the beach. Are there any other people there walking around? Any bushes, any trees at a distance? Look at the sky again. Are there any seagulls floating around? Some may be diving toward the ocean in their attempt to catch some fish for their meal. That's right. Isn't that interesting?

Now, I would like you to move on and experience that ocean beach with your sense of hearing. Listen to the sounds. That's right. The sounds of the ocean waves coming onto the beach, one after the other. That's right. The sounds of the seagulls as they float in the air. Perhaps the sound of a radio playing in the distance, or the sounds of people talking, if you wish. Now, go on and experience that ocean beach with your sense of touch. Allow yourself to touch the sand with your bare feet. I would like you to sense the texture of the granules of this sand. Walk toward the waters of the ocean, and as you do, notice the change in the firmness of the sand from dry to firm, wet sand as you approach the waves of the ocean. Get a little closer and allow your feet to be touched by the ocean waters as they come onto the beach. Allow yourself to sense the coolness and wetness on your feet from the ocean waters as compared with the rest of your body exposed to the sun . . . feeling the sun rays touching your body with dry warmth, creating inside a comfortable, warm feeling of healing. Keep on walking on the beach and notice if there is a breeze. Notice the air movement touching your hair and your face, clear and clean and comfortable. Keep on walking and notice whether you see on the beach some of the seashells that have been left from the last high tide. You may want to pick one of them up, touch it with your fingers. Notice the sand that covers the seashell. Allow yourself, if you wish, to wash the sand off the shell with the ocean waters. Now, notice the special design on the seashell. Isn't that interesting?

Keep on walking on the beach, and take a deep breath through your nose. Experience the ocean beach with your sense of smell. Notice the special smell of the ocean beach. A blend of fish, seaweed, and salt that you are so familiar with. That's right. Isn't that interesting? Keep on walking on the beach, and get closer, if you wish, to a place where there are lots of big rocks. That's where the waves are breaking with even greater force . . . and throwing into the air a cloud of mist that is made up of billions of tiny droplets of water. Some of them land on your face and on your lips, and quickly dry out, leaving a tiny film of salt on your lips. All you have to do now is experience this ocean beach of yours with your sense of taste, allowing your tongue to lick your lips. That's right. Go ahead, if you wish, and experience this special salty taste of the ocean beach. Now, notice that the more you experience this ocean beach with all your senses, the more relaxed and calm you have become without even noticing it happening.

All you have to do in the future is to focus on your special beach and experience it with all your senses—as if you are there. And now you know you can do this exercise on your own anytime you wish to. The more you do it, the easier and easier it becomes for you. The more you do it, the more talented and gifted you become in doing this exercise. Promoting a state of total calmness and relaxation in your mind, body, and spirit. That's right. Now the way to come out of this state of self-hypnosis is to count back from three to one and go right ahead. At three, you get ready. Two, with your eyelids closed, you look up with the eyes, and one, the eyes open, they come back into focus. You are becoming fully alert, awake, oriented and the inner calmness and relaxation continue to stay with you as long as you need.

Information Resources for Patients with Depression

- Burns D. *Feeling Good: The New Mood Therapy.* New York: William Morrow, 1980.
- Burns D. *The Feeling Good Handbook.* New York: Plume, 1989.
- Braiker H. *Getting Up When You're Feeling Down: A Woman's Guide to Overcoming and Preventing Depression.* New York: Putnam's, 1988.
- Cronkite K. *On the Edge of Darkness: Conversations about Conquering Depression.* New York: Doubleday, 1994.
- Depression Guideline Panel. *Depression Is a Treatable Illness: A Patient's Guide.* Clinical practice guideline no. 5, AHCPR publication no. 93–0553. Rockville, MD: Department of Health and Human Services, Public Health Service, Agency for Health Care Policy and Research, 1993.
- Dowling C. *You Mean I Don't Have to Feel this Way?* New York: Scribner's, 1991.
- Emery G. *Getting Undepressed: How a Woman can Change Her Life Through Cognitive Therapy.* New York: Simon and Schuster, 1988.
- Fieve R. *Prozac: Questions and Answers for Patients, Families, and Physicians.* New York: Avon Books, 1994
- Goldberg I. *Questions and Answers About Depression and Its Treatment.* Philadelphia: Charles Press, 1993.
- Kramer P. *Listening to Prozac: A Psychiatrist Explores Antidepressant Drugs and the Remaking of the Self.* New York: Viking, 1993.
- Styrom W. *Darkness Visible: A Memoir of Madness.* New York: Random House, 1990.
- Thompson T. *The Beast: A Reckoning with Depression.* New York: Putnam's, 1995.

References

1. Ballenger CB. Psychiatric morbidity and the menopause: survey of a gynaecological outpatient clinic. Br J Psychiatry 1977;131:83–83.
2. Byrne P. Psychiatric morbidity in a gynaecology clinic: an epidemiological survey. Br J Psychiatry 1984;144:28–34.
3. American Psychiatric Glossary. 7th ed. Washington, DC: American Psychiatric Press, 1994.
4. American Psychiatric Association. Diagnostic and Statistical Manual of Mental Disorders. 4th ed. Washington, DC: American Psychiatric Association, 1994.
5. Zung WW. A rating instrument for anxiety disorders. Psychosomatics 1971;12:371–379.
6. Weissman MM, Bland RC, Canino GJ, et al. The cross-national epidemiology of panic disorder. Arch Gen Psychiatry 1997;54:305–309.
7. Hale AS. Anxiety. BMJ 1997;314:1886–1889.
8. Schmidt LA, Greenberg BD, Holzman GB, et al. Treatment of depression by obstetrician-gynecologists: a survey study. Obstet Gynecol 1997;90:296–300.
9. Kessler RC, McGonagle KA, Zhao S, et al. Lifetime and 12-month prevalence of DSM-III-R psychiatric disorders in the United States: results from the National Comorbidity Survey. Arch Gen Psychiatry 1994;51:8–19.
10. Simpson HB, Nee JC, Endicott J. First-episode major depression: few sex differences in course. Arch Gen Psychiatry 1997;54:633–639.
11. National Center for Health Statistics. Advance Report of Final Mortality Statistics, 1987: Monthly Vital Statistics Report. Hyattsville, MD: Public Health Service, 1989:38(5 suppl).
12. Olfson M, Weissman MM, Leon AC, et al. Suicidal ideation in primary care. J Gen Intern Med 1996;11:447–453.
13. Zung WW, Richards CB, Short MJ. Self-rating depression scale in an outpatient clinic: further validation of the SDS. Arch Gen Psychiatry 1965;13:508–515.
14. Beck AT, Ward CH, Mendelson M, et al. An inventory for measuring depression. Arch Gen Psychiatry 1961;4:53–63.
15. Radloff LS. The CES-D Scale: a self-report depression scale for research in the general population. Appl Psychol Meas 1977;1:385–401.
16. Beck AT, Rush J, Shaw B, Emery G. Cognitive Therapy of Depression. New York: Guilford Press, 1979.
17. Beck AT. Cognitive therapy. In: Zein J, ed. The Evolution of Psychotherapy. New York: Brunner-Mazel, 1987:149–163.
18. Burns D. Feeling Good: The New Mood Therapy. New York: William Morrow, 1980.
19. Yapko MD. Breaking the Patterns of Depression. New York: Doubleday, 1997.
20. Torem M. Depression as illness and mood: the implications for diagnosis and treatment. Ohio State Med J 1983;79:792–795.
21. Shapiro CM, Dement WC. Impact and epidemiology of sleep disorders. BMJ 1993;306:1604–1607.

INDEX

Page numbers in *italic* represent figures; page numbers followed by a "t" represent tables.